FREE INTERNET UPDATES!!!

Mosby is pleased to provide drug updates via our web site to keep the cards you purchased current. These may be found at:

http://www.mosby.com/MERLIN/drug_card_updates/

The internet updates will contain:

1. recent new drugs that have become available since these cards have gone to press
2. additional established, less frequently used drugs not currently covered in the cards due to space limitations

You will also find links to other useful pharmacology web sites.

Check with us every few months for new drugs and other useful information!

Drug:

CATEGORY: Preg Cat:

BRAND NAME **DOSAGE FORMS**

DOSAGE:

USE/ACTION:

SIDE/ADVERSE EFFFCTS:

PHARMACOKINETICS:

INTERACTIONS: Drug:
Food:
Lab:

CONTRAINDICATIONS:

CC:

Note: Side/adverse effects: common in *italic;* serious in ***boldface italic.***

*Available in Canada only.

NURSING MANAGEMENT PRIORITIES
ADMINISTRATION:

EVALUATION:

EDUCATION:

OVERDOSE MANAGEMENT:

NOTES:

Mosby's 2000 Nursing Drug Cards

Joseph A. Albanese, B.S. in Pharm., M.S., Ph.D.
Professor Emeritus,
College of Staten Island,
City University of New York,
Staten Island, New York

Patricia A. Nutz, R.N., M.S.N., M.Ed.
Instructor,
School of Nursing, St. Francis Hospital,
New Castle, Pennsylvania

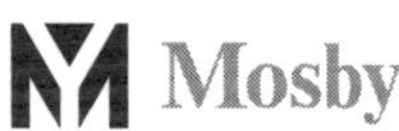

St. Louis Baltimore Boston Carlsbad Chicago Minneapolis New York Philadelphia Portland
London Milan Sydney Tokyo Toronto

Editor-in-Chief, Nursing: Sally Schrefer
Editor-in-Chief, Nursing Databases: N. Darlene Como
Senior Developmental Editor: Laurie Sparks
Project Manager: Patricia Tannian
Project Specialist: Suzanne C. Fannin
Design Manager: Gail Morey Hudson
Box Designer: Teresa Breckwoldt
Cover Art: Ken Joudrey

Tenth Edition

Mosby, Inc.
A Harcourt Health Sciences Company
11830 Westline Industrial Drive
St. Louis, Missouri 63146

Printed in the United States of America
Composition by Graphic World, Inc.
Printing/binding by Comfort Fiedler

NOTICE

Pharmacology is an ever-changing field. Standard safety precautions must be followed, but as new research and clinical experience broaden our knowledge, changes in treatment and drug therapy may become necessary or appropriate. Readers are advised to check the most current product information provided by the manufacturer of each drug to be administered to verify the recommended dose, the method and duration of administration, and contraindications. It is the responsibility of the treating physician, relying on experience and knowledge of the patient, to determine dosages and the best treatment for each individual patient. Neither the Publisher nor the editor assumes any liability for any injury and/or damage to persons or property arising from this publication.

International Standard Book Number ISBN 0-323-00795-3

99 00 01 02 03 / 9 8 7 6 5 4 3 2 1

Mosby's 2000 Nursing Drug Cards includes more than 770 generic and 1275 trade drugs. All drugs have been thoroughly updated to provide the most up-to-date content for nurses and nursing students administering these drugs in clinical settings. Unique features include the fundamentals of drug therapy cards, the drug class quickfacts section, the drug review guide, the management of ingested drug overdose cards, drug dosage calculations, and the pound and kilogram equivalents chart. Twenty-seven new individual drug cards and two new category cards have been added. In addition, new drugs have been added to existing individual, category, and drug cards, totaling 55 new drugs in this edition.

DRUG CARD EXPLANATION

CATEGORY: Classifies the drug by using chemical, pharmacologic, and/or therapeutic descriptors. **Rx:** Any drug that contains on the package the label: "Caution: Federal law prohibits dispensing without prescription." **OTC:** Any drug that can be sold legally over the counter (OTC) without a prescription. **Schedule Drug:** Controlled substance; any drug that is listed in Schedule C-II, C-III, C-IV, or C-V of the Comprehensive Drug Abuse Prevention and Control Act of 1970. Schedule C-II drugs have the greatest potential for misuse and addiction, whereas Schedule C-V drugs exhibit the least potential for misuse and addiction. Schedule C-I drugs have no accepted medical use and are illegal. Examples include diacetylmorphine (heroin), LSD, and mescaline. **Pregnancy Categories:** The purpose of the pregnancy categories is to establish a reasonable presumption for the possibility of drug-induced fetal harm and/or teratogenic effects. The categories established by the FDA are A, B, C, D, and X (NA indicates that an FDA category has not been assigned). Category A drugs represent relatively no risk; Category B, relatively no risk but not confirmed; Category C, potential risk, conclusive studies not available; Category D, therapeutic benefits must outweigh potential risks; and Category X, contraindicated during pregnancy. No drug was assigned a pregnancy category unless it was listed on the FDA labeling for the drug. **Nursing Management Priorities** include information regarding administration, evaluation, and education. Patient education, dietary management, lab test evaluation, and geriatric (G), pediatric (P), and obstetric (OB) special considerations are included when appropriate.

BRAND NAMES: Lists the proprietary (brand) name and manufacturer for the drug. The manufacturer of brand-name drugs is fluid and frequently changes because of company takeovers, mergers, and other current pharmaceutical economic factors. However, the brand name, drug dosage, and indications usually remain the same, regardless of the manufacturer. Most cards present a complete list of brand-name preparations. Abridged listings were used when the available proprietary preparations were too numerous to list. Drugs available only in Canada are marked with an asterisk (*). A footnote to this effect appears on all drug cards. Drugs not available in proprietary preparations are listed as available dosage forms without manufacturer identification.

COMBINATION PRODUCTS: Lists the formula(s) of the product(s), manufacturer(s), and available dosage form(s).

USE: Lists and describes the current medical use(s) of the drug. Nonlabeled use(s) of the drug (not approved by the FDA on the current labeling for the drug) or experimental use(s) are listed for selected drugs.

ACTION: Gives a brief description of the action(s) and effect(s) of the drug.

PHARMACOKINETICS: Lists available data as stated by the company that developed the drug, whenever possible. Data are variable and depend on the study, number and age of subjects, and normal or diseased population. Parameters for older drugs are usually limited in scope. **Absorption:** Passage of drug molecules from the site of administration into circulating body fluids. **Duration:** Total time of clinical drug activity obtained after administration. **Excretion:** Removal of the drug or its metabolites from the body. **Half-life:** Time required to reduce concentration of unchanged drug by 50% in the body. **Onset:** Time required to produce a measurable clinical drug effect after administration. **Peak:** Time required to produce the maximum serum/plasma levels after administration. **Protein Binding:** Occurs when the drug combines with a body protein (usually plasma albumin) to form a reversible drug-protein complex. Protein-bound drug molecules must dissociate to produce therapeutic activity.

DOSAGE: Gives the recommended oral and parenteral dose ranges, including elderly and pediatric dosages when appropriate. Whenever discrepancies existed in the literature, the FDA labeling for the specific drug was used as the final authority. Routes include IA, intraarticular; IM, intramuscular; IV, intravenous; IVPB, intravenous piggyback; PO, oral; RC, rectal; SC, subcutaneous; SL, sublingual; and TOP, topical.

CONTRAINDICATIONS: Cites specific patient conditions that preclude use of the drug. **Clinical Considerations (CC):** Lists specific circumstances that can cause the drug to be extremely dangerous or harmful to the patient. Explains what to do or what not to do in certain clinical circumstances.

SIDE/ADVERSE EFFECTS: Undesired effects produced by the drug. Those listed are condensed. Common side effects appear in *italics*; serious adverse effects appear in ***boldface italics.*** Abbreviations for side/adverse effects include CNS, central nervous system; CV, cardiovascular; EENT, eye, ear, nose, and throat; END, endocrine; GI, gastrointestinal; GU, genitourinary; HEM, hematologic; HEP, hepatic; INT, integumentary; MET, metabolic; MS, musculoskeletal; PSYCH, psychiatric; REN, renal; and RESP, respiratory.

INTERACTIONS: Drug: Limited to more serious reactions. **Laboratory (Lab):** Only listed if significant. **Food:** Only listed if important.

NURSING MANAGEMENT PRIORITIES: Nursing responsibilities associated with each drug are summarized under the following categories. **Administration:** Major nursing responsibilities related to preparation, administration, and storage. **Evaluation:** Major nursing responsibilities related to monitoring the specific drug's effects on the patient following administration. **Education:** Major nursing responsibilities related to considerations for patient education, including discharge teaching and patient teaching in the hospital or ambulatory care setting.

For category cards the nursing management also includes the following:

POTENTIAL NURSING DIAGNOSES ndx: Any NANDA nursing diagnoses that could be associated with drug administration. These are subdivided into **Therapeutic Effects:** Nursing diagnoses that may require use of a drug within the specific drug category (drug indications) and **Adverse Effects:** Nursing diagnoses that may result from the administration of a drug within the specific drug category (drug side effects).

OVERDOSE MANAGEMENT: Describes the recommended antidotal treatment for the drug.

We welcome comments from users so that we may continue to provide nursing-oriented drug information in as useful a manner as possible.

Joseph A. Albanese
Patricia A. Nutz

Selected manufacturer abbreviations

A-H	Allen & Hanburys	P-D	Parke-Davis
A-U	American-Urological	P-G	Procter & Gamble Pharmaceuticals
B-I	Boehringer Ingelheim	P-F	Purdue Frederick
B-M	Boehringer Mannheim	R-C	Reed & Carnrick
BM-ONC	Bristol-Myers Oncology	R-R	Reid-Rowell
B-MS	Bristol-Myers Squibb	RPR	Rhone-Poulenc Rorer
C-G	CibaGeneva Pharmaceuticals	S-W	Sanofi Winthrop
G-W	Glaxo Wellcome	S-S	Schiapparelli Searle
H-M-R	Hoechst Marion Roussel	SKB	SmithKline Beecham Pharmaceuticals
MAL	MAL	W-C	Warner Chilcott Laboratories
MJP	Mead Johnson Pharmaceuticals	W-A	Wyeth-Ayerst Laboratories

Symbols

α, β	Alpha, beta
t , y	Increase(d), decrease(d)
2°	Secondary; second-degree
1°	Primary; first-degree
▲, ∆, ◆	Alternate salt(s) of drug

Time

ac	Before meals
bid	Twice/day
d	Day
h	Hour
hs	Bedtime
m	Minute, meter
mo	Month
pc	After meals
prn	As needed
q	Every
qd	Daily
qid	Four times/day
qod	Every other day
tid	Three times/day
wk(s)	Week(s)
y/o	Years old
yr(s)	Year(s)

Miscellaneous

ABG	Arterial blood gas
ACE	Angiotensin-converting enzyme
ALT	Alanine aminotransferase
APTT	Activated partial thromboplastin time
ARC	AIDS-related complex
AST	Aspartate aminotransferase
BM	Bowel movement
BP	Blood pressure
BUN	Blood urea nitrogen
$\bar{c}$	With
cAMP	Cyclic adenosine monophosphate
CBC	Complete blood cell count
CHF	Congestive heart failure
CN	Cranial nerve
CO_2	Carbon dioxide
COPD	Chronic obstructive pulmonary disease
CR	Controlled-release
C&S	Culture and sensitivity
CSF	Cerebrospinal fluid
CVP	Central venous pressure
D/C	Discontinue
dig	Digitalis/digitalized
DS	Double strength
D_5W	5% dextrose in water

dx	Diagnosis
ECG	Electrocardiogram
EEG	Electroencephalogram
esp	Especially
FBS	Fasting blood sugar
F/E	Fluid/electrolyte
G	Geriatrics
gtt	Drops
H&H	Hemoglobin and hematocrit
hx	History
incl	Including
I&O	Intake and output
ICP	Intracranial pressure
IOP	Intraocular pressure
IPPB	Intermittent positive-pressure breathing
LA	Long-acting
LDH	Lactate dehydrogenase
LDL	Low-density lipoprotein
LE	Lupus erythematosus
LOC	Level of consciousness
μg	Microgram
MAO-I	Monoamine oxidase inhibitors
MI	Myocardial infarction
MIC	Minimum inhibitory concentration
NG	Nasogastric
NPN	Nonprotein nitrogen
NSAIA	Nonsteroidal antiinflammatory agent
N/V/D	Nausea/vomiting/diarrhea
OB	Obstetrics
OD	Overdose
P	Pediatrics
PDA	Patent ductus arteriosus
PPD	Purified protein derivative
ppt	Precipitate
pt(s)	Patient(s)
PT	Prothrombin time
PTT	Partial thromboplastin time
PVC	Premature ventricular contraction; polyvinyl chloride
RBC	Red blood cell
REM	Rapid eye movement (sleep)
ROM	Range of motion
Rx	Prescription
rx	Reaction
SA	Sinoatrial
SLE	Systemic lupus erythematosus
SR	Sustained release
T_3, T_4	Triiodothyronine, thyroxine
TCA	Tricyclic antidepressant
TSH	Thyroid-stimulating hormone
U	Unit
UA	Urinalysis
UOQ	Upper outer quadrant
URI	Upper respiratory (tract) infection
UTI	Urinary tract infection
VS	Vital signs
WBC	White blood cell count
w/in, w/out	Within, without

Bibliography

American Society of Health System Pharmacists: AHFS drug information, Bethesda, Md, 1999.

Clark W, Brater C, Johnson AR: *Medical pharmacology,* ed 13, St. Louis, 1992, Mosby.

Clayton BD, Stock Y: *Basic pharmacology for nurses,* ed 11, St Louis, 1997, Mosby.

Drug interaction viewer, Nutley, NJ, Roche Laboratories.

Gahart B: *1999 Intravenous medications,* ed 16, St Louis, 2000, Mosby.

Goodman LS, Gilman A, editors: *The pharmacological basis of therapeutics,* ed 9, New York, 1996, Macmillan.

Kastrup E, editor: *Facts and comparisons,* St Louis, current, Facts and Comparisons.

Kim MJ: *Pocket guide to nursing diagnoses,* ed 7, St Louis, 1997, Mosby.

Pharmaceutical manufacturers' current catalogs.

Physicians' desk reference, ed 53, Oradell, NJ, 1999, Medical Economics.

Professional drug package inserts from various pharmaceutical manufacturers.

Remington: *The science and practice of pharmacy,* ed 19, Easton, Pa, 1995, Mack.

USP DI, ed 19, United States Pharmacopeial Convention, Rockville, Md, 1999.

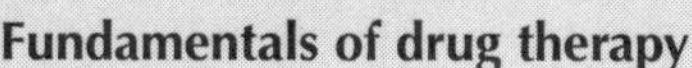

Fundamentals of drug therapy

PHARMACOLOGY & THE NURSE

A ***drug*** is a chemical that alters existing physiologic processes when introduced into the body ▪ ***Pharmacology*** is the study of the interaction of drugs on body cells ▪ Drugs act at ***receptors*** located in various tissues. When the drug molecule fits a specific receptor (like a ***key*** into a ***lock***), it produces a cellular response that may be ***therapeutic*** (desired) or ***adverse*** (harmful). A drug can act at more than one receptor in the body, thus producing a number of effects. A drug that stimulates a receptor is an ***agonist***; a drug that blocks a receptor, thus preventing a specific drug response, is an ***antagonist*** ▪ Many factors affect the drug's effect on body tissues incl age, sex, body weight, genetics, pathologic condition, & emotional response ▪ Many drugs used today achieve therapeutic effects in pt care. The ***nurse*** is the health team member who administers drugs & is best able to evaluate the pt's response to drug therapy ▪ Similar-acting drugs are grouped together in ***classifications*** or ***categories.*** This enables the health care provider to better understand how the drug produces its effects, both therapeutic & adverse, & to implement interventions to ensure therapeutic value of the drug c̄ minimal discomfort for the pt ▪ The ***nursing process*** provides a framework for ensuring safe, effective drug therapy for pts.

Assessment: Medication hx, allergy hx, medical hx/physical exam, results of diagnostic studies, **ndx** re: therapeutic & adverse effects. **Plan:** Pt outcomes re: drug therapy (therapeutic & adverse effects). **Intervention:** Administration of drugs to meet pt needs, drug teaching, specific drug-related measures, documentation of drug effects. **Evaluation:** Attainment of therapeutic effect.

PHARMACOKINETICS

Pharmacokinetics is the movement of the drug molecule throughout the body. This process comprises four phases: absorption, distribution, metabolism, & excretion ▪ ***Absorption*** refers to movement of the drug from the site of administration to systemic circulation. When a drug is absorbed it becomes ***bioavailable,*** or ready to exert action. The ***small intestine*** is the main organ of PO drug absorption ▪ For a PO drug to enter the bloodstream, it must first enter the hepatic portal system. Some drugs are extensively metabolized by the liver before reaching the systemic circulation & are thus said to exert a ***first-pass* phenomenon.** For these drugs, PO doses need to be much greater than IV doses ▪ ***Distribution*** involves movement of the drug molecule throughout the body to reach receptor sites. The ***blood*** is the major organ of drug distribution.

Drugs are readily distributed to tissues that are highly perfused, such as the heart, liver, kidneys, & brain. Factors affecting drug distribution incl plasma binding & blood-brain barrier. ***Plasma binding:*** Drug molecules attach to a plasma protein in the bloodstream & are transported to receptor sites in various body tissues. When the drug is "bound" to the plasma protein, it is unable to exert a drug effect. When the drug is "free" or "unbound" in the bloodstream, it is capable of interacting at receptor sites to produce a drug effect. ***Blood-brain barrier:*** A highly lipid membrane separates the central nervous system (CNS) from blood. Only nonionized, lipid-soluble drug molecules readily pass this blood-brain barrier; thus drugs used to treat CNS disorders must be lipid soluble to exert a therapeutic effect ▪ ***Metabolism,*** or ***biotransformation,*** refers to the alteration of drug molecules to a more water-soluble drug metabolite(s). The major organ of drug metabolism is the ***liver*** due to the vast number of microsomial enzymes ▪ ***Excretion*** involves elimination of drug/drug metabolite molecules from the body. The major organ of drug excretion is the ***kidney*** ▪ Any pathologic process affecting the liver or the kidney promotes drug accumulation in the body, thus producing drug ***toxicity.*** Also, the very young (due to developing, immature body systems) & the elderly (due to declining body system function) are predisposed to drug accumulation in the body & thus drug toxicity.

DRUG EFFECTS & INTERACTIONS

Every drug has a physiologic mechanism that it exerts at tissue receptors to produce a drug effect. This mechanism is referred to as a ***drug action*** ▪ Drug actions produce specific ***drug effects*** throughout the body. These effects are the outward manifestation of the drug action ▪ ***Therapeutic effect*** refers to the desired or intended effect for the specific drug therapy. Drugs may produce more than one therapeutic effect ▪ ***Adverse effect*** refers to each of the drug effects other than the desired, therapeutic effect. Adverse drug effects are often referred to as ***side effects,*** which are considered uncomfortable, undesired drug effects resulting from the drug molecule ▪ Adverse effects may be ***predictable*** or expected as a result of drug therapy. ***Unpredictable*** adverse effects may occur due to individual pt variables ▪ A ***hypersensitivity*** is a type of unpredictable drug side effect. It is a manifestation resulting from an allergic rx of the pt when taking a drug. However, a thorough patient/family clinical profile can reveal any known drug hypersensitivities. Drugs such as antibiotics & local anesthetics possess antigenic potential for allergic rxs ▪ An ***idiosyncratic*** rx is an individual pt variation that manifests by a drug response that is typically not produced by the drug. These idiosyncratic (atypical) rxs are due to inherited genetic factors that significantly alter the metabolism of a drug(s) when compared with the drug metabolism

of the general population. The metabolism (acylation) of the antitubercular isoniazid (INH) is a prime example of idiosyncratic drug rxs. Atypical INH acylation can be more rapid or slower than normal. Patients who rapidly metabolize INH (rapid acylators) require a greater than normal dose to achieve a satisfactory antimycobacterial effect. Accordingly, slow acylators are given a reduced dosage schedule to preclude toxicity & other adverse effects. A ***paradoxic*** rx is one that is opposite that which is normally expected to be produced by the drug in the body ▪ A ***teratogenic*** rx refers to abnormal fetal development that occurs when certain drugs cross the placenta. The Food and Drug Administration Drug Pregnancy Categories identify the significance of the teratogenicity of the drug on the fetus ▪ The action of one drug can be affected by its ***interaction*** with another drug or food in the body. Drug interactions may be beneficial to pt care; however, most interactions are undesirable & even harmful to the pt. OTC drugs, alcohol, tobacco, & various foods can produce potentially harmful drug interactions.

PREVENTING MEDICATION ERRORS

Safe, effective drug therapy depends on the responsibility, knowledge base, and accountability of the nurse administering medication to pts ▪ Always adhere to the "Five Rights of Medication Administration" to ensure safety in drug therapy (the right drug, right dose, right patient, right route, and right time). In addition, ***CAUTION*** should be used when administering medications to pts: ***C***heck expiration dates before administering any drug, ***A***ssess & document the pt's response after administering any medication, ***U***sed needles & syringes should be properly discarded, ***T***imes of drug administration should be closely checked & adhered to (esp prn medications), ***I***dentify pt by reading the wrist band & calling by name, ***O***nly the specific drug ordered (or a permissible legal substitute) should be administered, ***N***ever administer a drug that has been prepared by another nurse or that appears abnormal (discolored, precipitate) ▪ Using ***CAUTION*** & adhering to the "Five Rights of Medication Administration" ensures safety for the nurse in implementing drug therapy.

Drug class quickfacts

ANTIINFECTIVE AGENTS

Antibiotics: Resolve infection (compounds of living microbial or semisynthetic origin) ▪ Synthetic antiinfectives: Resolve infection (chemically synthesized).

CARDIOVASCULAR-RENAL SYSTEM

Antianginals: ↓ workload on heart (↑ O_2 supply to myocardium) ▪ Antiarrhythmics: Promote normal cardiac rate, rhythm ▪ Anticoagulants: Prevent new clots from forming ▪ Antihypertensives: ⬇ BP (vasodilators) ▪ Antihyperlipidemics: ⬇ blood cholesterol levels ▪ Antiplatelets: Promote blood flow (⬇ platelet organization) ▪ Diuretics: ⬆ urine output by kidney ▪ Positive inotropes: ⬆ strength & force of myocardial contractility ▪ Thrombolytics: Break down existing clots ▪ Uricosurics: Promote excretion of uric acid by kidney ▪ Vasopressors: ⬆ BP.

CENTRAL NERVOUS SYSTEM

Analgesics: Relieve pain (narcotics: central-acting; nonnarcotics: peripheral-acting) ▪ Anticonvulsants: Control seizure activity ▪ Antidepressants: Resolve depression, elevate mood ▪ Anxiolytics: ⬇ anxiety ▪ Barbiturates: ⬇ anxiety, insomnia, convulsive episodes (promote CNS depression) ▪ Muscle relaxants: ⬇ spasms; ⬆ musculoskeletal function ▪ NSAIDs: ⬇ pain, inflammation, fever.

ENDOCRINE SYSTEM

Glucocorticoids: ⬇ inflammation, immune response ▪ Insulin: ⬇ blood sugar ▪ PO hypoglycemics: ⬇ hyperglycemic manifestations ▪ Thyroid: Affects basal metabolic rate (BMR) (enhancers: ⬆; inhibitors: ⬇).

GASTROINTESTINAL SYSTEM

Antacids: Neutralize gastrointestinal (GI) tract activity ▪ Antidiarrheals: Resolve diarrhea; promote formed stool ▪ Antisecretories: ⬇ GI secretions ▪ Antiemetics: ⬇ N/V ▪ Antispasmodics: ⬇ GI spasms ▪ Laxatives: Relieve constipation; promote regular defecation.

IMMUNE SYSTEM

Biologic response modifiers: Promote immune system function, antitumor activity ▪ Biologics: Prevent specific disease (toxoids & vaccines) ▪ Colony-stimulating factors: ⬆ neutrophil production; prevent/resolve infection ▪ Immunosuppressants: Organ rejection prophylaxis (⬇ immune system function) ▪ Interferons: Promote immune system function; antiviral, antineoplastic effects.

REPRODUCTIVE SYSTEM

Androgens: Maintain male reproductive system ▪ Estrogens/progesterones: Maintain female reproductive system ▪ Oxytocics: ⬆ uterine contractility ▪ Uterine relaxants: ⬇ uterine spasms.

RESPIRATORY SYSTEM

Antiasthmatics: Promote bronchodilation ▪ Antihistamines: Relieve allergic rxs, cold symptoms ▪ Antitussives: ⬇ cough ▪ Decongestants: Promote patency of upper airway passages.

This review guide presents all of the drugs that are listed on the individual drug cards and a few drugs that are listed on selected category cards in a comprehensive drugs study guide outline. The drugs listed for each of the 13 major groupings use an integrated combination of physiologic systems & chemical, pathologic, pharmacologic, & therapeutic descriptors; thus vital clinical drug information & classifications are available in a comprehensive study guide. In addition, the various category cards should be used c̄ the guide because the category cards list all drugs currently available for each category of drugs.

ANTIINFECTIVE AGENTS

ANTIBIOTICS (MICROBIAL OR MICROBIAL/SEMISYNTHETIC ORIGIN): Antifungals: amphotericin B, nystatin. **Antituberculants:** kanamycin sulfate, rifabutin, rifampin, streptomycin sulfate. **Beta-lactams:** ***Cephalosporins:*** *First-generation:* cefadroxil, cefazolin sodium, cephalexin/hcl, cephapirin sodium, cephradine. *Second-generation:* cefaclor, cefamandole nafate, cefmetazole, cefonicid sodium, cefoxitin sodium, cefpodoxime proxetil, cefprozil monohydrate, ceftibuten, cefuroxime axetil/sodium. *Third-generation:* cefdinir, cefepime, cefixime, cefoperazone sodium, cefotaxime sodium, cefotetan disodium, ceftazidime, ceftizoxime sodium, ceftriaxone sodium. **Penicillins:** *Aminopenicillins:* amoxicillin trihydrate, amoxicillin trihydrate/clavulanate, ampicillin sodium/trihydrate. *Extended-spectrum:* mezlocillin sodium, piperacillin sodium, piperacillin sodium/tazobactam sodium, ticarcillin. *Natural:* penicillin g benzathine, penicillin g potassium, penicillin g procaine, penicillin v potassium. *Penicillinase-resistant:* cloxacillin sodium, dicloxacillin sodium, methicillin sodium, nafcillin sodium, oxacillin sodium. **Miscellaneous:** aztreonam, imipenem/cilastatin sodium, loracarbef, meropenem. **AMINOGLYCOSIDES:** amikacin sulfate, gentamicin sulfate, kanamycin sulfate, netilmicin sulfate, streptomycin sulfate, tobramycin sulfate. **MACROLIDES:** azithromycin, clarithromycin, dirithromycin, erythromycin base, E. estolate, E. ethylsuccinate, E. gluceptate, E. lactobionate, E. stearate. **RIFAMYCINS:** rifabutin, rifampin. **TETRACYCLINES:** doxycycline hyclate, minocycline hyclate, tetracycline hcl. **Miscellaneous:** bacitracin, chloramphenicol/palmitate/sodium succinate, fosfomycin, spectinomycin hcl, vancomycin hcl. **SYNTHETIC ANTIINFECTIVES: Antifungals:** fluconazole, flucytosine, itraconazole, ketoconazole, miconazole, terbinafine hcl. **Antiprotozoans:** atovaquone, metronidazole, pentamidine isethionate. **Antituberculars:** ethambutol hcl, isoniazid (see also category card #355). **Antiviral agents:** (see also category card #356): acyclovir/sodium, amantadine hcl, didanosine, foscarnet sodium, imiquimod, stavudine, zalcitabine, zidovudine. **Fluoroquinolones:** ciprofloxacin, grepafloxacin, levofloxacin, lomefloxacin, norfloxacin, ofloxacin, sparfloxacin. **Quinolones:** cinoxacin, nalidixic acid. **Sulfonamides:** co-trimoxazole (trimethoprim/sulfamethoxazole), sulfamethoxazole, sulfisoxazole. **Topical antifungals:** (see category card #383). **Miscellaneous:** nitrofurantoin, trimethoprim.

ANTINEOPLASTICS

These agents can be classified by their interaction on the life cycle (phase specificity) of the neoplastic cell. Antineoplastics capable of affecting a specific phase of the life cycle are termed *cycle-phase–specific* or *cell-cycle–specific*. Drugs that can interact with many or all life cycle phases are designated as *cycle-phase–nonspecific* or *cell cycle–nonspecific*. In addition, antineoplastics are also classified by their (1) mechanism of action, (2) source or origin, (3) chemical structure, or (4) any combination of the above. **Alkaloids** (Vinca): vinblastine, vincristine, vinorelbine ▪ **Alkylating agents:** busulfan, carboplatin, cisplatin, cyclophosphamide, melphalan ▪ **Antibiotic:** bleomycin sulfate ▪ **Antimetabolites:** Folic acid antagonist: methotrexate ▪ Purine antagonists: mercaptopurine ▪ Pyrimidine antagonists: cytarabine, fluorouracil, gemcitabrine hcl ▪ **Antimicrotubulars:** docetaxel, paclitaxel ▪ **Biologic response modifiers:** aldesleukin, interferon alfa 2a, interferon alfa 2b ▪ **Enzymes:** asparaginase, pegaspargase ▪ **Hormonals:** Antiestrogen: letrozole, tamoxifen, toremifene citrate ▪ Estrogenic: diethylstilbestrol ▪ Glucosteroid: prednisone ▪ **Immunoglobulin:** rituximab ▪ **Progestin:** medroxyprogesterone ▪ **Lymphokines** (Cytokines): aldesleu-kin, interferon alfa 2a, interferon alfa 2b ▪ **Mitotic inhibitors:** vinblastine, vincristine, vinorelbine ▪ **Vaccine:** BCG (intravesical).

AUTONOMIC NERVOUS SYSTEM

SYMPATHETIC NERVOUS SYSTEM: Sympathomimetics (adrenergics): α agents: dextroamphetamine sulfate, methoxamine hcl, phenylephrine hcl. **α-β agents:** ephedrine sulfate, epinephrine, metaraminol bitartrate, norepinephrine bitartrate. **β agents:** isoproterenol hcl, metaproterenol sulfate. **β-1 agents:** dobutamine hcl, dopamine. **β-2 agents:** albuterol sulfate, ritodrine hcl, salmeterol xinafoate, terbutaline hcl. **Sympatholytics (adrenergic blockers): α blockers:** ergotamine tartrate, phenoxybenzamine hcl, phentolamine mesylate. **α-1 blockers:** doxazosin mesylate, prazosin hcl, tamsulosin. **α-β blockers:** carvedilol, labetalol hcl. **β blockers:** carteolol hcl, nadolol, penbutolol sulfate, propranolol hcl, timolol maleate. **β-1 blockers:** acebutolol hcl, atenolol, metoprolol tartrate. **PARASYMPATHOMIMETICS (cholinergics, muscarinics). Cholinergics:** donepezil hcl, edrophonium chloride, neostigmine bromide, pilocarpine hcl, tacrine hcl. **PARASYMPATHOLYTICS (anticholinergics, antimuscarinics). Anticholinergics:** atropine sulfate, ipratropium bro-

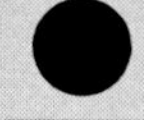

mide, propantheline bromide, scopolamine hbr, tolterodine tartrate.

CARDIOVASCULAR-RENAL SYSTEM

ANGINA: β blockers: nadolol, propranolol hcl. ***β-1 blockers:*** atenolol, metoprolol tartrate. **Calcium blockers:** diltiazem hcl, nicardipine hcl, nifedipine, verapamil hcl. **Nitrates:** isosorbide dinitrate, nitroglycerin. **ANTICOAGULANTS:** danaparoid sodium, heparin sodium, warfarin sodium. **ANTIPLATELET AGENTS:** aspirin, clopidrogrel bisulfate, dipyridamole, ticlopidine. **ARRHYTHMIAS: β blockers:** propranolol hcl. ***β-1 blockers:*** acebutolol. **Calcium blockers:** diltiazem hcl, verapamil hcl. **Cardiac glycosides:** digitoxin, digoxin. **Local anesthetics/derivatives:** flecainide hcl, lidocaine hcl, mexiletine hcl, procainamide hcl, tocainide hcl. **Quinidine salts:** quinidine gluconate/polygalacturonate/sulfate. **Other:** disopyramide phosphate. **CONGESTIVE HEART FAILURE: ACE-I:** captopril, enalapril maleate, lisinopril, quinapril hcl. **Cardiac glycosides:** digitoxin, digoxin. **Cardiac ionotropes:** amrinone lactate, milrinone lactate. **EDEMA: Diuretics:** ***Carbonic anhydrase inhibitors:*** acetazolamide/sodium. ***Loop:*** bumetanide, furosemide. ***Osmotic:*** mannitol. ***Potassium-sparing:*** amiloride hcl, spironolactone, triamterene. ***Thiazides:*** chlorothiazide, hydrochlorothiazide. ***Thiazidelike:*** metolazone. **HYPERTENSION: ACE-I:** captopril, enalapril maleate, enalaprilat, lisinopril, trandolapril. **Adrenergic activity:** ***α blockers:*** phenoxybenzamine hcl, phentolamine mesylate. ***α-1 blockers:*** doxazosin mesylate, prazosin hcl. ***α-2 agonist agents:*** clonidine hcl, guanabenz acetate, guanfacine hcl. ***α-β blockers:*** carvedilol, labetalol hcl. ***Alteration of catecholamine synthesis:*** methyldopa, methyldopate hcl. ***β blockers:*** carteolol hcl, nadolol, penbutolol sulfate, propranolol hcl, timolol maleate. ***β-1 blockers:*** acebutolol hcl, atenolol, metoprolol tartrate. ***Norepinephrine depletors:*** guanethidine monosulfate, reserpine. **Angiotensin II antagonist:** candesartan cilexetil, irbesartan, losartan potassium, valsartan. **Calcium blockers:** diltiazem hcl, nicardipine hcl, nifedipine, verapamil hcl. **Direct acting:** diazoxide, hydralazine hcl, minoxidil. **Diuretics:** ***Loop:*** bumetanide, furosemide. ***Potassium-sparing:*** spironolactone. ***Thiazides:*** chlorothiazide, hydrochlorothiazide. ***Other:*** antihypertensive combinations (see category card #351), nitroglycerin. **HYPERLIPIDEMIA: Bile acid sequestrants:** cholestyramine resin. **HMG-Co reductase inhibitors:** atorvastatin, fluvastatin, lovastatin, pravastatin sodium, simvastatin (see category card #369). **Other:** clofibrate. **MYOCARDIAL INFARCTION: ACE-I:** captopril. **β blockers:** propranolol hcl, timolol maleate. ***β-1 blockers:*** atenolol, metoprolol tartrate. **Tissue plasminogen activator:** alteplase recombinant, reteplase recombinant. **NEO-**

NATAL PULMONARY HYPERTENSION: tolazoline hcl. **PATENT DUCTUS ARTERIOSUS:** indomethacin sodium trihydrate. **PHEOCHROMOCYTOMA:** α **blockers:** phenoxybenzamine hcl, phentolamine. β **blocker:** propranolol hcl. **PROSTATITIS:** α**-1 blockers:** doxazosin mesylate, tamsulosin. **Testosterone inhibitor:** finasteride. **URICOSURICS:** probenecid. **URINARY ANALGESICS:** pentosan polysulfate sodium, phenazopyridine hcl. **URINARY BLADDER STABILIZER:** tolterodine tartrate. **VASCULAR HEADACHES:** α **blocker:** ergotamine tartrate, naratriptan, rizatriptan benzoate, sumatriptan succinate, zolmitriptan. *β* **blockers:** propranolol hcl, timolol maleate. **Serotonin receptor agonists:** naratriptan, rizatriptan, sumatriptan succinate, zolmitriptan. **VASOPRESSORS: Sympathomimetics (adrenergics):** *α* ***agents:*** methoxamine hcl, phenylephrine hcl. *α-β* ***agents:*** epinephrine, metaraminol bitartrate, norepinephrine bitartrate. *β* ***agents:*** isoproterenol hcl. ***β-1 agents:*** dobutamine hcl, dopamine. **VENTRICULAR DYSFUNCTION (LEFT):** captopril, enalapril maleate.

CENTRAL NERVOUS SYSTEM

ALZHEIMER'S DISEASE: donepezil hcl, tacrine hcl. **ANXIETY: Benzodiazepines:** alprazolam, chlordiazepoxide hcl, clorazepate dipotassium, diazepam, halazepam, lorazepam, oxazepam, prazepam. **Other:** buspirone hcl, doxepin hcl, hydroxyzine hcl. **ATTENTION DEFICIT HYPERACTIVITY DISORDER:** dexedrine sulfate. **CONVULSIVE DISORDERS: Barbiturates:** pentobarbital, phenobarbital. **Benzodiazepines:** clonazepam, clorazepate dipotassium, diazepam. **Carbonic anhydrase inhibitor:** acetazolamide. **Hydantoin:** phenytoin sodium. **Succinimide:** ethosuximide. **Other:** carbamazepine, valproate sodium, valproic acid (see also category card #346). **DEPRESSION: MAO-I:** phenelzine sulfate, tranylcypromine sulfate. **Tricyclics:** amitriptyline hcl, amoxapine, clomipramine hcl, doxepin hcl, imipramine hcl/pamoate, maprotiline hcl. **Selective serotonin reuptake inhibitors:** fluoxetine hcl, fluvoxamine maleate, paroxetine hcl, sertraline hcl. **Other:** bupropion hcl, mirtazapine, nefazodone hcl, trazodone hcl, venlafaxine. **EMETIC:** ipecac syrup. **INSOMNIA: Barbiturates:** pentobarbital sodium, phenobarbital. **Benzodiazepines:** estazolam, flurazepam hcl, quazepam, temazepam, triazolam. **Other:** zolpidem tartrate. **MANIC DEPRESSION:** lithium carbonate/citrate. **MIGRAINE:** ergotamine tartrate, naratriptan, rizatriptan benzoate, sumatriptan succinate, zolmitriptan. **MUSCLE RELAXANTS:** chlorzoxazone, cyclobenzaprine hcl. **NARCOLEPSY:** dextroamphetamine. **PAIN: Analgesic:** ***Central acting:*** tramadol hcl. ***NSAIAs:*** *Acetic acid derivatives:* diclofenac sodium, etodolac, sulindac. *Indole:* indomethacin/sodium/trihydrate. *Oxicam:* piroxicam. *Propionic acid derivatives:* fenoprofen calcium, flurbiprofen, ibuprofen, ketoprofen, naproxen/sodium, oxaprozin. *Salicylates:* aspirin, diflunisal. *Other:* acetaminophen, celecoxib, ketorolac tromethamine, nabumetone, tolmetin sodium. ***Narcotics (opiates, opioids):*** *Natural:* codeine phosphate/sulfate, morphine sulfate. *Synthetic agonists/antagonists:* butorphanol tartrate, nalbuphine hcl, pentazocine lactate/hcl. *Synthetic narcotic agonists:* meperidine hcl, methadone hcl, propoxyphene hcl/napsylate, oxycodone hcl. *Synthetic narcotic antagonist:* naloxone hcl. **PANIC DISORDER SYNDROME:** phenelzine sulfate. **PARKINSON'S DISEASE: Anticholinergics:** benztropine mesylate, biperiden hcl, procyclidine hcl, trihexyphenidyl hcl. **Antihistamine:** diphenhydramine hcl. **Dopaminergic:** ***Direct acting:*** bromocriptine mesylate. ***Indirect acting:*** amantadine hcl, pramipexole, tolcapone. ***Replacement:*** levodopa, levodopa-carbidopa. **PSYCHOTIC DISORDERS: Benzisoxazole:** risperidone. **Butyrophenones:** haloperidol/decanoate. **Dibenzodiazepine:** clozapine. **Dibenzoxazepine:** loxapine. **Phenothiazines:** ***Aliphatic:*** chlorpromazine hcl. ***Piperazine:*** fluphenazine decanoate/enanthate/hcl, perphenazine, perphenazine-amitriptyline hcl, prochlorperazine/edisylate/maleate. **Other:** olanzapine, quetiapine. **VOMITING: Anticholinergic:** scopolamine/ hbr. **Antidopaminergics:** ***Phenothiazines:*** chlorpromazine hcl, perphenazine, prochlorperazine/edisylate. ***Other:*** benzquinamide hcl, metoclopramide hcl, trimethobenzamide hcl. **Antihistamines:** diphenhydramine hcl, promethazine hcl. **Antiserotonergics:** granisetron hcl, ondansetron hcl.

ENDOCRINE SYSTEM

ADRENAL AGENTS: Adrenal cortex: ***Systemic glucosteroids:*** cortisone, dexamethasone, prednisone, triamcinolone. **Topical glucosteroids:** (see category card #334). **Adrenal medulla:** ***Adrenergics (sympathomimetics):*** epinephrine, norepinephrine. **OVARIAN AGENTS: Estrogens:** diethylstilbestrol, estradiol, estrogens conjugated. **Progestin:** medroxyprogesterone acetate. **Estrogen/progestins:** contraceptive products (see category card #375). **PANCREATIC AGENTS: Hypoglycemics:** ***Insulins:*** regular, lente, NPH, ultra-lente, regular/NPH mixture. ***Sulfonylureas:*** *First-generation:* acetohexamide, chlorpropamide, tolazamide, tolbutamide. *Second-generation:* glipizide, glyburide, miglitol. ***Biguanides:*** metformin. ***Oligosaccharides:*** acarbose, troglitazone. ***Other:*** repaglinide. **Hyperglycemic:** diazoxide. **PITUITARY/HYPOTHALAMUS: Anterior pituitary:** oxytocin, vasopressin. **TESTICULAR AGENTS: Androgen:** methyltestosterone. **Androgen inhibitor:** finasteride. **THYROID AGENTS: Antithyroids:** methimazole, propylthiouracil. **Thyroids:** levothyroxine sodium, liothyronine sodium, liotrix, thyroid extract.

GASTROINTESTINAL SYSTEM

ANTACIDS: (see category card #342). **ANTICHOLINERGICS/ANTISPASMODICS:** atropine sulfate, propantheline bromide, scopolamine hbr. **ANTIEMETICS:** benzquinamide hcl, granisetron hcl, ondansetron hcl. **ANTIDIARRHEALS:** diphenoxylate hcl/atropine sulfate, kaopectate preparations, loperamide hcl. **ANTISECRETORY: Anticholinergics:** (see anticholinergics/antispasmodics [previously mentioned] & category card #345). **Gastric acid pump inhibitor:** omeprazole. **H_2 blockers (H_2 antihistamines):** cimetidine, famotidine, nizatidine, ranitidine. **Prostaglandin E analog:** misoprostol. **LAXATIVES:** (see category card #372). **STIMULANT:** metoclopramide. **Other:** sucralfate.

HEMATOLOGIC SYSTEM

Iron salts, oprelvekin.

IMMUNE SYSTEM

BIOLOGICALS: Toxoids: diphtheria, DPT, tetanus. **Vaccines: *Bacterials:*** Baccilus of Calmette-Guérin (BCG), cholera, *Haemophilus* B, meningitis, plague, pneumococcus. ***Viral:*** hepatitis B, influenza, measles, mumps, polio, rabies, rubella, yellow fever. **COLONY-STIMULATING FACTORS:** filgrastim, sargramostim. **LYMPHOKINE (BIOLOGIC RESPONSE MODIFIER):** aldesleukin. **IMMUNOGLOBULIN:** rituximab. **IMMUNOSUPPRESSANTS: Corticosteroid:** prednisone. **Other:** azathioprine/sodium, cyclosporine. **INTERFERONS: Alfa:** alfa-2a, alfa-2b, alfa-n3. **Beta:** beta-1b. **Gamma:** gamma-1b.

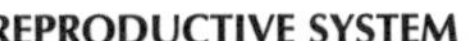

REPRODUCTIVE SYSTEM

FEMALE: Oxytocics: ergonovine maleate, methylergonovine maleate, oxytocin. **Sex hormones: *Estrogens:*** estradiol, estrogens conjugated, diethylstilbestrol. ***Progestin:*** medroxyprogesterone acetate. ***Estrogen/progestin:*** oral contraceptive products (see category card #375). ***Uterine relaxant:*** ritodrine hcl. **MALE: Sex hormones: *Androgen:*** methyltestosterone. ***Androgen inhibitor:*** finasteride.

RESPIRATORY SYSTEM

ANTIASTHMATICS: Anticholinergics: ipratropium bromide. **Bronchodilators: *Adrenergics:*** α-β *agents:* ephedrine sulfate, epinephrine. *β agents:* isoproterenol hcl, metaproterenol sulfate. *β-2 agents:* albuterol sulfate, salmeterol xinafoate, terbutaline hcl. ***Xanthines:*** aminophylline, theophylline. **Other:** cromolyn sodium, montelukast sodium, nedocromil sodium, zafirlukast, zileuton. **ANTIHISTAMINES:** astemizole, fexofenadine, loratadine, terfenadine (see also category card #348). **ANTITUSSIVE:** codeine sulfate. **EMBOLISM:** alteplase recombinant (tPA). **LUNG SURFACTANTS:** beractant, calfactant, colfosceril

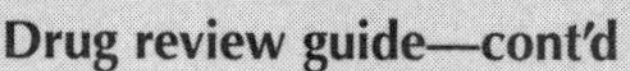

palmitate. **NASAL DECONGESTANT: Adrenergics:** (see also category card #334). α ***agents:*** phenylephrine hcl. α-β ***agents:*** ephedrine sulfate, epinephrine.

SKELETAL SYSTEM
ANTIOSTEOPOROSIS: alendronate sodium, calcium salts, raloxifene.

SPECIAL SENSES
GLAUCOMA: brimonidine tartrate, latanoprost, pilocarpine hcl.

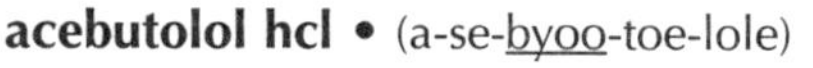

acebutolol hcl • (a-se-byoo-toe-lole)

CATEGORY: *β_1-adrenergic blocker:* antiarrhythmic, antihypertensive Rx; Preg Cat B

BRAND NAME	DOSAGE FORMS
Sectral (W-A)	Capsule: 200, 400mg

USE: Treatment of hypertension as sole agent or in combination c̄ other antihypertensives (esp thiazide diuretic) ▪ Treatment of ventricular premature beats. **ACTION:** Blocks access of catecholamine neurotransmitters to β_1 receptors located in heart; antihypertensive effect not determined.

PHARMACOKINETICS

PO absorption	Peak	Half-life	Protein binding	Excretion
90%	2.5h	3-4h	26%	30%-40% via urine, 50%-60% nonrenal

CONTRAINDICATIONS: Hypersensitivity, severe bradycardia, heart block >1°, overt cardiac failure, cardiogenic shock. **CC:** Abrupt D/C can ⬆ ischemic heart disease ▪ Possible cardiac failure c̄ ⬇ in myocardial contractility ▪ Use in pts c̄ bronchospastic diseases, diabetes, hypoglycemia, peripheral vascular disease requires caution ▪ Tachycardia of hyperthyroidism may be masked & abrupt D/C may induce thyrotoxicosis ▪ ⬇ Dosage in pt c̄ hepatic or renal dysfunction ▪ Avoid doses >800mg/d in geriatric pts.

DOSAGE

Adult *PO* Individualized dose starting c̄ 400mg/d. Usual range 400-800mg/d divided. Dose range for ventricular arrhythmia 600-1200mg/d divided

SIDE/ADVERSE EFFECTS: CNS: *fatigue, headache,* dizziness, insomnia, depression ▪ CV: bradycardia, ***heart failure,*** hypotension, chest pain ▪ EENT: abnormal vision ▪ GI: constipation, diarrhea, dyspepsia, flatulence, nausea ▪ GU: urinary frequency ▪ MS: arthralgia ▪ RESP: dyspnea.

INTERACTIONS: Drug: Use c̄ reserpine, other catecholamine-depleting drugs can result in serious adrenergic blockage ▪ Nonselective β adrenergics antagonize therapeutic response ▪ Use c̄ Ca blockers may prolong AV conduction ▪ Diabetics may require adjustment of antidiabetic agent(s).

NURSING MANAGEMENT PRIORITIES

ADMINISTRATION: Assess for hx of β-blocker hypersensitivity ▪ Assess BP, apical pulse; if <60/m hold drug, notify physician ▪ Assess hepatic function, I&O; may require ↓ dosage if impaired ▪ Do *not* administer in presence of respiratory distress (asthma, CHF, COPD) ▪ Avoid exposure to heat/moisture in storage ▪ Avoid abrupt withdrawal; D/C gradually ▪ Elderly may require ↑ dosage.

EVALUATION: Monitor hepatic, renal, respiratory status ▪ Monitor BP, pulse ▪ Monitor CBC, FBS (diabetics) ▪ Assess for CHF (dyspnea, peripheral edema, ↑ weight); notify physician ▪ Assess for depression ▪ May produce alteration in blood glucose levels; may mask signs of hypoglycemia.

EDUCATION: Take as directed by physician; do *not* skip doses ▪ May take w/out regard to food ▪ Procedure for checking radial pulse ▪ Check pulse before taking; if <60/m do *not* take drug, notify physician ▪ Do *not* D/C w/out notifying physician ▪ Check c̄ physician/pharmacist before taking OTC/Rx preparations ▪ Drowsiness/dizziness may occur; use caution when engaging in potentially hazardous activities ▪ Avoid changing positions (lying/sitting/standing) rapidly ▪ Diabetics: carefully monitor blood/urine glucose; observe for symptoms of hypoglycemia (headache, ↑ sweating, hunger, weakness) ▪ May experience ↑ sensitivity to cold ▪ Notify physician of respiratory distress or leg edema ▪ Notify physician/dentist of β blocker use before treatment ▪ Maintain optimum weight; follow low-Na^+ diet ▪ Keep scheduled appointments c̄ physician ▪ Store in tightly closed container ▪ Avoid ↑ exercise, temperature extremes, smoking ▪ Women: avoid breastfeeding.

NOTES:

acetaminophen (APAP) • (a-seat-a-mee-noe-fen)

CATEGORY: *Analgesic: p*-aminophenol, nonsalicylate analgesic OTC; Preg Cat B

BRAND NAMES
**Abenol*
Acephen
Aceta
Apacet
**Atasol*
**Campain*
**Exdol*
Feverall
Genapap
Genebs
Liquiprin
Mapap
Panadol
**Raunox*
**Robigesic*
Silapap
Tapanol
Tempra
Tylenol

COMBINATION PRODUCTS
Codeine/Acetaminophen Rx-C-III-Preg Cat C
Phenaphen c̄ Codeine (Robins) #2 (15/375mg), #3 (30/325mg), #4 (60/300mg), 650 c̄ Codeine (30/650mg)
Tylenol c̄ Codeine (McNeil) #1 (7.5/300mg), #2 (15/300mg), #3 (30/300mg), #4 (60/325mg)
Hydrocodone/Acetaminophen Rx-C-III-Preg Cat C
Anexsia (Mannheim) 5/500, 7.5/650
Vicodin (Knoll) (5/500mg), ES (7.5/750mg)
Zydone (Du Pont) (5/500mg)

DOSAGE FORMS
Caplet, capsule, chewable tablet, drops, elixir, liquid, suspension, suppository, tablet, wafer

USE: Analgesic for mild to moderate pain as sole agent or in combination c̄ other analgesics or narcotics ▪ Antipyretic for febrile states ▪ ⬇ Pain and fever associated c̄ DPT inoculations. **ACTION:** ⬆ Pain threshold; affects hypothalamic heat-regulating center, resulting in analgesia/antipyresis about equal to aspirin; exerts no antiinflammatory or uricosuric activity.

PHARMACOKINETICS

PO absorption	Peak	Half-life	Protein binding	Excretion
Almost complete	0.5-1.5h	1.5-3h	25%	80% excreted as conjugates in complete urine

CONTRAINDICATIONS: Hypersensitivity, known glucose-6-phosphate dehydrogenase deficiency. **CC:** Use by alcoholics may produce significant hepatotoxicity.

Note: Side/adverse effects: common in *italic;* serious in ***boldface italic.***

*Available in Canada only.

■ Continued ↑ fevers may indicate significant illness/infection ■ Use in children for >5d or in adults for >10d requires medical supervision.

DOSAGE

Pediatric *PO/Rectal* q4-6h	0-3mo 40mg	4-5y/o 240mg
	4-11mo 80mg	6-8y/o 320mg
	1-2y/o 120mg	9-10y/o 400mg
	2-3y/o 160mg	11-12y/o 480mg
Adult *PO*	325-650mg; do *not* exceed 4g/d, 2.6g/d c̄ long-term use	

SIDE/ADVERSE EFFECTS: HEM: anemia, leukopenia, neutropenia, pancytopenia; ***hemolytic anemia,*** methemoglobinemia (rare) ■ HEP: jaundice ■ INT: erythematous rxs, urticaria.

INTERACTIONS: Drug: PO anticoagulants can be displaced from protein storage sites; excessive use can enhance bleeding tendencies ■ Use c̄ phenothiazines may produce hypothermia. **Lab:** OTC blood glucose-testing kits can produce false-negative results.

NURSING MANAGEMENT PRIORITIES

ADMINISTRATION: Assess for hx of hypersensitivity ■ Shake suspensions well before administering ■ Administer c̄ food if GI irritation occurs ■ Store suppositories in refrigerator.

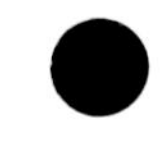

EVALUATION: Assess hepatic, renal status during long-term therapy ■ Assess for bleeding (GI, GU, skin/mucous membrane) c̄ long-term, high-dose therapy.

EDUCATION: Notify physician if rash develops; D/C drug ■ *Not* effective as antiinflammatory agent ■ Avoid use c̄ alcohol ■ Compliance c̄ prescribed dosage regimen.

OVERDOSE MANAGEMENT: Principal symptoms: sweating, gastric irritation, chills, cyanosis, oliguria, jaundice, coma, convulsions, death from respiratory failure ■ Treatment: removal of drug by emesis or gastric lavage followed by acetylcysteine to ↓ liver toxicity.

NOTES:

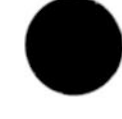

acetazolamide/acetazolamide sodium▲ • (a-seet-a-zole-a-mide)

CATEGORY: *Carbonic anhydrase inhibitor:* anticonvulsant, diuretic Rx; Preg Cat C

BRAND NAMES
Diamox (Lederle)
**Acetazolam (ICN)*

DOSAGE FORMS
Tablet: 125, 250mg
Injection (IM/IV)▲: 500mg/vial
Sequels: 500mg

USE: Adjunct for open-angle, 2° glaucoma ▪ Adjunct anticonvulsant & in treating of edema due to CHF ▪ Preop reduction of pressure in acute-angle glaucoma ▪ Acute mountain sickness. **ACTION:** Diuretic effect due to inhibition of carbonic anhydrase in renal tubules; results in moderate diuresis c̄ alkaline urine, which leads to systemic acidosis; in addition, reduction in aqueous humor of eye; anticonvulsant activity.

CONTRAINDICATIONS: Hypersensitivity, marked kidney/liver disease, low serum Na^+/K^+, hyperchloremic acidosis, adrenal gland failure. **CC:** Rare, fatal rxs are possible c̄ sulfonamides & their derivatives ▪ Cross-allergenicity c̄ sulfonamides & thiazides is possible.

DOSAGE

Glaucoma			8-30mg/kg/d divided
	Pediatric	*PO*	5-10mg/kg q6h
		IM/IV	250mg-1g/d divided
	Adult	*PO*	500mg repeated in 2-4h prn
		IM/IV	
Epilepsy			
	Pediatric/Adult	*PO*	8-30mg/kg/d; usual range 375mg-1g/d
Edema			5mg/kg/d
	Pediatric/Adult	*PO*	250-375mg/d (5mg/kg) on alternate days or for 2d c̄ day of rest

PHARMACOKINETICS

PO absorption	Tablet Onset	Tablet Peak	Tablet Duration	Sequel Onset	Sequel Peak	Sequel Duration	Excretion
Good	1h	2-4h	8-12h	2h	8-18h	18-24h	Unchanged via urine

Note: Side/adverse effects: common in *italic;* serious in ***boldface italic.*** *Available in Canada only.

Mountain sickness
Adult *PO* 0.5-1g/d in divided doses prn

SIDE/ADVERSE EFFECTS: CNS: drowsiness, confusion, *paresthesias, convulsions* ▪ EENT: transient myopia ▪ GI: anorexia, melena ▪ GU: polyuria, hematuria, glycosuria ▪ INT: urticaria, photosensitivity (rare) ▪ MET: acidotic states (long-term therapy).

INTERACTIONS: Drug: ↑ Dig toxicity due to hypokalemia; quinidine toxicity due to ↓ renal excretion ▪ Severe hypokalemia c̄ corticosteroids ▪ PO hypoglycemics may require dosage adjustment c̄ concurrent therapy ▪ Use c̄ ↑ aspirin requires caution. **Lab:** False-positive result is possible c̄ urinary proteins c̄ Albustix.

NURSING MANAGEMENT PRIORITIES

ADMINISTRATION: Assess for hx of sulfonamide-derivative hypersensitivity ▪ Diuretic: administer single PO dose in AM c̄ food ▪ Parenteral: reconstitute contents of vial (500mg) c̄ 5ml sterile H_2O for injection; use w/in 24h ▪ IM: painful; direct IV recommended ▪ Assess serum electrolytes ▪ Institute seizure precautions (epileptic) ▪ Maintain hydration ▪ Avoid abrupt withdrawal (anticonvulsant) ▪ Avoid exposure to heat/moisture during storage.

EVALUATION: Monitor F/E, hepatic, renal status ▪ Assess for fluid retention (I&O, daily weight) ▪ Assess for signs of sulfonamide toxicity (fever, rash, crystalluria, renal calculus) ▪ Assess for hyperglycemia (diabetics) ▪ Monitor IOP.

EDUCATION: Take as directed by physician; do *not* omit dose ▪ Take c̄ food; swallow SR capsules whole ▪ Drowsiness may occur; use caution in potentially hazardous activities ▪ Avoid changing positions (lying/sitting/standing) rapidly ▪ Eat foods high in K^+ (bananas, citrus fruits, raisins); avoid black licorice ▪ Symptoms of hypokalemia (anorexia, nausea, lethargy, muscle weakness, mental confusion, hypotension); D/C, notify physician of hypokalemia, tingling/tremors, sore throat, fever, skin rash, unusual bleeding/bruising ▪ May cause temporary visual disturbances (esp far vision) ▪ ↑ Fluid intake (8-10 glasses/d) ▪ Diabetics: carefully monitor blood/urine glucose ▪ Maintain optimum weight; avoid high-Na^+ substances ▪ Store in tightly closed container ▪ Avoid changing brand-name preparations ▪ Carry identification (MedicAlert) if epileptic.

NOTES:

acetohexamide/chlorpropamide • (a-seet-oh-hex-a-mide/ klor-proe-pa-mide)

CATEGORY: *Oral hypoglycemic:* antidiabetic 1st-generation sulfonylurea Rx; Preg Cat C

BRAND NAMES	DOSAGE FORMS
acetohexamide	
Dymelor (Lilly)	Tablet: 250, 500mg
chlorpropamide	
Diabinese (Pfizer)	Tablet: 100, 250mg
**Novopropamide* (Novopharm)*	Tablet: 250mg

USE: Management of type II (noninsulin-dependent) diabetes that cannot be controlled by diet alone. **ACTION:** Antidiabetic activity due to stimulation of insulin release from functioning β cells of pancreas.

PHARMACOKINETICS

PO absorption	Onset	Peak	Duration	Half-life	Excretion
acetohexamide					
Rapid	1h	3h	12-24h	1.3h	80%-90% via urine
chlorpropamide					
Rapid	1h	2-4h	24h or more	36h	80%-90% via urine

CONTRAINDICATIONS: Hypersensitivity, diabetic ketoacidosis c̄ or w/out coma. **CC:** Use can ↑ risk of cardiovascular mortality in comparison to diet or insulin treatment ▪ Pts require constant medical evaluation during treatment.

DOSAGE: Must be individualized. Adult *PO*

acetohexamide	Usual maintenance range 250mg-1.5g/d
chlorpropamide	Usual maintenance range 100-500mg/d

SIDE/ADVERSE EFFECTS: GI: *nausea, epigastric fullness,* heartburn ▪ HEM: ***aplastic anemia, agranulocytosis, leukopenia, hemolytic anemia,*** pancytopenia, ***thrombocytopenia*** ▪ INT: erythema, morbilliform/maculopapular eruptions, photosensitivity ▪ MET: hypoglycemia.

INTERACTIONS: Drug: Use c̄ alcohol, MAO-Is, β blockers, probenecid, salicylates, sulfonamides can significantly ↑ hypoglycemic effects ▪ Use c̄ anabolic steroids, chloramphenicol, guanethidine, PO anticoagulants, probenecid, salicylates, sulfinpyrazones, sulfonamides ↑ hy-

Note: Side/adverse effects: common in *italic;* serious in ***boldface italic.***

*Available in Canada only.

poglycemic effects ▪ Use c̄ adrenergics, corticosteroids, phenytoin, thiazides, thyroid preparations ⬇ hypoglycemic effects ▪ Use c̄ NSAIAs can ⬆ hypoglycemic effects ▪ Use c̄ alcohol can produce disulfiram-like rxs.

NURSING MANAGEMENT PRIORITIES

ADMINISTRATION: Assess for hx of hypersensitivity ▪ Maintenance dose <1g/d, administer as single AM dose c̄ breakfast; >1g, administer in AM & PM c̄ meals ▪ Avoid exposure to moisture in storage ▪ Elderly may require ⬇ dosage.

EVALUATION: Monitor hepatic, renal, hematologic status ▪ Monitor FBS ▪ Evaluate pt closely during 1st wk to assess effectiveness ▪ Monitor for signs of hypoglycemia/hyperglycemia.

EDUCATION: Compliance c̄ special diet therapy ▪ Blood/urine glucose/ketone testing procedure ▪ Symptoms of hypoglycemia (anxiety, headache, fatigue, nausea, sweating); notify physician immediately ▪ Always carry lump of sugar/candy for quick use if hypoglycemia occurs ▪ Avoid alcoholic beverages ▪ Check c̄ physician before taking OTC preparations ▪ Symptoms of hyperglycemia (excessive hunger, thirst, urination, rapid pulse, sweet-smelling breath, weight loss); notify physician immediately ▪ Need for good personal hygiene ▪ Carry medical identification (MedicAlert) ▪ Store in tightly closed containers ▪ Keep scheduled appointments c̄ physician/for blood glucose determinations ▪ Schedule periodic eye exams ▪ Maintain optimum body weight ▪ Avoid prolonged exposure to sunlight; use sunscreen, protective clothing ▪ Women: avoid breastfeeding ▪ PO hypoglycemic needs may change c̄ ⬆ stress, ⬆ exercise, ⬇ appetite; notify physician.

NOTES:

acyclovir/acyclovir sodium▲ • (ay-<u>sye</u>-kloe-veer)

CATEGORY: *Antiviral*: purine nucleoside analog

Rx; Preg Cat C

BRAND NAME
Zovirax (G-W)

DOSAGE FORMS
Capsule: 200mg
Powder for injection (IV)▲: 500mg/vial
Ointment: 5%
Suspension: 200mg/5ml
Tablet: 800mg

USE: Management of herpes genitalis (HSV-2), mucocutaneous herpes simplex (HSV-1) in immunocompromised pts ▪ Acute treatment of herpes zoster ▪ Treatment of chickenpox. **ACTION**: Antiviral activity due to interference $\bar{c}$ virus DNA polymerase & DNA replication in virus-infected host cells; selective for herpesvirus (HSV-1, HSV-2), varicella-zoster (VZV).

CONTRAINDICATIONS: Hypersensitivity. **CC:** IV powder for injection not intended for PO, SC, IM, topical use, or use in the eyes.

DOSAGE

Topical	Apply ointment q3h 6 times/d for 7d
Pediatric *IV*	250mg/m² administered at constant rate for 1h q8h for 7d for HSV-1 & HSV-2. For encephalitis & VZV 500mg/m² q8h for 10d
PO	Chickenpox: 20mg/kg (do *not* exceed 800mg) 4 times/d. Initiate at earliest symptoms Genital herpes: initial treatment of 200mg q4h 5 times/d for 10d. For suppressive therapy or recurrent infection 400mg bid for up to 12mo

PHARMACOKINETICS

PO absorption	Peak	Half-life	Protein binding	Excretion
15%-30%	1.5-2.5h	2-3.5h	9%-33%	Urine via tubular secretion, glomerular filtration primarily as unchanged drug

Adult	*IV*	5mg/kg administered at constant rate for 1h q8h for 7d for HSV-1 and HSV-2. For encephalitis & herpes zoster 10mg/kg q8h for 10d
	PO	Initial genital herpes: 200mg q4h 5 times/d for 10d Long-term suppression/recurrent disease: 400mg bid for up to 12mo or 200mg tid or 5 times/d Intermittent treatment: 200mg q4h 5 times/d for 5d Herpes zoster: 800mg q4h 5 times/d for 7-10d

SIDE/ADVERSE EFFECTS: CNS: agitation, confusion, hallucinations, lethargy, tremors, seizures/coma (all systemic) ▪ CV: *inflammation* or *phlebitis* at infusion site, hypotension ▪ INT: *burning/stinging* at application site (topical), rash, hives, pruritus.

INTERACTIONS: Drug: Probenecid will ⬇ urinary excretion of acyclovir, causing accumulation c̄ potential toxicity ▪ Use c̄ caution c̄ interferon/methotrexate; neurologic rxs may occur.

NURSING MANAGEMENT PRIORITIES

ADMINISTRATION: Parenteral: administer only by IV infusion over 1h; use infusion control device; avoid rapid/bolus dose; dilute 500mg vial c̄ 10ml sterile H_2O for injection (50mg/ml); shake vial well until solution is clear, stable for 12h (room temperature); further dilute c̄ dextrose/electrolyte solutions to ≥70mg (7mg/ml), use w/in 24h (room temperature); precipitate occurs c̄ refrigeration, will redissolve at room temperature ▪ PO suspension: shake well before pouring ▪ Topical: use glove to prevent herpes transmission ▪ Maintain hydration ▪ Avoid exposure to heat/moisture in storage ▪ Administer at *end* of hemodialysis.

EVALUATION: Monitor F/E, hepatic, renal status ▪ Assess for ⬆ BUN, serum creatinine (IV).

EDUCATION: Take exactly as directed by physician ▪ Take PO form c̄ food; shake suspension well before use ▪ Dizziness may occur; use caution in potentially hazardous activities ▪ ⬆ Fluid intake (8-10 glasses/d) ▪ Use condoms if sexually active ▪ Information on herpes (symptoms, hygiene, transmission) ▪ Women: avoid breastfeeding ▪ Store in tightly closed container ▪ Procedure for topical application.

NOTES:

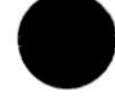

albuterol sulfate/terbutaline sulfate • (al-byoo-tear-ole/ter-byoo-ta-leen) 8

CATEGORY: *Sympathomimetic:* β_2 adrenergic, bronchodilator Rx; Preg Cat C-B

BRAND NAMES	DOSAGE FORMS
albuterol	
Proventil (Schering)	Aerosol: 90µg/dose Inhalation solution: 0.5% Nebulization solution: 0.083% Syrup: 2mg/5ml Repetab: 4mg Tablet: 2, 4mg
Ventolin (G-W)	Aerosol: 90µg/dose Inhalation solution: 0.5% Nebulization solution (Nebules): 0.083% Powder for inhalation (Rotocaps) 200µg Syrup: 2mg/5ml Tablet: 2, 4mg
terbutaline	
Brethaire (Geigy)	Aerosol: 0.2mg/dose
Brethine (Geigy)	Injection (SC): 1mg/ml Tablet: 2.5, 5mg
Bricanyl (HMR)	Injection (SC): 1mg/ml Tablet: 2.5, 5mg

USE: Treatment of bronchial asthma, reversible bronchospasm associated c̄ bronchitis/emphysema. **ACTION:** Sympathomimetic activity at β_2 receptors produces bronchodilation.

PHARMACOKINETICS

PO absorption	Onset	Peak	Excretion
albuterol			
Rapid	30m	2-3h	Via urine as metabolites
terbutaline			
35%-50%	30m	1-2h	Via urine primarily as unchanged drug

CONTRAINDICATIONS: Hypersensitivity. **CC:** Inhalation administration can result in life-threatening, paradoxic bronchospasm.

DOSAGE

albuterol

Children *PO*

2-6y/o	0.1mg/kg tid
6-12y/o	2mg 3-4 times/d

Adult/Children ≥12y/o		2-4mg 3-4 times/d
Adult/Children ≥4y/o		
	Aerosol	2 inhalations q4-6h
Adult/Children ≥12y/o		
	Solutions	2.5-mg inhalations 3-4 times/d
Adult/Children ≥4y/o		
	Powder	200-μg inhalations q4-6h

terbutaline

Adolescent 12-15y/o	*PO*	2.5mg q6h tid. Do *not* exceed 7.5mg/d
	Aerosol	2 inhalations q4-6h
Adult	*PO*	5mg q6h tid. Do *not* exceed 15mg/d
	SC	0.25mg. Repeat if no improvement w/in 15-30m. Do *not* exceed 0.5mg/4h
	Aerosol	2 inhalations q4-6h

SIDE/ADVERSE EFFECTS: CNS: nervousness, tremor, insomnia, headache, drowsiness ▪ CV: ↑ heart rate; palpitations, hypotension ▪ GI: N/V ▪ MS: muscle cramps ▪ Other: bronchospasm.

INTERACTIONS: Drug: Use c̄ nonselective β blockers (eg, propranolol) will antagonize bronchodilation ▪ Use c̄ MAO-I contraindicated ▪ Use c̄ other sympathomimetics best avoided.

NURSING MANAGEMENT PRIORITIES

ADMINISTRATION: Assess for hx of catecholamine hypersensitivity ▪ Assess BP, pulse before administration ▪ Administer c̄ food to ↓ GI irritation; may crush tablets ▪ Check dosages c̄ another RN.

EVALUATION: Monitor VS, esp heart rate ▪ Monitor I&O ▪ Diabetics: closely monitor blood glucose (hyperglycemia).

EDUCATION: Take c̄ food to ↓ GI distress; may crush tablets ▪ Take as ordered by physician; do *not* ↑ dose ▪ Procedure for radial pulse determination ▪ Keep scheduled appointments c̄ physician ▪ Check c̄ physician/pharmacist before taking OTC preparations ▪ Procedure for inhalation administration (do *not* puncture/incinerate aerosol container).

NOTES:

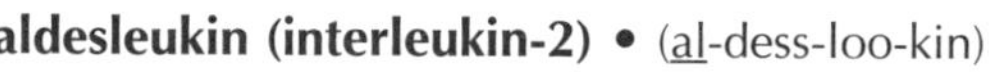

aldesleukin (interleukin-2) • (al-dess-loo-kin)

CATEGORY: *Lymphokine:* antineoplastic, biologic response modifier Rx; Preg Cat C

BRAND NAME	DOSAGE FORM
Proleukin (Chiron)	IV powder for injection: 22 million IV/vial

USE: Treatment of selected pts c̄ metastatic renal cell carcinoma ■ Can be used as a sole agent or in combination c̄ lymphokine-activated killer (LAK) cells obtained from pt. **ACTION:** Biosynthetic analog of human interleukin-2, an endogenous lymphokine produced by genetically engineered (recombinant DNA) *Escherichia coli.* Possesses complex antineoplastic & immunomodulating activity. Exact antineoplastic mechanism(s) not fully known. Aldesleukin antitumor activity is related to production & activation of killer cells.

PHARMACOKINETICS: Onset of tumor reduction is ≥4 wk c̄ a duration for up to 12mo after start of therapy.

CONTRAINDICATIONS: Hypersensitivity, pts c̄ abnormal pulmonary function & thallium stress tests, organ grafts, previous toxicities from aldesleukin treatment. **CC:** Administration requires experienced personnel & available cardiopulmonary/intensive care facilities if required ■ Use can cause capillary leak syndrome resulting in hypotension, ↓ organ perfusion, possible death ■ Use only in pts c̄ normal cardiac & pulmonary function ■ Use in pts who develop moderate/severe lethargy/ somnolence during treatment can become comatose ■ Possible exacerbation of undiagnosed/treated CNS metastases ■ Use can ↑ risk of infection due to ↓ neutrophil function ■ Treated pts should practice birth control ■ Use can induce thyroid impairment & replacement therapy may be required ■ Possible ↑ rejection in allograph transplant pts ■ Safety & efficacy in pts <18y/o not established.

DOSAGE

Adult *IV*	600,000 IU/kg dose by a 15-m infusion q8h for 14 doses. Schedule is repeated following a 9-d rest period

SIDE/ADVERSE EFFECTS: Produces an extensive array of rxs. All rxs listed are in descending percentage of occurrence (ended at the 10% level). CNS: mental status changes, dizziness, headache, sensory dysfunction ■ CV: hypotension, sinus tachycardia ■ GI: N/V/D, stomatitis, anorexia, ***bleeding*** ■ HEM: anemia, ***thrombocytopenia,*** leukopenia ■ HEP: ↑ in bilirubin, transaminases, alkaline phosphatase, jaundice ■ INT: pruritus, erythema, rash, dry skin, exfoliative dermatitis ▪ MET: hypomagnesemia, ***acidosis***, hypocalcemia, hypophosphatemia ▪ REN: ***anuria/oliguria,*** ↑ BUN, serum creatinine, proteinuria ▪ RESP: congestion, dyspnea, edema, ***failure*** ▪ Other: fever/chills, pain, fatigue, infection, weight gain.

INTERACTIONS: Drug: Use c̄ cardiotoxic, hepatotoxic, myelotoxic, nephrotoxic drugs can produce additive toxicity ▪ Use c̄ antihypertensives can result in ↑ hypertension.

NURSING MANAGEMENT PRIORITIES

ADMINISTRATION: Assess for hx of hypersensitivity ▪ Obtain CBC, differential & platelet counts, electrolytes, chest x-ray, stress thallium study before administration ▪ Assess hepatic, pulmonary, renal function; notify physician if impaired ▪ Assess for hx of seizures; use caution ▪ Administer via 15-m infusion q8h ▪ Dilute/reconstitute according to manufacturer's directions; refrigerate ▪ Use reconstituted preparations w/in 48h at room temperature; discard unused portion.

EVALUATION: Monitor VS, esp ↓ BP ▪ Monitor AST, ALT (hepatotoxicity) ▪ Monitor hematologic, renal function ▪ Monitor fluid retention (I&O, daily weight) ▪ Assess mental status (LOC, irritability) ▪ Avoid extravasation; assess for pain, redness at site ▪ Assess for hypovolemia (capillary leak syndrome) ▪ Assess organ transplant pts for graft rejection ▪ Monitor thyroid function; notify physician if impaired.

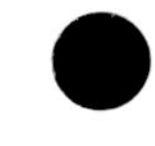

EDUCATION: Dizziness/drowsiness may occur; use caution c̄ ambulation ▪ Notify nurse/physician of abnormal rxs (fever, chills, lethargy) ▪ Avoid exposure to infection ▪ Women: avoid pregnancy, breastfeeding ▪ Use contraception if sexually active.

NOTES:

alendronate sodium • (a-len-dro-nate)

CATEGORY: *Antiosteoporosis agent:* biophosphonate

Rx; Preg Cat C

BRAND NAME
Fosamax (Merck)

DOSAGE FORMS
Tablet: 10, 40mg

USE: Treatment of osteoporosis in postmenopausal females. ▪ Treatment of Paget's disease in pts having excessive alkaline phosphatase levels (≥2 times the upper normal limit), asymptomatic and/or pts who are at further risk from complications of the disease. **ACTION:** Alendronate localizes at osteoclasts that are specific sites of bone resorption. Antiosteoporosis activity due to dose-dependent inhibition of osteoclast–mediated bone resorption resulting in an ⬆ in bone mass.

PHARMACOKINETICS: PO absorption is adequate after overnight fasting & administered at least 30m before breakfast or the first food of the day. Protein binding is about 78% & bone-incorporated drug is inactive & has a terminal elimination half-life of ≥10yrs. No metabolism of drug occurs.

CONTRAINDICATIONS: Hypersensitivity, delayed esophageal emptying time, hypocalcemia, pts unable to sit upright and/or stand for 30m after administration. **CC:** Therapeutic effect requires continuous treatment. Bone-incorporated drug is inactive ▪ Use can produce GI disease, esp esophageal ulcers, & use in pts c̄ existing conditions requires close supervision ▪ Concurrent hormonal replacement therapy not adequately studied ▪ Use in nursing mothers not currently recommended ▪ Safety & effectiveness in pediatric or male pts not established ▪ Pts c̄ impaired renal function can experience greater bone accumulation ▪ Currently not recommended in pts c̄ severe renal dysfunction.

DOSAGE

PO	Postmenopausal osteoporosis: 10mg/d Paget's disease: 40mg/d for 6mo

SIDE/ADVERSE EFFECTS: GI: abdominal pain, N/V/D, constipation, dyspepsia, flatulence, acid regurgitation, ***ulcers*** ▪ Other: headache, muscular pain, taste disturbances.

INTERACTIONS: Drug: Use c̄ aspirin & other ulcerogenic drugs can produce additive effects ▪ Calcium products can ⬇ alendronate absorption. **Lab:** Transient ⬇ in serum phosphate & calcium. **Food:** Coffee, orange juice, mineral water will ⬇ alendronate absorption.

NURSING MANAGEMENT PRIORITIES

ADMINISTRATION: Assess for hx of biphosphonate hypersensitivity ▪ Assess renal function; use c̄ caution if impaired ▪ Administer 1h ac c̄ full glass of H_2O ▪ Avoid administration w/in 2h of calcium-containing foods ▪ Maintain upright position for at least 30m after taking drug.

EVALUATION: Monitor renal, hepatic function ▪ Monitor serum calcium levels throughout therapy.

EDUCATION: Take at least 30m before the first food, beverage, or medication of the day c̄ full glass of H_2O ▪ Maintain adequate calcium & vitamin D intake ▪ Wait minimum of 30m before taking any other drug ▪ May alter taste sensation ▪ Avoid excessive cigarette smoking or use of alcohol ▪ Avoid lying down for at least 30m after taking drug.

NOTES:

allopurinol • (al-oh-pure-i-nole)

CATEGORY: *Antigout:* xanthine oxidase inhibitor Rx; Preg Cat C

BRAND NAMES / **DOSAGE FORMS**

BRAND NAMES	DOSAGE FORMS
**Alloprin (ICN)*	Tablet: 100, 200, 300mg
**Novopurinol (Novopharm)*	Tablet: 100, 200, 300mg
**Purinol (Horner)*	Tablet: 100, 200, 300mg
**Roucal (Rougier)*	Tablet: 100, 200, 300mg
Zyloprim (G-W)	Tablet: 100, 300mg

USE: Treatment of gout, uric acid neuropathy, recurrent uric acid stone formation ▪ Prevention of tissue urate deposition, renal calculi, uric acid nephropathy in pts c̄ leukemia, lymphomas, malignancies receiving chemotherapy ▪ Management of recurrent calcium oxalate calculi in pts c̄ daily uric acid excretion rates of over 800mg/d (males) & 750mg/d (females). **ACTION:** Antigout effect due to inhibition of xanthine oxidase, which converts purines into uric acid.

PHARMACOKINETICS

PO absorption	Peak	Half-life	Excretion
90%	1.5h	1-2h	80% via urine, 20% via feces

CONTRAINDICATIONS: Hypersensitivity. **CC:** D/C use c̄ first appearance of skin rash ▪ Initial stages of treatment can induce ⬆ gout attacks ▪ Rare cases of hepatotoxicity have been reported ▪ Use c̄ caution in nursing mothers due to presence of drug in milk ▪ Not indicated for asymptomatic hyperuricemia.

DOSAGE

Adult	*PO*	200-600mg/d c̄ maximum 800mg/d
Children	*PO*	
Secondary hyperuricemia		6-10y/o: 300mg/d and 150mg/d for <6y/o. Adjust dosage after 48h if needed

SIDE/ADVERSE EFFECTS: CNS: peripheral neuritis ▪ EENT: cataracts ▪ GI: N/V/D ▪ HEM: ***agranulocytosis,*** anemia, ***aplastic anemia,*** bone marrow depression ▪ HEP: vasculitis or necrotizing angiitis leading to irreversible hepatotoxicity/death ▪ INT: *rash,* ***exfoliative dermatitis,*** urticaria, ***Stevens-Johnson syndrome, toxic epidermal necrolysis.***

Note: Side/adverse effects: common in *italic;* serious in ***boldface italic.***

*Available in Canada only.

INTERACTIONS: Drug: Use c̄ azathioprine/mercaptopurine will significantly alter their biotransformation; dosage adjustment required ■ ↑ PO absorption of iron preparations ■ Use c̄ dicumarol may ↑ bleeding time.

NURSING MANAGEMENT PRIORITIES

ADMINISTRATION: Assess CBC, hepatic, renal function; may require ↓ dosage if impaired ■ Administer >300mg in divided doses ■ Administer pc ■ ↑ Fluid intake (3000ml/d).

EVALUATION: Monitor hepatic, renal status ■ Monitor CBC, serum uric acid, I&O ■ May produce ↓ serum glucose ■ Normal serum uric acid: 2.5-6mg/100ml.

EDUCATION: Drowsiness may occur; use caution when engaging in potentially hazardous activities ■ Take as directed by physician ■ Take pc ■ D/C, notify physician of rash/flulike symptoms ■ Used to prevent, *not* relieve, gout attacks ■ Avoid alcohol intake ■ ↑ Fluid intake (10-12 glasses/d) ■ Do *not* take c̄ iron preparations ■ Store in tightly closed container ■ Keep scheduled appointments for serum uric acid determinations ■ Women: avoid breastfeeding ■ Check c̄ physician before taking vitamin C preparations (↑ kidney stone formation) ■ Maintain optimum weight ■ ↓ Intake of high-purine foods (organ meats, legumes) ■ Full drug effects may require several mo of therapy.

NOTES:

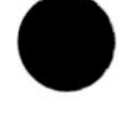

alprazolam/halazepam • (al-praz-oh-lam/hal-az-e-pam)

CATEGORY: *Benzodiazepine:* antianxiety agent, anxiolytic

Rx C-IV; Preg Cat D

BRAND NAMES	DOSAGE FORMS
alprazolam	
Xanax (Upjohn)	Tablet: 0.25, 0.5, 1mg
halazepam	
Paxipam (Schering)	Tablet: 20, 40mg

USE: Short-term treatment of anxiety (DSM-IV-R) ▪ Treatment of panic disorder c̄ or w/out agoraphobia (alprazolam). **ACTION:** Benzodiazepines appear to potentiate the inhibitory effects of gamma-aminobutyric acid (GABA)—mediated central neurotransmission. Anxiolytic activity due to depression of CNS at brainstem reticular formation, limbic, thalamic areas.

PHARMACOKINETICS

PO absorption	Peak	Half-life	Protein binding	Excretion
alprazolam				
Very good	1-2h	12-15h	80%	Via urine as unchanged drug, metabolites
halazepam				
Rapid	1-3h	14h	—	Via urine as metabolites (99%)

CONTRAINDICATIONS: Hypersensitivity, narrow-angle glaucoma ▪ Concurrent use c̄ ketoconazole, itraconazole. **CC:** Benzodiazepines are not indicated for psychiatric disorders, esp when anxiety is not a significant symptom ▪ Use can result in dependence; abrupt D/C can result in withdrawal symptoms incl seizures ▪ Use c̄ caution in pts c̄ hepatic or renal dysfunction ▪ Concurrent use c̄ ketoconazole, itraconazole due to inhibition of alprazolam.

DOSAGE

alprazolam

Anxiety		
Adult	*PO*	0.25-0.5mg tid. Do *not* exceed 4mg/d
Geriatric	*PO*	0.25mg bid or tid or higher if needed or tolerated
Panic disorder		
Adult	*PO*	0.5mg tid c̄ a range of 1-10mg/d

halazepam

Adult	*PO*	20-40mg 3-4 times/d
Geriatric	*PO*	20mg 1-2 times/d

SIDE/ADVERSE EFFECTS: CNS: *drowsiness, fatigue, ataxia,* paradoxic anxiety, hallucinations, hyperexcitation ▪ CV: hypotension ▪ HEM: neutropenia (rare).

Note: Side/adverse effects: common in *italic;* serious in ***boldface italic.***

*Available in Canada only.

INTERACTIONS: Drug: Use c̄ other CNS depressants produces additive effects ▪ Use c̄ MAO-I can produce serious toxic effects ▪ Use c̄ PO contraceptives, fluoexetine will ↑ alprazolam plasma concentration ▪ Use c̄ fluoxetine, oral contraceptives can ↑ alprazolam concentration.

NURSING MANAGEMENT PRIORITIES

ADMINISTRATION: Assess for hx of benzodiazepine hypersensitivity ▪ Avoid exposure to heat/moisture/light in storage ▪ Avoid abrupt withdrawal ▪ Have emergency support measures available ▪ Elderly may require ↓ dosage ▪ Ventilation of feelings, sympathetic listening contribute to relief of anxiety.

EVALUATION: Monitor renal, hepatic status ▪ Assess for symptoms of abrupt withdrawal (tremor, abdominal/muscle cramps, convulsions) c̄ prolonged use ▪ Check for signs of dependence c̄ prolonged therapy (↑ drug request) ▪ Monitor activity status (safety precautions) ▪ Assess for tolerance to therapeutic dose ▪ Assess for paradoxic rxs (CNS stimulation), esp elderly ▪ Check for depression; suicide precautions prn.

EDUCATION: Drowsiness may occur; use caution when engaging in potentially hazardous activities ▪ Avoid use c̄ alcohol, other CNS depressants ▪ Indiscriminate use may lead to dependence ▪ Do *not* keep at bedside ▪ Take as ordered by physician; do *not* ↑ dose ▪ Check c̄ physician/pharmacist before taking OTC preparations ▪ Women: avoid breastfeeding ▪ Use alternate methods (relaxation exercises, ventilation of feelings) to ↓ anxiety.

NOTES:

alteplase recombinant/reteplase recombinant • (all-teh-place/reh-teh-place)

CATEGORY: *Thrombolytic agent:* biosynthetic tissue plasminogen activator (tPA) Rx; Preg Cat C

BRAND NAMES	DOSAGE FORMS
alteplase recombinant	IV powder for injection:
Activase (Genetech)	20, 50, 100mg/vial
reteplase recombinant	IV powder for injection: 18.8mg
Retavase (B-M)	(10.81U)/vial

USE: *alteplase:* Management (lysis of thrombi) of acute MI ▪ Management of pulmonary embolism ▪ Management of acute ischemic stroke. *reteplase:* Management (lysis of thrombi) of acute MI. **ACTION:** Tissue plasminogen activator (tPA) is an enzyme that is part of the endogenous fibrinolytic mechanism of the circulatory system. tPA regulates conversion of inactive plasminogen in blood into plasmin, an active fibrinolytic enzyme that dissolves blood clots. Exogenous biosynthetic (bacterial recombinant DNA) tPA has the same activity as endogenous tPA & is used to dissolve serious blood clots.

PHARMACOKINETICS: alteplase: Drug has a short half-life & requires continuous IV infusion to produce clinical thrombolytic activity, which appears to be dose dependent. Approximately 50% of drug is cleared from plasma w/in 5m & 80% cleared w/in 10m after termination of infusion. Excretion of drug is via urine c̄ 80% excreted w/in 1.8h. reteplase: Drug has effective half-life of 13-16m. Excretion is via liver & kidney.

CONTRAINDICATIONS: Common: Active bleeding or known bleeding tendencies, arteriovenous malformation or aneurysm, hx of CVA, intracranial neoplasm, intercranial or intraspinal surgery/trauma, severe uncontrolled hypertension. alteplase: Additional for ischemic stroke: bleeding diathesis, hx of intracranial bleeding, hypertension 185 systolic or >110 diastolic, pretreatment evaluation c̄ evidence of intracranial bleeding, recent previous stroke, seizure at onset of stroke, suspicion of subarachnoid bleeding. **CC:** Possibility of bleeding from GI/GU/respiratory tract, intercranial, retroperitoneal & from surgical procedure sites, esp c̄ concurrent heparin use ▪ Use (coronary thrombolysis) may result in arrhythmias c̄ coronary reperfusion or cholesterol embolization ▪ Avoid IM injections, excess pt handling ▪ Following clinical conditions requires potential risk considerations before use & extreme caution during use: advanced age, cardiac conditions that include acute pericarditis, possible left heart thrombus, subacute bacterial endocarditis; cardiovascular disease, concurrent use of anticoagulants, hemostatic effects 2° to severe hepatic/renal disease, hypertension ≥180 systolic or >110 diastolic, pregnancy, previous puncture of noncompressible vessels, serious infection at AV cannula sites, recent GI/GU bleeding or any other potential bleeding condition, severe hepatic/renal impairment, recent surgery or trauma ▪ Additional for alteplase: doses of 150mg can cause an ↑ in intracranial bleeding ▪ Additional for reteplase: do not administer a second bolus dose if significant bleeding is occurring before administration.

DOSAGE: Adult *IV*

alteplase

Acute MI	3-hr infusion method:
>65kg	Total dose of 100mg over 3h. 1st h: 60-mg dose (6-10mg is given as bolus dose over 1-2m, remaining 50-54mg given by infusion). 2nd & 3rd h: subsequent maintenance infusion of 20mg/h
<65kg	Total dose of 1.25mg/kg infused over 3h. 1st h: 0.75mg/kg (0.045-0.075mg/kg as bolus dose over 1-2m, remaining 0.675-0.705mg/kg given by infusion). 2nd & 3rd h: subsequent maintenance infusion of 0.25mg/h
	Accelerated infusion method:
>65kg	Total dose of 100mg: 1st dose of 15mg as bolus dose followed by 50mg infused over next 30m, then 35mg infused over 1h
<65kg	Total dose of 100mg: 15-mg bolus dose followed by 0.75mg/kg infused over next 30m (do *not* exceed a total dose of 50mg) then 0.5mg/kg over 1h (do *not* exceed 35mg)
Acute ischemic stroke	0.9mg/kg infused over 1h $\bar{c}$ 10% of dose given as initial bolus over 1m. Do *not* exceed a total dose of 90mg
Pulmonary embolism	100mg infused over 2h

reteplase

Acute MI	10U + 10U double-bolus injection; 1st bolus (10U) given over 2m; 2nd 10U given 30m after 1st injection over 2m

SIDE/ADVERSE EFFECTS: CV: ***bleeding, reperfusion-related atrial/ventricular arrhythmias, venous thrombosis, embolism,*** hypotension ▪ GI: N/V ▪ Other: edema, anaphylactoid rxs.

INTERACTIONS: Drug: Use c̄ PO anticoagulants or heparin requires caution because of ⬆ bleeding tendencies ▪ Use c̄ platelet inhibitors (aspirin, dipyridamole, abciximab) & vitamin K antagonists can produce additive bleeding tendencies. **Lab:** Coagulation/fibrinolytic tests performed during treatment may be unreliable because drug is active in in-vitro conditions.

NURSING MANAGEMENT PRIORITIES

ADMINISTRATION: Assess for hx of hypersensitivity ▪ Assess CV status, coagulation studies ▪ Assess renal, hepatic function; use caution if impaired ▪ Assess for hx of internal bleeding, hypertension, anticoagulant use ▪ Reconstitute c̄ sterile H_2O for injection according to manufacturer's directions immediately before use, avoid excessive agitation ▪ Administer via infusion pump as soon as possible after onset of symptoms.

EVALUATION: Monitor CV function q15m until stabilized, then qh ▪ Assess for relief of chest pain; notify physician if pain persists or recurs ▪ Assess for bleeding; monitor coagulation studies continuously; apply manual pressure/pressure dressing to bleeding site; D/C infusion if bleeding is uncontrollable.

EDUCATION: Notify nurse/physician of abnormal rxs (difficult breathing, chest pain, irregular heartbeat, bleeding at IV insertion site).

NOTES:

amantadine hcl • (a-man-ta-deen)

CATEGORY: *Anti-Parkinson agent, antiviral*

Rx; Preg Cat C

BRAND NAME
Symmetrel (Du Pont)

DOSAGE FORMS
Capsule: 100mg
Syrup: 50mg/5ml

USE: Treatment of Parkinson's disease, drug-induced extrapyramidal rxs, CO-induced Parkinson's disease ▪ Prevention, treatment of influenza A virus respiratory tract infections. **ACTION:** Anti-Parkinson activity may be due to ↑ in dopamine release in brain; antiviral activity appears related to inhibition of viral replication, release of viral nuclei in host cells.

PHARMACOKINETICS

PO absorption	Peak	Half-life	Excretion
Good	4h	15h	Via urine as unchanged drug

CONTRAINDICATIONS: Hypersensitivity. **CC:** Pts c̄ hx of seizure disorders can experience ↑ in seizure activity ▪ Pts >65y/o require ↓ doses ▪ Risk of CHF c̄ use ▪ Caution required in pts c̄ liver disease.

DOSAGE

Pediatric	*PO*	Influenza: 1-9y/o 2-4mg/kg/d. Do *not* exceed 150mg/d 9-12y/o 100mg bid
Adult	*PO*	Parkinson's disease: usual range 100-200mg divided. 400mg/d may be necessary Influenza: 100-300mg/d divided

SIDE/ADVERSE EFFECTS: CNS: *depression,* dizziness, headache ▪ CV: ***CHF,*** *orthostatic hypotensive episodes,* peripheral edema ▪ GI: anorexia, N/V, constipation, dry mouth ▪ GU: *urinary retention* ▪ HEM: leukopenia, neutropenia ▪ INT: skin rash, eczematoid dermatitis ▪ PSYCH: *psychosis,* confusion, anxiety.

INTERACTIONS: Drug: Use c̄ anticholinergics will produce additive anticholinergic effects ▪ Use c̄ CNS stimulants is best avoided because of CNS additive effects.

NURSING MANAGEMENT PRIORITIES

ADMINISTRATION: Assess for hx of hypersensitivity ▪ Assess for CHF, fluid retention, renal impairment; requires

Note: Side/adverse effects: common in *italic;* serious in ***boldface italic.***

*Available in Canada only

↓ dosage ▪ Administer pc; do *not* administer hs (insomnia) ▪ Avoid abrupt withdrawal (may induce parkinsonian crisis); D/C drug gradually.

EVALUATION: Monitor CV, GI, GU, hepatic, neurologic, renal status ▪ Monitor VS ▪ Monitor I&O ▪ Assess for muscle weakness ▪ Observe for exaggerated anticholinergic effects (dry mouth, urinary retention) ▪ Observe for CNS stimulation/psychiatric manifestations; notify physician.

EDUCATION: Dizziness may occur; avoid engaging in potentially hazardous activities ▪ Avoid changing positions (lying/sitting/standing) rapidly ▪ Take as directed by physician ▪ Take pc ▪ Do *not* D/C w/out notifying physician ▪ May cause blurred vision ▪ Redness/mottling of skin may occur; will disappear after several wks of therapy ▪ Use sugarless gum/hard candy to diminish dry mouth ▪ Use calibrated measuring device for PO liquid forms ▪ Avoid alcohol intake ▪ Women: avoid breastfeeding ▪ Store in tightly closed container ▪ Safety precautions $\bar{c}$ ↑ activity ▪ Notify physician if Parkinson symptoms reappear (trembling, shuffling gait, rigidity) ▪ Full drug effects may require several days of therapy.

NOTES:

amiloride hcl • (a-mill-oh-ride)

CATEGORY: *Potassium-sparing diuretic*

Rx; Preg Cat B

BRAND NAME
Midamor (MSD)

DOSAGE FORM
Tablet: 5mg

COMBINATION PRODUCT
Moduretic (MSD) Amiloride 5mg/hydrochlorothiazide 50mg/tablet

USE: Adjunct (antikaliuretic) c̄ thiazides/other kaliuretic diuretics in treatment of CHF, hypertension. **ACTION**: Antikaliuretic mechanism not established; weak antihypertensive, diuretic, natriuretic activity.

PHARMACOKINETICS

PO absorption	Onset	Peak	Half-life	Excretion
50%	2h	6-10h	6-9h	Unchanged via urine (50%), feces (40%) in 72h

CONTRAINDICATIONS: Hypersensitivity, hyperkalemia, impaired renal function, potassium supplements. **CC:** Uncorrected hyperkalemia (>5.5mEq/L) c̄ drug use can be fatal ▪ Avoid use in diabetic pts if possible ▪ Use c̄ caution in pts c̄ cardiopulmonary disease due to risk of metabolic acidosis.

DOSAGE

Adult *PO* 5-10mg/d to prevent hypokalemia, c̄ 10-20mg/d for persistent cases. Moduretic dose usually 1-2 tablets/d

SIDE/ADVERSE EFFECTS: CNS: *headache*, dizziness ▪ GI: *N/V, anorexia*, abdominal pain ▪ GU: impotence, polyuria, dysuria, urinary frequency.

INTERACTIONS: **Drug:** Use c̄ lithium is best avoided because of ⬇ renal clearance ▪ Use c̄ antikaliuretic agents/potassium supplements produces significant hyperkalemia. **Lab:** D/C use for at least 3d in pts c̄ diabetes before glucose tolerance testing.

NURSING MANAGEMENT PRIORITIES

ADMINISTRATION: Assess renal function; do *not* administer if impaired ▪ Assess serum K^+ (normal: 3.5-5mEq/L); notify physician of ⬆ level ▪ Administer c̄ meals/milk on arising ▪ Maintain hydration ▪ Elderly may require ⬇ dosage.

Note: Side/adverse effects: common in *italic;* serious in ***boldface italic.***

*Available in Canada only

EVALUATION: Monitor F/E, hepatic, renal status ▪ Monitor BP ▪ Monitor serum K^+; do *not* administer if hyperkalemic ▪ Monitor fluid retention (I&O, daily weight).

EDUCATION: Expect ↑ urine output; have bathroom facilities easily accessible ▪ May cause weakness, lethargy ▪ Take as directed by physician even if symptom free; do *not* skip doses ▪ Take on waking, at same time qd ▪ Used to control, *not* cure, hypertension ▪ Notify physician of signs of hyperkalemia (difficult breathing, tingling extremities, nervousness, irregular heartbeat) ▪ Avoid changing positions (lying/sitting/standing) rapidly ▪ Avoid foods high in K^+ (bananas, citrus juices, raisins) ▪ Avoid high-Na^+ foods (canned soups, lunch meats, cheese) ▪ Notify physician of N/V/D ▪ Maintain optimum weight ▪ Store in tightly closed container ▪ Check c̄ physician before taking OTC/Rx preparations ▪ Notify physician/dentist of use before treatment.

NOTES:

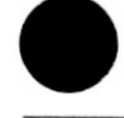

aminophylline • (am-i-noff-i-lin)

CATEGORY: *Bronchodilator:* antiasthmatic, xanthine drug

Rx; Preg Cat C

BRAND NAMES

Aminophylline (various)
**Corophyllin (Beecham)*
**Palaron (Fisons)*
Phyllocontin (P-F)

DOSAGE FORMS

Injection (IV), PO liquid, rectal solution, suppositories, tablets

USE: Treatment of asthma, reversible bronchospasm associated c̄ COPD. **ACTION:** Bronchodilation due to direct relaxation of respiratory smooth muscle; in addition, drug stimulates CNS, produces diuresis, has positive chronotropic/inotropic cardiac effect.

PHARMACOKINETICS

PO absorption	Peak	Protein binding	Excretion
Usually complete	1-2h	60%	90% as metabolites via urine

DOSAGE

Pediatric	*PO*	12mg/kg/24h in 4 divided doses
	Parenteral	For continuous infusion, loading dose 6mg/kg, then 1.2mg/kg/h for 12h, 1mg/kg/h beyond 12h for 6mo-9y/o. 1mg/kg/h for 12h, 0.8mg/kg/h for children 9-16y/o & young adult smokers
	Rectal	12mg/kg in 3-4 divided doses for suppositories/retention enema
Adult	*PO*	600-1600mg in 3-4 divided doses
	Parenteral	For continuous infusion, loading dose 0.6mg/kg, then 0.7mg/kg/h for 12h, 0.5mg/kg/h beyond 12h for nonsmokers. 0.6mg/kg/h for 12h, 0.3mg/kg/h for older pts
	Rectal	250-500mg 1-3 times/d. Retention enema 500mg 3-4 times/d

CONTRAINDICATIONS: Hypersensitivity to any xanthine bronchodilator, irritable rectum or lower colon (suppositories). **CC:** Significant toxicity occurs c̄ plasma levels >25µg/ml ▪ Status asthmaticus *not* responsive to PO administration.

SIDE/ADVERSE EFFECTS: CNS: headache, reflex hyperexcitability, clonic/tonic generalized convulsions, insomnia, nervousness ▪ CV: hypotension, tachycardia, ***ventricular arrhythmias,*** palpitations ▪ GI: N/V/D, epigastric pain ▪ GU: albuminuria, diuresis ▪ RESP: tachypnea.

Note: Side/adverse effects: common in *italic;* serious in ***boldface italic.***

*Available in Canada only.

INTERACTIONS: Drug: ↑ Serum levels c̄ allopurinol, cimetidine, erythromycin, PO contraceptives, flu vaccine ■ ↑ Excretion of lithium ■ Use c̄ propranolol will ↓ aminophylline excretion ■ Use c̄ adrenergic drugs will ↓ CNS stimulation. **Lab:** Bittner/colorimetric technique will produce false ↑ for serum uric acid levels.

NURSING MANAGEMENT PRIORITIES

ADMINISTRATION: Assess for hx of xanthine-derivative administration/hypersensitivity ■ PO: administer c̄ full glass of H_2O/food ■ Rectal: administer after evacuation ■ IV: dilute to 25mg/ml; administer *slowly* (25mg/m); do *not* mix in syringe c̄ other medications; use infusion control device; check compatibility c̄ other drugs ■ Do *not* administer discolored/precipitated solutions ■ Have emergency support equipment (IV) available ■ Maintain hydration (2000ml/d) ■ Heavy smokers may require ↑ dosage ■ Dosage adjustment must be made when switching from IV to PO.

EVALUATION: Monitor CV, F/E, hepatic, renal status ■ Monitor VS, ECG (IV), I&O ■ Monitor respiratory status, auscultate lungs, ABG ■ Observe for signs of toxicity (nausea, CNS stimulation, headache, diarrhea, arrhythmias); stop administration if present, notify physician ■ Monitor therapeutic blood levels: 10-20μg/ml (adult).

EDUCATION: Take as prescribed by physician at equal intervals ■ Dizziness may occur; avoid hazardous activities ■ Check c̄ physician before taking OTC preparations ■ Avoid caffeine, charcoal-broiled foods ■ ↑ Fluid intake (8-10 glasses/d) ■ Avoid changing brand-name preparations ■ Notify physician if experiencing rapid heartbeat, diarrhea, CNS stimulation ■ Keep scheduled appointments c̄ physician/for blood work ■ Retain suppository/rectal solution 30m.

OVERDOSE MANAGEMENT: Symptoms incl anorexia, nausea, restlessness, hyperthermia, convulsions, cardiac arrhythmias ■ Emergency treatment incl maintaining respiration c̄ oxygen, 5% dextrose for dehydration; controlling convulsions c̄ IV diazepam for short-acting barbiturates.

NOTES:

amitriptyline hcl • (a-mee-trip-ti-leen)

CATEGORY: *Tricyclic antidepressant:* mood elevator

Rx; Preg Cat C

BRAND NAMES
Elavil (Zeneca)

**Levate (ICN)*
**Meraril (Medic)*
**Novatriptyn (Novopharm)*

DOSAGE FORMS
IM injection: 10mg/ml
Tablet: 10, 25, 50, 75, 100, 150mg

COMBINATION PRODUCTS
Etrafon products (Schering)
Triavil products (MSD)
(see *Perphenazine*)

USE: Treatment of endogenous depression. **ACTION:** Antidepressant activity appears related to inhibition of norepinephrine reuptake in central adrenergic neurons.

PHARMACOKINETICS

PO absorption	Peak	Half-life	Excretion
Complete	4-12h	10-50h	Up to 50% via urine as metabolites in 24h

CONTRAINDICATIONS: Hypersensitivity, MAO-I therapy, MI (acute recovery period). **CC:** Use can produce arrhythmias, MI, stroke ▪ Caution required c̄ hx of ↑ IOP, narrow-angle glaucoma, seizures ▪ Use c̄ caution in nursing mothers due to presence of drug in milk

DOSAGE

Adolescent/Geriatric	*PO*	10mg tid, 20mg/h
Adult	*PO*	75-150mg/d divided
	IM	20-30mg qid

SIDE/ADVERSE EFFECTS: CNS: *drowsiness,* dizziness, headache, extrapyramidal symptoms, paresthesia (extremities), insomnia ▪ CV: ***arrhythmias,*** hypertension, orthostatic hypotension ▪ EENT: blurred vision, tinnitus ▪ GI: anorexia, N/V, dry mouth, constipation ▪ GU: urinary hesitancy ▪ INT: skin rash, photosensitivity, alopecia, jaundice ▪ PSYCH: disorientation, hallucinations ▪ Other: parotid swelling.

INTERACTIONS: Drug: Significant depressant effects c̄ alcohol ▪ Anticholinergics, chlorpromazine produce ↑ atropinelike effects; paralytic ileus could occur ▪ Significant

Note: Side/adverse effects: common in *italic;* serious in ***boldface italic.***

*Available in Canada only.

↑ in activity c̄ epinephrine, levarterenol, other adrenergic agents ▪ Significant antagonism to effects of reserpine, guanethidine-type antihypertensives ▪ Use c̄ MAO-I best avoided.

NURSING MANAGEMENT PRIORITIES

ADMINISTRATION: Assess for hx of TCA hypersensitivity, hepatic dysfunction, glaucoma ▪ PO: administer as single dose/d at hs c̄ food ▪ Institute suicide/safety precautions ▪ Parenteral: do *not* administer IV ▪ ↑ Dosage *slowly* ▪ Avoid abrupt withdrawal; D/C gradually ▪ Heavy smokers may require ↑ dosage.

EVALUATION: Monitor CV, hepatic, renal status ▪ Monitor VS (esp BP), CBC, hepatic function tests, fluid retention, constipation ▪ Assess for symptoms of abrupt withdrawal (nausea, headache, malaise).

EDUCATION: Dizziness/drowsiness may occur; use caution in potentially hazardous activities ▪ Avoid changing positions rapidly ▪ Avoid alcohol, other CNS depressants for up to 1wk after ending therapy ▪ Take PO forms c̄ food to ↓ GI irritation ▪ Take as directed by physician ▪ Use sugarless gum/hard candy to diminish dry mouth ▪ ↑ Fluids, bulk-containing foods ▪ Check c̄ physician before taking OTC/Rx preparations ▪ May produce peculiar taste ▪ Notify physician/dentist of use before treatment ▪ Store in tightly closed container ▪ Avoid exposure to direct sunlight/UV light (sun lamps); use sunscreen, protective clothing ▪ Notify physician of fever, sore throat, malaise ▪ May turn urine blue-green ▪ Keep scheduled appointments c̄ physician ▪ Full drug effects may require several wks of therapy.

NOTES:

amitriptyline hcl/perphenazine • (a-mee-trip-ti-leen/per-fen-a-zeen)

CATEGORY: *Fixed-combination antidepressant/antipsychotic* Rx; Preg Cat NA

BRAND NAMES	DOSAGE FORMS
Etrafon (Schering)	perphenazine/amitriptyline per tablet: 2mg/10mg, 2mg/25mg, 4mg/10mg (A), 4mg/25mg (Forte)
Triavil (Merck)	perphenazine/amitriptyline per tablet: 2mg/10mg, 2mg/25mg, 4mg/10mg, 4mg/25mg, 4mg/50mg

USE: Treatment of moderate/severe depression ▪ Agitation, depressed mood ▪ Depression c̄ severe anxiety/agitation ▪ Depression, anxiety c̄ chronic physical disease. **ACTION:** *See* amitriptyline hcl; perphenazine.

CONTRAINDICATIONS: Hypersensitivity, blood dyscrasias, bone marrow depression, comatose states, presence of large amounts of CNS depressants, subcortical brain damage, MAO-I, recovery phase following MI. **CC:** Antipsychotic drugs are associated c̄ extrapyramidal symptoms, tardive dyskinesia, neuroleptic malignant syndrome ▪ Antidepressant drug possesses anticholinergic activity; caution is required in pts c̄ glaucoma, ↑ IOP, urinary retention.

DOSAGE

Adult *PO*	Suggested starting dose, one 2/25 or 4/25mg tablet 3-4 times/d or one 4/25mg bid. Dosage must be adjusted to needs of pt. Full therapeutic response may require several wks

NURSING MANAGEMENT PRIORITIES

ADMINISTRATION: Assess for hx of phenothiazine/TCA hypersensitivity ▪ Assess for hx of hepatic disease; may require ↓ dosage ▪ Assess VS, esp BP ▪ Administer c̄ food ▪ Avoid abrupt withdrawal; D/C gradually ▪ Maintain hydration ▪ Heavy smokers may require dosage evaluation ▪ Elderly/debilitated may require ↓ dosage.

EVALUATION: Monitor hepatic, ophthalmic, renal status ▪ Monitor BP, CBC ▪ Assess for extrapyramidal symptoms (tics/spasms, trembling, shuffling gait) ▪ Assess for symptoms of abrupt withdrawal (nausea, dyskinesia, trembling, dizziness, headache, malaise) ▪ Assess for actual swallowing of PO forms.

EDUCATION: Dizziness/drowsiness may occur; use caution in potentially hazardous activities ▪ Avoid changing positions (lying/sitting/standing) rapidly ▪ Avoid use of alcohol, other CNS depressants ▪ Take c̄ meals to ↓ GI irritation ▪ Store in tightly closed, light-resistant container ▪ Use sugarless gum/hard candy to diminish dry mouth ▪ Constipation may occur; ↑ fluids, bulk-containing foods ▪ May turn urine pink/red/brown ▪ Women: avoid breast-feeding ▪ Notify physician/dentist of use before treatment ▪ Avoid exposure to direct sunlight, UV light (sunlamps); use sunscreen, protective clothing ▪ Notify physician of fever, sore throat, bruising/bleeding, headache, malaise ▪ Notify physician of extrapyramidal symptoms (tics/spasms, trembling, shuffling gait) ▪ Avoid ↑ exercise, temperature extremes ▪ Take as directed by physician; do *not* ↑ dose ▪ Check c̄ physician before taking OTC/Rx preparations ▪ Do *not* take antacids/antidiarrheals w/in 2h of drug ▪ Keep scheduled appointments c̄ physician ▪ Full drug effects may require several wks of therapy.

NOTES:

amoxapine • (a-mox-a-peen)

CATEGORY: *Tricyclic antidepressant:* mood elevator Rx; Preg Cat C

BRAND NAME
Asendin (Lederle)

DOSAGE FORMS
Tablet: 25, 50, 100, 150mg

USE: Treatment of endogenous, reactive, psychotic depression ▪ Treatment of depression accompanied by anxiety/agitation. **ACTION:** Antidepressant activity appears related to inhibition of norepinephrine reuptake in central adrenergic neurons.

PHARMACOKINETICS

PO absorption	Peak	Half-life	Protein binding	Excretion
Complete	90m	8h	90%	80% via urine, 20% via feces as metabolites

CONTRAINDICATIONS: Hypersensitivity, MAO-I therapy, MI (acute recovery period). **CC:** Use may induce neuroleptic malignant syndrome, tardive dyskinesia, arrhythmias, MI, stroke ▪ Caution required c̄ ↑ IOP, angle-closure glaucoma, urinary retention ▪ Use c̄ caution in nursing mothers due to presence of drug in milk.

DOSAGE

Adult	*PO*	≥50-100mg tid. Usual maintenance range 150-300mg/d
Geriatric	*PO*	≥25-50mg tid. Usual maintenance range 150-300mg/d

SIDE/ADVERSE EFFECTS: CNS: *drowsiness*, dizziness, headache, incoordination, tremors, extrapyramidal symptoms, paresthesia (extremities), insomnia ▪ CV: ***arrhythmias, MI, stroke, heart block,*** hypotension, orthostatic hypotension ▪ EENT: tinnitus ▪ END: testicular swelling, galactorrhea, breast enlargement ▪ GI: *dry mouth*, anorexia, N/V/D, cramps, constipation ▪ GU: urinary hesitancy ▪ HEM: ***agranulocytosis,*** eosinophilia, ***thrombocytopenia*** ▪ HEP: cholestatic jaundice ▪ INT: skin rash, photosensitivity, alopecia ▪ PSYCH: disorientation, hallucinations, exacerbation of psychosis ▪ Other: parotid swelling, ***neuroleptic malignant syndrome.***

INTERACTIONS: Drug: Significant depressant effects c̄ alcohol ▪ Anticholinergics, chlorpromazine produce ↑ atropinelike effects; paralytic ileus could occur ▪ Significant ↑ in activity c̄ epinephrine, levarterenol, other adrenergic agents ▪ Significant antagonism to effects of reserpine, clonidine, guanethidine-type antihypertensives ▪ Use c̄ MAO-I best avoided.

NURSING MANAGEMENT PRIORITIES

ADMINISTRATION: Assess for hx of TCA hypersensitivity ▪ Assess for impaired hepatic, renal function; hx of glaucoma, prostatic hypertrophy; may require ↓ dosage ▪ Administer c̄ food ▪ Institute suicide/safety precautions ▪ ↓ Dosage slowly, maintenance dose lowest dose that will maintain remission of depression ▪ Avoid abrupt withdrawal; D/C gradually ▪ Heavy smokers may require ↓ dosage ▪ Elderly may require ↓ dosage.

EVALUATION: Monitor CV, hepatic, renal status ▪ Monitor VS, esp BP ▪ Monitor CBC, esp long-term ▪ Monitor fluid retention (I&O, daily weight), constipation ▪ Assess for symptoms of abrupt withdrawal (nausea, headache, malaise) ▪ Assess for actual swallowing of PO forms.

EDUCATION: Dizziness/drowsiness may occur; use caution in potentially hazardous activities ▪ Avoid changing positions (lying/sitting/standing) rapidly ▪ Avoid alcohol, other CNS depressants for up to 1wk after therapy has ended ▪ Take c̄ food to ↓ GI irritation ▪ Take as directed by physician ▪ Use sugarless gum/hard candy to diminish dry mouth ▪ Constipation may occur; ↑ fluids, bulk-containing foods ▪ Check c̄ physician before taking OTC/Rx preparations ▪ May produce peculiar taste ▪ Notify physician/dentist of use before treatment ▪ Store in tightly closed container ▪ Avoid exposure to direct sunlight, UV light (sun lamps); use sunscreen, protective clothing ▪ Encourage recreational/diversional interests ▪ Notify physician of fever, sore throat, malaise ▪ Keep scheduled appointments c̄ physician ▪ Full drug effects may require several wks of therapy.

NOTES:

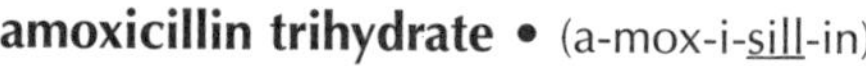

amoxicillin trihydrate • (a-mox-i-sill-in)

CATEGORY: *Aminopenicillin:* antibiotic

Rx; Preg Cat B

BRAND NAMES

Amoxil (SKB)
(Ayerst [Canada])
**Apo-Amoxi (Apotex)*
**Novamoxin (Novopharm)*
Trimox (Apothecon)

DOSAGE FORMS

Capsule, chewable tablet, powder for pediatric drops/ PO suspension

COMBINATION PRODUCTS

Augmentin (SKB)
**Clavulin (Beecham)*

amoxicillin/clavulanate
per tablet:
250mg/125mg,
500mg/125mg;
875mg/125mg
per chewable tablet:
125mg/31.5mg,
200mg/28.5mg
250mg/62.5mg;
400mg/57mg
per 5ml: 125mg/31.25mg,
200mg/28.5mg
250mg/62.5mg
400mg/57mg

USE: Treatment of auditory, GU, respiratory, GI tract infections caused by susceptible strains of *Escherichia coli, Haemophilus influenzae, Neisseria gonorrhoeae, Proteus mirabilis* ▪ Treatment of *Streptococcus faecalis, S. pneumoniae* infections ▪ Augmentin indicated for treatment of β-lactamase (penicillinase)–producing *E. coli, Enterobacter* spp, *H. influenzae, Moraxella catarrhalis, Staphylococcus aureus* infections. **ACTION:** Bactericidal activity due to inhibition of mucopeptide cell wall synthesis in susceptible organisms; clavulanic acid, chemical similar to penicillins, added to amoxicillin (Augmentin) to block activity of penicillinase (β-lactamase) against amoxicillin; thus amoxicillin (Augmentin) can be used to treat infections caused by penicillinase-producing organisms. Dosage for Augmentin based on amoxicillin content; essentially same as for amoxicillin.

PHARMACOKINETICS

PO absorption	Peak	Half-life	Protein binding	Excretion
74%-92%	1-2h	40-84m	20%	In urine in 6-8h

Note: Side/adverse effects: common in *italic;* serious in ***boldface italic.***

*Available in Canada only.

CONTRAINDICATIONS: Penicillin hypersensitivity. **CC:** Serious, fatal anaphylactic rxs have occurred c̄ penicillin use.

DOSAGE

Pediatric	*PO*	<20kg: 20-40mg/kg/d divided q8h
Adult	*PO*	250-500mg q8h. 3.5g c̄ 1g probenecid as single dose for gonorrhea

SIDE/ADVERSE EFFECTS: CV: edema ▪ GI: N/V/D, glossitis, stomatitis ▪ HEM: anemia, ***thrombocytopenia***, thrombocytopenic purpura, eosinophilia, leukopenia, ***agranulocytosis*** ▪ HEP: ↑ in serum AST ▪ INT: maculopapular rash, ***erythema multiforme, exfoliative dermatitis,*** urticaria ▪ MS: arthralgia ▪ Other: fever, laryngeal edema, ***anaphylaxis.***

INTERACTIONS: Drug: Antacids, antidiarrheal suspensions, ion-exchange resins ↓ PO absorption ▪ Concurrent use of bacteriostatic antibiotics c̄ any penicillin can produce antibiotic antagonism ▪ Antibiotics that ↓ intestinal flora may ↑ activity of PO anticoagulants.

NURSING MANAGEMENT PRIORITIES

ADMINISTRATION: Assess for hx of penicillin/cephalosporin hypersensitivity ▪ Obtain C&S before therapy ▪ Reconstitute powder for drops/PO suspension according to manufacturer's directions; use w/in 14d (room temperature or refrigerated) ▪ Shake drops/PO suspension well before using ▪ Avoid exposure to moisture in storage ▪ Have support equipment available for anaphylaxis.

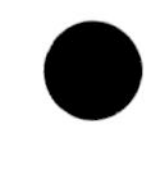

EVALUATION: Monitor pts c̄ allergies/asthma (high risk for hypersensitivity) ▪ Monitor renal, hepatic, hemopoietic status ▪ Observe for signs of superinfection (diarrhea, itching, coated tongue) ▪ Monitor VS, esp temperature.

EDUCATION: Complete full course of therapy (usually 10d) even if symptoms subside ▪ Can be taken c̄ meals; *best* on empty stomach ▪ Take at equal intervals around clock to maintain blood levels ▪ Diarrhea may occur ▪ Store in dry, tightly closed container ▪ Discard outdated preparations ▪ Maintain good personal hygiene (esp perineal, oral) ▪ ↑ Fluid intake (8-10 glasses/d) ▪ Women: avoid breastfeeding ▪ Notify physician of symptoms of allergic rx (fever, difficult breathing, rash) ▪ Carry identification (MedicAlert) if penicillin allergic.

NOTES:

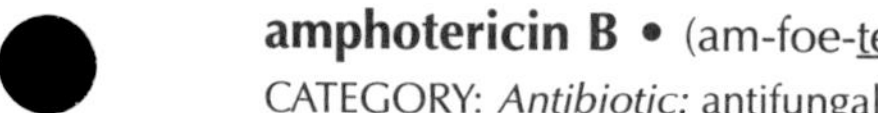

amphotericin B • (am-foe-ter-i-sin)

CATEGORY: *Antibiotic:* antifungal, antimonilial

Rx; Preg Cat B

BRAND NAMES	DOSAGE FORMS
Fungizone (B-MS)	Cream: 3% Lotion: 3% Powder for injection (IV): 50mg/vial Ointment: 3%
Abelcet (Liposome) *Amphotec (Sequus)*	IV lipid suspension injection: 5mg/ml

USE: Treatment of aspergillosis, coccidioidomycosis, cryptococcosis, disseminated moniliasis, histoplasmosis, mucormycosis, North American blastomycosis, sporotrichosis ▪ Treatment of invasive aspergillosis for pts c̄ renal impairment (amphotericin cholesteryl) ▪ Topical treatment of candidiasis (moniliasis). **ACTION:** Antifungal activity in susceptible fungi due to binding c̄ cell membrane sterols, resulting in leakage of vital intracellular fungal components.

PHARMACOKINETICS: Administered IV because of poor PO absorption; exhibits high protein binding (90%-95%), long half-life; excreted via kidneys over period of days.

CONTRAINDICATIONS: Hypersensitivity. **CC:** Potential benefits must be balanced against serious side effects.

DOSAGE

Pediatric/Adult *IV*	Initial daily dose 0.25mg/kg; total daily dosage may range from 1-1.5mg/kg; do *not* exceed total daily dose 1.5mg/kg, amphotericin cholesteryl: 3-6mg/kg given at an infusion rate of 1mg/kg/h
Pediatric/Adult *IV suspension*	5mg/kg/d as a single infusion
Topical	Apply several times/d

SIDE/ADVERSE EFFECTS: CNS: *headache*, vertigo, peripheral neuropathy, ***convulsions*** ▪ CV: local venous pain at injection site c̄ phlebitis, ***thrombophlebitis, arrhythmias, cardiac arrest*** ▪ EENT: diplopia, hearing loss ▪ GI: *N/V/D*, dyspepsia, epigastric pain ▪ GU: azotemia, hyposthenuria, tubular acidosis ▪ HEM: ***coagulation defects, thrombocytopenia,*** leukopenia, ***agranulocytosis*** ▪ HEP: ***acute liver failure*** (rare) ▪ MET: hypokalemia.

Note: Side/adverse effects: common in *italic;* serious in ***boldface italic.***

*Available in Canada only.

INTERACTIONS: Drug: Use c̄ doxacurium, gallamine, succinylcholine, tubocurarine, dig will ↑ their toxicity ▪ Use c̄ corticosteroids produces hypokalemia, severe superinfections ▪ Use c̄ nephrotoxic drugs produces additive toxicity.

NURSING MANAGEMENT PRIORITIES

ADMINISTRATION: Assess for hx of hypersensitivity ▪ Obtain C&S before therapy ▪ Assess renal function; may require ↓ dosage if impaired ▪ IV: reconstitute c̄ 10ml sterile H_2O for injection (5mg/ml), shake until clear; further dilute c̄ 5% dextrose (pH >4.2); use strict aseptic technique; infuse *slowly* (6h), protect from light, stable in dark for 24h at room temperature, 1wk refrigerated; may use in-line membrane filter of mean pore diameter >1μm; for hospital use only, observe pt closely ▪ Topical: rub liberal amounts on affected area; avoid occlusive dressings ▪ Do *not* administer discolored/precipitated solutions ▪ Store powder for injection in refrigerator; protect from light ▪ Avoid mixing c̄ saline solutions, antibiotics, or bacteriostatic agents.

EVALUATION: Monitor hepatic, renal status ▪ Monitor VS, esp temperature ▪ Observe injection site for signs of inflammation; rotate sites ▪ Monitor I&O ▪ D/C if BUN >40mg/100ml, serum creatinine >3mg/100ml ▪ Assess for signs of hypokalemia (anorexia, lethargy, muscle weakness, mental confusion); notify physician.

EDUCATION: Report any discomfort at infusion site *immediately* ▪ Procedure for topical application; avoid occlusive dressing ▪ Cream may discolor skin; lotion, ointment may discolor nails ▪ Discoloration of fabrics can be removed by washing c̄ soap & H_2O (cream, lotion) or standard cleaning fluid (ointment).

NOTES:

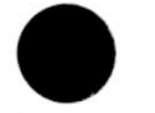

ampicillin sodium▲/ampicillin trihydrate • (am-pi-<u>sill</u>-in) 22

CATEGORY: *Aminopenicillin:* antibiotic Rx; Preg Cat B

BRAND NAMES

**Ampilean (Organon)*
**Apo-Ampi (Apotex)*
Omnipen (W-A)
Omnipen-N (W-A)
Polycillin-N▲ (Squibb)
Principen (Apothecon)
Totacillin-N▲ (SKB)

DOSAGE FORMS

Capsule, powder for injection (IM/IV) powder for PO suspension

COMBINATION PRODUCTS Rx

Unasyn (Roerig)	amipicillin Na/sulbactam Na per vial: 1g/0.5g, 2g/1g

USE: Treatment of auditory, GU, respiratory, GI tract infections caused by susceptible strains of *Escherichia coli, Haemophilus influenzae, Neisseria gonorrhoeae, N. meningitidis, Proteus mirabilis, Salmonella* spp, *Shigella* spp ▪ Treatment of subacute bacterial endocarditis, enterococci infections ▪ Drug of choice for treating typhoid fever *(Salmonella typhosa)* resistant to chloramphenicol.

ACTION: Bactericidal activity due to inhibition of mucopeptide cell wall synthesis in susceptible organisms.

PHARMACOKINETICS

PO absorption	Peak	Half-life	Protein binding	Excretion
30%-55%	1-2h	40-84m	20%-25%	Via urine

CONTRAINDICATIONS: Penicillin hypersensitivity. **CC:** Serious, fatal anaphylactic rxs have occurred c̄ penicillin use.

DOSAGE

Pediatric	*PO*	<20kg: 50-100mg/kg/d divided q6-8h >20kg: 250-500mg qid
	IM/IV	25-50mg/kg divided qid Meningitis: 100-200mg/kg/d in equal doses
Adult	*PO*	250-500mg qid Gonorrhea: single dose, 3.5g c̄ 1g probenecid
Adult	*IM/IV*	250-500mg q6h Meningitis: 8-14g in equal doses

SIDE/ADVERSE EFFECTS: CV: edema ▪ GI: N/V/D, glossitis, stomatitis ▪ HEM: anemia, ***thrombocytopenia,***

Note: Side/adverse effects: common in *italic;* serious in ***boldface italic.***

*Available in Canada only.

thrombocytopenic purpura, eosinophilia, leukopenia, ***agranulocytosis*** ▪ HEP: ↑ serum AST ▪ INT: maculopapular rash, ***erythema multiforme, exfoliative dermatitis,*** urticaria ▪ MS: arthralgia ▪ Other: fever, laryngeal edema, ***anaphylaxis.***

INTERACTIONS: Drug: Antacids, antidiarrheals, ion-exchange resins ↓ PO absorption ▪ Concurrent use of bacteriostatic antibiotics c̄ any penicillin can produce antibiotic antagonism ▪ Antibiotics that ↓ intestinal flora may ↑ activity of PO anticoagulants.

NURSING MANAGEMENT PRIORITIES

ADMINISTRATION: Assess for hx of penicillin/cephalosporin hypersensitivity ▪ Obtain C&S before therapy ▪ Reconstitute powder for drops/PO suspension/injection according to manufacturer's directions ▪ Shake drops/PO suspension well before using; use w/in 7d at room temperature, 14d refrigerated ▪ Handle solution carefully to avoid contact dermatitis ▪ Avoid exposure to moisture in storage ▪ Administer 1h ac/2h pc ▪ Have support equipment available for anaphylaxis.

EVALUATION: Monitor pts c̄ allergies/asthma ▪ Monitor VS, esp temperature; renal, hepatic, hematologic status ▪ Observe for signs of superinfection (diarrhea, itching, coated tongue) ▪ Monitor pts receiving anticoagulant therapy; may potentiate bleeding ▪ Differentiate characteristic drug rash, hypersensitivity rx.

EDUCATION: Complete full course of therapy (usually 10d) even if symptoms subside ▪ Take on empty stomach at equal intervals ▪ Diarrhea may occur ▪ Store in dry, tightly closed container ▪ Maintain good personal hygiene (esp perineal, oral), fluid intake (6-8 glasses/d) ▪ Use Clinistix/Diastix for urine testing ▪ Women: avoid breastfeeding ▪ Notify physician of symptoms of allergic rx (fever, difficult breathing, rash) ▪ Carry identification (MedicAlert) if penicillin allergic.

NOTES:

amrinone lactate/milrinone lactate • (am-ri-none/mill-rih-none)

CATEGORY: *Cardiac inotropic agent* Rx; Preg Cat C

BRAND NAMES	**DOSAGE FORMS**
amrinone lactate	
Inocor (S-W)	IV injection: 5mg/ml
milrinone lactate	
Primacor (S-W)	IV injection: 1mg/ml

USE: Short-term treatment of CHF. **ACTION:** Produces + inotropic effect that ↑ force/velocity of myocardial systolic contractions by inhibiting myocardial cyclic adenosine monophosphate phosphodiesterase activity, which ↑ cardiac cellular level of cAMP; does not inhibit Na-K-activated adenosine triphosphatase activity (produced by dig); produces direct relaxant effect on vascular smooth muscle.

PHARMACOKINETICS: *amrinone:* onset of 2-5m, peaks at all dosage levels in 10m, duration of 0.5h (0.75μg/kg) and 2h (3mg/kg). Half-life 3.6-8h, protein binding 10%-49% & excretion is via feces & urine primarily as unchanged drug. *milrinone:* onset of 5-15m c̄ a maximum cardiac effect at plasma concentrations of 150-250ng. Protein binding is 70% c̄ excretion via feces & urine primarily as unchanged drug.

CONTRAINDICATIONS: Hypersensitivity to drugs or bisulfites used or injection stabilizers (amrinone). **CC:** Possible allergic rx can occur due to sodium metabisulfite context (amrinone) ▪ Do not mix c̄ furosemide injection (amrinone) ▪ Do not dilute c̄ dextrose/glucose until time of administration (amrinone) ▪ Possible induction of atrial/ventricular arrhythmias ▪ Use c̄ caution in pts c̄ severe obstructive aortic or pulmonic valvular disease in the absence of surgical intervention.

DOSAGE: Adult *IV*

amrinone	0.75mg/kg slowly over 2-3m, then usual maintenance dose 5-10μg/kg/m. Do *not* exceed a total daily dose of 10mg/kg.
milrinone	Loading dose 50μg/kg over 10m. Maintenance infusion of 0.375-0.75μg/kg/m according to response.

SIDE/ADVERSE EFFECTS: CV: ***angina, arrhythmia, hypotension, thrombocytopenia*** ▪ GI: N/V, abdominal pain, anorexia, ▪ HEP: cell necrosis (amrinone) ↑ enzyme levels ▪ Other: chest pain, fever, headache, hypokalemia.

INTERACTIONS: Drug: Use $\bar{c}$ disopyramide produced excessive hypotension in one pt (amrinone) ▪ Drugs appear to be compatible $\bar{c}$ most CV drugs, anticoagulants, insulin, diazepam.

NURSING MANAGEMENT PRIORITIES

ADMINISTRATION: Assess for hx of hypersensitivity (incl bisulfites) ▪ Administer via infusion control device for continuous IV infusion ▪ Concurrent K^+ supplements may be ordered in hypokalemia ▪ Avoid exposure to light during storage ▪ Dilute $\bar{c}$ normal saline solution; use w/in 24h ▪ Avoid mixing $\bar{c}$ dextrose solutions ▪ Do *not* mix $\bar{c}$ IV furosemide (precipitation occurs).

EVALUATION: Monitor serum electrolytes (hypokalemia, hypercalcemia enhance toxicity), hemodynamic parameters ▪ Assess renal status; monitor I&O, daily weight ▪ Monitor VS, esp BP, heart rate ▪ Assess platelet count qd ▪ Check cardiac monitor for arrhythmia.

EDUCATION: Notify nurse/physician of rx (abnormal heartbeat, GI distress, bleeding).

NOTES:

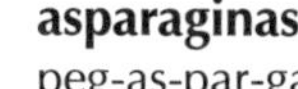

asparaginase/pegaspargase (peg-L-asparaginase) • (a-spar-a-gi-nase/ peg-as-par-gase)

CATEGORY: *Antineoplastic:* enzyme

Rx; Preg Cat C

BRAND NAMES	DOSAGE FORMS
asparaginase	
Elspar (Merck)	IM/IV powder for injection: 10,000 IU/vial
pegaspargase	
Oncaspar (RPR)	IM/IV injection: 750 IU/m

USE: In combination c̄ other agents for the treatment of responsive lymphocytic leukemia esp in children ▪ Use as a pale agent restricted to pts not suitable for combination therapy ▪ Pegaspargase indicated for pts who have developed asparaginase hypersensitivities. **ACTION:** L-asparaginase and its modified derivative pegaspargase (PEG-L-asparaginase) are bacterial enzymes that hydrolize the amino acid asparagine, an essential component for cellular protein synthesis, into inactive asparatic acid & ammonia. Selected neoplastic cells that lack asparagine synthetase enzyme are unable to synthesize the amino acid & are dependent on preformed exogenous asparagine for survival. The enzymatic destruction of asparagine from the plasma will result in an antineoplastic effect in asparagine-dependent cells. Pegaspargase has a longer plasma half-life & exhibits ↓ immunogenic potential (drug hypersensitivity).

PHARMACOKINETICS: Asparaginase has a plasma half-life of 8-30h & the amino acid asparagine usually reappears in plasma w/in 23-33d after D/C treatment. Pegaspargase has a plasma half-life of 2-5d. Both drugs exhibit no appreciable urinary excretion.

CONTRAINDICATIONS: Patients c̄ serious allergic rxs to treatment, hemorrhagic episodes c̄ previous therapy, pancreatitis. **CC:** Use can cause significant allergic rxs esp c̄ L-asparaginase (3%-73% of treated pts) ▪ Use should be restricted to qualified physicians ▪ Significant hepatotoxicity or pancreatitis may result from treatment.

DOSAGE

asparaginase

Children/ Adults *IV* 200 IU/kg/d for 28d as a single agent

pegaspargase
Children/
Adults ≥0.6m² IM/IV 2500 IV/m² q14d as a single agent

SIDE/ADVERSE EFFECTS: CNS: dizziness, headache, seizures/status epilepticus (PEG), Parkinson-like syndrome (asparaginase) ▪ CV: ***atrial/venous thrombosis,*** hemorrhage ▪ GI: anorexia, constipation, ***pancreatitis*** ▪ HEM: leukopenia, ***thrombocytopenia*** ▪ HEP: ***hepatotoxicity*** ▪ INT: skin rash, petechial rash, urticaria ▪ REN: hematuria ***hemorrhagic cystitis, renal failure*** ▪ Other: arthralgia, hyperglycemia/hypoglycemia, ***rare fatal hyperthermia.***

INTERACTIONS: Drugs: Use c̄ methotrexate will ⬇ its effectiveness ▪ Use c̄ vincristine may produce additive toxicity ▪ Use c̄ aspirin, anticoagulants can ⬆ bleeding tendencies. **Lab:** ⬆ ALT, AST, BUN, serum uric acid.

NURSING MANAGEMENT PRIORITIES

ADMINISTRATION: Check pt hx for recent course of radiation/antineoplastic agents ▪ Assess for pancreatitis; do *not* administer if present ▪ Administer antiemetic before therapy ▪ Provide emotional support ▪ Reconstitute according to manufacturer's directions, use w/in 8h of reconstitution & only if clear ▪ IV: (ASP) infuse over 30m via NSS or 5% dextrose IV solution (PEG) infuse over 1-2h in 100 ml NSS or 5% dextrose ▪ IM: do *not* exceed 2ml at a single injection site ▪ Avoid excessive agitation ▪ Administer intradermal skin test before initial administration & if > 1wk before doses.

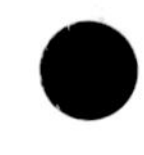

EVALUATION: Monitor hepatic, neurologic, renal function; CBC, esp WBC, platelets throughout therapy; notify physician if ⬇ ▪ Assess for infection, bleeding, anemia ▪ May produce hyperglycemia; monitor diabetics closely ▪ Assess hydration status (I&O, daily weight) ▪ Monitor for hepatic toxicity (jaundice, clay-colored stools) ▪ Monitor serum amylase levels; notify physician if ⬆ (pancreatitis) ▪ Assess for anaphylactic rxs; have support equipment available.

EDUCATION: ⬆ Fluid intake (8-10 glasses/d) ▪ Avoid exposure to infection ▪ Check c̄ physician before immunization ▪ Diet as tolerated; avoid spicy foods ▪ Maintain good oral hygiene; use soft-bristled toothbrush ▪ Notify physician of symptoms of bone marrow depression (fever, sore throat, bruising, bleeding, lethargy) & pancreatitis (N/V, severe abdominal pain) ▪ Dizziness/drowsiness may occur; use caution in potentially hazardous activities ▪ Notify physician of symptoms of allergic rx (fever, difficult breathing, rash).

NOTES:

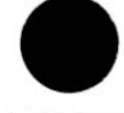

aspirin (acetylsalicylic acid) • (as-pir-in)

CATEGORY: *Salicylate:* analgesic, antiinflammatory, antipyretic, antiplatelet, NSAIA OTC/Rx

BRAND NAMES
**Apo-Asen (Apotex)*
ASA (Lilly)
Ascriptin (Rorer)
Bufferin (Bristol-Myers)
Ecotrin (SKB)
Empirin (G-W)
**Novasen (Novopharm)*

DOSAGE FORMS
Capsule, enteric tablets, suppository, tablet.

COMBINATION PRODUCTS
Codeine/Aspirin Rx-C-III-Preg Cat C
Generic #2 (15/325mg), #3 (30/325mg), #4 (60/325mg)
Empirin c̄ Codeine (G-W) #4 (60/325mg)

USE: Analgesic for mild/moderate pain as sole agent in combination c̄ other analgesics/narcotics ▪ Antipyretic ▪ Rheumatoid/osteoarthritis, other arthritic diseases ▪ Symptomatic treatment of rheumatic fever ▪ Prophylaxis of thrombosis-related diseases, esp coronary artery disease.
ACTION: Produces analgesia by ↑ pain threshold, ↓ synthesis of prostaglandins; antipyresis due to effects on hypothalamic heat-regulating center; antiinflammatory effect due to ↓ in prostaglandin synthesis, release; ↓ prothrombin synthesis, platelet adhesiveness.

PHARMACOKINETICS

Absorption PO/Rectal	Duration	Protein binding	Excretion
70%-100%	4-6h	88%	In urine as metabolites

CONTRAINDICATIONS: Hypersensitivity to any salicylate; active ulcers. **CC:** Use c̄ chickenpox/flulike symptoms in children/teenagers has been associated c̄ Reye's syndrome ▪ Avoid use in surgical pts.

DOSAGE

Pediatric *PO/Rectal*	
Analgesic	11-16mg/kg 4-6 times/d
Antirheumatic	16mg/kg 6 times/d to 10mg/kg 6 times/d
Rheumatic fever	90-130mg/kg/d divided q4-6h
Adult *PO/Rectal*	
Analgesic	325-650mg 4-6 times/d
Antirheumatic	1g 4-6 times/d. Do *not* exceed 10g/d
Antithrombotic	325-650mg 2-4 times/d
Rheumatic fever	4-8g/d divided q4-6h

SIDE/ADVERSE EFFECTS: CNS: tinnitus ▪ CV: hypoprothrombinemia ▪ GI: epigastric distress, nausea, ***bleeding ulcer*** ▪ HEP: ↑ serum AST, ALT ▪ INT: skin rash.

INTERACTIONS: Drug: Use c̄ large amounts of antacids best avoided ▪ Buffered aspirin better ▪ Use c̄ ulcerogenic drugs best avoided ▪ ↑ Activity of PO anticoagulants, antidiabetic agents ▪ ↓ Uricosuric effects of probenecid, sulfinpyrazone ▪ ↓ PO absorption, uricosuric action of indomethacin. **Lab:** False + for vanillylmandelic acid levels c̄ most techniques.

NURSING MANAGEMENT PRIORITIES

ADMINISTRATION: Assess for hx of salicylate hypersensitivity ▪ Administer c̄ food if GI irritation occurs ▪ Avoid large amounts of concurrent antacid suspensions ▪ Do *not* crush enteric-coated/timed-release preparations ▪ Avoid use in children c̄ chickenpox, flulike symptoms; may precipitate Reye's syndrome.

EVALUATION: Assess for bleeding (GI, GU, skin, mucous membrane) ▪ Diabetics: monitor for hypoglycemia ▪ Monitor for signs of OD (CNS disturbances, tinnitus, hyperventilation) ▪ Monitor pt receiving anticoagulant therapy; may potentiate bleeding.

EDUCATION: Check c̄ physician/pharmacist before taking OTC preparations ▪ Notify physician if signs of bleeding occur ▪ Take c̄ food/milk/antacids to ↓ GI irritation ▪ Swallow enteric-coated/timed-release preparations whole ▪ Notify physician of constant ringing in ears; D/C drug ▪ Avoid taking c̄ NSAIAs.

OVERDOSE MANAGEMENT: Remove drug by emesis or lavage followed by activated charcoal & a saline cathartic ▪ Maintain respiration & adequate blood volume c̄ IV fluids ▪ Treat alkalosis, acidosis, hyperkalemia, etc., as they arise.

NOTES:

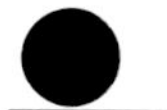

atenolol • (a-ten-oh-lole)

CATEGORY: *β-adrenergic blocker:* antianginal, antihypertensive Rx; Preg Cat A

BRAND NAME
Tenormin (Zeneca)

DOSAGE FORMS
Tablet: 50, 100mg
Injection (IV): 5mg/ml

COMBINATION PRODUCTS
Tenoretic (Zeneca) atenolol/chlorthalidone per tablet: 50mg/25mg, 100mg/25mg

USE: Treatment of hypertension as sole agent/in combination c̄ other antihypertensive agents (esp thiazide diuretic) ▪ Long-term management of angina ▪ To ↓ mortality in stable pts after MI. **ACTION:** Blocks access of catecholamine neurotransmitters to β_1 receptors located in heart; at higher doses, blockage of β_2 receptors will occur in bronchial tree, vascular smooth muscle; antihypertensive effect not determined.

PHARMACOKINETICS

PO absorption	Peak	Half-life	Protein binding	Excretion
50%	2-4h	6-7h	6%-16%	Via urine, feces as unchanged drug

CONTRAINDICATIONS: Hypersensitivity, serious bradycardia, heart block >1°. **CC:** Abrupt D/C can ↑ ischemic heart disease ▪ Possible cardiac failure c̄ ↓ myocardial contractility ▪ Tachycardia of hyperthyroidism may be masked, abrupt D/C may induce thyrotoxicosis ▪ Use c̄ brochospastic disease, diabetes, peripheral vascular disease requires caution.

DOSAGE

Adult	*PO*	
Hypertension		Starting dose of 50mg/d & ↑ to 100mg/d prn. Doses >100mg do not produce further results
Angina		Starting dose of 50mg/d & ↑ to 200mg/d prn
MI prevention		50mg given 10m after last IV dose followed by 50mg in 12h. Then 50-100mg/d for 6-9d or until discharge
	IV	5mg over 5m followed by another 5mg in 10m for initiation of MI prevention
Tenorectic	*PO*	Usual range 1-2 tablets/d

SIDE/ADVERSE EFFECTS: CNS: *dizziness, tiredness,* drowsiness, *depression* ▪ CV: *cold extremities,* bradycardia, postural hypotension ▪ GI: N/D, constipation, anorexia ▪ RESP: dyspnea, wheeziness.

INTERACTIONS: Drug: Use $\bar{c}$ reserpine, other catecholamine-depleting drugs can result in serious adrenergic blockage ▪ Nonselective β-adrenergics antagonize therapeutic response ▪ Use $\bar{c}$ furazolidone, general anesthetics, MAO-I best avoided.

NURSING MANAGEMENT PRIORITIES

ADMINISTRATION: Assess for hx of β-blocker hypersensitivity ▪ Assess BP, apical pulse; if <60/m hold drug, notify physician ▪ Assess hepatic function, I&O; may require ↓ dosage if impaired ▪ Do *not* administer in presence of respiratory distress (asthma, CHF, COPD) ▪ Avoid exposure to heat/moisture in storage ▪ Avoid abrupt withdrawal; D/C gradually ▪ Elderly may require ↓ dosage.

EVALUATION: Monitor hepatic, renal, respiratory status ▪ Monitor BP, pulse ▪ Monitor CBC, FBS (diabetics) ▪ Assess for depression ▪ May produce alteration in blood glucose levels; may mask signs of hypoglycemia.

EDUCATION: Take as directed by physician even if symptom free; do *not* skip doses ▪ May take w/out regard to food ▪ Do *not* D/C w/out notifying physician ▪ Procedure for checking radial pulse ▪ Check pulse before taking; if <60m do *not* take drug, notify physician ▪ Check $\bar{c}$ physician before taking OTC/Rx preparations ▪ Drowsiness may occur; use caution when engaging in potentially hazardous activities ▪ Avoid changing positions (lying/sitting/standing) rapidly ▪ Diabetics: carefully monitor blood/urine glucose; observe for symptoms of hypoglycemia (headache, ↑ sweating, hunger, weakness) ▪ May experience ↑ sensitivity to cold ▪ Notify physician of respiratory distress, leg edema ▪ Notify physician/dentist of β blocker use before treatment ▪ Maintain optimum weight; follow low-Na^+ diet ▪ Keep scheduled appointments $\bar{c}$ physician ▪ Store in tightly closed container ▪ Avoid ↑ exercise, temperature extremes, smoking ▪ Women: avoid breastfeeding.

NOTES:

atovaquone • (a-toe-vah-kwone)

CATEGORY: *Antiprotozoan:* antipneumocystis carinii Rx; Preg Cat C

BRAND NAME	DOSAGE FORM
Mepron (G-W)	Suspension: 750mg/5ml

USE: Treatment of mild to moderate *Pneumocystis carinii* (PCP) in pts intolerant to trimethoprim-sulfamethoxazole (TMP-SMZ). **ACTION:** Antipneumocystis activity not fully determined. May inhibit electron transport system of organism resulting in ⬇ ATP, nucleic acid synthesis.

PHARMACOKINETICS

PO absorption	Peak*	Half-life	Protein binding	Excretion
Low	1-8h	2.2-2.9d	99.9%	Via feces (>94%) as unchanged over 21d

* Drug exhibits a double peak. Second peak occurs 24-96h later.

DOSAGE

Adult *PO*	750mg c̄ food bid for 21d

CONTRAINDICATIONS: Hx or development of life-threatening hypersensitivity. **CC:** Not evaluated for PCP prophylaxis, for use in pts >65 y/o, pediatric pts ▪ Failure to administer c̄ food can limit therapeutic response due to ⬇ PO absorption.

SIDE/ADVERSE EFFECTS: CNS: *headache*, insomnia, dizziness, anxiety ▪ CV: hypotension ▪ EENT: sinusitis, rhinitis ▪ GI: *N/V/D*, abdominal pain, anorexia, oral monilia, dyspepsia ▪ INT: *rash*, pruritus ▪ Other: fever, cough, pain, asthenia, hypoglycemia.

INTERACTIONS: Drug: Use c̄ other high protein-bound drugs can result in displacement from inactive protein binding sites ▪ Use c̄ a rifamycin antibiotic will ⬇ atovaquone plasma concentration. **Food:** Failure to administer c̄ food may ⬇ therapeutic response.

NURSING MANAGEMENT PRIORITIES

ADMINISTRATION: Assess for hx of hypersensitivity ▪ Obtain C&S before therapy ▪ Assess renal function, may require ⬇ dosage if impaired ▪ Administer c̄ food.

EVALUATION: Monitor VS, CBC ▪ Diabetics: monitor blood glucose (hypoglycemia) ▪ Monitor renal function (nephrotoxicity); notify physician ▪ May ⬆ serum ALT, AST, creatinine, K^+; ⬇ Ca^{++}.

EDUCATION: Dizziness/drowsiness may occur; use caution in potentially hazardous activities ▪ Complete full course of therapy as directed by physician ▪ Take c̄ food ▪ Notify physician *immediately* of bleeding/bruising, difficult breathing, rash, severe GI distress ▪ Maintain good personal hygiene.

NOTES:

atropine sulfate • (a-troe-peen)

CATEGORY: *Anticholinergic:* antimuscarinic, parasympatholytic   Rx; Preg Cat C

AVAILABLE PREPARATIONS

Atropine sulfate (various)

Ophthalmic preparations; injection (IM/IV/SC), tablets

USE: Treat, manage, cause bradycardia, cardiospasm, colitis, dysmenorrhea, enuresis, GI spasm, inhibition of secretions, mydriasis/cycloplegia, pylorospasm, spastic/rigid states due to CNS injury, ureteral colic, urinary frequency ▪ Antidote for cholinergic drug OD & systemic-type insecticide ingestion. **ACTION:** Anticholinergic activity due to competition c̄ acetylcholine for muscarinic receptors at postganglionic fiber of parasympathetic nervous system.

PHARMACOKINETICS

	Peak	Half-life	Excretion
PO	1.5-4h	2-3h	75%-95% in urine, c̄ 50% as unchanged drug
IM	1.6-2h	2-3h	75%-95% in urine, c̄ 50% as unchanged drug

CONTRAINDICATIONS: Hypersensitivity; adhesions between iris, lens; advanced hepatic/renal impairment, asthma, hiatal hernia associated c̄ reflux esophagitis, intestinal atony, myasthenia gravis, narrow-angle glaucoma, obstructive GI/GU conditions, severe ulcerative colitis. **CC:** Use in high environmental temperatures may result in heat prostration.

DOSAGE

Pediatric	*PO*	0.01mg/kg q4-6h
Anticholinergic	*IM/IV/SC*	0.01mg/kg q4-6h
Antidote	*IV*	0.5-1mg followed by 0.5mg q10-15m until signs of atropine toxicity appear
		0.01-0.03mg/kg
Bradyarrhythmia	*IV*	3kg, 0.1mg; 7-9kg, 0.2mg;
Preop	*IM*	12-16kg, 0.3mg; 20-27kg, 0.4mg; 32kg, 0.5mg; 41kg, 0.6mg
		0.1-1.2mg q4-6h
Adult	*PO*	0.4-0.6mg q4-6h
Anticholinergic	*IM/IV/SC*	1-4mg followed by 1-2mg
Antidote	*IV*	q5-10m until signs of atropine toxicity appear

Bradyarrhythmia	*IV*	0.4-1mg
Hypotonic radiography	*IM*	1mg
Preop	*IM/SC*	0.4-1mg

SIDE/ADVERSE EFFECTS: CNS: mental confusion ▪ CV: tachycardia ▪ EENT: blurred vision, cycloplegia, mydriasis, ↑ IOP, photophobia ▪ GI: N/V, constipation, loss of taste, dysphagia ▪ GU: urinary retention ▪ INT: urticaria, skin rash ▪ Other: suppression of lactation/body secretions.

INTERACTIONS: Drug: Use c̄ antihistamines, phenothiazines, TCAs ↑ anticholinergic effects ▪ MAO-I ↑ activity by ↓ anticholinergic biotransformation.

NURSING MANAGEMENT PRIORITIES

ADMINISTRATION: Assess for hx of hypersensitivity ▪ Administer tablets ac/hs ▪ Have physostigmine available for OD ▪ Parenteral antidotal therapy: first dose IV injection; repeated doses IM ▪ Elderly may require ↓ dosage (paradoxic rxs).

EVALUATION: Monitor VS, esp heart rate; I&O ▪ Observe for anticholinergic effects.

EDUCATION: Advise pt of expected anticholinergic side effects (dry mouth, photophobia, constipation) ▪ Notify physician *immediately* of skin rash, flushing of skin, eye pain; D/C drug ▪ Avoid concurrent antacid administration ▪ Avoid strenuous work/exercise during hot, humid weather ▪ Use sugarless gum/hard candy to diminish dry mouth ▪ Avoid OTC cough/hay fever preparations ▪ Avoid potentially hazardous activities ▪ ↑ Fluid intake (10-12 glasses/d).

NOTES:

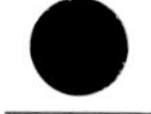

auranofin • (au-rane-oh-fin)

CATEGORY: *Antiinflammatory:* gold compound

Rx; Preg Cat C

BRAND NAME	DOSAGE FORM
Ridaura (SKB)	Capsule: 3mg

USE: Treatment of rheumatoid arthritis. **ACTION:** Antiinflammatory mechanism not determined.

PHARMACOKINETICS: Approximately 25% of gold absorbed, c̄ mean body half-life 80d; excretion of absorbed gold via urine (60%).

CONTRAINDICATIONS: Hx of gold-induced necrotizing enterocolitis, pulmonary fibrosis, exfoliative dermatitis, bone marrow aplasia, other severe blood dyscrasias. **CC:** Possible gold toxicity (up to 25% of gold content is absorbed) resulting in leukopenia, thrombocytopenia, bleeding ▪ Use in pts c̄ hepatocellular disease, inflammatory bowel disease, bone marrow depression requires extreme caution & careful consideration of potential gold toxicity.

DOSAGE

Adult *PO*	Initial dose 6mg/d given once or 3mg bid. May ⬆ to 9mg/d after 6mo if response is inadequate

SIDE/ADVERSE EFFECTS: GI: *loose stools or diarrhea, abdominal pain, nausea,* vomiting, constipation, anorexia, flatulence, *stomatitis* ▪ GU: proteinuria, hematuria ▪ HEM: anemia, ***leukopenia, thrombocytopenia***, eosinophilia ▪ HEP: jaundice, ⬆ enzyme levels ▪ INT: *rash, pruritus.*

INTERACTIONS: Drug: No significant rxs reported. **Lab:** Possible ⬆ response to tuberculin skin test.

NURSING MANAGEMENT PRIORITIES

ADMINISTRATION: Assess for hx of gold/heavy metal hypersensitivity ▪ Assess for hx of blood dyscrasia; do *not* administer ▪ Have emergency support equipment available.

EVALUATION: Monitor hepatic, renal status ▪ Monitor CBC, UA ▪ Assess joint function; comply $\bar{c}$ physical therapy ▪ False +: tuberculin skin test.

EDUCATION: Take exactly as directed by physician even if symptom free ▪ Notify physician of diarrhea, itching ▪ D/C, notify physician of signs of bleeding (bruising, red pinpoint rash, black tarry stools) ▪ Keep scheduled appointments $\bar{c}$ physician/for laboratory tests ▪ May produce changes in taste ▪ Maintain good oral hygiene; use soft-bristled toothbrush; avoid smoking, alcohol, acidic foods ▪ Check $\bar{c}$ physician before taking OTC/Rx preparations ▪ Full drug effect may require several mo of therapy.

NOTES:

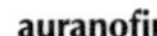

azathioprine/azathioprine sodium▲ • (ay-zah-thigh-oh-preen)

CATEGORY: *Immunosuppressive:* purine antagonist

Rx; Preg Cat D

BRAND NAME
Imuran (G-W)

DOSAGE FORMS
IV injection▲: 100mg (powder)/vial
Tablet: 50mg

USE: Adjunct for suppression of rejection in kidney transplants (renal homotransplantation) ▪ Treatment of active/erosive rheumatoid arthritis not responsive to more conventional therapy (aspirin, other NSAIAs). **ACTION:** Suppresses T-cell effects & cell-mediated hypersensitivities, alters antibody production. However, specific immunosuppressive activity for tissue transplants not determined. Has little effect on established transplant rejections & is metabolized in the body into mercaptopurine.

PHARMACOKINETICS

PO absorption	Peak	Protein binding	Excretion
Good	1-2h	30%	Via urine primarily as metabolites

CONTRAINDICATIONS: Hypersensitivity, treatment of rheumatoid arthritis during pregnancy or previous treatment c̄ alkylating agents due to risk of neoplasia. **CC:** Chronic use can result in oncogenic activity ▪ Use can result in severe leukopenia, infections, thrombocytopenia.

DOSAGE

Renal transplant

Children/Adult *IV/PO*	3-5mg/kg/d starting on day of transplant and/or 1-3d before procedure. ⬇ To a PO maintenance dose of 1-2mg/kg/d when possible

Arthritis

Adult *PO*	Usual starting dose 1mg/kg/d as single dose or divided twice/d. If no response, daily dose may be ⬆ by 0.5 mg/kg after 6-8wks. Further ⬆ of 0.5-2.5mg/kg/d may be required at 4-wk intervals. ⬇ To lowest effective maintenance dose as soon as possible. Dosage reduction schedule usually 0.5mg/kg/d q4wks. D/C treatment after 12wks if pt shows no response

Note: Side/adverse effects: common in *italic;* serious in ***boldface italic***.

▲Available in Canada only.

SIDE/ADVERSE EFFECTS: GI: N/V/D, abdominal pain ▪ HEM: Dose-related *leukopenia* & ***thrombocytopenia*** ▪ Other: ***hepatotoxicity, rare hepatic venoocclusive disease (renal transplants),*** oliguria, alopecia, arthralgia, skin rashes, negative nitrogen balance.

INTERACTIONS: Drug: Use c̄ allopurinol requires ⅓ to ¼ dosage ⬇ of azathioprine ▪ Radiation or other myelosuppressive drugs will result in ⬆ bone marrow depression ▪ Use of live vaccines not recommended.

NURSING MANAGEMENT PRIORITIES

ADMINISTRATION: Assess for hx of hypersensitivity ▪ PO: administer c̄ food to ⬇ GI irritation ▪ IV: add 10ml sterile H_2O; use w/in 24h; further dilute c̄ sterile saline or dextrose; infuse over 30-60m ▪ Assess renal function; ⬇ dosage if impaired ▪ Elderly may require ⬇ dosage.

EVALUATION: Monitor CBC ▪ Monitor hepatic, renal status ▪ Monitor I&O, daily weight ▪ Assess for edema in extremities.

EDUCATION: Avoid exposure to infection-producing situations ▪ ⬆ Fluid intake (8-10 glasses/d) ▪ Diarrhea may occur ▪ Notify physician/dentist of use before treatment ▪ Women: notify physician of possibility of pregnancy; avoid breastfeeding ▪ Keep scheduled appointments c̄ physician/for blood work ▪ Notify physician *immediately* of fever, sore throat, bruising/bleeding, abdominal pain, dark urine.

NOTES:

azithromycin • (a-zi-thro-my-sin)

CATEGORY: *Antibiotic:* macrolide antibiotic (semisynthetic) Rx; Preg Cat B

BRAND NAME
Zithromax (Pfizer)

DOSAGE FORMS
Capsule: 250mg
PO suspension: 100, 250mg/5ml
IV powder for injection: 500mg/vial
Tablet: 250, 500mg

USE: Treatment of lower & upper respiratory, skin, & sexually transmitted infections caused by susceptible strains of *Chlamydia pneumoniae, C. trachomatis, Haemophilus ducreyi* (chancroid), *H. influenzae, Legionella pneumophilia, Moraxella catarrhalis, Mycoplasma hominis, M. pneumoniae, Neisseria gonorrhoeae, Staphylococcus aureus, Streptococcus agalactiae, S. pneumoniae, S. pyogenes* ▪ Pediatric acute otitis media due to *H. influenzae, M. cartarrhalis, S. pneumonia;* pharyngitis, tonsillitis (PO suspension) ▪ Treatment of disseminated mycobacterium avium complex (MAC) c̄ rifabutin in advanced HIV infection. **ACTION:** Bacteriostatic activity due to inhibition of ribosomal protein synthesis in microorganisms.

PHARMACOKINETICS

PO absorption	Peak	Half-life	Protein binding	Excretion
40%	2.5h	68h	Up to 51%	Via feces (biliary) & urine as unchanged drug

CONTRAINDICATIONS: Hypersensitivity to drug, erythromycin, or any macrolide. **CC:** Allergic rxs have recurred after D/C w/out further drug exposure ▪ Use can result in pseudomembranous colitis ▪ Use in pts c̄ liver dysfunction requires caution.

DOSAGE

Adults/Children	
16 or over *PO*	500mg as single dose on day 1, then 250mg once/d 1h ac or 2h pc on days 2-5 (total dose of 1.5g)
MAC	1200mg once/wk
Chancroid	1g as a single dose
Gonorrhea	2g as a single dose
Nongonoccocal cervicitis urethritis	1g as a single dose

	IV	500mg infused over >60m for 1-2d followed by 250-500mg for 7-10d
Children	*PO*	
Otitis media		10mg/kg as a single dose on d1 (do not exceed a total dose of 500mg/d) then 5mg/kg for 4 more days (d2-5); do *not* exceed a total dose of 250mg/d
Pharyngitis/ tonsillitis		12mg/kg once/d for 5d

SIDE/ADVERSE EFFECTS: CNS: dizziness, headache, somnolence ▪ CV: chest pain, palpitations ▪ GI: N/V/D (highest dose: 1g), dyspepsia, flatulence, cholestatic jaundice, melena, ***pseudomembranous colitis*** ▪ GU: monilia, nephritis, vaginitis ▪ INT: rash, photosensitivity ▪ Other: angioedema, fatigue.

INTERACTIONS: Drug: Bacteriostatic antibiotics can antagonize effects of bactericidal antibiotics ▪ Use c̄ carbamazepine, cyclosporine, digoxin, ergot alkaloids, phenytoin, theophylline, triazolam can ↑ their toxicity ▪ Use c̄ astemizole, terfenadine not recommended. **Lab:** ↑ ALT, AST, serum creatinine phosphokinase.

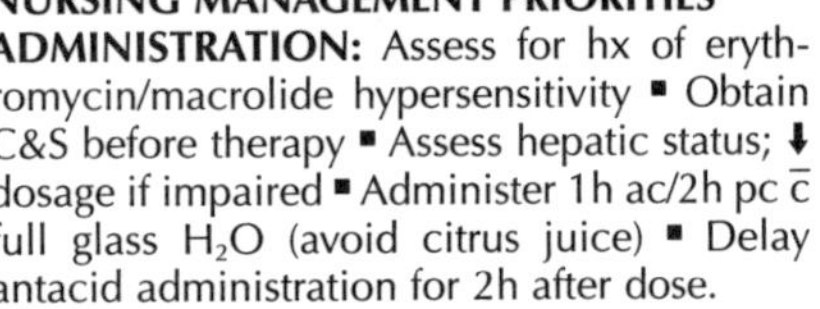

NURSING MANAGEMENT PRIORITIES

ADMINISTRATION: Assess for hx of erythromycin/macrolide hypersensitivity ▪ Obtain C&S before therapy ▪ Assess hepatic status; ↓ dosage if impaired ▪ Administer 1h ac/2h pc c̄ full glass H_2O (avoid citrus juice) ▪ Delay antacid administration for 2h after dose.

EVALUATION: Monitor VS, esp temperature; hepatic status ▪ Observe for signs of superinfection (diarrhea, perineal itching, oral ulcers).

EDUCATION: Complete full course of therapy ▪ Take on empty stomach; do *not* take c̄ citrus juice ▪ Take at equal intervals around clock to maintain blood levels ▪ Diarrhea may occur.

NOTES:

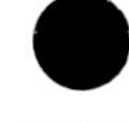

aztreonam • (az-tree-oh-nam)

CATEGORY: *Antibiotic:* monobactam, synthetic β-lactam Rx; Preg Cat B

BRAND NAME
Azactam (Squibb)

DOSAGE FORMS
Powder for injection (IM/IV): 500mg; 1, 2g

USE: Treatment of gynecologic, intraabdominal, lower respiratory, septicemia, skin & skin structure infections, UTIs caused by susceptible strains of *Citrobacter* spp, *Enterobacter cloacae, Escherichia coli, Haemophilus influenzae, Klebsiella oxytoca, K. pneumoniae, Proteus mirabilis, Pseudomonas aeruginosa, Serratia* spp. **ACTION:** Bactericidal activity due to inhibition of mucopeptide cell wall synthesis in susceptible organisms.

PHARMACOKINETICS

IM peak	Half-life	Protein binding	Excretion
1h	1.5-2h	56%	Complete w/in 12h primarily via urine

CONTRAINDICATIONS: Hypersensitivity. **CC:** Use can result in pseudomembranous colitis ▪ Use in pts c̄ hepatic or renal dysfunction requires caution ▪ Cross-allergenicity c̄ other β-lactam antibiotics is rare but requires caution when used in pts who are hypersensitive to β-lactam antibiotics ▪ Use can produce pseudomembranous colitis.

DOSAGE

Adult *IM/IV* 500mg-1g q8-12h. For moderate infection 1-2g q8-12h. For life-threatening infection 2g q6-8h IV. Dosage must be ↓ c̄ renal impairment

SIDE/ADVERSE EFFECTS: CNS: dizziness, confusion, headache, paresthesia ▪ CV: transient ventricular bigeminy, PVC, hypotension ▪ EENT: diplopia, tinnitus, nasal congestion ▪ GI: cramps, oral ulcers, taste change, ***pseudomembranous colitis*** ▪ HEM: anemia, pancytopenia, neutropenia ▪ HEP: ↑ AST, ALT, alkaline phosphatase ▪ INT: pruritus, purpura, ***erythema multiforme, exfoliative dermatitis,*** urticaria ▪ Other: breast tenderness, muscular aches, vaginal monilia.

INTERACTIONS: Drug: Use c̄ furosemide/probenecid can cause slight ↑ in serum aztreonam levels ▪ In *Enterobacter* & *Pseudomonas* infections, avoid concurrent use c̄ β-lactamase-inducing antibiotics such as cefoxitin.

NURSING MANAGEMENT PRIORITIES

ADMINISTRATION: Assess for hx of penicillin/cephalosporin hypersensitivity ▪ Obtain C&S before therapy ▪ IM/IV: reconstitute according to manufacturer's directions; shake well; discard unused solution.

EVALUATION: Monitor VS, esp temperature ▪ Monitor hepatic status ▪ Observe for signs of superinfection (diarrhea, perineal itching, oral ulcers) ▪ Check IV site carefully; monitor for phlebitis (red streak, heat, pain) ▪ Assess for ↑ serum creatinine; ↓ dose.

EDUCATION: Diarrhea may occur ▪ Maintain good personal hygiene (esp perineal, oral) ▪ Maintain fluid intake (6-8 glasses/d) ▪ Notify physician of symptoms of allergic rx (difficult breathing, rash) ▪ IM injection may be painful.

NOTES:

bacitracin/bacitracin sterile▲ • (bass-i-tray-sin)

CATEGORY: *Antibiotic:* polypeptide antibiotic Rx; Preg Cat NA

AVAILABLE PREPARATIONS
Bacitracin ointment, ophthalmic ointment (various)
Bacitracin powder for injection (various)

USE: Treatment of topical infections caused by susceptible organisms ▪ Treatment of pneumonia, empyema in infants caused by susceptible strains of staphylococci. **ACTION:** Bactericidal activity due to inhibition of mucopeptide cell wall synthesis in susceptible organisms.

PHARMACOKINETICS

IM absorption	Peak	Excretion
Complete	1-2h	Via urine

CONTRAINDICATIONS: Hypersensitivity. **CC:** Systemic use (IM) can cause tubular, glomerular necrosis resulting in renal failure.

DOSAGE

Infant *IM*	<2.5kg: 900U/kg/d in 2-3 divided doses
	>2.5kg: 1000U/kg/d in 2-3 divided doses

SIDE/ADVERSE EFFECTS: CV: ↑ blood levels w/out ↑ in dosage ▪ GI: N/V ▪ GU: ***nephrotoxicity*** c̄ albuminuria, cylinduria, azotemia ▪ INT: skin rash ▪ Other: local pain at IM injection site.

INTERACTIONS: Drug: Use c̄ nephrotoxic drugs such as aminoglycosides, colistimethate sodium, polymyxin B can result in significant toxicity ▪ Surgical neuromuscular blocking agent activity enhanced; can result in respiratory depression, paralysis.

NURSING MANAGEMENT PRIORITIES

ADMINISTRATION: Assess for hx of hypersensitivity (incl neomycin) ▪ Obtain C&S before therapy ▪ IM: dilute; administer *deep, slowly* into gluteal UOQ; refrigerate ▪ Do *not* administer IV ▪ Avoid application to severely burned areas ▪ Maintain alkaline urine ▪ Maintain hydration.

EVALUATION: Monitor renal status ▪ Assess for skin rash; notify physician, D/C use ▪ Monitor I&O (IM) ▪ Monitor serum for ↑ BUN, creatinine.

EDUCATION: Notify physician of changes in urination ▪ ↑ Fluid intake (8-10 glasses/d) ▪ IM injection may be painful ▪ Ophthalmic application: wash hands; sterile technique, do *not* contaminate tip of tube; do *not* share c̄ others; blurring of vision may occur ▪ D/C use, notify physician of burning, itching, difficult breathing.

NOTES:

benztropine mesylate • (<u>benz</u>-troe-peen)

CATEGORY: *Anti-Parkinson* agent: anticholinergic

Rx; Preg Cat C

BRAND NAME
Cogentin (Merck)

DOSAGE FORMS
Injection (IM/IV): 1mg/ml
Tablet: 0.5, 1, 2mg

USE: Adjunct to treatment of all forms of Parkinson's disease ▪ Management of extrapyramidal symptoms (except tardive dyskinesia) induced by antipsychotic agents. **ACTION:** Anti-Parkinson effect due to central anticholinergic inhibition of hyperactive cholinergic activity in striated fibers.

PHARMACOKINETICS: Not available.

CONTRAINDICATIONS: Hypersensitivity, glaucoma. **CC:** Use in high environmental temperatures may result in heat prostration.

DOSAGE

Adults *PO/IM/IV* — Parkinson's disease: 1-2mg/d c̄ range 0.5-6mg
Drug-induced extrapyramidal symptoms: 1-4mg/d or bid

SIDE/ADVERSE EFFECTS: EENT: blurred vision ▪ GI: dry mouth, dysphagia, constipation, N/V ▪ Other: allergic rxs (rare).

INTERACTIONS: Drug: Use c̄ antihistamines, phenothiazines, TCAs will produce ↑ anticholinergic effects ▪ Amantadine can significantly ↑ anticholinergic effects of benztropine.

NURSING MANAGEMENT PRIORITIES

ADMINISTRATION: Assess for hx of hypersensitivity ▪ Administer in divided doses c̄ meals, as single AM dose, or as single hs dose ▪ Avoid exposure to moisture during storage ▪ Avoid abrupt withdrawal ▪ Parenteral: avoid freezing ▪ Elderly may require ↓ dosage.

EVALUATION: Monitor GI, GU, CV status ▪ Assess for muscle weakness ▪ Observe for exaggerated anticholinergic effects ▪ Monitor VS ▪ Monitor I&O ▪ Assess IOP ▪ Assess for tolerance to therapeutic dose.

EDUCATION: Drowsiness may occur; use caution when engaging in potentially hazardous activities ▪ Avoid use c̄

Note: Side/adverse effects: common in *italic;* serious in ***boldface italic***.

*Available in Canada only.

alcohol, other CNS depressants ▪ Take c̄ meals ▪ Avoid extremes in exercise, hot climate ▪ Take as ordered by physician; do *not* ↑ dose ▪ Store in tightly closed container ▪ Schedule periodic eye exams ▪ Use sugarless gum/hard candy to diminish dry mouth ▪ Take antacid/antidiarrheal preparations at least 1h before or after taking drug ▪ Wear sunglasses to ↓ discomfort from bright light ▪ Avoid changing positions (lying/sitting/standing) rapidly ▪ Safety precautions c̄ ↑ activity ▪ Women: avoid breastfeeding ▪ Full drug effects may require several days of therapy.

NOTES:

beractant/calfactant/colfosceril palmitate • (bear-ac-tant/kal-fak-tant/coal-foss-er-ill)

CATEGORY: *Lung surfactant*

Rx; Preg Cat NA

BRAND NAMES	DOSAGE FORMS
beractant	Intratracheal suspension:
Survanta (Ross)	25mg/ml
calfactant	Intratracheal suspension:
Infasurf (Forest)	35mg/ml
colfosceril palmitate	Powder for intratracheal
Exosurf Neonatal (G-W)	suspension: 108mg/10ml vial

USE: Prophylaxis of respiratory distress syndrome (RDS) in susceptible infants ▪ Rescue treatment in infants c̄ RDS.

ACTION: Alleviate symptoms of neonatal RDS (hyaline membrane disease) by replacing deficient endogenous pulmonary surfactant. Both lung surfactants restore surface activity in lungs. This results in lower alveolar surface tension & ↑ alveoli, resistant to structural collapse at resting transpulmonary pressure.

Beractant is a natural pulmonary phospholipid containing surfactant obtained from bovine lung extract & modified c̄ the addition of colfosceril palmitate.

Calfactant is a natural exogenous pulmonary surfactant obtained from calf lung extracts that contains phospholipids, neutral lipids, fatty acids, & surfactant-associated proteins (SP-B, SP-C).

Colfosceril palmitate is a synthetic protein-free lung surfactant.

PHARMACOKINETICS: Available data are very limited. Administered surfactant becomes respiratory associated within a few h.

CONTRAINDICATIONS: None. **CC:** Only for intratracheal administration ▪ Use can rapidly effect oxygenation, lung compliance & may require modified O_2 therapy & ventilatory support ▪ Use can produce intracranial/pulmonary hemorrhage ▪ Monitor for drug reflux & mucous plug in endotracheal tube ▪ Do not suction after dosing unless clinically indicated ▪ Use can result in cyanosis, drug reflux, mucous plugs (calfactant).

DOSAGE

beractant

Intratracheal	4ml (100mg)/kg usually for 4 doses in the first 48h of life. Do *not* administer more frequently than q6h

calfactant	
Intratracheal	Prophylactic: 3ml/kg of birth weight administered as 2 doses of 1.5ml/kg as soon as possible Rescue: 3ml/kg of birth weight administered as 2 doses of 1.5ml/kg up to a total of 3 doses 12h apart.
colfosceril	5ml (54mg)/kg
Intratracheal	Prophylactic: give first dose as soon as possible after birth. Give second dose w/in 12h & third dose in 12h (24h after first dose). Further doses prn for infants on assisted respiration Rescue: 5ml/kg after RDS diagnosis, second dose 12h later if assisted ventilation is still required

SIDE/ADVERSE EFFECTS: CV: transient bradycardia, vasoconstriction, hypotension ▪ GI: ***necrotizing enterocolitis*** ▪ HEM: ***thrombocytopenia*** ▪ RESP: ***pulmonary hemorrhage,*** apnea, air leaks, hypocarbia, hypercarbia, post-treatment infections, hyperoxia.

INTERACTIONS: Drug: None currently reported.

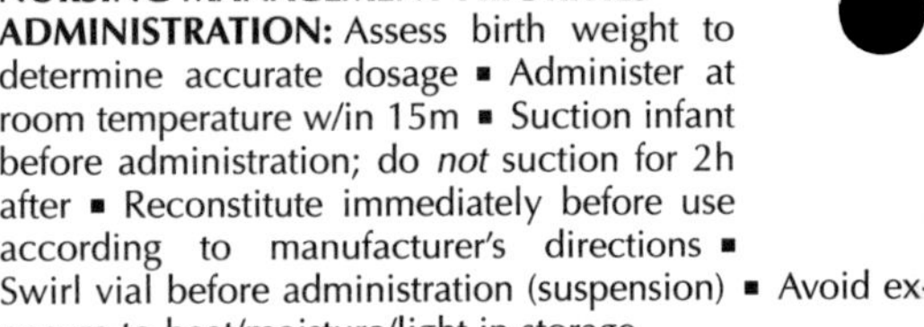

NURSING MANAGEMENT PRIORITIES

ADMINISTRATION: Assess birth weight to determine accurate dosage ▪ Administer at room temperature w/in 15m ▪ Suction infant before administration; do *not* suction for 2h after ▪ Reconstitute immediately before use according to manufacturer's directions ▪ Swirl vial before administration (suspension) ▪ Avoid exposure to heat/moisture/light in storage.

EVALUATION: Monitor VS, esp heart rate ▪ Monitor respiratory status.

EDUCATION: Notify physician of abnormal rx ▪ Explain procedure, rationale to family.

NOTES:

biperiden hcl/biperiden lactate▲/procyclidine hcl/trihexyphenidyl hcl • 36

(bye-per-i-den/proe-sike-leh-deen/trye-hex-ee-fen-i-dill)

CATEGORY: *Anti-Parkinson agent:* anticholinergic — Rx; Preg Cat C

BRAND NAMES	DOSAGE FORMS
biperiden	
Akineton (Knoll)	Injection (IM/IV)▲: 5mg/ml Tablet: 2mg
procyclidine	
Kemadrin (G-W)	Tablet: 5mg
trihexyphenidyl	
**Aparkane*	Tablet: 2, 5mg
**Apo-Trihex*	Tablet 2, 5mg
Artane (Lederle)	Elixir: 2mg/5ml SR capsule: 5mg Tablet: 2, 5mg

USE: Adjunct in treatment of all forms of Parkinson's disease ▪ Management of extrapyramidal symptoms (except tardive dyskinesia) induced by antipsychotic agents. **ACTION:** Anti-Parkinson effect due to central anti-cholinergic inhibition of hyperactive cholinergic activity in striated fibers.

PHARMACOKINETICS: biperiden: Good PO absorption; appears to peak after 1-1½h; metabolic path not fully determined. procyclidine: Not available. trihexyphenidyl: Rapid PO absorption c̄ onset of 1h, peak at 2-3h, duration of 6-12h. Excretion via urine as unchanged drug.

CONTRAINDICATIONS: Hypersensitivity, glaucoma, megacolon. **CC:** Use c̄ caution in pts c̄ arrhythmias & epilepsy.

DOSAGE

biperiden		
Adult	*PO*	Parkinson's disease: 2mg 3-4 times/d Extrapyramidal: 2mg 1-3 times/d
	IM/IV	Extrapyramidal: 2mg q½h until control is achieved; do *not* exceed 8mg/24h
procyclidine		
Adult	*PO*	Parkinson's disease: 2.5-5mg tid pc Extrapyramidal: 10-20mg/d divided
trihexyphenidyl		
Adult	*PO*	Parkinson's disease: 6-10mg/d divided Extrapyramidal: 5-15mg/d divided

Note: Side/adverse effects: common in *italic;* serious in ***boldface italic***

*Available in Canada only.

SIDE/ADVERSE EFFECTS: EENT: blurred vision ▪ GI: dry mouth, dysphagia, constipation, N/V ▪ GU: urinary retention ▪ Other: allergic rxs.

INTERACTIONS: Drug: Use c̄ antihistamines, phenothiazines, TCAs will ↑ anticholinergic effects ▪ Amantadine can significantly ↑ anticholinergic effects.

NURSING MANAGEMENT PRIORITIES

ADMINISTRATION: Assess for hx of hypersensitivity ▪ Administer in divided doses c̄ meals/pc ▪ Avoid exposure to moisture during storage ▪ Avoid abrupt withdrawal; D/C gradually ▪ Parenteral: avoid freezing ▪ Elderly may require ↓ dosage.

EVALUATION: Monitor CV, GI, GU status ▪ Assess for muscle weakness ▪ Observe for exaggerated anticholinergic effects ▪ Monitor VS ▪ Monitor I&O ▪ Assess IOP ▪ Assess for tolerance to therapeutic dose.

EDUCATION: Drowsiness may occur; use caution when engaging in potentially hazardous activities ▪ Avoid changing positions (lying/sitting/standing) rapidly ▪ Avoid use c̄ alcohol, other CNS depressants ▪ Take as ordered by physician ▪ Take c̄ meals/pc ▪ Avoid extremes in exercise, temperature ▪ Store in tightly closed container ▪ Schedule periodic eye exams ▪ Use sugarless gum/hard candy to diminish dry mouth ▪ Take antacid preparations at least 1h before/after taking drug ▪ Wear sunglasses to ↓ discomfort from bright lights ▪ Safety precautions c̄ ↑ activity ▪ Full drug effects may require several days of therapy.

NOTES:

bleomycin sulfate • (blee-oh-mye-sin)

CATEGORY: *Antineoplastic:* antibiotic

Rx; Preg Cat D

BRAND NAME
Blenoxane (BM-ONC)
(*Bristol [Canada]*)

DOSAGE FORMS
Powder for injection
(IM/IV/SC): 15, 30U/vial

USE: Palliative treatment of squamous cell carcinoma of head-mouth area, neck; response is poor in pts who have undergone radiation therapy ▪ Palliative treatment of lymphomas incl Hodgkin's disease, lymphosarcoma, reticulum cell sarcoma ▪ Palliative treatment of testicular carcinoma ▪ Treatment of malignant pleural effusion. **ACTION:** Antineoplastic activity appears to be related to inhibition of DNA, RNA, protein synthesis.

PHARMACOKINETICS: Short half-life; excreted via urine as unchanged drug (70%).

CONTRAINDICATIONS: Hypersensitivity. **CC:** Use requires qualified physicians ▪ Rare idiosyncratic rx (1%) resulting in hypotension, confusion, fever, chills, wheezing ▪ Use in pts c̄ compromised pulmonary function or renal dysfunction requires caution ▪ Pulmonary toxicities occur in 10% of treated pts ▪ Drug-induced nonspecific pneumonitis can progress to pulmonary fibrosis & death (about 1%).

DOSAGE
IM/IV/SC

Hodgkin's disease	0.25-0.5U/kg 1-2 times/wk; after 50% response, maintenance dose 1U qd or 5U/wk IV or IM
Other cancers	0.25-0.5U/kg 1-2 times/wk
Malignant pleural effusion	60U as a single bolus intrapleural injection

SIDE/ADVERSE EFFECTS: GI: N/V, anorexia, fever, chills ▪ INT: *most frequent (50%): alopecia, erythema,* hyperkeratosis, hyperpigmentation, nail changes, *pruritus, rash, stomatitis, striae, vesiculation* ▪ RESP: pulmonary toxicity (10%), dose or age related, esp c̄ high doses (>400U) or old age (70); pneumonitis, which can lead to fatal ***pulmonary fibrosis.***

INTERACTIONS: Drug: Use c̄ vinblastine has produced isolated Raynaud's disease in pts c̄ testicular carcinoma ▪ Use c̄ pulmotoxic/hepatotoxic drugs results in ↑ toxicity ▪ Use c̄ colony stimulating factor can ↑ risk of pulmonary toxicity.

Note: Side/adverse effects: common in *italic;* serious in ***boldface italic.***

[1]Available in Canada only.

NURSING MANAGEMENT PRIORITIES

ADMINISTRATION: Assess for hx of hypersensitivity ▪ Assess pulmonary function (chest x-ray, auscultation of lungs) ▪ Wear disposable surgical gloves, mask when preparing solutions ▪ IM or SC: dissolve in 1-5ml sterile or bacteriostatic H_2O, CaCl, or D_5W for injection ▪ IM: inject *deep, slowly* into gluteal UOQ; rotate sites ▪ IV: dissolve in 5ml NaCl or D_5W for injection; administer *slowly,* over 10m ▪ Reconstituted solutions are stable for 24h (room temperature) or 7d (refrigerated) ▪ Have support equipment available for anaphylaxis ▪ Administer antiemetic before therapy ▪ Provide emotional support.

EVALUATION: Monitor hepatic, renal, hemopoietic status ▪ Monitor breath sounds, respiratory function (chest x-ray) ▪ Assess for hyperthermia (fever, chills); administer antipyretic as ordered ▪ Assess for skin rash; D/C drug ▪ Assess for infection, bleeding, anemia ▪ Assess hydration status (I&O, daily weight).

EDUCATION: Notify physician *immediately* of cough, shortness of breath ▪ Check all OTC preparations c̄ physician/pharmacist before use ▪ Darkened skin may occur ▪ Avoid smoking (↑ pulmonary toxicity) ▪ ↑ Fluid intake (10-12 glasses/d) ▪ Avoid exposure to infection ▪ Diet as tolerated; avoid spicy foods ▪ Maintain good oral hygiene; use soft-bristled toothbrush ▪ Loss of hair may occur (reversible after therapy) ▪ Notify physician of symptoms of bone marrow depression (fever, sore throat, bruising, bleeding, lethargy) ▪ Encourage ventilation of feelings ▪ Women: avoid breastfeeding ▪ Use contraception if sexually active.

NOTES:

brimonidine tartrate • (brye-<u>moe</u>-ni-deen)

Category: *Antiglaucoma agent:* α_2-adrenergic agonist Rx; Preg Cat B

BRAND NAME
Alphagan (Allergan)

DOSAGE FORM
Ophthalmic solution: 0.2%

DOSAGE
Adult 1 gtt in affected eye(s) tid

USE: Treatment of open-angle glaucoma. **ACTION:** Antiglaucoma activity related to ⬇ in aqueous humor production and ⬆ in uveoscleral outflow. Peak ⬇ in IOP occurs 2h after dosing.

PHARMACOKINETICS

Peak plasma	Half-life	Excretion
1-4h	3h	Via urine

CONTRAINDICATIONS: Hypersensitivity, concurrent MAO-I therapy. **CC:** Use c̄ caution in pts c̄ severe cardiovascular disease, cerebral/coronary insufficiency, orthostatic hypotension, hepatic/renal impairment, Raynaud's disease, thromboangiitis obliterans ▪ Ophthalmic solution contains benzalkonium chloride as a preservative & pts c̄ soft contact lense should wait at least 15 min after dosing before inserting lenses ▪ Safety & efficacy in pediatric pts not established.

SIDE/ADVERSE Effects: Ocular: burning, hyperemia, blurring, conjunctival follicles, pruritus, corneal staining, photophobia, blepharitis, conjunctival hemorrhage, dryness ▪ Other: headache, upper respiratory smptoms.

INTERACTIONS: Drug: Use c̄ MAO-I is contraindicated ▪ Use c̄ CNS depressants can produce additive effects ▪ Use c̄ β blockers, cardiac glycosides requires caution.

NURSING MANAGEMENT PRIORITIES

ADMINISTRATION: Assess for hx of hypersensitivity ▪ Wash hands thoroughly before administration ▪ Avoid contamination of solution, dropper tip ▪ Apply pressure to lacrimal sac 1-2m after installation; instruct pt to keep eyes closed for 3-5m after insertion of gtt ▪ Avoid exposure to moisture/heat in storage.

EVALUATION: Monitor IOP ▪ Monitor hepatic, CV, renal function; use caution if impaired ▪ Assess for signs of contact allergy (burning, itching, ocular dryness); D/C drug, notify physician.

EDUCATION: Dizziness, drowsiness, blurred vision may occur; avoid potentially hazardous activities ▪ Take as ordered by physician; do *not* ↑ dose ▪ Notify physician *immediately* of eye irritation; D/C drug ▪ Keep scheduled appointments c̄ ophthalmologist ▪ Procedure for ophthalmic administration ▪ Soft contact lens wearers: insert 15m following instillation ▪ Women: avoid breast-feeding.

NOTES:

bromocriptine mesylate • (broe-moe-krip-teen)

CATEGORY: *Dopaminergic:* dopamimetic, prolactin inhibitor Rx; Preg Cat B

BRAND NAME
Parlodel (Sandoz)

DOSAGE FORMS
Capsule 5mg
Tablet 2.5mg
Snap Tabs: 2.5mg

USE: Treatment of idiopathic Parkinson's disease ▪ Short-term treatment of amenorrhea/galactorrhea associated c̄ hyperprolactinemia ▪ Prevention of lactation; some pts may experience mild/moderate rebound lactation ▪ Treatment of acromegaly. **ACTION:** Dopaminergic receptor activity, esp c̄ D-2 dopamine receptors in CNS, produces significant amelioration of hyperprolactinemia, Parkinson's disease; bromocriptine may cause symptoms of acromegaly to subside.

PHARMACOKINETICS

PO absorption	Peak	Protein binding	Excretion
28%	1-1.5h	90%-96%	Via bile (feces) as metabolites

CONTRAINDICATIONS: Hypersensitivity to drug/ergot alkaloids, uncontrolled hypertension, toxemia of pregnancy. **CC:** Possible relationship between use & hypertension, stroke, seizures, MI.

DOSAGE
Adult *PO*

Parkinson's disease	Initial dose 1.25mg bid. Dosage may ↑ q14-28d by 2.5mg/d. Do *not* exceed 100mg/d
Lactation	Therapy should start no sooner than 4h after delivery in pts c̄ stable VS. Usual dose 2.5mg bid for 14-21d
Acromegaly prevention	Initial dose 1.25-2.5mg/h c̄ food for 3d; c̄ 1.25-2.5mg increments q3-7d until satisfactory response obtained. Usual range 20-30mg/d. Do *not* exceed 100mg/d
Hyperprolactinemic indications	Initial dose 1.25-2.5mg/d. 2.5mg as tolerated may be added q3-7d. Usual dose 5-7.5mg/d c̄ a daily range of 2.5-15mg

SIDE/ADVERSE EFFECTS: CNS: *dizziness, headache,* fatigue, lethargy, ***epileptiform seizures,*** nightmares, confusion ▪ CV: hypotension, edema, palpitations ▪ EENT: nasal congestion, visual disturbances ▪ GI: *N/V/D,* cramps, anorexia, constipation, dyspepsia, dry mouth, metallic taste ▪ GU: urinary frequency ▪ Other: symptoms of ergotism.

INTERACTIONS: Drug: Use c̄ hypotensive agents can produce significant hypotension ▪ Use c̄ levodopa can ↑ frequency of visual/auditory hallucinations ▪ Phenothiazines can ↑ prolactin levels, are best avoided.

NURSING MANAGEMENT PRIORITIES

ADMINISTRATION: Assess for hx of ergot alkaloid hypersensitivity ▪ Avoid exposure to heat/moisture/light in storage ▪ Administer c̄ meals/milk ▪ Assess BP for stability before administration.

EVALUATION: Monitor hepatic/neuropsychiatric status ▪ Monitor VS, esp BP ▪ Pregnancy test at periodic intervals ▪ Assess serum FSH, LH, prolactin, urinary retention, pregnanediol prn ▪ Assess visual fields.

EDUCATION: Take c̄ meals ▪ Avoid alcohol ▪ May cause dizziness; use caution in potentially hazardous activities ▪ Avoid changing positions (lying/sitting/standing) rapidly ▪ Women: use birth control during therapy (unless for fertility); do *not* use PO contraceptives; avoid if breastfeeding ▪ Keep scheduled appointments c̄ physician ▪ May take >6wks for menses to recur ▪ Missed dose; if remembered >4h, do *not* take; do *not* double dose; resume regular dose schedule ▪ Store in tightly closed container ▪ Maintain good oral hygiene ▪ Use sugarless gum/hard candy to diminish dry mouth.

NOTES:

bumetanide • (byoo-met-a-nide)

CATEGORY: *Loop diuretic* Rx; Preg Cat C

BRAND NAME
Bumex (Roche)

DOSAGE FORMS
Injection (IM/IV): 0.25 mg/ml
Tablet: 0.5, 1mg

USE: Treatment of edema due to CHF, renal/hepatic dysfunction. **ACTION:** Diuretic activity due to excretion of H_2O, Na^+, Cl^-, other electrolytes by inhibiting tubular reabsorption, esp in medullary, cortical portions of ascending limb of loop of Henle.

DOSAGE

Adult	*PO*	0.5-2mg/d, to maximum 10mg
	IM/IV	0.5-1mg given at 2-3h intervals. Do *not* exceed 10mg/d

SIDE/ADVERSE EFFECTS: CNS: dizziness, encephalopathy, headache ▪ CV: *hypotension,* ECG changes ▪ EENT: impaired hearing ▪ GI: *nausea,* vomiting, abdominal pain ▪ INT: pruritus, hives ▪ MET: hypoglycemia, hyperuricemia, metabolic alkalosis ▪ MS: *muscle cramps,* pain, arthritic pain.

PHARMACOKINETICS

PO absorption	Onset	Peak	Duration	Half-life	Protein binding	Excretion
85%-95%	30-60m	1-2h	4-6h	1-1.5h	95%-96%	Via urine, feces as metablites, unchanged drug (45%)

CONTRAINDICATIONS: Hypersensitivity, hepatic coma, anuria, severe electrolyte depletion. **CC:** Excessive use can produce significant diuresis c̄ resulting electrolyte, water loss.

INTERACTIONS: Drug: Use c̄ neurotoxic drugs incl aminoglycosides, capreomycin, chloroquine, vancomycin can result in significant toxicity ▪ Induced hypokalemia ↑ dig toxicity ▪ Avoid use c̄ nephrotoxic drugs, lithium, indomethacin, probenecid ▪ Antihypertensives may require dosage adjustment ▪ Use c̄ corticosteroids can produce severe hypokalemia. **Lab:** Hyperuricemia reported in ≥18% during pt use.

NURSING MANAGEMENT PRIORITIES

ADMINISTRATION: Assess for hx of hypersensitivity (incl sulfonamides) ▪ Assess renal function; do *not* administer if severely impaired ▪ PO: administer c̄ food/milk on arising ▪ IV: use infusion w/in 24h after preparation; administer *slowly* (2m) ▪ Do *not* use discolored/precipitated solutions ▪ Assess serum K^+ (normal: 3.5-5mEq/L) ▪ Elderly may require ⬇ dosage ▪ Avoid exposure to light in storage ▪ IM: inject *deep, slowly* into gluteal UOQ.

EVALUATION: Monitor F/E, hepatic, renal status ▪ Monitor VS, esp BP, pulse ▪ Monitor serum for ⬆ BUN, creatinine, uric acid; ⬇ K^+ ▪ Diabetics: monitor blood glucose (hypoglycemia) ▪ Monitor fluid retention (I&O, daily weight) ▪ Monitor digitalized pts closely (⬇ K^+, ⬆ dig toxicity) ▪ Assess for ⬇ hearing (ototoxicity).

EDUCATION: Expect ⬆ urine output; have bathroom facilities easily accessible ▪ May cause weakness, lethargy ▪ Take PO forms c̄ food ▪ Take on waking, at same time qd ▪ Take even if symptom free ▪ Notify physician of signs of hypokalemia (muscle cramps, lethargy, nausea), hyponatremia (thirst, dry mouth, drowsiness) ▪ Avoid changing positions (lying/sitting/standing) rapidly ▪ Take as directed by physician; do *not* skip doses ▪ Eat foods high in K^+ (bananas, citrus juices, raisins); avoid black licorice ▪ Avoid high-Na^+ foods (canned soup, lunch meats, cheese) ▪ Maintain optimum weight ▪ Check c̄ physician before taking OTC/Rx preparations ▪ Diabetics: check blood/urine glucose carefully.

NOTES:

bupropion hcl • (byoo-proe-pee-on)

CATEGORY: *Antidepressant*

Rx; Preg Cat B

BRAND NAMES	**DOSAGE FORMS**
Wellbutrin (G-W)	Tablet: 75, 100mg
Zyban (G-W)	SR tablet: 150mg

USE: Treatment of depression. Avoid abrupt withdrawal of drug ▪ Smoking aid deterrent (SR tablet). **ACTION:** Antidepressant mechanism not established. Drug exhibits weak inhibition of dopamine, norepinephrine, serotonin & is devoid of MAO-I activity.

PHARMACOKINETICS

PO absorption	Peak	Half-life	Protein binding	Excretion
Good	2h	14h	80%	87% via urine, 10% via feces

CONTRAINDICATIONS: Hypersensitivity, seizure disorders, current or prior anorexia nervosa or bulimia, use of MAO-I. **CC:** Rare episodes of seizures (0.4%) occur, appear related to drug dosage, pt predisposing factors.

DOSAGE: Adult *PO*

Antidepressant	Initial dose 200mg/d with a usual daily dose of 300mg after 3d. Do *not* exceed a single dose of 150mg or a dose ↑ of 100mg/d in a 3d period. Maximum dose 450mg/d
Smoking aid deterrent	150mg/d for 3d then 300mg/d c̄ an interval of at least 8h between doses for 7-12wks. Do not exceed 300mg/d

SIDE/ADVERSE EFFECTS: CNS: *headache, migraine, insomnia,* dizziness, seizure disorders, neuropsychiatric disturbances, *agitation, tremor,* anxiety ▪ CV: edema, ECG abnormalities, rare phlebitis, tachycardia, cardiac arrhythmias ▪ ENT: visual & auditory disturbances ▪ GI: *dry mouth, N/V, constipation,* anorexia, rare colitis, bleeding ▪ GU: nocturia, menstrual complaints, male sexual dysfunction ▪ INT: rash, pruritus, dry skin, alopecia, hair color change ▪ Other: weight loss, dyspnea, gynecomastia, fatigue, arthritis.

INTERACTIONS: Drug: Use c̄ phenelzine ↑ toxicity ▪ Use c̄ L-dopa may produce ↑ in adverse effects ▪ Use c̄ drugs that ↓ seizure threshold best avoided ▪ Use c̄ carbamazepine, cimetidine, phenobarbital, phenytoin requires caution.

NURSING MANAGEMENT PRIORITIES

ADMINISTRATION: Assess for hx of hypersensitivity ▪ Assess neurologic status; may potentiate if impaired ▪ Assess for hx of bulimia, anorexia nervosa (↑ seizures) ▪ Administer first dose >14d after MAO-I therapy ▪ Assess hepatic, renal status; ↓ dosage if impaired ▪ Administer in 3 equally divided doses/d ▪ Institute safety, seizure precautions ▪ Institute suicide precautions ▪ Avoid abrupt withdrawal; D/C gradually ▪ Heavy smokers may require ↑ dosage ▪ Elderly may require ↓ dosage.

EVALUATION: Monitor CV, hepatic, renal status ▪ Monitor fluid retention (I&O, daily weight), constipation ▪ Assess for symptoms of abrupt withdrawal (nausea, headache, malaise) ▪ Assess for actual swallowing of PO forms ▪ May ↑ serum prolactin ▪ Assess for restlessness, agitation, insomnia after starting therapy; notify physician.

EDUCATION: Dizziness/drowsiness may occur; use caution in potentially hazardous activities ▪ Avoid use of alcohol, other CNS depressants for up to 1wk after end of therapy ▪ Take as directed by physician ▪ Use sugarless gum/hard candy to diminish dry mouth ▪ Constipation may occur; ↑ fluids, bulk-containing foods ▪ Check c̄ physician/pharmacist before taking OTC/Rx preparations ▪ Notify physician/dentist of use before treatment ▪ Store in tightly closed container ▪ Encourage recreational/diversional interests ▪ Notify physician of fever, sore throat, malaise ▪ Keep scheduled appointments c̄ physician ▪ Women: notify physician of pregnancy possibility; avoid breastfeeding ▪ Full drug effects may require several wks of therapy.

NOTES:

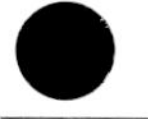

buspirone hcl • (byoo-spear-own)

CATEGORY: *Antianxiety agent:* anxiolytic

Rx; Preg Cat B

BRAND NAME
BuSpar (B-MS)

DOSAGE FORMS
Tablet: 5, 10mg

USE: Treatment of anxiety disorders ▪ Short-term relief of anxiety symptoms. **ACTION:** Antianxiety activity not determined. Drug has no anticonvulsant, muscle relaxant, sedative activity. Buspirone appears to be a midbrain modulator and has a role in serotonin, dopamine neurotransmission.

PHARMACOKINETICS

PO absorption	Peak	Half-life	Protein binding	Excretion
Almost complete	40-90m	2-4wks	95%	Via urine, feces primarily as metabolites

CONTRAINDICATIONS: Hypersensitivity. **CC:** Use c̄ MAO-I is dangerous ▪ Drug has no antipsychotic activity.

DOSAGE

Adult *PO* — Initial dose of 5mg tid. May ↑ to 5mg/d q2-3d. Do *not* exceed 60mg/d

SIDE/ADVERSE EFFECTS: CNS: *dizziness, drowsiness,* headache, *nervousness,* insomnia, lightheadedness, ↓ concentration, excitement, confusion, anger, hostility, paresthesia, tremor ▪ CV: palpitations, tachycardia ▪ GI: N/V/D, dry mouth, gastric distress ▪ INT: skin rash, sweating ▪ Other: blurred vision, muscle aches, numbness, fatigue, weakness.

INTERACTIONS: Drug: Use c̄ MAO-I not recommended.

NURSING MANAGEMENT PRIORITIES

ADMINISTRATION: Assess for hx of hypersensitivity ▪ Avoid exposure to moisture, light in storage ▪ Administer c̄ or w/out food; tablets may be crushed ▪ Elderly may require ↓ dosage ▪ Problem discussion, sympathetic listening contribute to relief of anxiety.

EVALUATION: Monitor renal, hepatic status ▪ Monitor activity status (safety precautions) ▪ Assess for tolerance to therapeutic dose ▪ Assess for paradoxic rxs (CNS stimulation), esp in elderly ▪ Check for depression; suicide precautions ▪ Monitor serum for ↑ AST, ALT.

EDUCATION: Drowsiness may occur; use caution in potentially hazardous activities ▪ Avoid changing positions (lying/sitting/standing) rapidly ▪ Avoid use c̄ alcohol, other CNS depressants ▪ Do *not* keep at bedside ▪ Use sugarless gum/hard candy to diminish dry mouth ▪ Take c̄ or w/out food; may crush tablets ▪ Take as directed by physician; do *not* ↑ dose ▪ Check c̄ physician/pharmacist before taking OTC preparations ▪ Women: avoid breastfeeding ▪ Practice relaxation exercises, ventilation of feelings ▪ Full drug effects may require several wks of therapy.

NOTES:

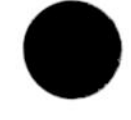

busulfan • (byoo-<u>sul</u>-fan)

CATEGORY: *Alkylating agent:* antineoplastic Rx; Preg Cat D

BRAND NAME	**DOSAGE FORM**
Myleran (G-W)	Tablet: 2mg

USE: Drug of choice for chronic myelocytic leukemia ▪ Treatment of polycythemia vera. **ACTION:** Antineoplastic activity due to alkylating effect on DNA replication; irreversible crosslinking of DNA strands results in disruption of DNA activity, inhibition of DNA replication, transcription of RNA; cytotoxic effect is produced, esp on myeloid elements.

PHARMACOKINETICS: Rapid PO absorption, c̄ blood levels appearing in 0.5-2h; extensively metabolized; up to 50% of single dose excreted in urine w/in 24h.

CONTRAINDICATIONS: Prior drug resistance; use only in adequately diagnosed chronic myelogenous leukemia. **CC:** Use requires qualified physicians, an established diagnosis of chronic myelogenous leukemia ▪ Use can result in bone marrow hypoplasia ▪ Use in premenopausal females can result in menopausal symptoms, amenorrhea, & ovarian suppression.

DOSAGE

Pediatric	*PO*	60-120μg/kg/d or 1.8mg/m²
Adult	*PO*	4-8mg/d; maintenance dose 1-3mg when remission period is <3mo

SIDE/ADVERSE EFFECTS: GI: N/V, *diarrhea*, glossitis ▪ GU: amenorrhea, gynecomastia ▪ HEM: dose-related myelosuppression resulting in ***thrombocytopenia***, pancytopenia ▪ INT: ***hyperpigmentation,*** anhidrosis, alopecia ▪ MET: hyperuricemia ▪ Other: ***interstitial pulmonary fibrosis.***

INTERACTIONS: Drug: Live vaccines contraindicated during therapy ▪ Radiation or other myelosuppressive drugs produce additive bone marrow depression.

NURSING MANAGEMENT PRIORITIES

ADMINISTRATION: Check hx for recent course of radiation or antineoplastic agents; report to physician ▪ Administer 1h ac/2h pc ▪ Avoid exposure to moisture during storage ▪ Administer antiemetic before therapy ▪ Provide emotional support.

EVALUATION: Monitor CBC throughout therapy ▪ Assess for infection, bleeding, anemia ▪ May produce ↑ serum uric acid level ▪ Monitor hepatic function ▪ Assess hydration status (I&O, daily weight).

EDUCATION: Store in dry, tightly closed container ▪ Take on empty stomach ▪ ↑ Fluid intake (10-12 glasses/d) ▪ Avoid exposure to infection ▪ Check c̄ physician before immunization (pt, family) ▪ Diet as tolerated; avoid spicy foods ▪ Maintain good oral hygiene; use soft-bristled toothbrush ▪ Notify physician of symptoms of bone marrow depression (fever, sore throat, bruising, bleeding, lethargy) ▪ Loss of hair may occur (reversible after therapy) ▪ Compliance c̄ prescribed dosage regimen ▪ Women: avoid breastfeeding ▪ Encourage ventilation of feelings ▪ Use contraception if sexually active.

NOTES:

butorphanol tartrate • (byoo-tor-fa-nole)

CATEGORY: *Analgesic:* opioid agonist/antagonist Rx; Preg Cat C

BRAND NAME
Stadol (MJP)

DOSAGE FORMS
Injection (IM/IV): 1, 2mg/ml
Nasal spray: 10mg/ml

USE: Relief of moderate/severe pain ▪ Peak analgesic activity in 30-60m (IM/IV) & 1-2h (spray) ▪ Preop medication & as a supplement to balanced anesthesia. **ACTION:** Analgesic mechanism not determined; possible site of activity may be subcortical areas of brain; narcotic agonist activity of 2mg approximately equivalent to 10-15mg morphine; narcotic antagonist activity equivalent to 1/40 that of naloxone.

DOSAGE

Adult *IV/IM*

Pain	2mg IM q3-4h or 1mg IV q3-4h. For severe pain 4mg IM or 2mg IV may be required
Preop	2mg IM 60-90m before surgery
Balanced anesthesia	Usual incremental dose 0.5-1mg IV
Nasal spray	1mg (1 spray) in one nostril. Repeat in 60-90m prn

PHARMACOKINETICS

Onset	Peak	Duration	Protein binding	Excretion
IV: 1-3m IM: 10-15m Spray: 15m	IM/IV: 20-40m Spray: 30-60m	3-4h	80%	85% via urine, 15% via feces

CONTRAINDICATIONS: Hypersensitivity. **CC:** Use in narcotic-dependent pts can produce withdrawal symptoms.

SIDE/ADVERSE EFFECTS: CNS: *sedation*, euphoria, hallucinations, dizziness, vertigo, headache ▪ CV: palpitations, BP changes ▪ EENT: blurred vision ▪ GI: vomiting, dry mouth ■ INT: rash, hives ■ RESP: respiratory depression ■ Other: *autonomic responses* (clammy sweating, flushing/warmth, sensitivity to cold).

INTERACTIONS: Drug: Use c̄ CNS depressant produces additive effects ■ Use in narcotic-dependent pts can produce withdrawal symptoms.

NURSING MANAGEMENT PRIORITIES

ADMINISTRATION: Assess for hx of opioid hypersensitivity ■ Check compatibility chart for mixing preop IM preparations ■ Do *not* administer if respirations are <12/m ■ IM: inject *deep* into muscle; rotate sites ■ IV: dilute; administer *slowly* ■ Do *not* administer SC ■ Have narcotic antagonist/support measures available ■ Avoid administration in pts c̄ suspected head injury ■ Administer *before* pt has intense pain ■ Avoid light/freezing in storage ■ Utilize + power of suggestion ■ Avoid abrupt withdrawal ■ Elderly may require ↓ dosage.

EVALUATION: Monitor respirations, circulatory function ■ Assess bowel function, abdominal distention ■ Assess renal function, urinary retention ■ Check for signs of dependence c̄ prolonged use (↑ drug request) ■ Assess for potentiation of CNS depressant effect ■ Assess for signs of OD (coma, pinpoint pupils, respiratory depression).

EDUCATION: Avoid changing positions (lying/sitting/standing) rapidly ■ Avoid excessive sensory stimulation ■ Keep bedrails up when nonambulatory ■ Obtain assistance prn when ambulatory ■ Turn, cough, deep breathe after surgery ■ Constipation may occur; ↑ fluid, bulk-containing foods ■ Avoid potentially hazardous activities ■ Avoid smoking while taking drug ■ Indiscriminate use may lead to dependence ■ Avoid alcohol, other CNS depressants.

OVERDOSE MANAGEMENT: naloxone hcl is specific antidote, in conjunction c̄ supportive therapy using oxygen, IV fluids, vasopressors.

NOTES:

calcium salts • (kal-see-um)

CATEGORY: *Antacid:* mineral supplement OTC/Rx

Calcium Carbonate
CATEGORY: *Antacid*: mineral supplement OTC

DOSAGE FORMS: Tablet: various strengths: 1g 1-3 times/d PO

Calcium Chloride
CATEGORY: *Electrolyte*: mineral Rx; Preg Cat C

DOSAGE FORMS: Injection (IV): 10%
1g calcium chloride = 13.6mEq calcium

USE: Treatment of acute hypocalcemic tetany 2° to array of causes ▪ Cardiac resuscitation.

DOSAGE

IV 500mg/g; subsequent dose schedule dependent on response
Cardiac resuscitation: ≥200mg injected into ventricular cavity

Calcium Gluconate
CATEGORY: *Electrolyte*: mineral

DOSAGE FORMS: Injection (IV): 10%
Tablet: various strengths (OTC)
1g of calcium = 4.5mEq calcium

USE: Calcium supplement esp in pregnancy, lactation ▪ Treatment of hypocalcemic conditions ▪ Antidote for magnesium, oxalic acid, carbon tetrachloride, fluoride, strontium. **ACTION:** Calcium is required for tissue growth/maintenance, regulation of physiologic activities; nerve transmission, muscular contraction, blood coagulation, renal function; involved c̄ activating enzymes, cell membrane & capillary permeability, neurotransmitter & hormone activity, maintenance of teeth & skeletal system.

DOSAGE

Pediatric	*PO*	125mg/kg 1-4 times/d
	IV	500mg/kg
Adult	*PO*	1-15g qd
	IV	500mg-2g

CONTRAINDICATIONS: Hypercalcemia, ventricular fibrillation, lithiasis. **CC:** Extravasation c̄ IV administration can result in severe tissue necrosis.

SIDE/ADVERSE EFFECTS: CNS: tingling sensations c̄ parenteral administration, depression of nerve functions ▪ CV: ***cardiac arrhythmias*** ▪ GI: anorexia, abdominal pain, N/V, constipation c̄ PO administration ▪ Other: hypercalcemia, azotemia, renal calculi, depression of muscle function.

INTERACTIONS: Drug: Use c̄ dig can produce cardiac arrhythmias ▪ Use c̄ tetracycline is contraindicated.

NURSING MANAGEMENT PRIORITIES

ADMINISTRATION: PO forms: take 2h ac/3h pc (antacid), 1h pc (electrolyte replacement), c̄ meals (antihyperphosphatemic); do *not* administer w/in 1-2h of other PO medication; do *not* administer c̄ milk ▪ PO suspension: shake well before pouring; high-Na^+ content ▪ Assess for Chvostek, Trousseau signs (hypocalcemia) ▪ IV: warm to body temperature; administer *slowly* (1ml/m) into large vein; use infusion control device, cardiac monitoring; maintain supine position for 1h after administration ▪ Do *not* administer calcium chloride IM/SC, calcium gluconate IM ▪ ⬇ Sensory stimulation if hypocalcemic ▪ Consult dietitian for dietary restrictions.

EVALUATION: Monitor VS, esp BP ▪ Monitor bowel function (constipation) ▪ Observe for signs of hypercalcemia (⬇ muscle tone, confusion, fatigue); D/C drug, notify physician ▪ Check IV insertion site carefully; avoid extravasation ▪ Monitor activity (safety precautions); pad bedrails if hypocalcemic ▪ Monitor serum calcium level (normal: 8.5-10.5mg/dl) ▪ Monitor serum phosphate level (normal: 3-4.5mg/dl).

EDUCATION: Chew tablets thoroughly before swallowing ▪ Do *not* take c̄ milk ▪ PO suspension: shake well before pouring ▪ Follow dietitian's suggestions of foods to avoid ▪ Notify physician *immediately* of nausea, muscle weakness, confusion; D/C drug ▪ Keep scheduled appointments c̄ physician/for blood work ▪ Constipation may occur; ⬆ fluids, use prescribed stool softener.

NOTES:

candesartan cilexetil/irbesartan • (can-deh-sar-tan/ear-beh-sar-tan)

CATEGORY: *Antihypertensive:* angiotensin II antagonist — Rx; Preg Cat C/D+

BRAND NAMES	DOSAGE FORMS
candesartan	
Atacand (Astra)	Tablet: 4, 8, 16, 32mg
irbesartan	
Avapro (B-MS)	Tablet: 75, 150, 300mg

USE: Treatment of hypertension as sole agent/in combination c̄ other antihypertensives. **ACTION:** Antihypertensive effect due to suppression of angiotensin II, a potent vasoactive hormone in renin-angiotensin-aldosterone system, by selectively blocking effects of angiotensin II on angiotensin II receptors (AT_1), resulting in ⬇ peripheral arterial resistance, ⬇ aldosterone secretion. Drug does not block conversion of angiotensin I by ACE into angiotensin II, has little affinity for angiotensin II (AT_2) receptors. Maximum antihypertensive effects occur in 3-6wks.

CONTRAINDICATIONS: Hypersensitivity. **CC:** African-Americans exhibit a slight ⬇ in clinical efficacy ▪ D/C during pregnancy as soon as possible ▪ Correct volume-depletion conditions before use or initiate c̄ ⬇ dosage ▪ Safety & efficacy in pts <18y/o not established

DOSAGE: Adult *PO*

candesartan	Initial dose of 16mg once/d c̄ a usual range of 8-32mg/d
irbesartan	Initial dose of 150mg once/d. Maximum daily dose is 300mg

SIDE/ADVERSE EFFECTS: CNS: dizziness, headache ▪ GI: N/V/D, abdominal pain, dyspepsia ▪ RESP: URI, cough ▪ Other: fatigue, back pain.

PHARMACOKINETICS

	PO absorption	Peak	Half-life	Protein binding	Excretion
candesartan	Low	3-4h	9h	99%	Via urine, feces
irbesartan	High	1.5-2h	11-15h	90%	Via urine, feces

Note: Side/adverse effects: common in *italic;* serious in ***boldface italic.***

*Available in Canada only.
+1st trimester, C, 2nd & 3rd trimesters, D.

INTERACTIONS: Drug: No significant rxs reported. **Lab:** Very low incidence of hyperuricemia c̄ candesartan. **Food:** Meals slow down PO absorption.

NURSING MANAGEMENT PRIORITIES

ADMINISTRATION: Assess for hx hypersensitivity ■ Assess BP; notify physician of extremes ■ Assess renal function; may require ↓ dosage if impaired & volume depleted ■ Diuretics may be D/C for 2-3d before beginning drug to avoid hypotension ■ Administer consistently c̄ or w/out food ■ Assess serum Na^+ (normal: 135-145mEq/L) ■ Assess for rapid ↓ in BP w/in 3h after administration of first dose (c̄ hyponatremia) ■ Avoid abrupt withdrawal; D/C gradually.

EVALUATION: Monitor VS, esp BP ■ Monitor CBC (esp WBC, differential) throughout therapy ■ Monitor electrolyte status (↑ K^+, ↓ Na^+) ■ Monitor I&O, daily weight ■ Monitor renal function (proteinuria); notify physician ■ Assess for edema in extremities.

EDUCATION: Dizziness may occur; use caution in potentially hazardous activities ■ Avoid changing positions (lying/sitting/standing) rapidly ■ Notify physician of fever, sore throat, bruising/bleeding, swelling of feet/legs ■ Take as ordered by physician even if symptom free; do *not* skip doses ■ Take consistently c̄ or w/out food ■ Do not D/C w/out notifying physician ■ Check c̄ physician/pharmacist before taking OTC/Rx preparations ■ Avoid high-Na^+ foods (canned soups, lunch meats, cheese) ■ Avoid high-K^+ foods (bananas, citrus juices, raisins) ■ Check c̄ physician/pharmacist before using salt substitutes ■ Avoid ↑ exercise, temperature extremes, smoking ■ Used to control, *not* cure, hypertension ■ Maintain optimum weight ■ Keep scheduled appointments c̄ physician; have BP checked regularly ■ Women: notify physician of pregnancy possibility; avoid breastfeeding ■ Full drug effects may require several wks of therapy.

NOTES:

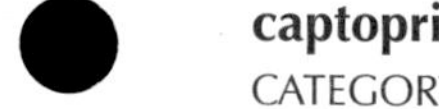

captopril • (kap-toe-pril)

CATEGORY: *Antihypertensive:* angiotensin inhibitor

Rx; Preg Cat C/D†

BRAND NAME
Capoten (B-MS)

DOSAGE FORMS
Tablet: 12.5, 25, 50, 100mg

COMBINATION PRODUCTS Rx

Capozide (B-MS) captopril/HCT per tablet: 25mg/15mg, 25mg/25mg, 50mg/15mg, 50mg/25mg. Dosage must be individualized starting c̄ 25mg/15mg tablet

USE: Treatment of hypertension as sole agent or c̄ other antihypertensives ▪ Treatment of heart failure usually in combination c̄ a diuretic & dig ▪ Treatment of diabetic neuropathy (proteinuria >500mg/d) c̄ type I insulin diabetes ▪ Treatment of left ventricular dysfunction after MI.

ACTION: Antihypertensive activity appears related to suppression of renin-angiotensin-aldosterone system by competitive inhibition of ACE, which produces angiotensin II from angiotensin I, resulting in ⬇ of peripheral arterial resistance, ⬇ in aldosterone secretion.

PHARMACOKINETICS

PO absorption no food	Peak	Half-life	Protein binding	Excretion
75%	1h	2h	25%-30%	95% via urine in 24h as metabolites (60%), unchanged drug (40%)

CONTRAINDICATIONS: Hypersensitivity. D/C during pregnancy as soon as possible. **CC:** Risk of anaphylactoid rxs, angioedema, agranulocytosis, neutropenia c̄ use.

DOSAGE: Adult *PO*

Hypertension	Start c̄ 25mg bid or tid. ⬆ Slowly to 50 or 100mg bid or tid. Usual dose range 25-150mg bid or tid. Do *not* exceed 450mg/d
Heart failure	Initial dose of 25mg tid 1h ac. Usual range 50-100mg tid. Do *not* exceed 450mg/d

Note: Side/adverse effects: common in *italic;* serious in ***boldface italic.***

*Available in Canada only.
†1st trimester, C; 2nd & 3rd trimesters, D.

Diabetic neuropathy	25mg tid ac, adjust
Left ventricular dysfunction	50mg tid ac is optimal dose

SIDE/ADVERSE EFFECTS: CV: hypotension, tachycardia, chest pain, palpitations, ***MI*** (rare), CHF, Raynaud syndrome ■ GU: proteinuria ■ HEM: ***agranulocytosis, neutropenia,*** anemia, ***thrombocytopenia*** ■ INT: rash, pruritus, angioedema ■ Other: reversible loss of taste.

INTERACTIONS: Drug: Aspirin, indomethacin, other NSAIAs may antagonize therapeutic response ■ Use potassium-sparing diuretics c̄ caution due to hyperkalemia. **Lab:** ↑ In liver transaminases, alkaline phosphatase, serum bilirubin.

NURSING MANAGEMENT PRIORITIES

ADMINISTRATION: Assess for hx of hypersensitivity ■ Assess BP; notify physician of extremes ■ Assess renal function; may require ↓ dosage if impaired ■ May crush, administer c̄ liquid; *best* on empty stomach (1h ac) ■ Assess serum Na^+ (normal: 135-145mEq/L); notify physician of abnormalities ■ Assess for rapid ↓ in BP w/in 3h after administration of 1st dose (occurs c̄ hyponatremia) ■ SLE, elderly may require ↓ dosage ■ Avoid abrupt withdrawal; D/C gradually.

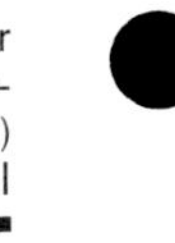

EVALUATION: Monitor VS, esp BP ■ Monitor CBC (esp WBC, differential) throughout therapy ■ Monitor electrolyte status (↑ K^+; ↓ Na^+) ■ Monitor I&O, daily weight ■ Monitor renal function (proteinuria); notify physician ■ Assess for loss of taste ■ Assess for edema in extremities.

EDUCATION: Dizziness may occur; use caution when engaging in potentially hazardous activities ■ Avoid changing positions (lying/sitting/standing) rapidly ■ Notify physician of fever, sore throat, bruising/bleeding, swelling of feet/legs ■ Take as ordered by physician even if symptom free; do *not* skip doses ■ Take 1h ac ■ Do *not* D/C w/out notifying physician ■ Check c̄ physician/pharmacist before taking OTC/Rx preparations ■ Avoid high-Na^+ foods (canned soups, lunch meats, cheese) ■ Avoid high-K^+ foods (bananas, citrus juices, raisins) ■ Check c̄ physician before using salt substitutes ■ Avoid ↑ exercise, temperature extremes, smoking ■ Loss of taste may occur ■ Tablets may smell like sulfur ■ Used to control, *not* cure, hypertension ■ Maintain optimum weight ■ Keep scheduled appointments c̄ physician; have BP checked regularly ■ Women: avoid breastfeeding ■ Full drug effects may require several wks of therapy.

NOTES:

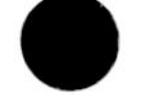

carbamazepine • (kar-ba-maz-e-peen)

CATEGORY: *Anticonvulsant:* analgesic

Rx; Preg Cat D

BRAND NAMES

Tegretol (Novartis)

Tegretol-XR (Novartis)

**Mazepine (ICN)*

DOSAGE FORMS

Tablet: 100, 200mg
Suspension: 200mg/5ml
Extended-release tablets: 100, 200, 400mg

USE: Treatment of partial seizures c̄ complex symptoms, grand mal, mixed seizure patterns in pts who have not responded to treatment c̄ other agents ▪ Pain associated c̄ trigeminal, glossopharyngeal neuralgia. **ACTION:** Anticonvulsant activity not determined; analgesic activity in trigeminal neuralgia due to ⬇ of synaptic activity in trigeminal nucleus.

CONTRAINDICATIONS: Hypersensitivity to drug, TCAs, previous bone marrow depression. **CC:** Possible agranulocytosis, aplastic anemia. Not indicated for minor pain ▪ Use c̄ caution in pts c̄ glaucoma, hx of adverse hematologic rxs, dormant/latent psychosis.

DOSAGE

Epilepsy

Children/ Adult *PO*	>12y/o: 200mg bid on d1. ⬆ Weekly by adding up to 200mg/d. Usual maintenance dose 800-1200mg/d. Do *not* exceed 1200mg/d in children, 1600mg in adults. 6-12y/o: 100mg bid on d1. ⬆ Weekly by adding up to 100mg/d. Usual maintenance dose 400-800mg/d. Do *not* exceed 1000mg/d
Neuralgia Adult *PO*	100mg bid on d1. ⬆ Slowly by adding up to 200mg/d. Do *not* exceed 1200mg/d

PHARMACOKINETICS

PO absorption	Peak	Half-life	Protein binding	Excretion
Adequate	4-5h	25-65h 5-20h in multiple doses	76%	Via urine (72%), feces (28%) as metabolites

Note: Side/adverse effects: common in *italic;* serious in ***boldface italic.***

*Available in Canada only.

SIDE/ADVERSE EFFECTS: CNS: *dizziness, drowsiness,* headache, abnormal involuntary movements, peripheral neuritis, paresthesias ▪ CV: edema, arrhythmias, hypotension, CHF, A-V block, thrombophlebitis ▪ EENT: blurred vision, transient diplopia, nystagmus, tinnitus, lens opacities ▪ GI: N/V/D, gastric distress, abdominal pain, anorexia, constipation, dry mouth ▪ GU: acute urinary retention, oliguria, azotemia, impotence ▪ HEM: ***aplastic anemia, agranulocytosis, thrombocytopenia,*** eosinophilia ▪ HEP: cholestatic/***hepatocellular jaundice***, hepatitis ▪ INT: pruritic/erythematous rashes, urticaria, ***Stevens-Johnson syndrome***, photosensitivity, ***exfoliative dermatitis,*** LE, alopecia, ***erythema multiforme***/nodosum, purpura ▪ MS: leg cramps, aching muscle/joints ▪ RESP: dyspnea, pneumonitis, pneumonia.

INTERACTIONS: Drug: Use c̄ doxycycline, phenytoin, warfarin, theophylline significantly ↓ their half-lives ▪ Avoid use c̄ MAO-I ▪ Use c̄ other bone marrow depressants can produce significant bone marrow toxicity.

NURSING MANAGEMENT PRIORITIES

ADMINISTRATION: Assess for hx of hypersensitivity (incl TCAs) ▪ Assess hepatic, hematologic status ▪ Administer c̄ meals ▪ PO suspension: shake well before using ▪ Avoid abrupt withdrawal ▪ Institute strict seizure precautions if drug is abruptly withdrawn ▪ Elderly may require ↓ dosage.

EVALUATION: Monitor occurrence/characteristics of seizures ▪ Monitor hepatic, hematologic status ▪ Monitor for ↑ IOP ▪ Monitor elderly for CNS, cardiac effects ▪ Monitor PT if taking PO anticoagulants; may ↓ effects ▪ May ↑ urine glucose, albumin; ↓ thyroid function tests ▪ Assess for skin rash; notify physician, D/C drug ▪ Monitor activity status (safety precautions) ▪ Assess for symptoms of abrupt withdrawal (tremors, abdominal/muscle cramps, convulsions) ▪ Therapeutic blood level: 4-12μg/ml.

EDUCATION: Do *not* omit daily dose ▪ Do *not* use for general pain relief ▪ Take c̄ meals ▪ Keep scheduled appointments for periodic eye exams ▪ Women: avoid breastfeeding ▪ Diabetics: may ↑ urine sugar; monitor blood sugar ▪ Dizziness/drowsiness may occur; use caution in potentially hazardous activities ▪ Avoid use c̄ alcohol, other CNS depressants ▪ Avoid changing positions (lying/sitting/standing) rapidly ▪ Use sugarless gum/hard candy to diminish dry mouth ▪ Avoid exposure to direct sunlight, UV light ▪ Notify physician of fever, sore throat, bruising/bleeding ▪ Safety precautions may be instituted (bedrails) ▪ Do *not* smoke after taking drug ▪ Carry medical identification (MedicAlert) ▪ Notify physician/dentist of use before treatment.

NOTES:

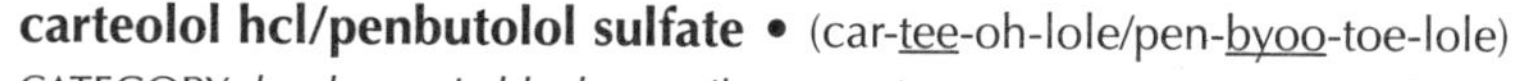

carteolol hcl/penbutolol sulfate • (car-tee-oh-lole/pen-byoo-toe-lole)

CATEGORY: *b-adrenergic blocker:* antihypertensive   Rx; Preg Cat C

BRAND NAMES	**DOSAGE FORMS**
carteolol	
Cartrol (Abbott)	Tablet: 2.5, 5mg
penbutolol	
Levatol (Schwarz)	Tablet: 20mg

USE: Treatment of hypertension as a sole agent or c̄ other antihypertensive agents (esp thiazide diuretics). **ACTION:** Blocks access of catecholamine neurotransmitters to β_1, β_2 receptors, resulting in bronchial constriction, ↓ heart rate, myocardial contractility ▪ Antihypertensive effect not determined.

PHARMACOKINETICS

PO absorption	Peak	Half-life	Protein binding	Excretion
carteolol				
Complete	1-3h	6h	23%-30%	50%-70% as unchanged drug via urine
penbutolol				
Complete	1.5-3h	5h	80%-98%	Via urine as unchanged drug and metabolites

CONTRAINDICATIONS: Hypersensitivity, asthma, cardiogenic shock, sinus bradycardia, greater than 1° heart block; CHF, severe bradycardia (carteolol). **CC:** Abrupt D/C can ↑ ischemic heart disease ▪ Possible cardiac failure c̄ ↓ myocardial contractility ▪ Tachycardia of hyperthyroidism may be masked, abrupt D/C may induce thyrotoxicosis ▪ Use c̄ caution c̄ bronchospastic disease, diabetes, peripheral vascular disease.

DOSAGE

Normal renal function

Adult *PO*

carteolol	Initial single dose of 2.5mg/d c̄ gradual ↑ to single dose of 5mg or 10mg/d. Usual maintenance range 2.5-5mg once/d
penbutolol	10-40mg once/d. Usual dose 20mg/d

SIDE/ADVERSE EFFECTS: CNS: somnolence, paresthesia, anxiety, dizziness, headache, abnormal dreams, bradycardia, cold extremities, chest pain, tiredness ▪ CV: angina, arrhythmia, palpitations, 2° heart block ▪ GI: N/V/D, constipation, dyspepsia, flatulence ▪ GU: impotence, urinary frequency, UTI ▪ HEM: agranulocytosis, thrombocytopenic purpura ▪ INT: pruritus, rash, sweating ▪ MS: *muscle* *cramps*, arthritis, gout ■ RESP: nasal congestion, pharyngitis, bronchospasm, respiratory distress ■ Other: *asthenia*, blurred vision, conjunctivitis, tinnitus.

INTERACTIONS: Drug: Use c̄ reserpine, other catecholamine-depleting drugs can result in serious adrenergic blockage ■ Nonselective β-adrenergics may antagonize therapeutic response ■ Use of general anesthetics, MAO-I best avoided ■ Use c̄ IV Ca blockers may prolong AV conduction time (carteolol) ■ Diabetics may require dosage adjustments of antidiabetic agent ■ NSAIAs may ↓ antihypertensive action of β blockers.

NURSING MANAGEMENT PRIORITIES

ADMINISTRATION: Assess for hx of hypersensitivity ■ Assess apical pulse; if <60/m hold drug, notify physician ■ Assess respiratory function; do *not* administer if impaired ■ Administer consistently c̄ or w/out food ■ Elderly may require ↓ dosage ■ Avoid abrupt withdrawal; D/C gradually.

EVALUATION: Monitor VS, esp BP (lying/standing), heart rate ■ Monitor I&O, daily weight ■ Assess peripheral circulation ■ Diabetics: closely monitor blood glucose (hypoglycemia) ■ Assess for edema in extremities ■ Monitor hepatic, CV, renal, hemopoietic status c̄ long-term use.

EDUCATION: Dizziness may occur; use caution in potentially hazardous activities ■ Avoid changing positions (lying/sitting/standing) rapidly ■ Procedure for checking radial pulse ■ Check pulse before taking; if <60/m do *not* take drug, notify physician ■ Take as ordered by physician, even if symptom free; do *not* change dose ■ Take consistently c̄ or w/out food ■ Used to control, *not* cure, hypertension ■ Avoid use c̄ alcohol ■ Avoid ↑ exercise, temperature extremes, smoking ■ Notify physician of muscle cramps, difficult breathing, cold extremities, leg edema ■ Keep scheduled appointments c̄ physician; have BP checked regularly ■ Maintain optimum weight ■ Avoid high-Na^+ foods (canned soups, lunch meats, cheese) ■ Check c̄ physician/pharmacist before taking OTC preparations ■ Notify physician/dentist of use before treatment ■ Do *not* D/C w/out checking c̄ physician ■ Carry medical identification (MedicAlert) if hypertensive ■ Do *not* abstain from food >12h (low blood sugar).

NOTES:

cefaclor • (sef-a-klor)

CATEGORY: *Cephalosporin* (2nd generation): antibiotic — Rx; Preg Cat B

BRAND NAME
Ceclor (Lilly)

DOSAGE FORMS
PO suspension: 125, 187, 250, 375mg/ml
Capsule: 250, 500mg
CD tablets: 375, 500mg

DOSAGE

Pediatric	*PO*	20mg/kg/d in divided doses q8h. For severe infections, 40mg/kg/d in divided doses q8h (otitis media)
Adult	*PO*	250mg q8h, range 1-4g/d

USE: Treatment of infections caused by susceptible strains of *Escherichia coli,* group A β-hemolytic streptococci, *Haemophilus influenzae, Klebsiella* spp, staphylococci. **ACTION:** Bactericidal activity due to inhibition of mucopeptide cell wall synthesis in susceptible organisms.

PHARMACOKINETICS

PO absorption	Peak	Half-life	Excretion
Good	30-60m	0.6-0.9h	Via urine as unchanged drug

CONTRAINDICATIONS: Hypersensitivity to any cephalosporin. **CC:** Use can produce pseudomembranous colitis ▪ Use in penicillin-allergic pts requires caution.

SIDE/ADVERSE EFFECTS: GI: N/V, *diarrhea,* symptoms of ***pseudomembranous colitis*** ▪ GU: vaginitis ▪ HEM: eosinophilia ▪ HEP: transitory ↑ in AST, ALT, BUN ▪ INT: pruritus, urticaria, morbilliform eruptions, ***erythema multiforme.***

INTERACTIONS: Drug: Bacteriostatic antibiotics can antagonize bactericidal activity ▪ Use c̄ PO anticoagulants may ↑ their activity ▪ Use c̄ aminoglycosides may produce additive nephrotoxicity ▪ Use c̄ probenecid will ↓ renal excretion. **Lab:** Possible false + c̄ Coombs' test.

NURSING MANAGEMENT PRIORITIES
ADMINISTRATION: Assess for hx of cephalosporin/penicillin hypersensitivity ▪ Obtain C&S before therapy ▪ Assess renal function; ↓ dosage if impaired ▪ Administer

1h ac/2h pc ▪ PO suspension: reconstitute powder according to manufacturer's directions; shake well before using; store reconstituted portion in refrigerator for 14d ▪ Avoid exposure to moisture/light during storage.

EVALUATION: Monitor VS, esp temperature ▪ Monitor hepatic, renal status ▪ Monitor CBC ▪ Urine glucose: false + c̄ Clinitest; use Clinistix/Diastix.

EDUCATION: Complete full course of therapy (usually 10d) even if symptoms subside ▪ Can be taken c̄ meals, but *best* on empty stomach ▪ Take at equal intervals around clock to maintain blood levels ▪ Diarrhea may occur ▪ PO suspension: refrigerate; shake well before use ▪ Store in dry, tightly closed container ▪ Discard outdated preparations ▪ Maintain good personal hygiene (esp perineal, oral) ▪ ↑ Fluid intake (8-10 glasses/d) ▪ Use Clinistix/Diastix for urine testing ▪ Notify physician of symptoms of allergic rx (fever, difficult breathing, rash) ▪ Carry identification (MedicAlert) if cephalosporin allergic.

NOTES:

cefadroxil • (sef-a-drox-ill)

CATEGORY: *Cephalosporin* (1st generation): antibiotic   Rx; Preg Cat B

BRAND NAME
Duricef (B-MS)
(Bristol [Canada])

DOSAGE FORMS
Capsule: 500mg
PO suspension: 125, 250, 500mg/5ml
Tablet: 1g

USE: Treatment of infections caused by susceptible strains of *Escherichia coli*, group A β-hemolytic streptococci, *Klebsiella* spp, *Proteus mirabilis*, staphylococci. **ACTION:** Bactericidal activity due to inhibition of mucopeptide cell wall synthesis in susceptible organisms.

PHARMACOKINETICS

PO absorption	Peak	Half-life	Excretion
Complete	1.5h	1-2h	90% via urine in 24h as unchanged drug

CONTRAINDICATIONS: Hypersensitivity to any cephalosporin. **CC:** Use can produce pseudomembranous colitis ▪ Use in penicillin-allergic pts requires caution.

DOSAGE

Pediatric	*PO*	30mg/kg/d in divided doses q12h
Adult	*PO*	1-2g/d as single dose or divided bid

SIDE/ADVERSE EFFECTS: GI: N/V, *diarrhea*, symptoms of ***pseudomembranous colitis*** ▪ GU: vaginitis ▪ HEM: eosinophilia ▪ HEP: transitory ↑ in AST, ALT, BUN ▪ INT: pruritus, urticaria, morbilliform eruptions, ***erythema multiforme***.

INTERACTIONS: Drug: Bacteriostatic antibiotics can antagonize bactericidal activity ▪ Use c̄ PO anticoagulants may ↑ their activity ▪ Use c̄ aminoglycosides may produce additive nephrotoxicity ▪ Use c̄ probenecid will ↓ renal excretion. **Lab:** Possible false + c̄ Coombs' test.

NURSING MANAGEMENT PRIORITIES
ADMINISTRATION: Assess for hx of cephalosporin/penicillin hypersensitivity ▪ Obtain C&S before therapy ▪ Assess renal function; ↓ dosage if impaired ▪ Administer 1h ac/2h pc ▪ PO suspension: reconstitute powder according to manufacturer's directions; shake well before

using; store reconstituted portion in refrigerator for 14d ▪ Avoid exposure to moisture/light during storage.

EVALUATION: Monitor VS, esp temperature ▪ Monitor hepatic, renal status ▪ Monitor CBC ▪ Urine glucose: false + c̄ Clinitest; use Clinistix/Diastix.

EDUCATION: Complete full course of therapy (usually 10d) even if symptoms subside ▪ Can be taken c̄ meals, but *best* on empty stomach ▪ Take at equal intervals around clock to maintain blood levels ▪ Diarrhea may occur ▪ PO suspension: refrigerate; shake well before use ▪ Store in dry, tightly closed container ▪ Discard outdated preparations ▪ Maintain good personal hygiene (esp perineal, oral) ▪ ↑ Fluid intake (8-10 glasses/d) ▪ Use Clinistix/Diastix for urine testing ▪ Notify physician of symptoms of allergic rx (fever, difficult breathing, rash) ▪ Carry identification (MedicAlert) if cephalosporin allergic.

NOTES:

cefazolin sodium • (sef-a-zoe-lin)

CATEGORY: *Cephalosporin* (1st generation): antibiotic — Rx; Preg Cat B

BRAND NAMES	DOSAGE FORMS
Ancef (SKB)	Powder for injection (IM/IV): 0.25-, 0.5-, 1-, 5-, 10-g vials
Kefzol (Lilly)	Powder for injection (IM/IV): 0.25-, 0.5-, 1-, 10-, 20-g vials
Zolicef (Squibb)	Powder for injection (IM/IV): 0.5-, 1-g vials

USE: Treatment of infections caused by susceptible strains of *Enterobacter aerogenes, Escherichia coli,* group A β-hemolytic streptococci, *Haemophilus influenzae, Klebsiella* spp, *Proteus mirabilis,* staphylococci (incl penicillinase-producing strains), *Streptococcus pneumoniae.*
ACTION: Bactericidal activity due to inhibition of mucopeptide cell wall synthesis in susceptible organisms.

PHARMACOKINETICS

IM peak	Half-life	Excretion
0.5-1h	1-2.2h	100% via urine in 24h as unchanged drug

CONTRAINDICATIONS: Hypersensitivity to any cephalosporin. **CC:** Use can produce pseudomembranous colitis ▪ Use in penicillin-allergic pts requires caution.

DOSAGE

Pediatric	*IM/IV*	25-50mg/kg/d in 3-4 doses. Severe infections, 100mg/kg/d
Adult	*IM/IV*	Usual range 250mg-1g q8-12h. Severe infections, dosage given q6-8h. Life-threatening infections, 1-1.5g q6h

SIDE/ADVERSE EFFECTS: GI: Symptoms of ***pseudomembranous colitis,*** *N/V* ▪ HEM: neutropenia, ***thrombocytopenia, hemolytic anemia*** ▪ INT: maculopapular rash, urticaria ▪ MS: pain, induration c̄ repeated IM injection ▪ Other: ***thrombophlebitis at IV site.***

INTERACTIONS: Drug: Bacteriostatic antibiotics can antagonize bactericidal activity ▪ Use c̄ PO anticoagulants may ↑ their activity ▪ Use c̄ aminoglycosides may produce additive nephrotoxicity ▪ Use c̄ probenecid will ↓ renal excretion. **Lab:** Possible false + c̄ Coombs' test.

NURSING MANAGEMENT PRIORITIES

ADMINISTRATION: Assess for hx of cephalosporin/penicillin hypersensitivity ▪ Obtain C&S before therapy ▪ Assess renal function; ↓ dosage if impaired ▪ IM: reconstitute according to manufacturer's directions; administer by *deep, slow* injection into gluteal UOQ ▪ IV: dilute according to manufacturer's directions; inject *slowly* (3-5m); avoid aminoglycoside administration in same site ▪ Do *not* administer discolored/precipitated solution; yellow-amber color does *not* indicate ↓ potency ▪ Thaw frozen preparations completely at room temperature; do *not* refreeze; stable 24h at room temperature, 10d refrigerated; do *not* use if cloudy/precipitated ▪ Use reconstituted preparations w/in 24h at room temperature, 96h refrigerated ▪ Have support equipment available for anaphylaxis ▪ Surgical prophylaxis: D/C w/in 24h after surgery ▪ Na^+ content: 2.2mEq (48mg)/g; calculate in Na^+-restricted diets ▪ Maintain hydration.

EVALUATION: Monitor VS, esp temperature ▪ Monitor renal, hepatic, hemopoietic status ▪ Observe for signs of superinfection (diarrhea, itching, oral ulcers).

EDUCATION: Use Clinistix/Diastix for urine testing ▪ Women: avoid breastfeeding ▪ Diarrhea may occur ▪ Maintain good personal hygiene (esp perineal, oral) ▪ ↑ Fluid intake (8-10 glasses/d) ▪ Notify nurse/physician of symptoms of allergic rx (difficult breathing, rash) ▪ Carry identification (MedicAlert) if cephalosporin allergic ▪ IM injection may be painful.

NOTES:

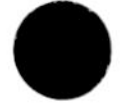

cefdinir • (sef-deh-near)

CATEGORY: *Cephalosporin* (3rd generation): antibiotic — Rx; Preg Cat B

BRAND NAME
Omnicef (P-D)

DOSAGE FORMS
Capsule: 300mg
PO suspension: 125mg/5ml

USE: Treatment of acute exacerbation of chronic bronchitis, community-acquired pneumonia, acute otitis media, sinusitis, pharyngitis, skin & skin structure, tonsillitis caused by susceptible strains of *Haemophilus influenzae, H. parainfluenzae, Moraxella catarrhalis, Staphylococcus aureus, Streptococcus pneumoniae.* **ACTION:** Bactericidal activity due to inhibition of mucopeptide cell wall synthesis in susceptible organisms.

PHARMACOKINETICS

PO absorption	Protein binding	Excretion
Good	60%-70%	Via urine primarily as unchanged drug

CONTRAINDICATIONS: Hypersensitivity to any cephalosporin. **CC:** Use can produce pseudomembranous colitis ▪ Use in penicillin-allergic pts requires caution due to possible cross-sensitivity.

DOSAGE: PO

Pediatric 6mo-12y/o	
Maxillary sinusitis, otitis media	7mg/kg q12h or 14mg/kg q24h for 10d
Pharyngitis, tonsillitis	7mg/kg q12h for 5-10d or 14mg/kg q24h for 10d
Skin/skin structure infection	7mg/kg q12h for 10d
Adult/Children ≥13y/o	
Bronchitis	300mg q12h for 10d
Maxillary sinusitis	300mg q12h or 600mg q24h for 10d
Pharyngitis, tonsillitis	300mg q12h for 5-10d or 600mg q12h for 10d
Skin/skin structure infection	300mg q12h for 10d

SIDE/ADVERSE EFFECTS: CNS: headache, dizziness ▪ GI: N/V/D, symptoms of ***pseudomembranous colitis,*** anorexia, thrush ▪ GU: vaginitis, candidiasis ▪ HEM: transitory ↑ in AST, eosinophilia, leukopenia, ***thrombocytopenia, hemolytic anemia*** ▪ INT: rash, urticaria, pruritus ▪ Other: asthenia, chills, fever, malaise.

INTERACTIONS: Drug: Bacteriostatic antibiotics can antagonize bactericidal activity ■ Use c̄ PO anticoagulants may ↑ their activity ■ Use c̄ aminoglycosides may produce additive nephrotoxicity ■ Use c̄ probenecid will ↓ renal excretion ■ Use c̄ iron foods/supplements will ↓ PO absorption. **Lab:** Possible false + c̄ nitroprusside test for ketones.

NURSING MANAGEMENT PRIORITIES

ADMINISTRATION: Assess for hx of cephalosporin/penicillin hypersensitivity ■ Obtain C&S before therapy ■ Assess renal function; ↓ dosage if impaired ■ Administer 1h ac/2h pc; may administer c̄ food to ↓ GI irritation ■ PO suspension: reconstitute powder according to manufacturer's directions; shake well before using; refrigerate reconstituted drug ■ Avoid exposure to moisture/light in storage ■ Maintain hydration.

EVALUATION: Monitor VS, esp temperature ■ Monitor hepatic, renal status ■ Monitor CBC ■ Urine glucose: false + c̄ Clinitest; use Clinistix/Diastix.

EDUCATION: Complete full course of therapy (usually 10d) even if symptoms subside ■ Can be taken c̄ meals; *best* on empty stomach ■ Take at equal intervals around clock to maintain blood levels ■ Diarrhea may occur ■ PO suspension: refrigerate; shake well before use; stable 10d after reconstitution ■ Store in dry, tightly closed, light-resistant container ■ Discard outdated preparations ■ Maintain good personal hygiene (esp perineal, oral) ■ ↑ Fluid intake (8-10 glasses/d) ■ Use Clinistix/Diastix for urine testing ■ Notify physician of symptoms of allergic rx (fever, difficult breathing rash) ■ Carry identification (MedicAlert) if cephalosporin allergic ■ Women: avoid breastfeeding.

NOTES:

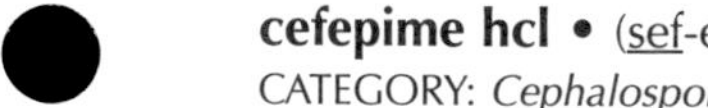

cefepime hcl • (sef-eh-peem)

CATEGORY: *Cephalosporin* (3rd generation): antibiotic Rx; Preg Cat B

BRAND NAME
Maxipime (B-MS)

DOSAGE FORMS
Powder for injection (IM/IV): 500-mg, 1-, 2-g vials

USE: Treatment of UTI including pyelonephritis caused by susceptible strains of *Escherichia coli, Klebsiella pneumoniae, Proteus mirabilis* ▪ Treatment of pneumonia caused by susceptible strains of *Enterobacter* spp, *K. pneumoniae, Pseudomonas aeruginosa, Streptococcus pneumoniae* ▪ Treatment of skin/skin structure infections caused by methicillin susceptible *Staphylococcus aureus; Streptococcus pyogenes* ▪ Empiric treatment of febrile neutropenic pts. **ACTION:** Bactericidal activity due to inhibition of mucopeptide cell wall synthesis in susceptible organisms; high resistance to most bacterial beta-lactamases.

PHARMACOKINETICS

Peak		Half-life	Protein binding	Excretion
IM	IV			
1-2	0.5h	2h	20%	Via urine primarily as unchanged drug (85%)

CONTRAINDICATIONS: Hypersensitivity to any cephalosporin. **CC:** Use may produce pseudomembranous colitis ▪ Use in penicillin-allergic pts requires caution ▪ Drug is excreted in very low concentration in breast milk ▪ Safety & efficacy in pts <12y/o not established ▪ Dosage in pts c̄ renal insufficiency requires a lower dose based on manufacturer's schedule ▪ Normal dosing schedule in pts c̄ renal insufficiency can result in encephalopathy.

DOSAGE

Adult	*IM*	0.5-1g q12h for 7-10d for mild to moderate UTI
	IV	1-2g q12h for 10d for moderate to severe infections & 2g q8h for empiric treatment for febrile neutropenic pts

SIDE/ADVERSE EFFECTS: GI: N/V/D, colitis, oral moniliasis, ***pseudomembranous colitis*** ▪ GU: moniliasis, vaginitis ▪ INT: rash, pruritus ▪ Other: headache, fever, ***phlebitis at IV site.***

INTERACTIONS: Drug: Bacteriostatic antibiotics can antagonize bactericidal effect ▪ Use c̄ PO anticoagulants

Note: Side/adverse effects: common in *italic;* serious in ***boldface italic.***

*Available in Canada only.

may ↑ their activity ▪ Use c̄ aminoglycosides may produce additive nephrotoxicity ▪ Use c̄ probenecid will ↓ renal excretion. **Lab:** False glucose + c̄ Clinitest tablets ▪ Possible false + c̄ Coombs' test ▪ ↑ In Serum ALT (SGPT), AST (SGOT).

NURSING MANAGEMENT PRIORITIES

ADMINISTRATION: Assess for hx or cephalosporin/penicillin hypersenstivity ▪ Obtain C&S before therapy ▪ Assess renal function; ↓ dosage if severely impaired ▪ IM: reconstitute according to manufacturer's directions; administer by *deep, slow* injection into gluteal UOQ ▪ IV: dilute according to manufacturer's directions; administer over 30m, avoid concurrent drug administration at same site ▪ Do *not* administer discolored/precipitated solutions; yellow-amber color does *not* indicate ↓ potency ▪ Use reconstituted preparations w/in 24h at room temperature, 7d refrigerated ▪ Have support equipment available for anaphylaxis ▪ Maintain hydration.

EVALUATION: Monitor VS, esp temperature ▪ Monitor renal, hepatic hemopoietic status ▪ Urine glucose: false + c̄ Clinitest; use Clinistix/Diastix ▪ Observe for signs of superinfection (diarrhea, itching, oral ulcers).

EDUCATION: Use Clinistix/Diastix for urine testing ▪ Women: avoid breastfeeding ▪ Diarrhea may occur ▪ Maintain good personal hygiene (esp perineal, oral) ▪ ↑ Fluid intake (8-10 glasses/d) ▪ Notify physician of symptoms of allergic rx (difficult breathing, rash) ▪ Carry identification (MedicAlert) if cephalosporin allergic ▪ IM injection may be painful.

NOTES:

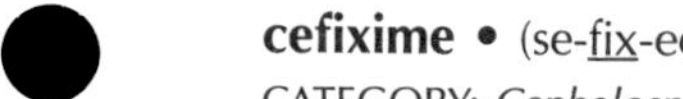

cefixime • (se-fix-eem)

CATEGORY: *Cephalosporin* (3rd generation): antibiotic   Rx; Preg Cat B

BRAND NAME
Suprax (Lederle)

DOSAGE FORMS
PO suspension: 100mg/5ml
Tablet: 200, 400mg

USE: Treatment of otitis media, respiratory infections, UTIs caused by susceptible strains of *Escherichia coli*, group A β-hemolytic streptococci, *Haemophilus influenzae, Moraxella catarrhalis, Proteus mirabilis* ▪ Treatment of otitis media requires use of PO suspension (peak is 25%-50% higher). **ACTION:** Bactericidal activity due to inhibition of mucopeptide cell wall synthesis in susceptible organisms.

PHARMACOKINETICS

PO absorption	Peak	Half-life	Protein binding	Excretion
40%-50%	2-6h	3-4h	65%	Via urine in 24h

CONTRAINDICATIONS: Hypersensitivity to any cephalosporin. **CC:** Use can produce pseudomembranous colitis ▪ Use in penicillin-allergic pts requires caution.

DOSAGE

Pediatric	*PO*	8mg/kg/d as a single dose or 4mg/kg q12h
Adult	*PO*	400mg/d as a single dose or 200mg q12h

SIDE/ADVERSE EFFECTS: CNS: headache, dizziness ▪ GI: *N/V/D,* symptoms of ***pseudomembranous colitis*** ▪ GU: vaginitis, candidiasis, ***toxic nephropathy*** ▪ HEM: transitory eosinophilia, leukopenia, thrombocytopenia, ***aplastic anemia*** ▪ HEP: transitory ↑ in AST, ALT, BUN ▪ INT: rash, urticaria, pruritus, ***erythema multiforme, Stevens-Johnson syndrome, toxic epidermal necrolysis*** ▪ Other: fever, + direct Coombs' test.

INTERACTIONS: Drug: Bacteriostatic antibiotics can antagonize bactericidal activity ▪ Use c̄ PO anticoagulants may ↑ their activity ▪ Use c̄ aminoglycosides may produce additive nephrotoxicity ▪ Use c̄ probenecid will ↓ renal excretion. **Lab:** Possible false + c̄ Coombs' test.

Note: Side/adverse effects: common in *italic;* serious in ***boldface italic.***

*Available in Canada only.

NURSING MANAGEMENT PRIORITIES

ADMINISTRATION: Assess for hx of cephalosporin/penicillin hypersensitivity ▪ Obtain C&S before therapy ▪ Assess renal function; ↓ dosage if impaired ▪ Administer 1h ac/2h pc; may administer c̄ food to ↓ GI irritation ▪ PO suspension: reconstitute powder according to manufacturer's directions; shake well before using; refrigerate reconstituted drug ▪ Avoid exposure to moisture/light in storage ▪ Maintain hydration.

EVALUATION: Monitor VS, esp temperature ▪ Monitor hepatic, renal status ▪ Monitor CBC ▪ Urine glucose: false + c̄ Clinitest; use Clinistix/Diastix.

EDUCATION: Complete full course of therapy (usually 10d) even if symptoms subside ▪ Can be taken c̄ meals; *best* on empty stomach ▪ Take at equal intervals around clock to maintain blood levels ▪ Diarrhea may occur ▪ PO suspension: refrigerate; shake well before use; stable 14d after reconstitution ▪ Store in dry, tightly closed, light-resistant container ▪ Discard outdated preparations ▪ Maintain good personal hygiene (esp perineal, oral) ▪ ↑ Fluid intake (8-10 glasses/d) ▪ Use Clinistix/Diastix for urine testing ▪ Notify physician of symptoms of allergic rx (fever, difficult breathing, rash) ▪ Carry identification (MedicAlert) if cephalosporin allergic ▪ Women: avoid breastfeeding.

NOTES:

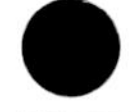

cefmetazole • (sef-met-a-zol)

CATEGORY: *Cephalosporin* (2nd generation): antibiotic Rx; Preg Cat B

BRAND NAME
Zefazone (Upjohn)

DOSAGE FORMS
IV powder for injection: 1, 2g vials
Frozen: 1, 2g/50ml injection

USE: Treatment of infections caused by susceptible strains of *Bacteroides* spp, *Clostridium perfringens, Escherichia coli, Haemophilus influenzae* (nonpenicillinase-producing), *Klebsiella* spp, *Morganella morganii, Proteus* spp, *Providencia stuartii,* staphylococci (incl penicillinase-producing), *Streptococcus* spp ▪ Preop prophylaxis to ⬇ incidence of abdominal/vaginal hysterectomy, cesarean section, cholecystectomy, colorectal surgery infections. **ACTION:** Bactericidal activity due to inhibition of mucopeptide cell wall synthesis in susceptible organisms.

CONTRAINDICATIONS: Hypersensitivity (cross-hypersensitivity can occur in up to 10% of pts c̄ penicillin allergies). **CC:** Use can produce pseudomembranous colitis ▪ Use in penicillin-allergic pts requires caution.

DOSAGE: Adult *IV* (Must be ⬇ in renal impairment)

Infection — Usual dose 2g q6-12h for 5-14d. Mild to moderate: 2g q8h (6g/d). Severe to life-threatening: 2g q6h (8g/d)
Urinary 2g q12h (4g/d)

Surgical prophylaxis
Hysterectomy
Abdominal — 1g 30-90m before surgery, repeated 8 & 16h later
Vaginal — 2g as single dose 30-90m before surgery or 1g 30-90m before surgery, repeated 8 & 16h later

PHARMACOKINETICS

Max	IV (2g q6h) trough	Plasma half-life	Protein binding	Excretion
138mg/ml	6mg/ml	1.2h	65%	85% via urine in 12h as unchanged drug

C-section	2g as single dose after clamping cord or 1g after clamping cord & repeated 8 & 16h later
Cholecystectomy (high risk)	1g 30-90m before surgery & repeated 8 & 16h later
Colorectal	2g as single dose 30-90m before surgery & repeated 8 & 16h later

SIDE/ADVERSE EFFECTS: CNS: headache, hot flashes ▪ CV: ***shock,*** hypotension ▪ EENT: color perception alteration ▪ GI: diarrhea (3.6%), nausea (1%), vomiting, pain, bleeding, candidiasis, ***pseudomembranous colitis*** (mild to life threatening) ▪ INT: rash (1.1%), pruritus, generalized erythema ▪ Local: pain, swelling at site of administration, phlebitis, ***thrombophlebitis*** ▪ RESP: pleural effusion, dyspnea, epistaxis ▪ Other: joint pain/inflammation, fever, vaginitis, superinfection.

INTERACTIONS: Drug: Alcohol can cause a disulfiram-like reaction ▪ Bacteriostatic antibiotics can antagonize bactericidal activity ▪ Use c̄ PO anticoagulants may ⬆ activity ▪ Use c̄ aminoglycosides may produce additive nephrotoxicity ▪ Use c̄ probenecid ⬇ renal excretion. **Lab:** Possible false + c̄ Coombs' test.

NURSING MANAGEMENT PRIORITIES

ADMINISTRATION: Assess for hx of cephalosporin/penicillin hypersensitivity ▪ Obtain C&S before therapy ▪ Assess renal function; ⬇ dosage if impaired ▪ Reconstitute & dilute according to manufacturer's directions; administer IVPB over 30-60m ▪ Do *not* administer discolored/precipitated solutions; yellow-amber color does *not* indicate ⬇ potency ▪ Use reconstituted IV preparations w/in 24h at room temperature, 7d refrigerated ▪ Have support equipment available for anaphylaxis ▪ Avoid exposure to light in storage ▪ Maintain hydration.

EVALUATION: Monitor VS, esp temperature ▪ Monitor renal, hepatic, hemopoietic status ▪ Urine glucose: false + c̄ Clinitest; use Clinistix/Diastix ▪ Observe for signs of superinfection (diarrhea, itching, oral ulcer) ▪ Check IV site closely (phlebitis) ▪ Monitor prothrombin levels; assess for bleeding.

EDUCATION: Use Clinistix/Diastix for urine testing ▪ Women: avoid breastfeeding ▪ Diarrhea may occur ▪ Avoid use c̄ alcohol ▪ Maintain good personal hygiene (esp perineal, oral) ▪ ⬆ Fluid intake (8-10 glasses/d) ▪ Notify nurse/physician of symptoms of allergic rx (difficult breathing, rash, fever, bleeding, diarrhea) ▪ Carry identification (MedicAlert) if cephalosporin allergic.

NOTES:

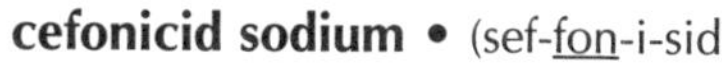

cefonicid sodium • (sef-fon-i-sid)

CATEGORY: *Cephalosporin* (2nd generation): antibiotic Rx; Preg Cat B

BRAND NAME
Monocid (SKB)

DOSAGE FORMS
Powder for injection (IM/IV): 1-, 10-g vials

USE: Treatment of infections caused by susceptible strains of *Escherichia coli,* group A β-hemolytic *Streptococcus, Haemophilus influenzae, Klebsiella pneumoniae, Proteus mirabilis, Staphylococcus aureus* (incl penicillinase-producing strains), *S. epidermidis, S. agalactiae, Streptococcus pneumoniae.* **ACTION:** Bactericidal activity due to inhibition of mucopeptide cell wall synthesis in susceptible organisms; exhibits good resistance to β-lactamases (penicillinase, cephalosporinase).

PHARMACOKINETICS

IM peak	Half-life	Protein binding	Excretion
1.3h	4.5h	>90%	99% via urine in 24h as unchanged drug

CONTRAINDICATIONS: Hypersensitivity to any cephalosporin. **CC:** Use may produce pseudomembranous colitis ▪ Use in penicillin-allergic pts requires caution.

DOSAGE
Adult *IM/IV* 1g q24h. For severe infections, 2g q24h

SIDE/ADVERSE EFFECTS: GI: diarrhea, symptoms of ***pseudomembranous colitis*** ▪ GU: moniliasis, vaginitis ▪ HEM: neutropenia, leukopenia ▪ HEP: ↑ AST, ALT, LDH, alkaline phosphatase ▪ Other: pain, induration at IM site; ***phlebitis at IV site***.

INTERACTIONS: Drug: Bacteriostatic antibiotics can antagonize bactericidal activity ▪ Use $\bar{c}$ PO anticoagulants may ↑ their activity ▪ Use $\bar{c}$ aminoglycosides may produce additive nephrotoxicity ▪ Use $\bar{c}$ probenecid will ↓ renal excretion. **Lab:** Possible false + $\bar{c}$ Coombs' test.

NURSING MANAGEMENT PRIORITIES
ADMINISTRATION: Assess for hx of cephalosporin/penicillin hypersensitivity ▪ Obtain C&S before therapy ▪ Assess renal function; ↓ dosage if impaired ▪ Reconstitute

c̄ sterile H_2O for injection: 2ml/500mg, 2.5ml/1g ▪ IM: administer by *deep, slow* injection into gluteal UOQ ▪ IV: inject *slowly* (3-5m); avoid aminoglycoside administration at same site; may administer IVPB ▪ Do *not* administer discolored/precipitated solutions; yellow-amber color does *not* indicate ⬇ potency ▪ Use reconstituted preparations w/in 24h at room temperature or 72h refrigerated ▪ Have supportive equipment available for anaphylaxis ▪ Surgical prophylaxis: D/C w/in 24h after surgery ▪ Na^+ content: 3.7mEq (85mg)/g; calculate in Na^+-restricted diets ▪ Avoid exposure to heat/light in storage ▪ Maintain hydration.

EVALUATION: Monitor VS, esp temperature ▪ Monitor renal, hepatic, hemopoietic status ▪ Observe for signs of superinfection (diarrhea, itching, oral ulcers) ▪ Urine glucose: false + c̄ Clinitest; use Clinistix/Diastix.

EDUCATION: Use Clinistix/Diastix for urine testing ▪ Women: avoid breastfeeding ▪ Diarrhea may occur ▪ Maintain good personal hygiene (esp perineal, oral) ▪ ⬆ Fluid intake (8-10 glasses/d) ▪ Notify nurse/physician of symptoms of allergic rx (difficult breathing, rash) ▪ Carry identification (MedicAlert) if cephalosporin allergic ▪ IM injection may be painful.

NOTES:

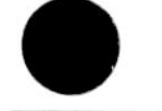

cefoperazone sodium • (sef-oh-per-a-zone)

CATEGORY: *Cephalosporin* (3rd generation): antibiotic Rx; Preg Cat B

BRAND NAME
Cefobid (Roerig)
(Pfizer [Canada])

DOSAGE FORMS
Powder for injection (IM/IV):
1-, 2-, 10-g vials
Frozen: 1, 2g/50-ml injection

USE: Treatment of infections caused by susceptible strains of *Bacteroides* (incl *B. fragilis), Clostridium* spp, *Enterobacter* spp, *Enterococcus* spp, *Escherichia coli,* group A β-hemolytic streptococci, *Haemophilus influenzae, Klebsiella pneumoniae, Neisseria gonorrhoeae, Proteus* spp (indole[+]/[−]), *Pseudomonas aeruginosa,* staphylococci (incl penicillinase-producing strains), *Streptococcus agalactiae, S. pneumoniae.* **ACTION:** Bactericidal activity due to inhibition of mucopeptide cell wall synthesis in susceptible organisms; good resistance to β-lactamases (penicillinase, cephalosporinase).

PHARMACOKINETICS

IM peak	Half-life	Protein binding	Excretion
1-2h	1.6-2.6h	82%-93%	Mainly via feces, 30% via urine

CONTRAINDICATIONS: Hypersensitivity to any cephalosporin. **CC:** Use can produce pseudomembranous colitis ▪ Use in penicillin-allergic pts requires caution.

DOSAGE
Adult *IM/IV* 2-4g/d in divided doses q12h. Severe infections, 6-12g/d in 2, 3, 4 doses

SIDE/ADVERSE EFFECTS: GI: N/V/D, symptoms of ***pseudomembranous colitis*** ▪ GU: moniliasis, vaginitis ▪ HEM: neutropenia, eosinophilia ▪ INT: rash, pruritus ▪ Other: pain at IM site, ***phlebitis at IV site***.

INTERACTIONS: Drug: Use c̄ alcohol may produce disulfiram rx ▪ Bacteriostatic antibiotics can antagonize bactericidal activity ▪ Use c̄ PO anticoagulants may ↑ their activity ▪ Use c̄ aminoglycosides may produce additive nephrotoxicity ▪ Use c̄ probenecid will ↓ renal excretion. **Lab:** Possible false + c̄ Coombs' test.

NURSING MANAGEMENT PRIORITIES
ADMINISTRATION: Assess for hx of cephalosporin/penicillin hypersensitivity ▪ Obtain C&S before therapy ▪ Assess for hx of bleeding disorder; avoid use ▪ Assess he-

Note: Side/adverse effects: common in *italic;* serious in ***boldface italic.***

*Available in Canada only.

patic function; ↓ dosage if impaired ▪ IM: reconstitute according to manufacturer's directions ▪ IV: dilute c̄ 2.8-5ml suitable diluent recommended by manufacturer; do *not* administer bolus ▪ Allow solution to stand after reconstitution; vigorous shaking may be required ▪ Do *not* administer discolored/precipitated solution; yellow-amber color does *not* indicate ↓ potency ▪ Use reconstituted preparations w/in 24h at room temperature, 5d refrigerated ▪ Na^+ content: 1.5mEq (34mg)/g; calculate in Na^+-restricted diets ▪ Maintain hydration.

EVALUATION: Monitor VS, esp temperature ▪ Monitor renal, hepatic, hemopoietic status ▪ Urine glucose: false + c̄ Clinitest; use Clinistix/Diastix ▪ False +: urine protein testing ▪ Monitor coagulation studies (PT); drug may potentiate bleeding ▪ Observe for signs of superinfection (diarrhea, itching, oral ulcers).

EDUCATION: Use Clinistix/Diastix for urine testing ▪ Women: avoid breastfeeding ▪ Diarrhea may occur ▪ Maintain good personal hygiene (esp perineal, oral) ▪ ↑ Fluid intake (8-10 glasses/d) ▪ Notify nurse/physician of symptoms of allergic rx (difficult breathing, rash) ▪ Carry identification (MedicAlert) if cephalosporin allergic ▪ IM injection may be painful ▪ Avoid alcohol intake ▪ Report any signs of bleeding immediately.

NOTES:

cefotaxime sodium • (sef-oh-taks-eem)

CATEGORY: *Cephalosporin* (3rd generation): antibiotic

Rx; Preg Cat B

BRAND NAME
Claforan (H-M-R)
(Roussel [Canada])

DOSAGE FORMS
Powder for injection (IM/IV): 1-, 2-, 10-g vials
Frozen: 1, 2g in 5% dextrose

USE: Treatment of infections caused by susceptible strains of *Bacteroides* (incl *B. fragilis*), *Citrobacter* spp, *Clostridium* spp, *Enterobacter* spp, *Enterococcus* spp, *Escherichia coli,* group A β-hemolytic streptococci, *Haemophilus influenzae, Klebsiella* spp, *Morganella morganii, Neisseria gonorrhoeae, Peptococcus* spp, *Peptostreptococcus* spp, *Proteus mirabilis, P. vulgaris, Providencia rettgeri, Serratia marcescens, Staphylococcus* (incl penicillinase-producing strains), *S. epidermidis, Streptococcus pneumoniae.* **ACTION:** Bactericidal activity due to inhibition of mucopeptide cell wall synthesis in susceptible organisms; drug exhibits good resistance to penicillinases, cephalosporinases.

PHARMACOKINETICS

IM peak	Half-life	Protein binding	Excretion
30m	1h	30%-50%	60% via urine in 6h as metabolites, unchanged drug

CONTRAINDICATIONS: Hypersensitivity to any cephalosporin. **CC:** Use may produce pseudomembranous colitis ▪ Use in penicillin-allergic pts requires caution.

DOSAGE

Pediatric	*IM/IV*	0-1wk: 50mg/kg IV q12h 1-4wks: 50mg/kg IV q8h 1mo-12y/o: 50-180mg/kg IM/IV in 4-6 equal doses. Do *not* exceed 12g/d
Adult	*IM/IV*	1-2g q12h. Moderate infections, 1-2g IV q8h, 2g IV q6-8h. Serious infections, 2g IV q4h

SIDE/ADVERSE EFFECTS: CNS: headache ▪ GI: colitis, N/V/D, ***symptoms of pseudomembranous colitis*** ▪ GU: moniliasis, vaginitis ▪ HEM: granulocytosis, eosinophilia, neutropenia ▪ HEP: ↑ AST, ALT, LDH, alkaline phosphatase ▪ INT: rash, pruritus ▪ Other: fever, local IV/IM site pain, induration, tenderness.

INTERACTIONS: Drug: Bacteriostatic antibiotics can antagonize bactericidal activity ▪ Use c̄ PO anticoagulants may ↑ their activity ▪ Use c̄ aminoglycosides may produce additive nephrotoxicity ▪ Use c̄ probenecid ↓ renal excretion. **Lab:** Possible false + c̄ Coombs' test.

NURSING MANAGEMENT PRIORITIES

ADMINISTRATION: Assess for hx of cephalosporin/penicillin hypersensitivity ▪ Obtain C&S before therapy ▪ Assess renal function; ↓ dosage if severely impaired ▪ IM: reconstitute according to manufacturer's directions; administer 2g in divided doses at different sites by *deep, slow* injection into gluteal UOQ ▪ IV: dilute according to manufacturer's directions, inject *slowly* (3-5m); avoid aminoglycoside administration at same site; may administer IVPB ▪ Do *not* administer discolored/precipitated solutions; yellow-amber color does *not* indicate ↓ potency ▪ Use reconstituted preparations w/in 24h at room temperature, 10d refrigerated, 13wks frozen ▪ Have support equipment available for anaphylaxis ▪ Surgical prophylaxis: D/C w/in 24h after surgery ▪ Na^+ content: 2.2mEq (51mg)/g; calculate in Na^+-restricted diets ▪ Maintain hydration.

EVALUATION: Monitor VS, esp temperature ▪ Monitor renal, hepatic, hemopoietic status ▪ Urine glucose: false + c̄ Clinitest; use Clinistix/Diastix ▪ Observe for signs of superinfection (diarrhea, itching, oral ulcers).

EDUCATION: Use Clinistix/Diastix for urine testing ▪ Women: avoid breastfeeding ▪ Diarrhea may occur ▪ Maintain good personal hygiene (esp perineal, oral) ▪ ↑ Fluid intake (8-10 glasses/d) ▪ Notify physician of symptoms of allergic rx (difficult breathing, rash) ▪ Carry identification (MedicAlert) if cephalosporin allergic ▪ IM injection may be painful.

NOTES:

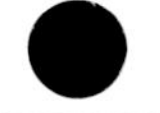

cefotetan disodium • (se-fo-tih-tan)

CATEGORY: *Cephalosporin* (3rd generation): antibiotic   Rx; Preg Cat B

BRAND NAME
Cefotan (Stuart)

DOSAGE FORMS
Powder for injection (IM/IV): 1-, 2-, 10-g vials
Frozen: 1, 2g/50-ml injection

USE: Treatment of infections caused by susceptible strains of *Bacteroides* spp, *Escherichia coli, Fusobacterium* spp, *Haemophilus influenzae, Klebsiella* spp, *Morganella morganii, Neisseria gonorrhoeae, Peptococcus* spp, *Peptostreptococcus* spp, *Proteus mirabilis, P. vulgaris, Staphylococcus aureus* (incl penicillinase producing), *S. epidermidis, Streptococcus pneumoniae, S. pyogenes* ▪ Surgical infection prophylaxis. **ACTION:** Bactericidal activity due to inhibition of mucopeptide cell wall synthesis in susceptible organisms.

PHARMACOKINETICS

Peak IM	Peak IV	Half-life	Protein binding	Excretion
1-3h	5-30m	3-4.6h	88%	51%-81% via urine, unchanged in 24h

CONTRAINDICATIONS: Hypersensitivity to any cephalosporin. **CC:** Use may produce pseudomembranous colitis ▪ Use in penicillin-allergic pts requires caution.

DOSAGE

Adult *IM/IV* 500mg-1g q12h. Severe infections may require 2g q12h IV. For life-threatening infection 3g q12h IV. Do *not* exceed 6g/d. Dosage must be ⬇ c̄ renal impairment

SIDE/ADVERSE EFFECTS: GI: N/V/D, symptoms of ***pseudomembranous colitis*** ▪ GU: vaginitis ▪ HEM: eosinophilia ▪ HEP: transitory ⬆ in AST, ALT, BUN ▪ INT: pruritus, urticaria, morbilliform eruptions, ***erythema multiforme.***

INTERACTIONS: Drug: Bacteriostatic antibiotics can antagonize bactericidal activity ▪ Use c̄ PO anticoagulants may ⬆ their activity ▪ Use c̄ aminoglycosides may produce additive nephrotoxicity ▪ Use c̄ probenecid ⬇ renal excretion. **Lab:** Possible false + c̄ Coombs' test.

NURSING MANAGEMENT PRIORITIES

ADMINISTRATION: Assess for hx of cephalosporin/penicillin hypersensitivity ▪ Obtain C&S before therapy ▪ Assess for hx of impaired renal function; ↓ dosage ▪ IM: reconstitute according to manufacturer's directions; administer by *deep, slow* injection into gluteal UOQ ▪ IV: dilute c̄ sterile H_2O for injection; administer *slowly* (3-5m); avoid aminoglycoside administration at same site; may administer IVPB ▪ Do *not* administer discolored/precipitated solutions; yellow-amber color does *not* indicate ↓ potency ▪ Use reconstituted preparations w/in 18h at room temperature, 7d refrigerated ▪ Have support equipment available for anaphylaxis ▪ Na^+ content: 2.3mEq (54mg)/g; calculate in Na^+-restricted diets ▪ Maintain hydration.

EVALUATION: Monitor VS, esp temperature ▪ Monitor renal, hepatic, hematologic status ▪ Urine glucose: false + c̄ Clinitest; use Clinistix/Diastix ▪ Observe for signs of superinfection (diarrhea, perineal itching, oral ulcers) ▪ Check IV site carefully; monitor for phlebitis (red streak, heat, pain).

EDUCATION: Use Clinistix/Diastix for urine testing ▪ Women: avoid breastfeeding ▪ Diarrhea may occur ▪ Maintain good personal hygiene (esp perineal, oral) ▪ Maintain fluid intake (6-8 glasses/d) ▪ Notify physician of symptoms of allergic rx (difficult breathing, rash) ▪ Carry identification (MedicAlert) if cephalosporin allergic ▪ IM injection may be painful.

NOTES:

cefoxitin sodium • (se-fox-i-tin)

CATEGORY: *Cephalosporin* (2nd generation): antibiotic Rx; Preg Cat B

BRAND NAME
Mefoxin (Merck)
(Frosst [Canada])

DOSAGE FORMS
Powder for injection (IM/IV): 1-, 2-, 10-g vials
Frozen: 1, 2g in 5% dextrose injection

USE: Treatment of infections caused by susceptible strains of *Bacteroides* spp, *Clostridium* spp, *Escherichia coli*, group B streptococci, *Haemophilus influenzae, Neisseria gonorrhoeae, Peptococcus* spp, *Peptostreptococcus* spp, *Proteus mirabilis, Proteus* spp (indole +), *Providencia* spp, staphylococci (incl penicillinase strains), *Streptococcus pneumoniae.* **ACTION:** Bactericidal activity due to inhibition of mucopeptide cell wall synthesis in susceptible organisms.

PHARMACOKINETICS

IM peak	Half-life	Protein binding	Excretion
20-30m	64.8m	55%-75%	85% via urine in 6h as unchanged drug

CONTRAINDICATIONS: Hypersensitivity to any cephalosporin. **CC:** Use may produce pseudomembranous colitis ▪ Use in penicillin-allergic pts requires caution.

DOSAGE

Pediatric	*IM/IV*	80-160mg/kg/d in 4-6 equal doses
Adult	*IM/IV*	1-2g q6-8h. Severe infection, 1g q4h or 2g q6-8h (IV). Life-threatening infection, 2g q4h or 3g q6h (IV)

SIDE/ADVERSE EFFECTS: GI: symptoms of ***pseudomembranous colitis***, N/V ▪ HEM: neutropenia, ***thrombocytopenia, hemolytic anemia*** ▪ INT: maculopapular rash, urticaria ▪ Other: pain, induration c̄ repeated IM injection; ***thrombophlebitis at IV site*** c̄ 3-g dose given over 6h.

INTERACTIONS: Drug: Bacteriostatic antibiotics can antagonize bactericidal activity ▪ Use c̄ PO anticoagulants may ↑ their activity ▪ Use c̄ aminoglycosides may produce additive nephrotoxicity ▪ Use c̄ probenecid will ↓ renal excretion. **Lab:** Possible false + c̄ Coombs' test.

NURSING MANAGEMENT PRIORITIES

ADMINISTRATION: Assess for hx of cephalosporin/penicillin hypersensitivity ▪ Obtain C&S before therapy ▪ Assess renal function; ↓ dosage if impaired ▪ IM: reconstitute c̄ 2ml sterile H_2O for injection or 0.5% or 1% lidocaine HCl injection (w/out epinephrine) ▪ IV: dilute c̄ sterile H_2O for injection; inject *slowly* (3-5m); avoid aminoglycoside administration at same site ▪ Do *not* administer discolored/precipitated solutions; yellow-amber color does *not* indicate ↓ potency ▪ Thaw frozen preparations completely at room temperature; do *not* refreeze; stable 24h at room temperature, 48h refrigerated ▪ Use reconstituted preparations w/in 24h at room temperature, 7d refrigerated, 30wks frozen ▪ Have support equipment available for anaphylaxis ▪ Surgical prophylaxis: D/C w/in 24h after surgery ▪ Na^+ content: 2.3mEq (54mg)/g; calculate in Na^+-restricted diets ▪ Avoid alkaline or strong acid solutions ▪ Maintain hydration.

EVALUATION: Monitor VS, esp temperature ▪ Monitor renal, hepatic, hemopoietic status ▪ Observe for signs of superinfection (diarrhea, itching, oral ulcers).

EDUCATION: Use Clinistix/Diastix for urine testing ▪ Women: avoid breastfeeding ▪ Diarrhea may occur ▪ Maintain good personal hygiene (esp perineal, oral) ▪ ↑ Fluid intake (8-10 glasses/d) ▪ Notify nurse/physician of symptoms of allergic rx (difficult breathing, rash) ▪ Carry identification (MedicAlert) if cephalosporin allergic ▪ IM injection may be painful.

NOTES:

cefpodoxime proxetil • (sef-poe-dox-eem)

CATEGORY: *Cephalosporin* (2nd generation): antibiotic — Rx; Preg Cat B

BRAND NAME
Vantin (Upjohn)

DOSAGE FORMS
PO suspension: 50, 100mg/5ml
Tablet: 100, 200mg

USE: Treatment of upper respiratory, lower respiratory, urinary, skin, skin structure infections/sexually transmitted diseases caused by susceptible strains of *Escherichia coli, Haemophilus influenzae* (incl β-lactamase-producing otitis media only), *Klebsiella pneumoniae, Moraxella catarrhalis, Neisseria gonorrhoeae* (incl penicillinase-producing strains), *Proteus mirabilis, Staphylococcus aureus* (incl penicillinase-producing strains), *S. saprophyticus, Streptococcus pyogenes.* **ACTION:** Bactericidal activity due to inhibition of mucopeptide cell wall synthesis in susceptible organisms.

PHARMACOKINETICS

PO absorption	Peak	Half-life	Protein binding	Excretion
50%	2-3h	3.5h	22%-33%	Via urine primarily as unchanged drug

CONTRAINDICATIONS: Hypersensitivity to any cephalosporin. **CC:** Use may produce pseudomembranous colitis ▪ Use in penicillin-allergic pts requires caution.

DOSAGE: *PO*

Children 6mo-12y/o	
Otitis media, pharyngitis/tonsillitis	5mg/kg q12h (200mg/d maximum) for 10d
Adult/Children ≥ 13y/o	
Gonorrhea	Single dose of 200mg
Pharyngitis/tonsillitis	100mg q12h for 10d
Pneumonia	200mg q12h for 14d
Skin/skin structure	400mg q12h for 7-14d
UTI	100mg q12h for 7d

SIDE/ADVERSE EFFECTS: CNS: headache, dizziness, anxiety ▪ GI: N/V/D, abdominal pain, taste changes, ***pseudomembranous colitis*** ▪ GU: vaginal fungal infections, genital pruritus ▪ HEM: *agranulocytosis,* eosinophilia ▪ HEP: ↑ ALT ▪ INT: fungal skin infections, skin scaling, rash ▪ Other: fever, eye twitching.

INTERACTIONS: Drug: Use c̄ antacids (high doses), H_2-blockers ↓ peak plasma levels ▪ Use c̄ anticholinergics delays peak plasma levels ▪ Use c̄ PO anticoagulants may ↑ their activity ▪ Bacteriostatic antibiotics can antagonize bactericidal activity ▪ Use c̄ probenecid ↓ renal excretion. **Lab:** Possible false + c̄ Coombs' test.

NURSING MANAGEMENT PRIORITIES

ADMINISTRATION: Assess for hx of cephalosporin/penicillin hypersensitivity ▪ Obtain C&S before therapy ▪ Administer c̄ food ▪ PO suspension: reconstitute powder according to manufacturer's directions; shake well before using; store reconstituted portion in refrigerator for 14d ▪ Avoid exposure to moisture/light in storage ▪ Maintain hydration.

EVALUATION: Monitor VS, esp temperature ▪ Monitor hepatic, renal status ▪ Monitor CBC ▪ Urine glucose: false + c̄ Clinitest; use Clinistix/Diastix ▪ Observe for signs of superinfection (diarrhea, itching, oral ulcers) ▪ Monitor prothrombin levels; assess for bleeding.

EDUCATION: Complete full course of therapy (usually 10d) even if symptoms subside ▪ Take c̄ food ▪ Take at equal intervals around clock to maintain blood levels ▪ Diarrhea may occur ▪ PO suspension: refrigerate; shake well before use ▪ Store in dry, tightly closed, light-resistant container ▪ Discard outdated preparations ▪ Maintain good personal hygiene (esp perineal, oral) ▪ ↑ Fluid intake (8-10 glasses/d) ▪ Use Clinistix/Diastix for urine testing ▪ Notify physician of symptoms of allergic rx (fever, difficult breathing, rash) ▪ Carry identification (MedicAlert) if cephalosporin allergic ▪ Women: avoid breastfeeding.

NOTES:

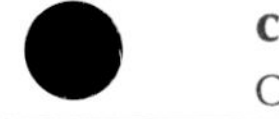

cefprozil monohydrate • (sef-proe-zill)

CATEGORY: *Cephalosporin* (2nd generation): antibiotic

Rx; Preg Cat B

BRAND NAME
Cefzil (B-MS)

DOSAGE FORMS
PO suspension:
125, 250mg/5ml
Tablet: 250, 500mg

USE: Treatment of upper respiratory, lower respiratory, skin, skin structure infections caused by susceptible strains of *Haemophilus influenzae, Moraxella catarrhalis, Staphylococcus aureus* (incl penicillinase-producing strains), *Streptococcus pneumoniae, S. pyogenes*. **ACTION:** Bactericidal activity due to inhibition of mucopeptide cell wall synthesis in susceptible organisms.

PHARMACOKINETICS

PO absorption	Peak	Half-life	Protein binding	Excretion
95%	1.5h	1.3h	36%	Via urine primarily as unchanged drug

CONTRAINDICATIONS: Hypersensitivity to any cephalosporin. **CC:** Use may produce pseudomembranous colitis ▪ Use in penicillin-allergic pts requires caution.

DOSAGE: *PO*

Children 6mo-12y/o	15mg/kg q12h for 10d
Adult/Children >13y/o	500mg q24h for URI, 500mg q12h for LRI, 250-500mg q12-24h for skin, skin structure infections

SIDE/ADVERSE EFFECTS: CNS: dizziness, headache, nervousness ▪ GI: *N/V/D,* abdominal pain ▪ GU: vaginitis, genital pruritus, moniliasis ▪ HEM: eosinophilia, ↓ leukocytes ▪ HEP: ↑ AST, ALT, bilirubin, rare cholestatic jaundice ▪ INT: rash, urticaria ▪ Other: ↑ BUN, serum creatinine.

INTERACTIONS: Drug: Use c̄ PO anticoagulants may ↑ their activity ▪ Bacteriostatic antibiotics can antagonize bactericidal activity ▪ Use c̄ aminoglycosides can produce ↑ nephrotoxicity ▪ Use c̄ probenecid will ↓ renal excretion. **Lab:** Possible false + c̄ Coombs' test.

NURSING MANAGEMENT PRIORITIES

ADMINISTRATION: Assess for hx of cephalosporin/penicillin hypersensitivity ▪ Obtain C&S before therapy ▪ Assess renal function; ↓ dosage if impaired ▪ Administer 1h ac/2h pc ▪ PO suspension: reconstitute powder according to manufacturer's directions; shake well before use; store reconstituted portion in refrigerator for 14d ▪ Avoid exposure to moisture/light in storage ▪ Maintain hydration.

EVALUATION: Monitor VS, esp temperature ▪ Monitor hepatic, renal status ▪ Monitor CBC ▪ Urine glucose: false + c̄ Clinitest; use Clinistix/Diastix ▪ Observe for signs of superinfection (diarrhea, itching, oral ulcers) ▪ Monitor prothrombin levels; assess for bleeding.

EDUCATION: Complete full course of therapy (usually 10d) even if symptoms subside ▪ Can be taken c̄ meals; *best* on empty stomach ▪ Take at equal intervals around clock to maintain blood levels ▪ Diarrhea may occur ▪ PO suspension: refrigerate; shake well before use ▪ Store in dry, tightly closed, light-resistant container ▪ Discard outdated preparations ▪ Maintain good personal hygiene (esp perineal, oral) ▪ ↑ Fluid intake (8-10 glasses/d) ▪ Use Clinistix/Diastix for urine testing ▪ Notify physician of symptoms of allergic rx (fever, difficult breathing, rash) ▪ Carry identification (MedicAlert) if cephalosporin allergic.

NOTES:

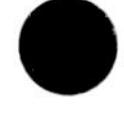

ceftazidime • (sef-tay-zi-deem)

CATEGORY: *Cephalosporin* (3rd generation): antibiotic — Rx; Preg Cat B

BRAND NAMES	DOSAGE FORMS
Fortaz (Glaxo)	Powder for injection (IM/IV): 500mg; 1, 2, 6g Frozen: 1, 2g in D_5W injection
Tazicef (SKB)	Powder for injection: 1, 2, 6g
Tazidime (Lilly)	Powder for injection (IM/IV): 500mg; 1, 2, 6g

USE: Treatment of infections caused by susceptible strains of *Bacteroides* spp, *Citrobacter* spp, *Enterobacter* spp, *Escherichia coli, Haemophilus influenzae, Klebsiella* spp, *Neisseria meningitidis, Proteus mirabilis, Pseudomonas* spp, *Serratia* spp, *Staphylococcus aureus, Streptococcus pneumoniae, S. pyogenes.* **ACTION:** Bactericidal activity due to inhibition of mucopeptide cell wall synthesis in susceptible organisms.

PHARMACOKINETICS

Peak IM	Peak IV	Half-life	Protein binding	Excretion
1h	0.5h	2h	10%	80%-90% via urine unchanged in 24h

CONTRAINDICATIONS: Hypersensitivity to any cephalosporin. **CC:** Use may produce pseudomembranous colitis ▪ Use in penicillin-allergic pts requires caution.

DOSAGE

Pediatric	*IV*	
Neonate		30 mg/kg q12h
Infants/Children		30-50mg/kg q8h. 6g/d may be required c̄ cystic fibrosis, meningitis, immunodeficiency
Adult	*IM/IV*	250mg-1g q8-12h. For bone/joint infections, usually 2g q12h IV. For serious and life-threatening infection, 2g q8h IV. Dosage must be ↓ in renal impairment

SIDE/ADVERSE EFFECTS: GI: N/V/D, symptoms of ***pseudomembranous colitis*** ▪ GU: vaginitis ▪ HEM: eosinophilia ▪ HEP: transitory ↑ in AST, ALT, BUN ▪ INT: pruritus, urticaria, morbilliform eruptions, ***erythema multiforme.***

Note: Side/adverse effects: common in *italic;* serious in ***boldface italic.***

*Available in Canada only.

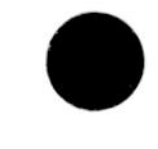

INTERACTIONS: Drug: Bacteriostatic antibiotics can antagonize bactericidal activity ▪ Use c̄ PO anticoagulants may ↑ their activity ▪ Use c̄ aminoglycosides may produce additive nephrotoxicity ▪ Use c̄ probenecid ↓ renal excretion. **Lab:** Possible false + c̄ Coombs' test.

NURSING MANAGEMENT PRIORITIES

ADMINISTRATION: Assess for hx of cephalosporin/penicillin hypersensitivity ▪ Obtain C&S before therapy ▪ Assess renal status; ↓ dosage if impaired ▪ IM: reconstitute according to manufacturer's directions; administer by *deep, slow* injection into gluteal UOQ ▪ IV: dilute c̄ sterile H_2O for injection; administer *slowly* (3-5m); avoid aminoglycoside administration at same site; may administer IVPB ▪ Do *not* administer discolored/precipitated solutions; yellow-amber color does *not* indicate ↓ potency ▪ Frozen preparations: thaw completely at room temperature; do *not* refreeze; stable 24h at room temperature, 7d refrigerated ▪ Use reconstituted preparations w/in 18h at room temperature, 7d refrigerated ▪ Have support equipment available for anaphylaxis ▪ Na^+ content: 2.3mEq (54mg)/g; calculate in Na^+-restricted diets ▪ Maintain hydration.

EVALUATION: Monitor VS, esp temperature ▪ Monitor renal, hepatic, hematologic status ▪ Urine glucose: false + c̄ Clinitest; use Clinistix/Diastix ▪ Observe for signs of superinfection (diarrhea, perineal itching, oral ulcers) ▪ Check IV site carefully; monitor for phlebitis (red streak, heat, pain).

EDUCATION: Use Clinistix/Diastix for urine testing ▪ Women: avoid breastfeeding ▪ Diarrhea may occur ▪ Maintain good personal hygiene (esp perineal, oral) ▪ Maintain fluid intake (6-8 glasses/d) ▪ Notify physician of symptoms of allergic rx (difficult breathing, rash) ▪ Carry identification (Medic-Alert) if cephalosporin allergic ▪ IM injection may be painful.

NOTES:

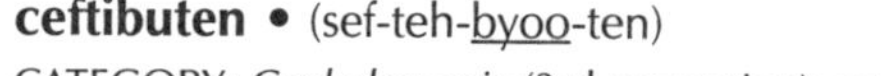

ceftibuten • (sef-teh-byoo-ten)

CATEGORY: *Cephalosporin* (3rd generation): antibiotic Rx; Preg Cat B

BRAND NAME
Cedax (Schering)

DOSAGE FORMS
Capsule: 400mg
PO suspension: 90, 180mg/5ml

USE: Acute exacerbations of chronic bronchitis due to *Haemophilus influenzae, Moraxella catarrhalis* (including β-lactamase-producing strains), *Streptococcus pneumoniae* (penicillin-susceptible strains) ▪ Acute otitis media due to *H. influenzae, M. catarrhalis* (including β-lactamase producing strains), *S. pyogenes* ▪ Pharyngitis/tonsillitis due to *S. pyogenes.* **ACTION:** Bactericidal activity due to inhibition of mucopeptide cell wall synthesis in susceptible organisms.

PHARMACOKINETICS

PO absorption	Half-life	Protein binding	Excretion
Rapid	Up to 23h	65%	Via urine, feces

CONTRAINDICATIONS: Hypersensitivity to any cephalosporins. **CC:** Use may produce pseudomembranous colitis ▪ Use in penicillin-allergic pts requires caution ▪ PO suspension contains 1g of sucrose/5ml.

DOSAGE: Dosage must be ⬇ with renal impairment.

Pediatric	*PO*	9mg/kg/d for 10d
Adult	*PO*	400mg/d for 10d

SIDE/ADVERSE EFFECTS: GI: abdominal pain, N/V/D, dyspepsia, taste changes, ***pseudomembranous colitis*** ▪ GU: vaginitis ▪ HEM: eosinophilia ▪ HEP: ⬆ AST, ALT, BUN ▪ INT: rash, urticaria, ***toxic epidermal necrolysis*** ▪ Other: headache, nasal congestion, somnolence.

INTERACTIONS: Drug: Bacteriostatic antibiotics can antagonize bactericidal activity ▪ Use c̄ PO anticoagulants may ⬆ their activity ▪ Use c̄ aminoglycosides may produce additive nephrotoxicity ▪ Use c̄ probenecid ⬇ renal execution ▪ Use c̄ ranitidine can ⬆ plasma concentrations. **Lab:** Possible false + c̄ Coombs' test.

NURSING MANAGEMENT PRIORITIES

ADMINISTRATION: Assess for hx of cephalosporin/penicillin hypersensitivity ▪ Obtain C&S before therapy ▪ Assess renal function; ⬇ dosage if impaired ▪ Administer c̄ meals to ⬇ GI distress (capsules); 2h ac/1h pc (suspension) ▪ PO suspension: reconstitute powder according to manufacturer's directions; shake well before using; store reconstituted portion in refrigerator for 14d ▪ Avoid exposure to moisture/light in storage.

EVALUATION: Monitor VS, esp temperature ▪ Monitor hepatic, renal status ▪ Monitor CBC ▪ Urine glucose: false + c̄ Clinitest; use Clinistix/Diastix.

EDUCATION: Complete full course of therapy (usually 10d) even if symptoms subside ▪ Capsules: take c̄ meals; PO suspension: take on empty stomach (2h ac/1h pc) ▪ Take at equal intervals around clock to maintain blood levels ▪ Diarrhea may occur ▪ Store in dry, tightly closed container ▪ Discard outdated preparations ▪ Maintain good personal hygiene (esp perineal, oral) ▪ ⬆ Fluid intake (8-10 glasses/d) ▪ Use Clinistix/Diastix for urine testing ▪ Notify physician of symptoms of allergic rx (fever, difficult breathing, rash) ▪ Carry identification (MedicAlert) if cephalosporin allergic.

NOTES:

ceftizoxime sodium • (sef-ti-zox-eem)

CATEGORY: *Cephalosporin* (3rd generation): antibiotic

Rx; Preg Cat B

BRAND NAME

Cefizox (Fujisawa)

DOSAGE FORMS

Powder for injection (IM/IV): 1-, 2-, 10-g vials

Frozen: 1, 2g in D_5W solution

USE: Treatment of infections caused by susceptible strains of *Bacteroides* (incl *B. fragilis), Enterobacter* spp, *Escherichia coli,* group A β-hemolytic streptococci, *Haemophilus influenzae, Klebsiella* spp, *Morganella morganii, Neisseria gonorrhoeae, Peptococcus* spp, *Peptostreptococcus* spp, *Proteus mirabilis, P. vulgaris, Providencia rettgeri, Pseudomonas* spp, *Serratia* spp, staphylococci (incl penicillinase-producing strains), *Staphylococcus epidermidis, Streptococcus pneumoniae.* **ACTION:** Bactericidal activity due to inhibition of mucopeptide cell wall synthesis in susceptible organisms; good resistance to β-lactamases (penicillinase, cephalosporinase).

PHARMACOKINETICS

IM peak	Half-life	Protein binding	Excretion
0.5-1.5h	1.7h	30%	Via urine in 24h as unchanged drug

CONTRAINDICATIONS: Hypersensitivity to any cephalosporin. **CC:** Use may produce pseudomembranous colitis ▪ Use in penicillin-allergic pts requires caution.

DOSAGE

Pediatric	*IM/IV*	>6mo: 50mg/kg q6-8h. May be ↑ 200mg/kg/d if needed
Adult	*IM/IV*	500mg-2g q8-12h. Life-threatening infections, 3-4g q8h

SIDE/ADVERSE EFFECTS: GI: N/V/D, symptoms of ***pseudomembranous colitis*** ▪ GU: moniliasis, vaginitis ▪ HEM: anemia, leukopenia, neutropenia, ***thrombocytopenia*** ▪ INT: rash, pruritus ▪ Other: pain, induration at IM site, ***phlebitis at IV site***.

INTERACTIONS: Drug: Bacteriostatic antibiotics can antagonize bactericidal activity ▪ Use c̄ PO anticoagulants may ↑ their activity ▪ Use c̄ aminoglycosides may produce additive nephrotoxicity ▪ Use c̄ probenecid will ↓ renal excretion. **Lab:** Possible false + c̄ Coombs' test.

NURSING MANAGEMENT PRIORITIES

ADMINISTRATION: Assess for hx of cephalosporin/penicillin hypersensitivity ▪ Obtain C&S before therapy ▪ Assess renal function; ↓ dosage if impaired ▪ IM: reconstitute according to manufacturer's directions; administer 2g as divided doses at different sites by *deep, slow* injection into gluteal UOQ ▪ IV: dilute c̄ sterile H_2O for injection; administer *slowly* (3-5m); avoid aminoglycoside administration at same site; may administer IVPB ▪ Do *not* administer discolored/precipitated solutions; yellow-amber color does *not* indicate ↓ potency ▪ Thaw frozen preparations completely at room temperature; do *not* refreeze; stable 24h at room temperature, 10d refrigerated ▪ Use reconstituted preparations w/in 8h at room temperature, 48h refrigerated ▪ Have support equipment available for anaphylaxis ▪ Na^+ content: 2.6mEq (60mg)/g; calculate in Na^+-restricted diets ▪ Avoid exposure to light in storage ▪ Maintain hydration.

EVALUATION: Monitor VS, esp temperature ▪ Monitor renal, hepatic, hemopoietic status ▪ Urine glucose: false + c̄ Clinitest; use Clinistix/Diastix ▪ Observe for signs of superinfection (diarrhea, itching, oral ulcers).

EDUCATION: Use Clinistix/Diastix for urine testing ▪ Women: avoid breastfeeding ▪ Diarrhea may occur ▪ Maintain good personal hygiene (esp perineal, oral) ▪ ↑ Fluid intake (8-10 glasses/d) ▪ Notify nurse/physician of symptoms of allergic rx (difficult breathing, rash) ▪ Carry identification (MedicAlert) if cephalosporin allergic ▪ IM injection may be painful.

NOTES:

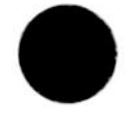

ceftriaxone sodium • (sef-try-ax-own)

CATEGORY: *Cephalosporin* (3rd generation): antibiotic Rx; Preg Cat B

BRAND NAME
Rocephin (Roche)

DOSAGE FORMS
IM/IV Powder: 0.25-, 0.5-, 1-, 2-, 10-g vial
Frozen: 1, 2g in dextrose injection

USE: Treatment of infections caused by susceptible strains of *Enterobacter* spp, *Escherichia coli,* group A β-hemolytic streptococci, *Haemophilus influenzae, H. parainfluenzae, Klebsiella* spp, *Morganella morganii, Neisseria gonorrhoeae, N. meningitidis, Proteus mirabilis, P. vulgaris, Pseudomonas aeruginosa, Serratia marcescens, Staphylococcus aureus* (incl penicillinase-producing strains), *S. epidermidis, Streptococcus pneumoniae.* **ACTION:** Bactericidal activity due to inhibition of mucopeptide cell wall synthesis in susceptible organisms.

PHARMACOKINETICS

IM peak	Half-life	Protein binding	Excretion
2h	5.8-8.7h	95%	33%-67% via urine as unchanged drug, remainder in feces as metabolites

CONTRAINDICATIONS: Hypersensitivity to any cephalosporin. **CC:** Use may produce pseudomembranous colitis ▪ Use in penicillin-allergic pts requires caution.

DOSAGE

Pediatric	*IM/IV*	50-75mg/kg divided q12h. For meningitis, 100mg/kg divided q12h
Adult	*IM/IV*	1-2g/d as single dose or divided. Do *not* exceed 4g/d

SIDE/ADVERSE EFFECTS: CNS: headache ▪ GI: N/V/D, taste impairment ▪ GU: moniliasis, vaginitis ▪ HEM: eosinophilia, thrombocytosis, leukopenia, anemia, neutropenia, ***thrombocytopenia*** ▪ HEP: ↑ AST, ALT, alkaline phosphatase, bilirubin ▪ INT: pruritus ▪ Other: pain, induration at IM site, phlebitis at IV site.

INTERACTIONS: Drug: Use c̄ alcohol may produce disulfiram rx ▪ Use c̄ PO anticoagulants may ↑ their activity ▪ Bacteriostatic antibiotics can antagonize bactericidal activity ▪ Use c̄ probenecid will ↓ renal excretion. **Lab:** Possible false + c̄ Coombs' test.

NURSING MANAGEMENT PRIORITIES

ADMINISTRATION: Assess for hx of cephalosporin/penicillin hypersensitivity ▪ Obtain C&S before therapy ▪ Assess renal function; ↓ dosage if impaired ▪ IM: reconstitute according to manufacturer's directions; administer by *deep, slow* injection into gluteal UOQ ▪ IV: dilute according to manufacturer's directions; avoid aminoglycoside administration at same site; may administer IVPB ▪ Frozen preparations: thaw completely at room temperature; do *not* refreeze ▪ Do *not* administer discolored/precipitated solutions; yellow-amber color does *not* indicate ↓ potency ▪ Use reconstituted IM/IV preparations w/in 3d at room temperature, 10d refrigerated ▪ Have support equipment available for anaphylaxis ▪ Surgical prophylaxis: D/C w/in 24h after surgery ▪ Na^+ content: 3.6mEq (83mg)/g; calculate in Na^+-restricted diets ▪ Avoid exposure to heat/light in storage ▪ Maintain hydration.

EVALUATION: Monitor VS, esp temperature ▪ Monitor renal, hepatic, hemopoietic status ▪ Urine glucose: false + c̄ Clinitest; use Clinistix/Diastix ▪ Observe for signs of superinfection (diarrhea, itching, oral ulcers) ▪ Monitor PT.

EDUCATION: Use Clinistix/Diastix for urine testing ▪ Women: avoid breastfeeding ▪ Diarrhea may occur ▪ Maintain good personal hygiene (esp perineal, oral) ▪ ↑ Fluid intake (8-10 glasses/d) ▪ Notify physician of symptoms of allergic rx (difficult breathing, rash) ▪ Carry identification (MedicAlert) if cephalosporin allergic ▪ IM injection may be painful.

NOTES:

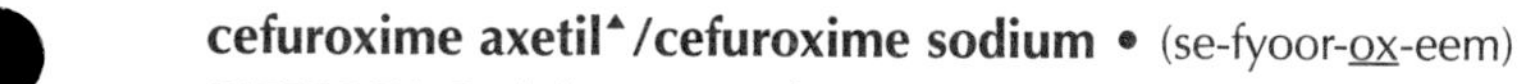

cefuroxime axetil▲/cefuroxime sodium • (se-fyoor-ox-eem)

CATEGORY: *Cephalosporin* (2nd generation): antibiotic Rx; Preg Cat B

BRAND NAMES	DOSAGE FORMS
Ceftin▲ (A-H)	Tablet: 125, 250, 500mg
Kefurox (Lilly)	IM/IV powder: 0.75-, 1.5-, 7.5-g vial
Zinacef (Glaxo)	IM/IV powder: 0.75-, 1.5-g vial Frozen: 0.75, 1.5g

USE: Treatment of infections caused by susceptible strains of *Enterobacter aerogenes, Escherichia coli,* group A β-hemolytic streptococci, *Haemophilus influenzae, Klebsiella pneumoniae, Neisseria gonorrhoeae, N. meningitidis, Staphylococcus aureus* (incl penicillinase-producing strains), *Streptococcus pneumoniae.* **ACTION:** Bactericidal activity due to inhibition of mucopeptide cell wall synthesis in susceptible organisms; drug exhibits good resistance to some β-lactamases.

PHARMACOKINETICS

IM peak	Half-life	Protein binding	Excretion
15-60m	1-2h	35%-50%	89%-100% via urine in 24h as unchanged drug

CONTRAINDICATIONS: Hypersensitivity to any cephalosporin. **CC:** Use may produce pseudomembranous colitis ▪ Use in penicillin-allergic pts requires caution.

DOSAGE

Pediatric	*IM/IV*	50-100mg/kg/d divided q6-8h >3mo; For meningitis, 200-240mg/kg/d divided q6-8h. ↓ To 100mg/kg/d after clinical improvement
Adult	*IM/IV*	0.75-1.5g q8h. For serious infections, 1.5g q6h

SIDE/ADVERSE EFFECTS: GI: N/V/D, symptoms of ***pseudomembranous colitis*** ▪ GU: moniliasis, vaginitis ▪ HEM: ↓ hematocrit/hemoglobin, neutropenia, leukopenia ▪ HEP: ↑ AST, ALT, LDH, alkaline phosphatase, bilirubin ▪ Other: pain, induration at IM site, ***phlebitis at IV site.***

INTERACTIONS: Drug: Bacteriostatic antibiotics can antagonize bactericidal activity ▪ Use c̄ PO anticoagulants may ↑ their activity ▪ Use c̄ aminoglycosides may produce additive nephrotoxicity ▪ Use c̄ probenecid ↓ renal excretion. **Lab:** Possible false + c̄ Coombs' test.

Note: Side/adverse effects: common in *italic;* serious in ***boldface italic.***

▲Available in Canada only.

NURSING MANAGEMENT PRIORITIES

ADMINISTRATION: Assess for hx of cephalosporin/penicillin hypersensitivity ▪ Obtain C&S before therapy ▪ Assess renal function; ↓ dosage if impaired ▪ IM: reconstitute c̄ 3.6ml sterile H_2O for injection; shake suspension well; administer by *deep, slow* injection into gluteal UOQ ▪ IV: dilute according to manufacturer's directions; inject *slowly* (3-5m); avoid aminoglycoside administration at same site; may administer IVPB ▪ Frozen preparations: thaw completely at room temperature; do *not* refreeze ▪ Do *not* administer discolored/precipitated solutions; yellow-amber color does *not* indicate ↓ potency ▪ Use reconstituted preparations w/in 24h at room temperature, 48h refrigerated ▪ Have support equipment available for anaphylaxis ▪ Surgical prophylaxis: D/C w/in 24h after surgery ▪ Na^+ content: 2.4mEq (55mg)/g; calculate in Na^+-restricted diets ▪ Avoid exposure to light in storage ▪ Maintain hydration ▪ PO: administer c̄ food; do *not* crush tablet (bitter); swallow whole.

EVALUATION: Monitor VS, esp temperature ▪ Monitor renal, hepatic, hemopoietic status ▪ Urine glucose: false + c̄ Clinitest; use Clinistix/Diastix ▪ Blood glucose: false − c̄ ferricyanide methods ▪ Observe for signs of superinfection (diarrhea, itching, oral ulcers).

EDUCATION: Use Clinistix/Diastix for urine testing ▪ Women: avoid breastfeeding ▪ Diarrhea may occur ▪ Maintain good personal hygiene (esp perineal, oral).

NOTES:

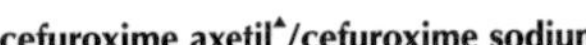

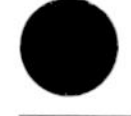

celecoxib • (sell-eh-sox-ib)

CATEGORY: *Antiinflammatory:* NSAIA

Rx; Preg Cat C

BRAND NAME	**DOSAGE FORM**
Celebrex (Searle/Pfizer)	Capsule: 100mg

USE: Treatment of rheumatoid arthritis/osteoarthritis ▪ Celecoxib exhibits ⬇ GI effects in comparison to other NSAIAs ▪ Bacterial, fungal, viral infections can ⬇ therapeutic effects. **ACTION:** Antiinflammatory activity appears related to inhibition of prostaglandin synthesis.

PHARMACOKINETICS

PO absorption	Peak	Half-life	Protein binding	Excretion
Good	3h	11.2h	97%	Via feces, urine primarily as metabolites

CONTRAINDICATIONS: Hypersensitivity, aspirin/other NSAIAs/sulfonamide hypersensitivity. **CC:** Use can ⬆ risk of GI bleeding, ulcers, perforation ▪ Use during late pregnancy may cause premature ductus arteriosus closure & should be avoided ▪ Use in dehydrated pts requires caution ▪ Celecoxib is excreted in rat breast milk & requires careful clinical consideration for use in nursing mothers ▪ Safety & efficacy in pts <18y/o not established.

DOSAGE: Adult *PO*

Osteoarthritis	200mg/d divided or as single dose
Rheumatoid arthritis	100-200mg/d

SIDE/ADVERSE EFFECTS: CNS: headache, dizziness, neuralgia ▪ CV: peripheral edema, ⬆ hypertension, angina, tachycardia, ***rare MI*** ▪ GI: dyspepsia, abdominal pain, N/V/D, flatulence, ***GI bleeding, ulcers,*** taste changes ▪ HEM: rare ***thrombocytopenia*** ▪ INT: alopecia, rash, rare photosensitivity ▪ RESP: pharyngitis, sinusitis, infection, dyspnea ▪ Urogenital: infection, prostatic disorder, dysmenorrhea, dysuria, hematuria ▪ Other: leg cramps, back pain, glaucoma, impaired vision.

INTERACTIONS: Drug: Use c̄ ACE-I can ⬇ their effects ▪ Use c̄ natriuretic diuretics can ⬇ their effects ▪ Use c̄ fluconazole, lithium may require ⬇ celecoxib doses due to ⬆ plasma levels of the two drugs ▪ Antacids can ⬇ plasma levels of celecoxib. **Lab:** ⬆ Levels of SGOT, SGPT. **Food:**

Meals c̄ ↑ fat content can ↓ peak levels from 1-2h & ↑ fatal drug absorption.

NURSING MANAGEMENT PRIORITIES

ADMINISTRATION: Assess for hx of NSAIA, sulfonamide hypersensitivity ▪ Avoid administration to pts c̄ hx of asthma, bleeding disorders, salycilate hypersensitivity ▪ Assess for hx of peptic ulcer; use c̄ caution ▪ Assess hematologic, renal, hepatic function; use caution if impaired ▪ Administer c̄ food/milk to ↓ GI irritation ▪ Elderly may require ↓ dosage.

EVALUATION: Monitor hepatic, renal status c̄ prolonged use ▪ Monitor I&O, daily weight ▪ Assess for edema in extremities ▪ Assess for visual disturbances; D/C drug, notify physician.

EDUCATION: Dizziness/drowsiness may occur; use caution in potentially hazardous activities ▪ Take c̄ food/milk to ↓ GI distress ▪ Take as ordered by physician, do *not* ↑ dose ▪ Notify physician *immediately* of bleeding, ↓ urine output, swelling of feet/legs, lethargy, GI distress, jaundice, visual disturbance ▪ Avoid taking c̄ aspirin/other NSAIAs ▪ Avoid use c̄ alcohol ▪ Check c̄ physician/pharmacist before taking OTC preparations ▪ Notify physician/dentist of use before treatment ▪ May produce alteration in taste ▪ Store in tightly closed container ▪ Schedule eye exams c̄ prolonged use ▪ Full drug effects may require several wks of therapy.

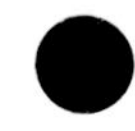

NOTES:

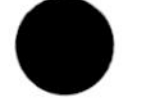

cephalexin/cephalexin hcl▲ • (sef-a-lex-in)

CATEGORY: *Cephalosporin* (1st generation): antibiotic

Rx; Preg Cat B

BRAND NAMES
**Ceporex (Glaxo)*
Keflex (Dista)
Keftab▲ (Dista)
**Novolexin (Novopharm)*

DOSAGE FORMS
Capsule: 250, 500mg
PO suspension: 125, 250mg/5m
Tablet: 500mg
Tablet: 1g

USE: Treatment of infections caused by susceptible strains of *Escherichia coli*, group A β-hemolytic streptococci, *Haemophilus influenzae, Klebsiella* spp, *Neisseria catarrhalis, Proteus mirabilis,* staphylococci, *Streptococcus pneumoniae.* **ACTION:** Bactericidal activity due to inhibition of mucopeptide cell wall synthesis in susceptible organisms.

PHARMACOKINETICS

PO absorption	Peak	Half-life	Protein binding	Excretion
Rapid	1h	0.5-1.2h	5%-15%	90% via urine in 8h as unchanged drug

CONTRAINDICATIONS: Hypersensitivity to any cephalosporin. **CC:** Use may produce pseudomembranous colitis ▪ Use in penicillin-allergic pts requires caution.

DOSAGE

Pediatric	*PO*	25-50mg/kg divided. For severe infections, 75-100mg/kg/d divided
Adult	*PO*	250mg q6h, c̄ range 1-4g/d

SIDE/ADVERSE EFFECTS: CNS: dizziness, fatigue, headache ▪ GI: N/V, dyspepsia, abdominal pain, symptoms of ***pseudomembranous colitis*** ▪ GU: vaginitis, vaginal discharge, moniliasis ▪ HEM: eosinophilia, neutropenia ▪ HEP: ↑ AST, ALT ▪ INT: urticaria, rash, angioedema ▪ Other: ***anaphylaxis.***

INTERACTIONS: Drug: Bacteriostatic antibiotics can antagonize bactericidal activity ▪ Use c̄ PO anticoagulants may ↑ their activity ▪ Use c̄ aminoglycosides may produce additive nephrotoxicity ▪ Use c̄ probenecid will ↓ renal excretion. **Lab:** Possible false + c̄ Coombs' test.

Note: Side/adverse effects: common in *italic;* serious in ***boldface italic.***

*Available in Canada only.

NURSING MANAGEMENT PRIORITIES

ADMINISTRATION: Assess for hx of cephalosporin/penicillin hypersensitivity ▪ Obtain C&S before therapy ▪ Assess renal function; ↓ dosage if impaired ▪ Administer 1h ac/2h pc ▪ PO suspension: reconstitute powder according to manufacturer's directions; shake well before using; store reconstituted portion for 14d in refrigerator ▪ Avoid exposure to moisture/light in storage.

EVALUATION: Monitor VS, esp temperature ▪ Monitor hepatic, renal status ▪ Monitor CBC ▪ Urine glucose: false + c̄ Clinitest; use Clinistix/Diastix.

EDUCATION: Complete full course of therapy (usually 10d) even if symptoms subside ▪ Can be taken c̄ meals; *best* on empty stomach ▪ Take at equal intervals around clock to maintain blood levels ▪ Diarrhea may occur ▪ PO suspension: refrigerate; shake well before use ▪ Store in dry, tightly closed, light-resistant container ▪ Discard outdated preparations ▪ Maintain good personal hygiene (esp perineal, oral) ▪ ↑ Fluid intake (8-10 glasses/d) ▪ Use Clinistix/Diastix for urine testing ▪ Notify physician of symptoms of allergic rx (fever, difficult breathing, rash) ▪ Carry identification (MedicAlert) if cephalosporin allergic ▪ Procedure for pediatric gtt administration.

NOTES:

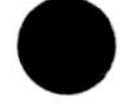

cephapirin sodium • (sef-a-pye-rin)

CATEGORY: *Cephalosporin* (1st generation): antibiotic — Rx; Preg Cat B

BRAND NAME
Cefadyl (Apothecon)

DOSAGE FORMS
Powder for injection (IM/IV): 0.5-, 1-, 2-, 4-, 20-g vials

USE: Treatment of infections caused by susceptible strains of α-*Streptococcus viridans, Escherichia coli,* group A β-hemolytic streptococci, *Haemophilus influenzae, Klebsiella* spp, *Proteus mirabilis,* staphylococci (incl penicillinase-producing strains), *Streptococcus pneumoniae.* **ACTION:** Bactericidal activity due to inhibition of mucopeptide cell wall synthesis in susceptible organisms.

PHARMACOKINETICS

IM peak	Half-life	Protein binding	Excretion
30m	36m	44%-50%	70%-94% via urine in 6h

CONTRAINDICATIONS: Hypersensitivity to any cephalosporin. **CC:** Use may produce pseudomembranous colitis ▪ Use in penicillin-allergic pts requires caution.

DOSAGE

Pediatric	*IM/IV*	40-80mg/kg in 4 equal doses
Adult	*IM/IV*	500mg-1g q4-6h. Severe infection may require 12g/d

SIDE/ADVERSE EFFECTS: GI: symptoms of ***pseudomembranous colitis*** ▪ HEM: neutropenia, ***thrombocytopenia,*** anemia ▪ INT: maculopapular rash, urticaria ▪ MS: pain, induration c̄ repeated IM injection ▪ Other: ***thrombophlebitis at IV site.***

INTERACTIONS: Drug: Bacteriostatic antibiotics can antagonize bactericidal activity ▪ Use c̄ PO anticoagulants may ↑ their activity ▪ Use c̄ aminoglycosides may produce additive nephrotoxicity ▪ Use c̄ probenecid will ↓ renal excretion. **Lab:** Possible false + c̄ Coombs' test.

NURSING MANAGEMENT PRIORITIES

ADMINISTRATION: Assess for hx of cephalosporin/penicillin hypersensitivity ▪ Obtain C&S before therapy ▪ Assess renal function; ↓ dosage if impaired ▪ IM: reconstitute according to manufacturer's directions; administer by *deep, slow* injection into gluteal UOQ ▪ IV: dilute according to manufacturer's directions; inject *slowly* (3-5m); avoid aminoglycoside administration at same site; may administer IVPB ▪ Do *not* administer precipitated solutions; color change does *not* indicate ↓ potency ▪ Use reconstituted preparations (depending on diluent) w/in 12-48h at room temperature, 10d refrigerated ▪ Have support equipment available for anaphylaxis ▪ Surgical prophylaxis: D/C w/in 24h after surgery ▪ Na^+ content: 2.4mEq (54mg)/g: calculate in Na^+-restricted diets ▪ Maintain hydration.

EVALUATION: Monitor VS, esp temperature ▪ Monitor renal, hepatic, hemopoietic status ▪ Observe for signs of superinfection (diarrhea, itching, oral ulcers) ▪ Urine glucose: false + $\bar{c}$ Clinitest; use Clinistix/Diastix.

EDUCATION: Use Clinistix/Diastix for urine testing ▪ Women: avoid breastfeeding ▪ Diarrhea may occur ▪ Maintain good personal hygiene (esp perineal, oral) ▪ ↑ Fluid intake (8-10 glasses/d) ▪ Notify nurse/physician of symptoms of allergic rx (difficult breathing, rash) ▪ Carry identification (MedicAlert) if cephalosporin allergic ▪ IM injection may be painful.

NOTES:

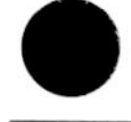

cephradine • (sef-ra-deen)

CATEGORY: *Cephalosporin* (1st generation): antibiotic Rx; Preg Cat B

BRAND NAME
Velosef (Apothecon)

DOSAGE FORMS
Capsule: 250, 500mg
PO suspension: 125, 250mg/5ml
Powder for injection (IM/IV): 0.25, 0.5, 1, 2g

USE: Treatment of infections caused by susceptible strains of *Escherichia coli*, group A β-hemolytic streptococci, *Haemophilus influenzae, Klebsiella* spp, *Proteus mirabilis*, staphylococci (incl penicillinase-producing strains), *Streptococcus pneumoniae*. **ACTION:** Bactericidal activity due to inhibition of mucopeptide cell wall synthesis in susceptible organisms.

PHARMACOKINETICS

PO absorption	Peak	Half-life	Protein binding	Excretion
Rapid	1h	1-2h	8%-17%	90% via urine in 6h as unchanged drug

CONTRAINDICATIONS: Hypersensitivity to any cephalosporin. **CC:** Use may produce pseudomembranous colitis ▪ Use in penicillin-allergic pts requires caution.

DOSAGE

Pediatric	*PO*	25-50mg/kg divided q6-12h. For otitis media, 75-100mg/kg/d divided q6-12h. Do *not* exceed 4g/d
	IM/IV	50-100mg/kg divided qid
Adult	*PO*	250-500mg q6h may be required
	IM/IV	2-4g/d divided qid. Do *not* exceed 4g/d

SIDE/ADVERSE EFFECTS: GI: N/V/D, symptoms of ***pseudomembranous colitis*** ▪ GU: vaginitis ▪ HEM: eosinophilia ▪ HEP: ↑ AST, ALT, BUN ▪ INT: pruritus, urticaria, morbilliform eruptions, ***erythema multiforme***.

INTERACTIONS: Drug: Bacteriostatic antibiotics can antagonize bactericidal activity ▪ Use c̄ PO anticoagulants may ↑ their activity ▪ Use c̄ aminoglycosides may produce additive nephrotoxicity ▪ Use c̄ probenecid ↓ renal excretion. **Lab:** Possible false + c̄ Coombs' test.

NURSING MANAGEMENT PRIORITIES

ADMINISTRATION: Assess for hx of cephalosporin/ penicillin hypersensitivity ▪ Obtain C&S before therapy ▪ Assess renal function; ↓ dosage if impaired ▪ PO: administer 1h ac/2h pc ▪ PO suspension: reconstitute powder according to manufacturer's directions; shake well before using; store reconstituted portion for 7d at room temperature, 14d in refrigerator ▪ IM: reconstitute according to manufacturer's directions; administer by *deep, slow* injection into gluteal UOQ; stable 2h at room temperature, 24h refrigerated ▪ IV: dilute according to manufacturer's directions; inject *slowly* (3-5m); avoid aminoglycoside administration at same site; may administer IVPB, stable 10h at room temperature, 48h refrigerated ▪ Do *not* mix c̄ other injectable antibiotics; avoid Ca^{++} solutions ▪ Do *not* administer precipitated solutions; color change does *not* indicate ↓ potency ▪ Have support equipment available for anaphylaxis ▪ Na^+ content: 6mEq (136mg)/g; calculate in Na^+-restricted diets ▪ Maintain hydration.

EVALUATION: Monitor VS, esp temperature ▪ Monitor hepatic, renal status ▪ Monitor CBC ▪ Urine glucose: false + c̄ Clinitest; use Clinistix/Diastix.

EDUCATION: Complete full course of therapy (usually 10d) even if symptoms subside ▪ Can be taken c̄ meals; *best* on empty stomach ▪ Take at equal intervals around clock to maintain blood levels ▪ Diarrhea may occur ▪ PO suspension: refrigerate; shake well before using ▪ Store in dry, tightly closed container ▪ Discard outdated preparations ▪ Maintain good personal hygiene (esp perineal, oral) ▪ ↑ Fluid intake (8-10 glasses/d) ▪ Use Clinistix/ Diastix for urine testing ▪ Notify physician of symptoms of allergic rx (fever, difficult breathing, rash) ▪ Carry identification (MedicAlert) if cephalosporin allergic.

NOTES:

chlorambucil • (klor-am-byoo-sill)

CATEGORY: *Alkylating agent:* antineoplastic

Rx; Preg Cat D

BRAND NAME
Leukeran (G-W)

DOSAGE FORM
Tablet: 2mg

USE: Treatment of chronic lymphocytic leukemia, malignant lymphomas incl lymphosarcoma, giant follicular lymphoma, Hodgkin's disease. **ACTION:** Antineoplastic activity due to alkylating effect on DNA replication.

PHARMACOKINETICS

PO absorption	Peak	Half-life	Protein binding	Excretion
Complete	1h	1.5h	99%	Very slow via urine as parent drug, metabolites

CONTRAINDICATIONS: Hypersensitivity, prior drug resistance. **CC:** Use can produce severe bone marrow depression, carcinogenic activity.

DOSAGE

Pediatric/Adult *PO* — 0.1-0.2mg/kg as single daily dose for 3-6wks. Usual maintenance dose 0.03-0.1mg/kg/d

SIDE/ADVERSE EFFECTS: GI: *N/V/D,* oral ulcers ▪ GU: sterile cystitis ▪ HEM: ***bone marrow depression*** resulting in neutropenia, thrombocytopenia ▪ HEP: hepatotoxicity ▪ MET: hyperuricemia ▪ Other: ***pulmonary fibrosis,*** drug fever.

INTERACTIONS: Drug: Live vaccines contraindicated during therapy ▪ Radiation/other myelosuppressive drugs will produce additive bone marrow depression.

NURSING MANAGEMENT PRIORITIES

ADMINISTRATION: Assess for hx of hypersensitivity (incl melphalan) ▪ Check hx for recent course of radiation or antineoplastic therapy; report to physician ▪ Avoid exposure to moisture/light in storage ▪ Administer antiemetic before therapy ▪ Force fluids (3000ml/d) ▪ Provide emotional support.

EVALUATION: Monitor CBC throughout therapy ▪ Assess for infection, bleeding, anemia ▪ Assess for ↑ serum uric acid levels ▪ Monitor hepatic function during therapy ▪ Assess hydration status (I&O, daily weight).

EDUCATION: Store in dry, tightly closed, light-resistant container ▪ ↑ Fluid intake (10-12 glasses/d) ▪ Avoid exposure to infection ▪ Check c̄ physician before immunization (pt, family) ▪ Diet as tolerated; avoid spicy foods ▪ Maintain good oral hygiene; use soft-bristled toothbrush ▪ Notify physician of symptoms of bone marrow depression (fever, sore throat, bruising, bleeding, lethargy) ▪ Loss of hair may occur (reversible after therapy) ▪ Compliance c̄ prescribed dosage regimen ▪ Women: avoid breastfeeding ▪ Encourage ventilation of feelings ▪ Use contraception if sexually active ▪ ↓ Fertility in both sexes.

NOTES:

chloramphenicol/chloramphenicol palmitate▲/ chloramphenicol sodium succinate△ • (klor-am-fen-i-kole)

CATEGORY: *Antibiotic*

Rx; Preg Cat NA

BRAND NAMES

Chloromycetin (P-D)
**Chloroptic (Allergan)*
**Fenical (Alcon)*
**Isopto Fenicol (Alcon)*
**Minims (S&N)*
**Novochlorocap (Novopharm)*
**Pentamycetin (Pentagone)*

DOSAGE FORMS

Capsules, ophthalmic drops, ointments, otic drops, PO suspension▲, powder for injection (IV)△, topical cream.

USE: Drug of choice for typhoid fever ▪ Treatment of serious infections caused by susceptible strains of *Haemophilus influenzae & Rickettsia*, lymphogranuloma, psittacosis ▪ Cystic fibrosis regimens ▪ Other susceptible organisms resistant to all other appropriate antimicrobial drugs. **ACTION:** Antimicrobial activity due to inhibition of protein synthesis in susceptible organisms, usually a bacteriostatic effect.

PHARMACOKINETICS

PO absorption	Peak	Half-life	Excretion
Rapid	1-3h	1.5-4.1h	Via urine, feces as metabolites, unchanged drug

CONTRAINDICATIONS: Hypersensitivity, previous chloramphenicol toxicity, any minor infections. **CC:** Fatal blood dyscrasias have occurred c̄ short-term & extended use ▪ Use should be limited to serious infections not responsive to other less toxic antiinfective agents ▪ Use in newborns can cause gray baby syndrome.

DOSAGE

Neonatal	*IV*	25mg/kg/d in 4 doses
Pediatric	*PO*	50mg/kg/d in 4 doses
	IV	50mg/kg/d in 4 doses
Adult	*PO*	50-100mg/kg/d in 4 doses
	IV	50mg/kg/d in 4 doses. Severe infections may require 100mg/kg/d, ⬇ as soon as possible as directed

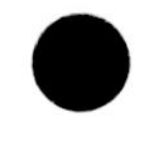

SIDE/ADVERSE EFFECTS: CNS: headache, mild depression, optic/peripheral neuritis ▪ GI: N/V/D, glossitis, stomatitis, enterocolitis ▪ HEM: ***aplastic anemia***, hypoplastic anemia, ***thrombocytopenia***, granulocytopenia, irreversible bone marrow depression ▪ Other: fatal gray baby syndrome in newborn; ⬇ dosage will usually preclude this syndrome.

INTERACTIONS: Drug: Use c̄ PO anticoagulants ⬆ their effects ▪ Avoid use c̄ other bone marrow depressants ▪ Use may ⬇ effects of vitamin B_{12}, folic acid, iron preparations in anemic pts.

NURSING MANAGEMENT PRIORITIES

ADMINISTRATION: Assess for hx of hypersensitivity ▪ Assess hematologic, hepatic, renal function ▪ Obtain C&S before therapy ▪ PO: administer on empty stomach (1h ac/2h pc) c̄ full glass H_2O ▪ IV: dilute; administer *slowly* (over 1m) ▪ Topical: wash, dry area thoroughly before application ▪ Otic: do *not* contaminate dropper ▪ Switch from parenteral to PO dosage form as soon as possible ▪ Na^+ content: 72mg/g; calculate in Na^+-restricted diets.

EVALUATION: Monitor VS, esp temperature; blood glucose in diabetics (hypoglycemia) ▪ Observe for signs of superinfection (diarrhea, perineal itching, oral ulcers) ▪ Assess for bleeding, eye pain, rash; D/C drug, notify physician ▪ Therapeutic blood level: 5-20µg/ml.

EDUCATION: Complete full course of therapy even if symptoms subside ▪ PO: take on empty stomach at equal intervals around clock to maintain blood levels ▪ Unpleasant taste may occur c̄ IV injection ▪ Use Clinistix/Diastix for urine testing ▪ Diarrhea may occur ▪ Maintain fluid intake (6-8 glasses/d) ▪ Notify physician of symptoms of allergic rx (fever, difficult breathing, rash), sore throat, bruising/bleeding ▪ Women: avoid breastfeeding.

NOTES:

chloramphenicol/chloramphenicol palmitate▲/chloramphenicol sodium succinate▲

chlordiazepoxide/chlordiazepoxide hcl▲ • (klor-dye-az-e-pox-ide)

CATEGORY: *Benzodiazepine:* antianxiety agent, anxiolytic Rx C-IV; Preg Cat NA

BRAND NAMES
Libritabs ▲ *(Roche)*
Librium (Roche)

DOSAGE FORMS
Tablet: 10, 25mg
Capsule: 5, 10, 25mg powder for injection (IM/IV): 20mg/ml

COMBINATION PRODUCTS Rx

Librax (Roche)	chlordiazepoxide HCl/clidinium bromide per capsule: 5mg/2.5mg
Limbitrol (Roche)	chlordiazepoxide HCl/amitriptyline HCl per tablet: 5mg/12.5mg
Limbitrol DS (Roche)	chlordiazepoxide HCl/amitriptyline HCl per tablet: 10mg/25mg

USE: Treatment of anxiety, alcoholism withdrawal symptoms. **ACTION:** Benzodiazepines appear to potentiate inhibitory effects of gamma aminobutyric acid (GABA) in central-mediated neurotransmission. Anxiolytic activity due to depression of CNS at brainstem reticular formation, limbic, thalamic areas.

PHARMACOKINETICS

PO absorption	Half-life	Excretion
Very good	24-48h	Via urine as unchanged drug, metabolites

CONTRAINDICATIONS: Hypersensitivity. **CC:** Use can result in dependence, abrupt D/C can result in withdrawal rxs incl seizures ▪ Use not recommended during first trimester of pregnancy ▪ Benzodiazepines are not indicated for psychiatric disorders esp when anxiety is not significant symptom.

DOSAGE

Pediatric	*PO*	>6y/o: 5mg 2-4 times/d. May ↑ to 10mg 2-3 times/d
Adult	*PO*	Mild/moderate anxiety: 5-10mg 3-4 times/d
		Severe anxiety: 20-25mg 3-4 times/d
	IM/IV	Severe anxiety: 50-100mg followed by 25mg 3-4 times/d

Adult	*IM/IV*	Preop: 50-100mg IM before surgery Alcoholism: 50-100mg. May be repeated 2-4h prn. Do *not* exceed 300mg/24h
Combination products		1-2 capsules/tablets 3-4 times/d

SIDE/ADVERSE EFFECTS: CNS: drowsiness, ataxia, confusion (esp in geriatric, debilitated pts), extrapyramidal symptoms, EEG pattern changes ■ HEM: ***agranulocytosis*** ■ HEP: jaundice, liver dysfunction.

INTERACTIONS: Drug: Use c̄ other CNS depressants produces additive effects ■ Use c̄ MAO-I can produce serious toxic effects.

NURSING MANAGEMENT PRIORITIES

ADMINISTRATION: Assess for hx of benzodiazepine hypersensitivity ■ Do *not* mix parenteral preparations due to incompatibility ■ IM: add 2ml special diluent to contents of ampule; avoid excessive pressure in injecting diluent to prevent bubbles; agitate gently until all powder is dissolved; inject *deep, slowly* into UOQ ■ IV: add 5ml sterile H_2O for injection/normal saline solution, agitate until all powder is dissolved; do *not* use this solution for IM administration ■ Parenteral: keep pt recumbent for 3h ■ Avoid exposure to moisture/light in storage (PO form) ■ Prepare parenteral solutions immediately before administration; discard unused portion ■ Avoid abrupt withdrawal ■ Have emergency support measures available ■ Elderly may require ↓ dosage ■ Problem discussion, sympathetic listening contribute to relief of anxiety.

EVALUATION: Monitor renal, hepatic status ■ Assess for symptoms of abrupt withdrawal (tremors, abdominal/muscle cramps, convulsions) c̄ prolonged use ■ Check for signs of dependence (↑ drug request) ■ Monitor activity status (safety precautions) ■ Assess for tolerance to therapeutic dose ■ Assess for paradoxic rxs (CNS stimulation), esp in elderly ■ Check for depression; suicide precautions prn ■ Monitor serum for ↑ alkaline phosphatase, AST, ALT ■ False + pregnancy test (Gravindex).

EDUCATION: Drowsiness may occur; use caution in potentially hazardous activities ■ Avoid use c̄ alcohol, other CNS depressants ■ Indiscriminate use may lead to dependence ■ Do *not* keep at bedside ■ Take as ordered by physicians; do *not* ↑ dose ■ Check c̄ physician/pharmacist before taking OTC preparations ■ Women: avoid breastfeeding ■ Practice relaxation exercises, ventilation of feelings.

NOTES:

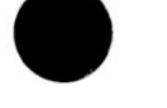

chlorothiazide/chlorothiazide sodium▲/hydrochlorothiazide •

(klor-oh-thye-a-zide/hye-droe-klor-oh-thye-a-zide)

CATEGORY: *Thiazide diuretic:* antihypertensive

Rx; Preg Cat NA

BRAND NAMES	DOSAGE FORMS
chlorothiazide	
Diuril (Merck) (Frosst [Canada])	PO suspension: 250mg/5ml Injection (IV)▲: 0.5g/vial Tablet: 250, 500mg
hydrochlorothiazide	
Esidrix (C-G)	Tablet: 25, 50
HydroDIURIL (Merck)	Tablet: 25, 50, 100mg
Oretic (Abbott)	Tablet: 25, 50mg

USE: Treatment of hypertension as sole agent/ in combination c̄ other antihypertensives ▪ Treatment of edema due to renal dysfunction ▪ Adjunct in treating edema due to CHF, hepatic cirrhosis, corticosteroids/ estrogen therapy. **ACTION:** Diuretic activity due to inhibition of Na^+ reabsorption, primarily in ascending limb of loop of Henle & early distal tubule of nephron; K^+, bicarbonate, other ions excreted w/out significant alteration of urine pH; antihypertensive activity due to ⬇ of peripheral vascular resistance.

CONTRAINDICATIONS: Hypersensitivity due to any thiazide, other sulfonamide-derivative drugs, anuria. **CC:** IV chlorothiazide use *not* recommended for infants, children.

DOSAGE

chlorothiazide

Pediatric	*PO*	<6mo: 15mg/lb/d in 2 doses <2y/o: 125-375mg/d in 2 doses 2-12y/o: 375mg-1g/d in 2 doses
Adult	*PO*	0.5-2g, usually divided
	IV	0.5-1g/d divided

PHARMACOKINETICS

	PO absorption	Onset	Peak	Duration	Excretion
chlorothiazide	Incomplete	2h	4h	6-12h	Via urine as unchanged drug
hydrochlorothiazide	Good	2h	4h	6-12h	Via urine as unchanged drug

Note: Side/adverse effects: common in *italic;* serious in ***boldface italic.***

▲Available in Canada only.

Pediatric	*PO*	<6 mo: 1.5 mg/lb/d in 2 doses <2 y/o: 12.5-37.5 mg/d in 2 doses 2-12y/o: 37.5-100 mg/d in 2 doses
Adult	*PO*	25-200 mg/d, usually divided

SIDE/ADVERSE EFFECTS: CNS: *dizziness*, vertigo, paresthesia, headache ▪ EENT: blurred vision, xanthopsia ▪ GI: anorexia, gastric irritation, N/V/D, jaundice ▪ HEM: ***agranulocytosis, aplastic anemia***, leukopenia, ***thrombocytopenia*** ▪ INT: purpura, urticaria, photosensitivity ▪ MET: hypokalemia, glycosuria, hyperglycemia ▪ MS: *fatigue, leg cramps* ▪ RESP: respiratory distress. ▪ Other: necrotizing angiitis

INTERACTIONS: Drug: ↑ Dig toxicity due to hypokalemia ▪ Use c̄ corticosteroids ↑ hypokalemia ▪ Antidiabetic agents may require dose adjustment ▪ Use c̄ diazoxide can produce significant diabetogenic effects ▪ Use c̄ lithium requires monitoring lithium levels. **Food:** Excessive consumption of licorice ↑ hypokalemia.

NURSING MANAGEMENT PRIORITIES

ADMINISTRATION: Assess for hx of thiazide/sulfonamide hypersensitivity ▪ Administer c̄ food/milk on arising ▪ Do *not* administer SC/IM ▪ IV: reconstitute c̄ 18ml sterile H_2O for injection, shake to dissolve; compatible c̄ D_5W, NaCl solutions; administer *slowly* (2m); stable for 24h at room temperature; *not* compatible c̄ whole blood/derivatives ▪ Assess serum K^+ (normal: 3.5-5mEq/L) ▪ Elderly may require ↓ dosage.

EVALUATION: Monitor VS, esp BP, pulse; serum for ↑ BUN, creatinine, uric acid; ↓ K^+; fluid retention (I&O, daily weight) ▪ Diabetics: closely monitor blood glucose (hyperglycemia).

EDUCATION: Expect ↑ urine output; have bathroom facilities easily accessible ▪ May cause lethargy ▪ Take PO forms c̄ food ▪ Take on waking, at same time qd ▪ Take even if symptom free ▪ Notify physician of signs of hypokalemia (muscle cramps, lethargy, nausea) ▪ Avoid changing positions (lying/sitting/standing) rapidly ▪ Take as directed by physician; do *not* skip doses ▪ Eat foods high in K^+ (bananas, fruit juices); avoid black licorice ▪ Avoid high-Na^+ foods ▪ Avoid exposure to direct sunlight, UV light ▪ Diabetics: check blood/urine glucose ▪ Avoid smoking ▪ Use sugarless gum/hard candy to diminish dry mouth.

NOTES:

chlorotrianisene • (klor-oh-trye-an-i-seen)

CATEGORY: *Estrogenic agent*

Rx; Preg Cat X

BRAND NAME
TACE (MMD)
(Merrell [Canada])

DOSAGE FORMS
Capsule: 12, 25mg

USE: Prevention of postpartum breast enlargement ▪ Treatment of moderate/severe symptoms associated c̄ menopause ▪ Treatment of atrophic vaginitis, kraurosis, female hypogonadism, prostatic cancer. **ACTION:** Estrogens are required for development & maintenance of female reproductive system, 2° sex characteristics.

PHARMACOKINETICS: Not available.

CONTRAINDICATIONS: Known/suspected pregnancy, estrogen-dependent neoplasia, breast cancer except in appropriately selected pts; abnormal genital bleeding, active thrombophlebitis, thromboembolic disorders or c̄ hx that was estrogen associated (except for breast/prostatic cancer treatment). **CC:** Estrogenic agents have been reported to ↑ risk of endometrial cancer, gallbladder disease.

DOSAGE

Adult *PO*

Postpartum breast enlargement: 12mg qid for 7d or 50mg q6h for 6 doses or 72mg bid for 2d. First dose w/in 8h after delivery
Menopause: 12-25mg/d administered cyclically (3wks on, 1wk off). Attempts to D/C/taper dosage should be made at 3-6mo intervals
Atrophic vaginitis, kraurosis vulvae: 12-25mg/d administered cyclically for 30-60d
Hypogonadism: 12-25mg/d for 21d
Prostatic cancer: 12-25mg/d

SIDE/ADVERSE EFFECTS: CNS: headache, migraine, dizziness, mental depression ▪ EENT: intolerance to contact lens, steepening of corneal curvature ▪ GI: N/V, abdominal cramps, bloating ▪ GU: amenorrhea, breakthrough bleeding, dysmenorrhea, candidiasis, change in menstrual flow, spotting, ↑ uterine fibromyoma size ▪ INT: melasma, ***erythema multiforme***, erythema nodosum, alopecia, hirsutism, urticaria ▪ Other: weight changes, edema, ↓ carbohydrate tolerance, porphyria exacerbation.

INTERACTIONS: Drug: Use c̄ TCAs may result in toxic rxs.

NOTES:

NURSING MANAGEMENT PRIORITIES

ADMINISTRATION: Assess for hx of estrogen hypersensitivity ▪ Administer c̄ food ▪ Do *not* crush capsule; administer whole ▪ Avoid abrupt withdrawal ▪ Avoid exposure to heat/moisture in storage.

EVALUATION: Monitor hepatic, renal status ▪ Monitor BP ▪ Assess for endometrial cancer (Pap test, physical exam) ▪ Monitor PT; may ↓ anticoagulant effect ▪ Diabetics: careful urine testing; may ↓ antidiabetic drug effect ▪ Assess for behavior changes, depression ▪ Monitor pt weight; observe for edema.

EDUCATION: Review package insert c̄ pt ▪ Nausea may occur during first 2wks of therapy ▪ Women: avoid pregnancy, breastfeeding ▪ Breast self-exam (incl male pts) ▪ Avoid smoking (↑ CV complications) ▪ Take c̄ food ▪ Notify physician/dentist of use before treatment ▪ Keep scheduled appointments c̄ physician ▪ Avoid direct sunlight/UV light ▪ D/C drug, notify physician if pregnancy suspected ▪ Notify physician *immediately* of chest/leg pain, unusual vaginal bleeding, difficult breathing, slurred speech ▪ Men: enlarged breasts, impotence are reversible after therapy ▪ Check weight, swelling in feet/legs daily.

chlorpromazine*/chlorpromazine hcl • (klor-proe-ma-zeen)

CATEGORY: *Phenothiazine:* antipsychotic, neuroleptic Rx; Preg Cat NA

BRAND NAME
Thorazine (SKB)

DOSAGE FORMS
Injection, concentrate, suppository*, capsule, syrup, tablet

USE: Treatment of psychotic states, pediatric behavioral problems ▪ Treatment of intractable hiccups, acute intermittent porphyria, nausea. **ACTION:** Antipsychotic activity appears associated c̄ ↓ neural transmission in central dopamine-dependent pathways, resulting in tranquilizing effect in psychotic pts; drug also exhibits anti-α adrenergic, anticholinergic, antiemetic, antiserotonin, ganglionic blocking activity.

PHARMACOKINETICS: PO onset of 30-40m, peak in 4-6h.

CONTRAINDICATIONS: Hypersensitivity, comatose states, bone marrow depression, presence of large amounts of CNS depressants. **CC:** Extended use will produce extrapyramidal systems, tardive dyskinesia.

DOSAGE

Psychiatric			
	Pediatric	*PO*	50-200mg/d
		IM	≤5y/o: 40mg/d; 5-12y/o: 75mg/d
	Adult	*PO*	30-1000mg or more/d
		IM	25mg, then 25-50mg in 1h
Nausea/vomiting			
	Pediatric	*PO*	0.25mg/lb q4-6h
		IM/Rectal	0.25mg/lb q6-8h
	Adult	*PO*	10-25mg q4-6h
		IM	25mg, then 25-50mg q3-4h
		Rectal	100mg q6-8h
Hiccups			
	Adult	*PO*	25-50mg 3-4 times/d
		IM	25-50mg 3-4 times/d
Porphyria			
	Adult	*PO*	25-50mg 3-4 times/d
		IM	25mg 3-4 times/d
Preop			
	Pediatric	*PO*	0.25mg/lb 2-3h before surgery
		IM	0.25mg/lb 1-2h before surgery
	Adult	*PO*	25-50mg 2-3h before surgery
		IM	12.5-25mg 1-2h before surgery

SIDE/ADVERSE EFFECTS: CNS: drowsiness, extrapyramidal rxs, tardive dyskinesia ▪ CV: postural hypotension, tachycardia, ECG changes in Q, T waves ▪ EENT: blurred vision, corneal/lenticular changes, epithelial keratopathy, nasal congestion ▪ END: lactation, moderate breast enlargement in female pts ▪ HEM: ***agranulocytosis***, eosinophilia, leukopenia, ***hemolytic anemia***, thrombocytopenic purpura ▪ HEP: cholestatic jaundice ▪ INT: urticaria, photosensitivity ▪ PSYCH: adverse behavioral changes ▪ Other: fever, hyperpyrexia, neuroleptic malignant syndrome, hypothermia.

INTERACTIONS: Drug: Aluminum-magnesium antacid preparations ↓ absorption ▪ Use c̄ narcotics, barbiturates, other CNS depressants ↑ CNS depression ▪ Guanethidine, related antihypertensives antagonized.

NURSING MANAGEMENT PRIORITIES

ADMINISTRATION: Assess for hx of phenothiazine hypersensitivity ▪ Assess VS, esp BP ▪ PO: administer c̄ food; do *not* crush/break SR capsules ▪ PO concentrate: dilute before administration c̄ >60ml fluid ▪ Syrup: shake well before using ▪ IM: inject *slowly, deep* into UOQ; keep pt lying down for 30m after injection ▪ Avoid SC injection ▪ IV: dilute according to manufacturer's directions; inject 1mg/m; maintain pt in supine position for 30m ▪ Discard discolored/precipitated solution ▪ Avoid exposure to moisture/light in storage ▪ Store suppositories at room temperature ▪ Avoid skin contact c̄ liquid forms (contact dermatitis) ▪ Avoid abrupt withdrawal ▪ Maintain hydration ▪ Elderly/debilitated may require ↓ dosage.

EVALUATION: Monitor hepatic, ophthalmic, renal status ▪ Monitor BP, CBC, fluid retention (I&O, daily weight), constipation ▪ Assess for extrapyramidal rx ▪ Seizure precautions in pts c̄ hx of convulsive disorders ▪ Long-term therapy: assess for jaundice, agranulocytosis.

EDUCATION: Dizziness/drowsiness may occur; use caution in potentially hazardous activities ▪ Avoid changing positions (lying/sitting/standing) rapidly ▪ Avoid use of alcohol, other CNS depressants ▪ Store in tightly closed, light-resistant container ▪ Use sugarless gum/hard candy to diminish dry mouth ▪ Constipation may occur; ↑ fluids, bulk-containing foods ▪ May turn urine pink/red/brown ▪ Avoid contact c̄ liquid forms ▪ Women: avoid breastfeeding ▪ Take PO forms c̄ food; swallow SR capsules whole ▪ Avoid exposure to direct sunlight, UV light ▪ Notify physician of fever, sore throat, bruising/bleeding, tics/spasms, trembling, shuffling gait ▪ Avoid ↑ exercise, temperature extremes ▪ Check c̄ physician before taking OTC preparations ▪ Do *not* take antacids/antidiarrheals w/in 2h of drug ▪ Full drug effects may require several wks of therapy.

chlorthalidone • (klor-thal-i-doan)

CATEGORY: *Diuretic:* antihypertensive

Rx; Preg Cat B

BRAND NAMES

**Apo-Chlorothalidone (Apotex)*
Hygroton (RPR) (Geigy [Canada])
Thalitone (Horus)
**Novothalidone (Novopharm)*
**Uridon (ICN)*

DOSAGE FORMS

Tablet: 15, 25, 50, 100mg

USE: Treatment of hypertension as sole agent/in combination c̄ other antihypertensives ▪ Treatment of edema due to renal dysfunction ▪ Adjunct in treating edema due to CHF, hepatic cirrhosis, corticosteroid, or estrogen therapy ▪ Investigational treatment of systolic hypertension. **ACTION:** Diuretic activity due to excretion of H_2O, Na^+, Cl^-, other electrolytes by inhibiting tubular reabsorption.

PHARMACOKINETICS

PO absorption	Onset	Duration	Half-life	Protein binding	Excretion
Good	2.6h	Up to 72h	40h	75%	Via urine primarily as unchanged drug

CONTRAINDICATIONS: Hypersensitivity due to any thiazide or other sulfonamide-derivative drugs, anuria. **CC:** Use c̄ caution in pts c̄ hx of bronchial asthma, liver, renal disease.

DOSAGE

Pediatric	*PO*	2mg/kg 3 times/wk
Adult	*PO*	50-100mg qd or 100mg on alternate days; 200mg qd may be needed

Note: Side/adverse effects: common in *italic;* serious in ***boldface italic.***

*Available in Canada only.

SIDE/ADVERSE EFFECTS: CNS: drowsiness, vertigo, paresthesia, headache ▪ EENT: blurred vision, xanthopsia ▪ GI: anorexia, gastric irritation, N/V/D, jaundice, ***pancreatitis*** ▪ HEM: ***agranulocytosis, aplastic anemia***, leukopenia, ***thrombocytopenia*** ▪ INT: purpura, urticaria, photosensitivity ▪ MET: ***hypokalemia***, glycosuria, hyperglycemia ▪ MS: *fatigue, leg cramps* ▪ Other: necrotizing angiitis, respiratory distress.

INTERACTIONS: Drug: ↑ Dig toxicity due to hypokalemia ▪ Use c̄ corticosteroids produces ↑ hypokalemia ▪ Antidiabetic agents may require dose adjustments ▪ Use c̄ diazoxide can produce significant diabetogenic effects.

NURSING MANAGEMENT PRIORITIES

ADMINISTRATION: Assess for hx of hypersensitivity (incl sulfonamides) ▪ Assess renal function; do *not* administer if impaired ▪ Administer c̄ food or milk on arising ▪ Assess serum K^+ (normal: 3.5-5mEq/L) ▪ Elderly may require ↓ dosage.

EVALUATION: Monitor F/E, hepatic, renal status ▪ Monitor VS, esp BP, pulse ▪ Monitor serum for ↑ BUN, creatinine, uric acid, ↓ K^+ ▪ Diabetics: closely monitor blood glucose (hyperglycemia) ▪ Monitor fluid retention (I&O, daily weight) ▪ Monitor digitalized pts closely (↓ K^+: ↑ dig toxicity).

EDUCATION: Expect ↑ urine output; have bathroom facilities easily accessible ▪ May cause weakness, lethargy ▪ Take c̄ food ▪ Take on waking, at same time qd ▪ Take even if symptom free ▪ Used to control, *not* cure, hypertension ▪ Notify physician of signs of hypokalemia (muscle cramps, lethargy, nausea) ▪ Avoid changing positions (lying/sitting/standing) rapidly ▪ Take as directed by physician; do *not* skip doses ▪ Eat foods high in K^+ (bananas, fruit juices, raisins); avoid black licorice ▪ Avoid high-Na^+ foods (canned soups, lunch meats, cheese) ▪ Maintain optimum weight ▪ Avoid exposure to direct sunlight/UV light ▪ Diabetics: check blood/urine glucose carefully ▪ Avoid smoking ▪ Use sugarless gum/hard candy to diminish dry mouth.

NOTES:

chlorzoxazone/cyclobenzaprine hcl • (klor-zox-a-zone/sye-kloe-ben-za-preen)

CATEGORY: *Skeletal muscle relaxant*

Rx; Preg Cat NA/B

BRAND NAMES	**DOSAGE FORMS**
chlorzoxazone	
Paraflex (McNeil)	Tablet: 250mg
Parafon Forte DSC (McNeil)	Tablet: 500mg
cyclobenzaprine	
Flexeril (Merck)	Tablet: 10mg

USE: Adjunct to relief of discomfort associated c̄ acute painful muscular conditions. **ACTION:** Exact mechanism of action not determined. Drugs are CNS depressants that appear to act primarily w/in spinal cord. Cyclobenzaprine is structurally similar to TCAs & possesses anticholinergic activity.

PHARMACOKINETICS

PO absorption	Onset	Peak	Duration	Excretion
chlorzoxazone				
Complete	1h	3-4h	3-4h	Via urine as metabolites
cyclobenzaprine				
Complete	1h	—	12-24h	Via feces, urine as metabolites

CONTRAINDICATIONS: Hypersensitivity. In addition, cyclobenzaprine is contraindicated c̄ arrhythmias, heart block/conduction disturbances, recovery phase of MI, concurrent use c̄ MAO-I or w/in 14d of their discontinuance. **CC:** chlorzoxazone: Use has been associated c̄ rare cases of serious hepatocellular toxicity ▪ cyclobenzaprine: TCAs have been reported to produce arrhythmias, MI, stroke.

DOSAGE

chlorzoxazone		
Pediatric	*PO*	125-500mg 3-4 times/d according to age, weight
Adult	*PO*	250-500mg 3-4 times/d or 750mg 3-4 times/d. Maintenance dose after improvement, 250mg 3-4 times/d
Parafon Forte		
Adult	*PO*	1 tablet (caplet) 3-4 times/d
cyclobenzaprine		
Adult	*PO*	10mg tid c̄ a range of 20-40mg/d for 2-3wks. Do *not* exceed 60mg/d

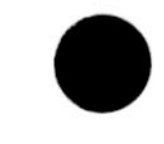

SIDE/ADVERSE EFFECTS: CNS: drowsiness, dizziness ▪ GI: some disturbances, rare bleeding ▪ INT: rash, petechiae, ecchymoses; angioneurotic edema ▪ Other: urine discoloration, malaise, hepatotoxicity.

INTERACTIONS: Drug: chlorzoxapine: Use c̄ CNS depressants will result in additive depression. cyclobenzaprine: Use/sequential use (w/in 14d) c̄ MAO-I may cause significant hyperpyretic rx ▪ Use c̄ anticholinergics, CNS depressants produces additive effects ▪ Use c̄ guanethidinelike drugs produces ⬇ antihypertensive effects.

NURSING MANAGEMENT PRIORITIES

ADMINISTRATION: Assess for hx of hypersensitivity ▪ Administer c̄ meals; tablets can be crushed/mixed c̄ food/liquid ▪ Avoid exposure to moisture in storage ▪ Elderly may require ⬇ dosage.

EVALUATION: Monitor hepatic status ▪ Monitor activity status (safety precautions) ▪ Assess for sensitivity rx (urticaria, skin redness, itching), liver dysfunction (jaundice, dark urine); D/C if present.

EDUCATION: Drowsiness may occur; use caution when engaging in potentially hazardous activities ▪ Avoid use c̄ alcohol, other CNS depressants ▪ Take c̄ food to ⬇ GI distress ▪ Rest, physical therapy will promote comfort ▪ May turn urine orange or red-purple.

OVERDOSE MANAGEMENT: Principal symptoms: N/V, loss of muscle movement/deep tendon reflexes, respiratory depression ▪ Emergency treatment: remove drug by lavage or emesis, followed by activated charcoal; maintain respiration; administer IV fluids; maintain adequate BP; analeptic drugs are of no value.

NOTES:

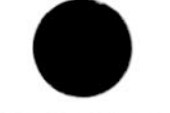

cholestyramine resin • (koe-less-tear-a-meen)

CATEGORY: *Antilipemic:* ion-exchange resin

Rx; Preg Cat C

BRAND NAMES

Questran (B-MS) (Bristol [Canada])

Questran Light (Bristol)

DOSAGE FORMS

Powder: 378-g cans, 9-g single-dose packets (9g powder contains 4g resin)

Tablet: 1g

5-g single-dose packets

Powder: 210g/can

USE: Adjunct management of type II hyperlipoproteinemia (LDL) ▪ Relief of pruritus associated c̄ partial biliary obstruction. **ACTION:** Resin binds bile acids in intestine to form insoluble complex, preventing reabsorption; loss of bile acids leads to ↑ oxidation of cholesterol, ↓ serum levels of cholesterol, β lipoproteins.

PHARMACOKINETICS: Drug not absorbed.

CONTRAINDICATIONS: Hypersensitivity, complete biliary obstruction or where bile is not secreted into the intestine. **CC:** Light powder formulations contain 16.8mg of phenylalanine per 5g & are not suitable for use c̄ phenylkentonuria pts.

DOSAGE

Adult *PO*

Light powder	10-20g/d in 2 divided doses or administered in 1-6 divided doses qd. Do *not* exceed 30g/d
Regular powder	18-36g/d in 2 divided doses or administered in 1-6 divided doses qd. Do *not* exceed 36g/d
Tablet	8-16/d in 2 divided doses or administered in 1-6 divided doses qd. Do *not* exceed 24g/d

SIDE/ADVERSE EFFECTS: CNS: headache ▪ EENT: tinnitus, night blindness ▪ GI: *constipation*, N/V, anorexia, flatulence, bleeding, bloating, steatorrhea ▪ MS: osteoporosis ▪ Other: burnt odor to urine, urticaria.

INTERACTIONS: Drugs: All drugs should be administered 1h before/4-6h after cholestyramine administration ▪ ↓ Fat-soluble vitamin absorption c̄ extremely high doses.

NURSING MANAGEMENT PRIORITIES

ADMINISTRATION: Assess for hx of hypersensitivity ▪ Assess serum cholesterol, triglyceride levels ▪ Administer ac ▪ Place dose on surface of 4-6oz liquid, allow to stand for several minutes while swirling glass; stir, administer to pt; rinse glass c̄ more liquid, administer ▪ Avoid exposure to heat/light in storage ▪ Administer other medication 1h before/4-6h after.

EVALUATION: Monitor GI status ▪ Monitor elderly for GI irritation ▪ Monitor PT if taking PO anticoagulants; may potentiate bleeding ▪ Digitalized pts: maintain dig levels during therapy, after D/C (⬇ absorption) ▪ Monitor serum triglyceride levels.

EDUCATION: Constipation/bad taste may occur ▪ Take ac ▪ Mix c̄ liquid, take drug; rinse glass c̄ liquid, drink; *never* take dry ▪ Follow prescribed diet (antihyperlipidemic) ▪ Check c̄ physician before taking any medication/OTC preparations ▪ Notify physician of changes in bowel function, bruising, bleeding ▪ ⬆ Fluid intake (8-10 glasses/d), ⬆ fiber in diet ▪ Do *not* skip doses ▪ Store in original container ▪ Take other medications 1h before/4-6h after.

NOTES:

Drug:

CATEGORY: Preg Cat:

BRAND NAME **DOSAGE FORMS** **DOSAGE:**

USE/ACTION:

SIDE/ADVERSE EFFECTS:

PHARMACOKINETICS:

INTERACTIONS: Drug:
Food:
Lab:

CONTRAINDICATIONS:

CC:

Note: Side/adverse effects; common in *italic*; serious in ***boldface italic.***

*Available in Canada only.

NURSING MANAGEMENT PRIORITIES
ADMINISTRATION:

NOTES:

EVALUATION:

EDUCATION:

OVERDOSE MANAGEMENT:

cisplatin • (sis-pla-tin)

CATEGORY: *Alkylating agent:* antineoplastic Rx; Preg Cat D

BRAND NAMES
Platinol (BM-ONC)
(Bristol [Canada])
Platinol AQ (BM-ONC)

DOSAGE FORMS
Powder for injection (IV)
10, 50mg/vial
Injection: 1mg/ml in 50-, 100-mg multidose vials

USE: Treatment of metastatic tumors of testes/ovaries, advanced bladder cancer. **ACTION:** Antineoplastic activity due to alkylating effect on DNA replication; bifunctional activity causes interstrand cross-linking of DNA.

PHARMACOKINETICS: Initial half-life 25-49m; postdistribution half-life 58-73h; approximately 27%-40% of drug excreted via urine in 5d.

CONTRAINDICATIONS: Hypersensitivity to drug/platinum, myelosuppression, renal/hearing impairment. **CC:** Use requires qualified physician ▪ Severe cumulative myelosuppression & renal toxicity ▪ High emetogenic activity ▪ Use multidose injection formulation c̄ caution to preclude overdosage; inform physician if dose >100mg/m²/cycle.

DOSAGE

Pediatric/Adult *IV*

Testicular cancer	20mg/m²/d for 5d q3wks for 3 courses, c̄ bleomycin sulfate 30U IV weekly on day 2 of each wk for 12 consecutive doses, vinblastine sulfate 0.15-0.2mg/kg IV on days 1, 2 q3wks for 4 courses
Ovarian cancer	Single agent: 100mg/m² once q4wks Therapy: 50mg/m² once q3wks, c̄ doxorubicin 50mg/m² IV once q3wks on day 1
Bladder cancer	50-70mg/m² IV once q3-4wks

SIDE/ADVERSE EFFECTS: CNS: peripheral neuropathy ▪ EENT: *ototoxicity* (up to 31% of pts c̄ single dose) ▪ GI: N/V, anorexia ▪ GU: dose-related ***nephrotoxicity*** (most limiting), more pronounced c̄ repeated treatment, hyperuricemia ▪ HEM: *leukopenia,* ***thrombocytopenia.***

Note: Side/adverse effects: common in *italic;* serious in ***boldface italic***

*Available in Canada only.

INTERACTIONS: Drug: Live vaccines contraindicated during therapy ▪ Radiation, other myelosuppressive drugs produce additive bone marrow depression ▪ Ototoxic/nephrotoxic drugs produce additive toxicity.

NURSING MANAGEMENT PRIORITIES

ADMINISTRATION: Reconstitute powder for injection c̄ 10ml sterile H_2O (10-mg vial) or 50ml (50-mg vial); produces 1mg/ml dilution ▪ Reconstituted solution stable for 20h at room temperature; do *not* refrigerate (precipitation) ▪ Administer antiemetic before therapy ▪ Administer IV fluids, mannitol 4h before, 24h after therapy to ensure urine output 100ml/h ▪ Administer by infusion over 6-8h ▪ Avoid using needles/IV sets c̄ aluminum-containing parts; precipitate will form c̄ drug contact ▪ Provide emotional support.

EVALUATION: Assess for hearing dysfunction ▪ Check IV site closely; avoid extravasation ▪ Assess serum for ↑ BUN, AST, ALT, creatinine ▪ Monitor neurologic, hepatic, renal function ▪ Assess for anaphylactic rxs; have support equipment available ▪ Monitor CBC throughout therapy, esp platelets ▪ Assess for ↑ serum uric acid levels ▪ Assess for infection, bleeding, anemia ▪ Assess hydration status (I&O, daily weight).

EDUCATION: ↑ Fluid intake (10-12 glasses/d) ▪ Avoid exposure to infection ▪ Check c̄ physician before immunization (pt, family) ▪ Diet as tolerated; avoid spicy foods ▪ Maintain good oral hygiene; use soft-bristled toothbrush ▪ Notify physician of symptoms of bone marrow depression (fever, sore throat, bruising, bleeding, lethargy) ▪ Report hearing difficulties to physician at once ▪ Women: avoid breastfeeding ▪ Encourage ventilation of feelings ▪ Use contraception if sexually active.

NOTES:

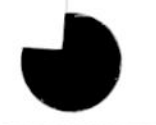

clarithromycin • (klah-rith-roe-mye-sin)

CATEGORY: *Antibiotic:* macrolide antibiotic (semisynthetic) Rx; Preg Cat C

BRAND NAME
Biaxin (Abbott)

DOSAGE FORMS
Tablet: 250, 500mg
PO suspension: 125, 250mg/5ml

USE: Treatment of infections caused by susceptible strains of *Haemophilus influenzae, Moraxella catarrhalis, Mycoplasma pneumoniae, Staphylococcus aureus, Streptococcus pneumoniae, S. pyogenes* ▪ Disseminated mycobacterial infections due to *Mycobacterium avium* & *M. intracellulare.* ▪ In combination c̄ omeprazole for treatment of duodenal ulcers associated c̄ *Helicobacter pylori.*
ACTION: Bacteriostatic activity due to inhibition of ribosomal protein synthesis in microorganisms.

PHARMACOKINETICS

PO absorption	Peak	Half-life	Excretion
50%	2h	3-7h	Via urine, feces as unchanged drug, metabolites

CONTRAINDICATIONS: Hypersensitivity to drugs or other macrolide antibiotics, terfenadine c̄ preexisting cardiac disorders. **CC:** Use during pregnancy should be limited to clinical infections for which no alternative treatment is appropriate ▪ Use can produce pseudomembranous colitis ▪ Use in pts c̄ severe renal impairment requires a ⬇ dosage schedule ▪ Treatment of mycobacterial infections should be life-long if clinical & mycobacterial improvement are present.

DOSAGE

Pediatric	*PO*	15mg/kg/d divided q12h for 10d. For mycobacterium infections, 7.5 mg/kg bid not to exceed 1g/d
Adults/Children ≥12y/o	*PO*	250mg q12h. Lower respiratory tract infections, acute sinusitis, mycobacterium infections usually require 500mg q12h
Ulcers		500mg tid c̄ 40mg of omeprazole qAM for 14d, then 20mg omeprazole qAM for 14 more days

Note: Side/adverse effects: common in *italic;* serious in ***boldface italic.***

*Available in Canada only.

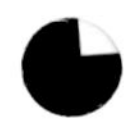

SIDE/ADVERSE EFFECTS: CNS: headache ▪ GI: N/D, abnormal taste, dyspepsia, abdominal discomfort/pain, ***pseudomembranous colitis***.

INTERACTIONS: Drug: Bacteriostatic antibiotics can antagonize effects of bactericidal antibiotics ▪ Use c̄ carbamazepine, dig, PO anticoagulants, theophylline can ↑ their toxicity ▪ Use c̄ astemizole not recommended ▪ Use c̄ cisapride can produce fatal cardiac arrhythmias. **Lab:** ↑ Alkaline phosphatase, ALT, AST, LDH serum levels.

NURSING MANAGEMENT PRIORITIES

ADMINISTRATION: Assess for hx of macrolide hypersensitivity, incl erythromycin ▪ Obtain C&S before therapy ▪ May administer w/out regard to meals ▪ Shake suspension well before administering ▪ Elderly, pts c̄ severe renal impairment may require ↓ dosage.

EVALUATION: Monitor VS, esp temperature ▪ Monitor renal status; may require ↓ dosage if severely impaired ▪ Observe for signs of superinfection (diarrhea, perineal itching, oral ulcers).

EDUCATION: Complete full course of therapy ▪ May be taken w/out regard to meals ▪ Take at equal intervals around clock to maintain blood levels ▪ Diarrhea may occur ▪ Women: avoid breastfeeding.

NOTES:

clofibrate • (kloe-fye-brate)

CATEGORY: *Antilipemic:* antilipidemic agent

Rx; Preg Cat C

BRAND NAMES
Atromid-S (W-A)
**Claripex (ICN);*
**Novofibrate (Novopharm)*

DOSAGE FORM
Capsule: 500mg

USE: Drug of choice for type III hyperlipoproteinemia ▪ Treatment of types IV/V hyperlipoproteinemia. **ACTION:** Antilipemic mechanism not determined.

PHARMACOKINETICS

PO absorption	Protein binding	Excretion
Good	>95%	Via urine primarily as metabolites

CONTRAINDICATIONS: Hypersensitivity, pregnant/nursing mothers, significant hepatic/renal dysfunction, primary biliary cirrhosis. **CC:** Drug exhibits rodent tumorigenicity activity ▪ Use can ⬆ risk of cholelithiasis, malignancies ▪ Use c̄ PO anticoagulants usually requires a 50% ⬇ in dosage.

DOSAGE

Adult *PO* — Usual dose 2g/d divided

SIDE/ADVERSE EFFECTS: CNS: drowsiness, dizziness, headache ▪ CV: ***cardiac arrhythmias*** ▪ GI: *nausea,* V/D, upset, gallstones, stomatitis, polyphagia ▪ GU: impotence, dysuria, hematuria, proteinuria, ⬇ urine output ▪ HEM: leukopenia ▪ INT: rash, pruritus, urticaria, alopecia ▪ MS: myalgia, arthralgia.

INTERACTIONS: Drug: Use c̄ PO anticoagulants ⬆ their activity, requires dosage adjustment ▪ Furosemide may displace clofibrate from inactive storage sites.

NURSING MANAGEMENT PRIORITIES

ADMINISTRATION: Assess for hx of hypersensitivity ▪ Assess serum cholesterol, triglyceride levels ▪ Administer c̄ meals to ⬇ GI distress ▪ Assess hepatic, renal function; use c̄ caution if impaired ▪ Avoid exposure to light in storage.

Note: Side/adverse effects: common in *italic;* serious in ***boldface italic***

*Available in Canada only.

EVALUATION: Monitor hepatic, renal status ▪ Monitor serum triglyceride levels ▪ Diabetics: closely monitor blood glucose (hypoglycemia) ▪ Monitor pt taking PO anticoagulants; may potentiate bleeding.

EDUCATION: Take c̄ meals to ↓ GI irritation ▪ Take as ordered by physician; do *not* change dose ▪ Check c̄ physician/pharmacist before taking OTC preparations ▪ Follow diet low in animal fats, triglycerides ▪ Women: use contraception for up to 2mo after therapy is ended if sexually active ▪ Diabetics: hypoglycemia (anxiety, headache, fatigue, nausea, sweating) may occur; take sugar, notify physician ▪ Notify physician *immediately* of "flulike" symptoms (fever, sore throat, weakness) ▪ Avoid use c̄ alcohol, barbiturates, narcotics ▪ Keep scheduled appointments c̄ physician/for blood work.

NOTES:

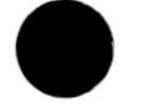

clomipramine hcl • (kloe-mip-ra-meen)

CATEGORY: *Tricyclic antidepressant:* antiobsessional

Rx; Preg Cat C

BRAND NAME
Anafranil (C-G)

DOSAGE FORMS
Capsule: 25, 50, 75mg

USE: Treatment of obsession and/or compulsions in obsessive-compulsive disorder (OCD). Long-term effectiveness (>10wks) not currently evaluated, but treatment has lasted for at least 1yr in selected pts. **ACTION:** Exact mechanism of anticompulsive activity not determined but appears related to serotonergic neural transmission. Drug inhibits serotonin reuptake.

PHARMACOKINETICS

PO absorption	Peak	Half-life	Protein binding	Excretion
Good	2-6h	19-37h	97%	Via urine, glucuronic metabolites, & other metabolites

CONTRAINDICATIONS: Hypersensitivity, MAO-I therapy, MI (acute recovery period). **CC:** Use c̄ caution in pts c̄ hx of seizures or other predisposing factors.

DOSAGE

Children/ Adolescent	*PO*	Initial dose 25mg/d c̄ gradual ↑ during the first 2wks. Do *not* exceed 3mg/kg and/or 100mg/d. Follow by gradual ↑ *not* to exceed 3mg/kg or 200mg/d (whichever is smaller). Maintenance dose lowest effective dose that can be given once/d at hs
Adult	*PO*	Initial dose 25mg/d c̄ gradual ↑ (2wks) to 100mg/d. Follow by gradual ↑ to 250mg/d. Maintenance dose lowest effective dose that can be given once/d at hs

SIDE/ADVERSE EFFECTS: CNS: somnolence, dizziness, tremor, nervousness, myoclonus, seizures ▪ CV: postural hypotension, tachycardia, palpitation ▪ GI: anorexia, constipation, nausea, dyspepsia, ↑ appetite, dry mouth ▪ INT: rash, pruritus, ↑ sweating ▪ Other: abnormal vision, tinnitus, weight gain, myalgia, micturition disorder, male sexual dysfunction.

INTERACTIONS: Drug: Significant depressant effects c̄ alcohol, other CNS depressants ▪ Use c̄ warfarin, digoxin can ↑ their effects by displacement from protein storage sites ▪ Use c̄ anticholinergics may produce ↑ atropinelike effects ▪ Use c̄ drugs that ↓ seizure threshold is best avoided.

NURSING MANAGEMENT PRIORITIES

ADMINISTRATION: Assess for hx of TCA hypersensitivity, hepatic dysfunction, glaucoma ▪ Assess VS, esp BP ▪ Administer c̄ food to ↓ GI irritation ▪ Avoid exposure to moisture/light in storage ▪ Avoid abrupt withdrawal; D/C *gradually* ▪ Maintain hydration ▪ Elderly/debilitated may require ↓ dosage ▪ ↑ Dosage *slowly* ▪ Heavy smokers may require ↑ dosage.

EVALUATION: Monitor CV, hepatic, ophthalmic, renal status ▪ Monitor BP, CBC, fluid retention (I&O, daily weight), constipation ▪ Assess mental status ▪ Assess for extrapyramidal symptoms (tics/spasms, trembling, shuffling gait) ▪ Institute seizure precautions in pts c̄ hx of convulsive disorders ▪ Assess for symptoms of abrupt withdrawal (nausea, headache, malaise) ▪ Assess IOP.

EDUCATION: Dizziness/drowsiness may occur; use caution in potentially hazardous activities ▪ Avoid changing positions (lying/sitting/standing) rapidly ▪ Avoid use c̄ alcohol, other CNS depressants for up to 1wk after therapy ▪ Take c̄ food ▪ Take as ordered by physician ▪ Constipation may occur; ↑ fluids, bulk-containing foods ▪ Store in tightly closed, light-resistant container ▪ Use sugarless gum/hard candy to diminish dry mouth ▪ Maintain fluid intake (6-8 glasses/d) ▪ Avoid exposure to direct sunlight, UV light (sunlamps); use sunscreen, protective clothing ▪ Notify physician of fever, sore throat, malaise ▪ Notify physician of extrapyramidal symptoms (tics/spasms, trembling, shuffling gait) ▪ Avoid ↑ exercise, temperature extremes ▪ Avoid smoking ▪ Check c̄ physician/pharmacist before taking OTC preparations ▪ Schedule periodic eye exams ▪ Full drug effects may require several wks of therapy ▪ Men: breast enlargement may occur ▪ May interfere c̄ sexual functioning.

NOTES:

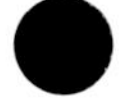

clonazepam • (kloe-na-ze-pam)

CATEGORY: *Benzodiazepine:* anticonvulsant

Rx C-IV; Preg Cat NA

BRAND NAMES
Klonopin (Roche)
**Rivotril (Roche)*

DOSAGE FORMS
Tablet: 0.5, 1, 2mg
Tablet: 0.5, 2mg

USE: Treatment of Lennox-Gastaut syndrome, akinesia, myoclonic seizures; may be useful in petit mal. **ACTION:** Anticonvulsant activity appears to be on subcortical level & in limbic system; about 30% of pts show loss of anti-convulsant activity.

DOSAGE

Pediatric	*PO*	Up to 10y/o or 30kg: initial dose 0.01-0.03mg/kg/d in 2-3 divided doses. ↑ By no more than 0.25-0.5mg q3d to maintenance dose 0.1-0.2mg/kg/d
Adult	*PO*	Initial dose *not* to exceed 1.5mg/d in 3 divided doses. ↑ By 0.5-1mg q3d until seizures are controlled or adverse effects preclude further use. Do *not* exceed 20mg/d

PHARMACOKINETICS

PO absorption	Onset	Peak	Duration	Half-life	Excretion
Very good	20-60m	1-2h	6-12h	18-50h	Via urine as metabolites

CONTRAINDICATIONS: Hypersensitivity, narrow-angle/significant glaucoma. **CC:** Use can produce dependence; abrupt D/C can result in withdrawal symptoms ▪ Breast-feeding during treatment should be avoided.

SIDE/ADVERSE EFFECTS: CNS: drowsiness (50%), ataxia (30%), behavior problems (25%), choreiform movements, ***coma,*** respiratory depression, hallucinations, psychosis, suicide attempts, dysarthria ▪ CV: palpitations, ankle/facial edema ▪ EENT: abnormal eye movement, diplopia ▪ GI: anorexia, coated tongue, dry mouth, gastritis, nausea ▪

Note: Side/adverse effects: common in *italic;* serious in ***boldface italic.***

*Available in Canada only.

HEM: anemia, leukopenia, ***thrombocytopenia***, eosinophilia ▪ HEP: hepatomegaly ▪ MS: muscle weakness.

INTERACTIONS: Drug: Use c̄ other CNS depressants produces additive effects ▪ Use c̄ MAO-I, TCAs produces sedation.

NURSING MANAGEMENT PRIORITIES

ADMINISTRATION: Assess for hx of benzodiazepine hypersensitivity ▪ Divide daily dose into 3 equal doses; if not possible, administer largest dose before hs ▪ Avoid use in pts c̄ glaucoma ▪ Avoid exposure to heat/moisture/light in storage ▪ Avoid abrupt withdrawal; institute strict seizure precautions if drug is abruptly withdrawn ▪ Have emergency support measures available ▪ Elderly may require ⬇ dosage.

EVALUATION: Assess for status epilepticus, hypoxia when therapy is D/C ▪ Assess serum for ⬆ alkaline phosphatases, transaminases ▪ Monitor occurrence/characteristics of seizures ▪ Monitor hemopoietic, renal, hepatic status ▪ Assess for symptoms of abrupt withdrawal (tremors, abdominal/muscle cramps, convulsions) c̄ prolonged use ▪ Check for signs of dependence (⬆ drug request) ▪ Monitor activity status (safety precautions) ▪ Assess for tolerance to therapeutic dose ▪ Assess for paradoxic rxs (CNS stimulation), esp in elderly ▪ Check for depression; suicide precautions prn.

EDUCATION: May cause ⬆ salivation ▪ Carry medical identification (MedicAlert) ▪ Women: avoid breastfeeding ▪ Drowsiness may occur; use caution in potentially hazardous activities ▪ Avoid use c̄ alcohol, other CNS depressants ▪ Indiscriminate use may lead to dependence ▪ Do *not* keep at bedside ▪ Take as ordered by physician; do *not* omit daily dose ▪ Check c̄ physician/pharmacist before taking OTC preparations ▪ Store in tightly closed, light-resistant container.

NOTES:

clonidine hcl • (kloe-ni-deen)

CATEGORY: *Antihypertensive:* α_2 agonist — Rx; Preg Cat C

BRAND NAMES	DOSAGE FORMS
Catapres (B-I)	Tablet: 0.1, 0.2, 0.3mg Transdermal system (TTS): 1, 2, 3
**Dixarit (B-I)*	Tablet: 0.025mg
Duraclon (Fujisawa)	Injection: 100μg/ml

COMBINATION PRODUCTS
Combipres 0.1, 0.2, 0.3 (see category card #350)

USE: Treatment of hypertension as sole agent/in combination c̄ other antihypertensive drugs. ▪ Treatment of severe cancer pain (epidural infusion) in combination c̄ opiates.
ACTION: Antihypertensive effect appears related to central α_2-adrenergic activity, which results in inhibition of bulbar sympathetic cardioaccelerator, sympathetic vasoconstriction centers.

PHARMACOKINETICS

PO absorption	Peak	Half-life	Excretion
Good	3-5h	12-16	Via kidney, feces primarily as metabolites

CONTRAINDICATIONS: Hypersensitivity. **CC:** Use c̄ caution in pts c̄ cerebrovascular/coronary insufficiency, recent MI & renal disease ▪ Drug ↑ growth hormone release but does not induce chronic elevations c̄ long-term use ▪ Tolerance can develop & may require reevaluation of treatment ▪ Transdermal patch can cause skin rash & application sites should be rotated.

DOSAGE

Adult *PO*	Initial dose 0.1mg bid. Usual maintenance dose range 0.2-0.8mg/d. Maximum effect dose 2.4mg/d
Epidural infusion	30-40μg/h
Transdermal	Apply patch TTS-1 (0.1mg/d), TTS-2 (0.2mg/d), or TTS-3 (0.3mg/d) q7d
Combipres	1 tablet bid

SIDE/ADVERSE EFFECTS: CNS: *drowsiness, sedation,* headache, vivid dreams, anxiety, mental depression ▪ CV: CHF, Raynaud's phenomenon, ECG changes (usually ventricular trigeminy), ***AV block*** ▪ EENT: nasal dryness, ocular irritation ▪ GI: *dry mouth,* constipation, anorexia, vomiting, parotid pain ▪ GU: urinary retention, impo-

Note: Side/adverse effects: common in *italic;* serious in ***boldface italic***

*Available in Canada only.

tence ▪ INT: rash, hives, alopecia, pruritus ▪ Other: ***angioneurotic edema.***

INTERACTIONS: Drug: Use c̄ alcohol, other CNS depressants produces additive depression.

NURSING MANAGEMENT PRIORITIES

ADMINISTRATION: Assess for hx of hypersensitivity ▪ Assess renal function; may require ⬇ dose if impaired ▪ Assess BP; if *hypotensive*, hold drug, notify physician ▪ Avoid abrupt withdrawal; D/C gradually ▪ Use c̄ diuretics will ⬆ antihypertensive effect ▪ Elderly may require ⬇ dosage.

EVALUATION: Monitor VS, esp BP ▪ Monitor I&O, daily weight ▪ Observe for mental depression; D/C drug, notify physician ▪ Assess for edema in extremities ▪ Schedule ophthalmic exams (retinopathy) ▪ Observe for signs of tolerance; notify physician.

EDUCATION: Drowsiness/dizziness may occur; use caution in potentially hazardous activities ▪ Avoid changing positions (lying/sitting/standing) rapidly ▪ Notify physician of fever, sore throat, bruising/bleeding ▪ Take as ordered by physician even if symptom free; do *not* skip doses ▪ Take last dose just before hs ▪ Do *not* D/C w/out notifying physician ▪ Check c̄ physician/pharmacist before taking OTC/Rx preparations ▪ Avoid use c̄ alcohol, CNS depressants ▪ Avoid high-Na^+ foods (canned soups, lunch meats, cheese) ▪ Avoid ⬆ exercise, temperature extremes, smoking ▪ Used to control, *not* cure, hypertension ▪ Maintain optimum weight ▪ Keep scheduled appointments c̄ physician/for eye exams ▪ Use sugarless gum/hard candy to diminish dry mouth ▪ Carry identification (MedicAlert) if taking antihypertensives ▪ Procedure for transdermal patch application: apply to hairless body area q7d; wash site c̄ soap, H_2O; dry thoroughly before applying; use firm pressure to ensure adherence to skin; rotate sites; do *not* apply to scarred or irritated area.

NOTES:

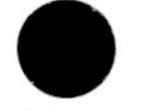

clopidrogrel bisulfate • (kloe-pid-roe-grel)

CATEGORY: *Platelet inhibitor:* anticoagulant Rx; Preg Cat B

BRAND NAME
Plavix (Sanofi)

DOSAGE FORM
Tablet: 75mg

USE: Prophylaxis of MI, stroke, vascular death in pts c̄ atherosclerosis documented by recent MI, stroke, established arterial disease. **ACTION:** Drug selectively & irreversibly binds to adenosine diphosphate (ADP) platelet receptor resulting in inhibition of platelet aggregation. Also, clopidrogrel inhibits platelet aggregation by blocking amplification of platelet activation by released ADP. The drug is inactive & must be metabolized into its active metabolite. Platelets exposed to active metabolite are inactive for their entire lifespan. Platelet inhibition occurs w/in 2h after a single dose. Platelet activity & bleeding time return to their original baseline values c̄ cessation of treatment in 5-6d.

PHARMACOKINETICS

PO absorption	Peak plasma	Half-life	Protein binding	Excretion
Approx. 50%	2h	8h	94%-98%	Via urine & feces as metabolites

CONTRAINDICATIONS: Hypersensitivity, active bleeding conditions. **CC:** Use c̄ caution in pts c̄ impaired liver function ▪ Use c̄ caution in pts c̄ potential bleeding conditions, incl surgery, trauma ▪ Drug must be D/C 7d before surgery ▪ Safety & efficacy not established for pediatric pts; use can cause rare cases of myelotoxicity.

DOSAGE

Adult	*PO*	75mg once/d regardless of meals

SIDE/ADVERSE EFFECTS: CNS: depression, headache, dizziness, ***rare intracranial hemorrhage*** ▪ CV: edema, hypertension ▪ GI: N/V/D, abdominal pain, dyspepsia, peptic/duodenal ulcers, ***hemorrhage*** ▪ HEM: ***rare agranulocytosis,*** neutropenia, purpura ▪ INT: rash, pruritus ▪ RESP: infection, pain, dyspnea, rhinitis, bronchitis ▪ Other: arthralgia, hypercholesterolemia, back pain, UTI.

INTERACTIONS: Drug: Use c̄ NSAIAs can produce additive GI bleeding ▪ Use c̄ aspirin, warfarin requires caution ▪ High doses of clopidrogrel may interfere c̄ metabolism of fluvastatin, NSAIAs, phenytoin, tamoxifen, tolbutamide, torsemide, warfarin.

NURSING MANAGEMENT PRIORITIES

ADMINISTRATION: Assess for hx of hypersensitivity ▪ Assess hepatic, renal function; use caution if impaired ▪ Administer c̄ food to ⬇ GI irritation.

EVALUATION: Monitor CBC ▪ Monitor hepatic, renal status ▪ Observe pt for signs of ⬆ bleeding, incl abdominal/lumbar pain, headache.

EDUCATION: Dizziness may occur; use caution in potentially hazardous activities ▪ Notify physician *immediately* of fever, sore throat, unusual bleeding/bruising, blood detected in urine/stool ▪ Take c̄ food ▪ Use soft-bristled toothbrush; electric razor/depilatory for hair removal ▪ Diarrhea may occur ▪ Avoid exposure to infection-producing situations ▪ Notify physician/dentist of drug use before treatment ▪ Women: avoid breastfeeding ▪ Check c̄ physician/pharmacist before taking OTC preparations.

NOTES:

clorazepate dipotassium • (klor-az-e-pate)

CATEGORY: *Benzodiazepine:* antianxiety, anxiolytic

Rx C-IV; Preg Cat NA

BRAND NAMES
Tranxene (Abbott)
Tranxene-SD (Abbott)
Tranxene-SD Half Strength (Abbott)

DOSAGE FORMS
Tablet: 3.75, 7.5, 15mg
Tablet: 22.5mg
Tablet: 11.25mg

USE: Treatment of anxiety, acute alcohol withdrawal ▪ Adjunct in management of partial seizures. **ACTION:** Benzodiazepines appear to potentiate the inhibitory effects of gamma aminobutyric acid (GABA) in central-mediated neurotransmission. Anxiolytic activity due to depression of CNS at brainstem reticular formation, limbic, thalamic areas.

PHARMACOKINETICS: Drug converted to nordiazepam (active metabolite) after PO absorption; excretion via urine, feces.

CONTRAINDICATIONS: Hypersensitivity, narrow-angle glaucoma. **CC:** Not indicated for depressive neuroses, psychotic disorders ▪ Use can produce dependence, abrupt D/C can result in withdrawal symptoms ▪ Use during pregnancy is best avoided ▪ Benzodiazepines are not indicated for psychiatric disorders esp when anxiety is not a significant symptom ▪ Use c̄ caution in pts c̄ hepatic or renal dysfunction.

DOSAGE

Anxiety		
Adult	*PO*	Start c̄ 30mg/d divided, adjust gradually to 15-60mg/d
Geriatric	*PO*	Start c̄ 7.5-15mg/d divided
Alcoholism		
Day 1		30mg followed by 30-60mg divided
Day 2		45-90mg divided
Day 3		22.5-45mg divided
Day 4		15-30mg divided Gradually ↓ dose to 7.5-15mg/d. D/C when pt is stable
Seizures		
Pediatric	*PO*	9-12y/o: Up to 7.5mg bid, adjust by 7.5-mg increments weekly to maximum 60mg/d
Adult	*PO*	Start c̄ 7.5mg tid, adjust by 7.5-mg increments weekly to maximum 90mg/d

SIDE/ADVERSE EFFECTS: CNS: *drowsiness, fatigue, ataxia* ▪ CV: hypotension ▪ HEM: neutropenia (rare) ▪ PSYCH: paradoxic anxiety, hallucinations, hyperexcited states.

INTERACTIONS: Drug: Use c̄ other CNS depressants produces additive effects ▪ Use c̄ MAO-I can produce serious toxic effects.

NURSING MANAGEMENT PRIORITIES

ADMINISTRATION: Assess for hx of benzodiazepine hypersensitivity ▪ Avoid exposure to heat/moisture/light in storage ▪ Avoid abrupt withdrawal ▪ Have emergency support measures available ▪ Elderly may require ⬇ dosage ▪ Problem discussion, sympathetic listening contribute to relief of anxiety.

EVALUATION: Monitor renal, hepatic status ▪ Assess for symptoms of abrupt withdrawal (tremors, abdominal/muscle cramps, convulsions) c̄ prolonged use ▪ Check for signs of dependence (⬆ drug request) ▪ Monitor activity status (safety precautions) ▪ Assess for tolerance to therapeutic dose ▪ Assess for paradoxic rxs (CNS stimulation), esp in elderly ▪ Check for depression; suicide precautions prn.

EDUCATION: Drowsiness may occur; use caution in potentially hazardous activities ▪ Avoid use c̄ alcohol, other CNS depressants ▪ Seizures: do *not* omit daily dose ▪ Indiscriminate use may lead to dependence ▪ Do *not* keep at bedside ▪ Take as ordered by physician; do *not* ⬆ dose ▪ Women: avoid breastfeeding ▪ Check c̄ physician/pharmacist before taking OTC preparations ▪ Practice relaxation exercises; ventilation of feelings.

NOTES:

cloxacillin sodium/dicloxacillin sodium • (klox-a-sill-in)

CATEGORY: *Penicillinase-resistant penicillin:* antibiotic

Rx; Preg Cat B

BRAND NAMES

cloxacillin
**Apo-Cloxi (Apotex)*
**Bactopen (SKB)*
Cloxapen (SKB)
**Orbenin (Ayerst)*

dicloxacillin
Dycill (SKB)
Dynapen (Apothecon)
Pathocil (W-A)

DOSAGE FORMS

cloxacillin	Capsule, 250, 550mg
	PO suspension 125mg/5ml
dicloxacillin	Capsule, 125, 250, 500mg
	PO suspension 62.5mg/5ml

USE: Treatment of infections due to susceptible penicillinase-producing staphylococci. **ACTION:** Bactericidal activity due to inhibition of mucopeptide cell wall synthesis in susceptible organisms.

CONTRAINDICATIONS: Hypersensitivity to any penicillin. **CC:** Serious, fatal anaphylaxis has occurred even c̄ PO dosage forms of penicillin ▪ Possible cross-allergenicity c̄ cephalosporins ▪ Resistant to any penicillinase-resistant penicillin should be interpreted as resistance to all; cross resistance c̄ cephalosporins occurs frequently.

DOSAGE

cloxacillin

Pediatric	*PO*	<20kg: ≥50-100mg/kg/d divided, q6h >20kg: ≥250-500mg q6h
Adult	*PO*	≥250-500mg q6h

dicloxacillin

Pediatric	*PO*	<20kg: ≥12.5-25mg/kg/d divided
Adult	*PO*	125-≥250mg q6h

PHARMACOKINETICS

	PO absorption	Peak	Half-life	Protein binding	Excretion
cloxacillin	37%-68%	0.5-2h	0.4-0.8h	90%-96%	Via urine as unchanged drug, metabolites
dicloxacillin	35%-76%	0.5-2h	0.7h	93%-96%	

SIDE/ADVERSE EFFECTS: CNS: neuropathy usually associated c̄ high parenteral doses ▪ GI: *N/V/D, epigastric distress,* black hairy tongue, flatulence, smell/taste disturbances ▪ GU: ***interstitial nephritis*** (rare) usually associated c̄ methicillin ▪ HEM: anemia, eosinophilia, leukopenia, neutropenia, ***thrombocytopenia*** ▪ HEP: ↑ serum AST, ALT, LDH ▪ INT: rash, pruritus, urticaria ▪ MS: arthralgia ▪ Other: fever, ***anaphylaxis***.

INTERACTIONS: Drug: Bacteriostatic antibiotics c̄ any penicillin can lead to antibiotic antagonism ▪ PO anticoagulant therapy may require dose adjustment.

NURSING MANAGEMENT PRIORITIES

ADMINISTRATION: Assess for hx of penicillin/cephalosporin hypersensitivity ▪ Obtain C&S before therapy ▪ Use reconstituted solution w/in 14d refrigerated; shake well before administering ▪ Administer 1h ac/2h pc ▪ Do *not* administer bacteriostatic agents w/in 1h ▪ Avoid exposure to moisture in storage ▪ Have support equipment available for anaphylaxis.

EVALUATION: Monitor pts c̄ allergies/asthma (risk for hypersensitivity) ▪ Monitor renal, hepatic, hemopoietic status ▪ Monitor VS, esp temperature ▪ Observe for signs of superinfection (diarrhea, perineal itching, oral ulcers).

EDUCATION: Complete full course of therapy (usually 10d) even if symptom free ▪ Take on empty stomach (1h ac/2h pc) at equal intervals around clock to maintain blood levels ▪ Do *not* take c̄ acid beverages (orange juice, carbonated beverage); take c̄ H_2O ▪ Diarrhea may occur ▪ Store in dry, tightly closed container ▪ Discard outdated preparations ▪ Maintain good personal hygiene (esp perineal, oral) ▪ Maintain fluid intake (6-8 glasses/d) ▪ Notify physician of symptoms of allergic rx (fever, difficult breathing, rash) ▪ Carry identification (MedicAlert) if penicillin allergic.

NOTES:

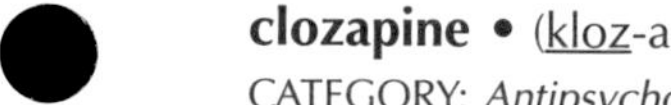

clozapine • (kloz-a-peen)

CATEGORY: *Antipsychotic:* neuroleptic

Rx; Preg Cat B

BRAND NAME
Clozaril (Sandoz)

DOSAGE FORMS
Tablet 25, 100mg

USE: Treatment of severe schizophrenia that is unresponsive to standard antipsychotic regimens. **ACTION:** Antipsychotic activity appears associated c̄ ↓ dopaminergic pathways, esp in limbic area, resulting in tranquilizing effect in psychotic pts. Drug is relatively free of extrapyramidal symptoms & exhibits antiadrenergic, anticholinergic, antihistaminic, & antiserotonin activity.

PHARMACOKINETICS

PO absorption	Peak	Half-life	Protein binding	Excretion
Good	2.5h	4-12h	95%	50% via urine, 30% via feces as metabolites

CONTRAINDICATIONS: Hypersensitivity, comatose states or severe CNS depression, bone marrow depression, severe granulocytopenia, hx of clozapine-induced agranulocytosis. **CC:** Use should be restricted to selected pts due to serious risk of potentially life-threatening agranulocytosis ▪ Use can induce seizures (up to 5%), neuroleptic malignant syndrome, tardive dyskinesia.

DOSAGE

Adults *PO* Initial dose 25mg once or twice/d c̄ increments of 25-50mg/d until 300 450mg is reached by the end of 2wks. Usual range 330-900mg/d with a usual dose of 600mg/d. Do *not* exceed 900mg/d

SIDE/ADVERSE EFFECTS: CNS: drowsiness, sedation, seizures, headache, tremor, syncope, sleep disorders, agitation, restlessness ▪ CV: tachycardia, hypotension, hypertension, chest pain, ECG changes ▪ GI: salivation, constipation, N/V, abdominal discomfort, dry mouth ▪ HEM: agranulocytosis, leukopenia, neutropenia ▪ Other: fever, rash, visual disturbances, weight gain.

INTERACTIONS: Drug: Use c̄ other CNS depressants will ↑ CNS depression ▪ Use c̄ warfarin, digoxin can ↑ their effects by displacement from protein storage sites ▪ Use c̄ anticholinergic drugs may ↑ atropine-like effects ▪ Use c̄ antihypertensives may ↑ hypotensive effect ▪ Avoid use c̄ other bone marrow depressants.

Note: Side/adverse effects: common in *italic;* serious in ***boldface italic.***

*Available in Canada only.

NURSING MANAGEMENT PRIORITIES

ADMINISTRATION: Assess VS, esp BP ▪ Administer c̄ food/full glass of H_2O or milk ▪ Avoid exposure to moisture/light in storage ▪ Avoid abrupt withdrawal; D/C gradually ▪ Maintain hydration ▪ Elderly/debilitated may require ↓ dosage.

EVALUATION: Monitor hepatic, ophthalmic, renal status ▪ Monitor BP, CBC; fluid retention (I&O, daily weight), constipation ▪ Assess mental status ▪ Assess for extrapyramidal symptoms (tics/spasms, trembling, shuffling gait) ▪ Institute seizure precautions in pts c̄ hx of convulsive disorders ▪ Long-term therapy: assess for jaundice, agranulocytosis ▪ Assess for symptoms of abrupt withdrawal (nausea, dyskinesia, trembling, dizziness) ▪ Assess IOP.

EDUCATION: Dizziness/drowsiness may occur; use caution in potentially hazardous activities ▪ Avoid changing positions (lying/sitting/standing) rapidly ▪ Avoid use c̄ alcohol, other CNS depressants ▪ Take as ordered by physician ▪ Take c̄ food ▪ Constipation may occur; ↑ fluids, bulk-containing foods ▪ Store in tightly closed, light-resistant container ▪ Use sugarless gum/hard candy to diminish dry mouth ▪ Maintain fluid intake (6-8 glasses/d) ▪ Avoid exposure to direct sunlight, UV light (sunlamps); use sunscreen, protective clothing ▪ Notify physician of fever, sore throat, bruising/bleeding ▪ Notify physician of extrapyramidal symptoms (tics/spasms, trembling, shuffling gait) ▪ Avoid ↑ exercise, temperature extremes ▪ Avoid smoking ▪ Check c̄ physician/pharmacist before taking OTC preparations ▪ Schedule periodic eye exams ▪ Full drug effects may require several wks of therapy.

NOTES:

codeine phosphate/codeine sulfate • (koe-deen)

CATEGORY: *Narcotic:* opium alkaloid

Rx C-II; Preg Cat C

AVAILABLE PREPARATIONS

Codeine phosphate (various)
Codeine sulfate (various)

DOSAGE FORMS: Hypodermic tablet: 15, 30, 60mg; injection: 15, 30, 60mg/ml; tablet: 15, 30, 60mg

Codeine phosphate has greater water solubility than does codeine sulfate.

USE: Relief of moderate pain as sole agent/in combination c̄ nonnarcotic analgesics ▪ Antitussive (usually present in cough formulations). **ACTION:** Narcotics produce analgesia, euphoria, sedation; codeine is a most popular antitussive & is included in many cough formulations; equianalgesic doses of codeine, morphine produce similar depression of respiration; 60mg codeine is approximately equal to 10mg morphine in analgesic activity.

PHARMACOKINETICS

PO absorption	Onset	Duration	Excretion
Good	15-30m	4-6h	Via urine primarily as metabolites

CONTRAINDICATIONS: Hypersensitivity; use c̄ extreme caution in head injuries. **CC:** Use can produce dependence; abrupt D/C can result in withdrawal symptoms.

DOSAGE

Pediatric *PO/SC/IM/IV* (IV not recommended)

Analgesic	6-11y/o: 5-10mg q4-6h. Do *not* exceed 60mg/d
Antitussive	2-5y/o: 2.5-5mg q4-6h. Do *not* exceed 30mg/d

Adult/Children ≥12y/o

Analgesic	15-60mg 3-4 times/d
Antitussive	10-20mg q4-6h. Do *not* exceed 120mg/d

SIDE/ADVERSE EFFECTS: CNS: *sedation, lightheadedness*, euphoria, dysphoria, tremors, disorientation, ↓ convulsive threshold ▪ CV: hypotension, palpitations, flushing of face ▪ EENT: miosis ▪ GI: *N/V*, dry mouth, constipation, biliary tract spasm ▪ GU: urine retention ▪ INT: pruritus, urticaria ▪ RESP: ***respiratory depression***.

INTERACTIONS: Drug: Use c̄ alcohol, antihistamines, barbiturates, benzodiazepines, methotrimeprazine, phenothiazines, other CNS depressants produces additive CNS depression; dosage ↓ may be required ▪ Use c̄ TCAs may produce additive respiratory depression.

NURSING MANAGEMENT PRIORITIES

ADMINISTRATION: Assess for hx of opioid hypersensitivity ▪ Assess quality, intensity, location of pain ▪ Store under double lock/key; document use accurately ▪ Check compatibility for mixing c̄ other drugs in solution ▪ Do *not* administer if respirations are <12/m ▪ IM: inject *deep* into muscle; rotate sites ▪ IV: dilute; administer *slowly*; keep pt supine for 2h ▪ Have narcotic antagonist (naloxone), support measures available ▪ Avoid administration in pts c̄ suspected head injury ▪ Administer *before* pt experiences intense pain ▪ Use + power of suggestion ▪ Avoid abrupt withdrawal; D/C gradually ▪ Elderly may require ↓ dosage.

EVALUATION: Monitor respirations, circulatory function ▪ Assess bowel function, abdominal distention ▪ Assess renal function, urinary retention ▪ Check for signs of dependence (↑ drug request) ▪ Assess for potentiation of CNS depressant effect ▪ Assess for N/V; administer antiemetic ▪ Assess for signs of OD (coma, pinpoint pupils, respiratory depression) ▪ SC: check for tissue irritation ▪ May produce ↑ CSF pressure.

EDUCATION: Avoid changing positions (lying/sitting/standing) rapidly ▪ Avoid excessive sensory stimulation ▪ Keep bedrails up when nonambulatory ▪ Turn, cough, deep breathe after surgery ▪ Constipation may occur; ↑ fluids, bulk-containing foods ▪ Avoid potentially hazardous activities ▪ Avoid smoking ▪ Take as ordered by physician; do *not* ↑ dose ▪ Indiscriminate use may lead to severe dependence ▪ Avoid use c̄ alcohol, other CNS depressants ▪ Women: avoid breastfeeding ▪ Notify physician/dentist of use before treatment.

OVERDOSE MANAGEMENT: *See* Narcotics.

NOTES:

colchicine • (kol-chi-seen)

CATEGORY: *Antigout agent*

Rx; Preg Cat D

BRAND NAME
Colchicine (various)

DOSAGE FORMS
Injection (IV): 1mg/2ml
Tablet: 0.5, 0.6mg

COMBINATION PRODUCT
ColBenemid (Merck)

colchicine/probenecid per tablet: 0.5mg/500mg

USE: Drug of choice for treating acute attacks of gout ▪ Prevention of gout attacks. **ACTION:** Complete mechanism not determined; antigout activity related to inhibition of leukocyte metabolism; ↓ in lactic acid production in polymorphonuclear leukocytes results in retarding urate acid crystal deposition in joints; powerful inhibitor of cell mitosis, extremely toxic, no effect on uric acid excretion.

PHARMACOKINETICS: Well absorbed PO, short plasma half-life, leukocyte half-life is about 60h; considerable enterohepatic recycling; excretion via feces as unchanged drug, metabolites.

CONTRAINDICATIONS: Hypersensitivity. **CC:** Hepatic, renal impairment can ↑ toxicity ▪ Possible effect on male spermatogenesis.

DOSAGE

Adult	*PO*	Initial dose 0.6-1.2mg, then 0.6mg q1-2h until pain is relieved or until N/V/D develop. Prophylactic dose 0.6mg 1-4 times/wk or 0.6-1.2mg/d in more severe cases
	IV	Initial dose 2mg, then 0.5mg q6h until condition improves. Do *not* exceed total of 4mg/d
ColBenemid		
Adult	*PO*	1-2 tablets for 1wk, then 1 bid. Do *not* exceed 4/d

SIDE/ADVERSE EFFECTS: GI: *N/V/D,* abdominal pain ▪ HEM: ***agranulocytosis, thrombocytopenia, aplastic anemia*** ▪ INT: alopecia, purpura ▪ Other: peripheral neuritis, chromosomal aberrations.

INTERACTIONS: Drug: Use c̄ adrenergics, CNS depressants enhances effects ▪ Possible malabsorption syndrome for vitamin B_{12}.

Note: Side/adverse effects: common in *italic;* serious in ***boldface italic.***

*Available in Canada only.

NURSING MANAGEMENT PRIORITIES

ADMINISTRATION: Assess for hx of hypersensitivity ▪ PO: administer c̄ food/milk to ↓ GI distress ▪ Assess serum uric acid (normal: 3-7mg/dl) ▪ Assess hepatic, cardiac, hematologic, renal function; use c̄ caution if impaired ▪ IV: administer *slowly* (2-5m); do *not* dilute/inject c̄ D_5W, bacteriostatic solutions (precipitation) ▪ Do *not* use discolored/precipitated solutions ▪ Do *not* administer IM/SC ▪ ↑ Fluid intake (3000ml/d) ▪ Avoid exposure to light in storage ▪ Elderly may require ↓ dosage.

EVALUATION: Monitor I&O, CBC ▪ Observe for signs of toxicity (N/D, abdominal pain); D/C drug, notify physician ▪ Check IV site carefully; avoid extravasation.

EDUCATION: Take c̄ food or milk ▪ Used to stop acute gout attack; always carry ▪ D/C drug if experiencing signs of toxicity (N/D, abdominal cramps); notify physician ▪ Limit purine dietary intake (organ meats, gravy, legumes) ▪ ↑ Fluid intake (10-12 glasses/d) ▪ Notify physician of fever, sore throat, bruising/bleeding, black/tarry stools ▪ Maintain optimum weight; *gradual* ↓ ▪ Avoid use c̄ alcohol ▪ Notify physician/dentist of use before therapy.

NOTES:

cortisone acetate • (<u>kor</u>-ti-sone)

CATEGORY: *Glucosteroid:* corticosteroid

Rx; Preg Cat NA

BRAND NAME

Cortone Acetate (Merck) (Upjohn [Canada])

DOSAGE FORMS

IM suspension: 50mg/ml
Tablet: 25mg (also 5mg in Canada)

USE: Treatment of adrenocorticoid deficiency, adrenogenital syndrome, other endocrine disorders; allergic states; collagen, dermatologic, GI, respiratory diseases; hematologic, ophthalmologic, rheumatic disorders ▪ Treatment of tubercular meningitis, neurologic or myocardial involvement associated c̄ trichinosis ▪ Remission of proteinuria in nephrotic syndrome, acute exacerbation of multiple sclerosis ▪ Palliative management of leukemia, lymphomas. **ACTION:** Glucosteroids cause wide variety of pharmacologic activity; two major effects are potent antiinflammatory effect, inhibition of immune response.

PHARMACOKINETICS: PO administration usually produces peak effect in 2h, duration about 1.5d.

CONTRAINDICATIONS: Systemic fungal infections, hypersensitivity, administration of live vaccines c̄ immunosuppressive doses. **CC:** Abrupt D/C can result in 2° adrenocortical deficiency ▪ Corticosteroids can mask symptoms of infection & activate latent amebiasis ▪ Extended use can result in glaucoma, subcapsular cataracts ▪ Use during pregnancy requires evaluation of benefits versus hazards & ↑ risk of cleft palate, spontaneous abortion, fetal growth retardation.

DOSAGE

Pediatric	*PO*	0.7-10mg/kg/d
Adult	*PO/IM*	25-300mg/d

SIDE/ADVERSE EFFECTS: CNS: ***convulsions,*** headache, psychic impairment, mood swings, vertigo; pseudotumor cerebri may develop after treatment ▪ CV: edema due to Na^+ retention, CHF, hypertension ▪ EENT: ↑ IOP, glaucoma, posterior subcapsular cataracts, exophthalmos ▪ END: cushingoid states, growth suppression in children, menstrual irregularities, 2° adrenocortical/pituitary unresponsiveness, hyperglycemia, carbohydrate intolerance ▪ GI: peptic ulcer c̄ ***possible perforation, pancreatitis,*** abdominal distention, ulcerative esophagitis ▪ INT: poor wound healing, fragile skin, petechiae/ecchymoses, facial erythema, ↑ sweating, urticaria, hirsutism ▪ MET: negative nitrogen balance, hypokalemic alkalosis ▪ MS: muscle weakness c̄ loss of mass, pathologic fracture of long bones, osteoporosis.

INTERACTIONS: Drug: Severe hypokalemia can occur $\bar{c}$ diuretics (nonpotassium-sparing) ▪ Use $\bar{c}$ ulcerogenic drugs (aspirin, indomethacin) can produce additive effects ▪ Use $\bar{c}$ antidiabetic agents may require higher doses of antidiabetic drugs. **Food:** Excessive consumption of licorice can ↑ risk of hypokalemia.

NURSING MANAGEMENT PRIORITIES

ADMINISTRATION: Assess for hx of hypersensitivity ▪ Administer single daily/alternate-day dose *before* 9AM; multiple doses at equal intervals ▪ PO: administer $\bar{c}$ food, milk, antacid ▪ Do *not* administer IV ▪ IM: shake well; do *not* mix, dilute, freeze; inject *deep* into gluteal UOQ (avoid deltoid); rotate sites ▪ Avoid abrupt withdrawal ▪ Avoid exposure to heat/light in storage ▪ Elderly may require ↓ dosage; monitor BP.

EVALUATION: Monitor VS, esp BP ▪ Diabetics: closely monitor blood/urine glucose (hyperglycemia) ▪ Assess mental/emotional status; avoid TCAs if depression induced ▪ Monitor serum electrolytes (esp K^+, Na^+), vision/IOP, stool for occult blood $\bar{c}$ prolonged use ▪ Monitor hydration status (I&O, daily weight).

EDUCATION: Take $\bar{c}$ food/milk (single dose *before* 9AM; multiple doses at equal intervals) ▪ Take as ordered by physician; do *not* ↑ dose ▪ Eat foods high in K^+, protein; avoid black licorice ▪ Follow low-Na^+ diet ▪ Check $\bar{c}$ physician before immunization (pt, family) ▪ Avoid exposure to infection ▪ Report following symptoms *immediately* to physician: anorexia, difficult breathing, weakness, dizziness; may appear during periods of ↑ stress, trauma ▪ Notify physician of black/tarry stools, slow wound healing, blurred vision, bruising/bleeding, weight gain, emotional changes ▪ Diabetics: closely monitor blood/urine glucose ▪ Store in tightly closed, light-resistant container ▪ Do *not* D/C drug w/out checking $\bar{c}$ physician ▪ Keep scheduled appointments $\bar{c}$ physician/for blood work/for eye exams ▪ Women: avoid breastfeeding ▪ Body image changes (full face, ↑ facial hair, ↑ fat deposit) may occur $\bar{c}$ prolonged use (reversible after therapy).

NOTES:

co-trimoxazole • (koe-trye-mox-a-zole)

CATEGORY: *Fixed-combination sulfonamide:* antiinfective — Rx; Preg Cat C

COMBINATION PRODUCTS

**Apo-Sulfatrim (Apotex)*
Bactrim (Roche)
**Novotrimel (Novopharm)*
**Protrin (Pro-Dec)*
**Roubac (Rougier)*
Septra (G-W)

CONTRAINDICATIONS: Hypersensitivity, pregnancy at term, nursing mothers, infants <2mo of age (except in treatment of congenital toxoplasmosis), folate-deficient megaloblastic anemia, urinary acidifier use. **CC:** Not indicated for streptococcal pharyngitis ▪ D/C at first appearance of skin rash or other significant adverse effects.

DOSAGE FORMS

	IV	PO suspension	Pediatric suspension	Tablet	DS tablet
Sulfamethoxazole (SMZ)	80mg/ml	200mg/5ml	200mg/5ml	400mg	800mg
Trimethoprim (TMP)	16mg/ml	40mg/5ml	40mg/5ml	80mg	160mg

USE: Treatment of UTIs caused by susceptible strains of *Enterobacter* spp, *Escherichia coli, Klebsiella* spp, *Morganella morganii, Proteus mirabilis, P. vulgaris* ▪ Treatment of pediatric otitis media, acute exacerbation of adult chronic bronchitis caused by susceptible strains of *Haemophilus influenzae, Streptococcus pneumoniae* ▪ Treatment of shigellosis caused by susceptible strains of *Shigella flexneri, S. sonnei* ▪ Treatment/prophylaxis of *Pneumocystis carinii* pneumonitis (PCP). **ACTION:** Bactericidal activity due to inhibition of two successive steps of folic acid synthesis.

DOSAGE

Pediatric	*PO*	
Ear, urinary infection		8mg/kg TMP, 40mg/kg SMZ in 24h in 2 doses/d for 10d
Shigellosis		8mg/kg TMP, 40mg/kg SMZ in 24h in 2 doses/d for 5d
Pneumonitis		20mg/kg TMP, 100mg/kg SMZ in 24h in 4 doses/d for 14d
Adult	*PO*	
Urinary infection, bronchitis		2 tablets, 1 DS tablet, 20ml suspension q12h for 10-14d

Note: Side/adverse effects: common in *italic;* serious in ***boldface italic.***

*Available in Canada only.

Shigellosis	2 tablets, 1 DS tablet, 20ml suspension, q12h for 5d
Pneumonitis	20mg/kg TMP, 100mg/kg SMZ in 24h in 4 doses/d for 14d
Pediatric/Adult *IV*	
Urinary infection	Based on TMP content 8-10mg/kg/d in 2-4 equal doses for 14d
Shigellosis	8-10mg/kg/d in 2-4 equal doses for 5d
PCP *IV/PO*	15-20mg/kg/d in 2-4 equal doses. Prophylactic dose: 160mg TMP q24h

SIDE/ADVERSE EFFECTS: CNS: headache, peripheral neuritis, ataxia, ***convulsions*** ▪ GI: N/V/D, anorexia, abdominal pain, stomatitis ▪ GU: crystalluria, toxic nephrosis ▪ HEM: ***agranulocytosis, aplastic anemia, hemolytic anemia,*** thrombocytopenic purpura, methemoglobinemia, hypoprothrombinemia, leukopenia ▪ INT: rash, pruritus, ***Stevens-Johnson syndrome, epidermal necrolysis, exfoliative dermatitis,*** photosensitivity ▪ MET: ↑ Serum transaminase, creatinine, BUN ▪ MS: arthralgia ▪ Other: serum sickness, allergic myocarditis, periorbital edema.

INTERACTIONS: Drug: Avoid *p*-aminobenzoic preparations during therapy ▪ ↑ Activity of PO hypoglycemics, methotrexate, phenytoin.

NURSING MANAGEMENT PRIORITIES

ADMINISTRATION: Assess for hx of sulfonamide hypersensitivity; furosemide, thiazide diuretics ▪ Obtain C&S before therapy ▪ Maintain hydration ▪ Administer 1h ac/2h pc c̄ full glass H_2O ▪ Avoid use in group A β-hemolytic streptococcal infections ▪ Shake suspension well before administering ▪ IV: dilute (5ml amp/125ml) D_5W; administer w/in 2h after diluting; administer over 60-90m; flush lines at end of infusion to remove residual; store infusion at room temperature, do *not* refrigerate ▪ Do *not* administer IM rapidly or by bolus injection ▪ Do *not* mix c̄ other drugs/solutions.

EVALUATION: Monitor hepatic status, temperature, CBC, UA, I&O.

EDUCATION: Complete full course of therapy ▪ Take on empty stomach c̄ full glass H_2O; if upset stomach occurs, take c̄ food ▪ Take at equal intervals around clock ▪ ↑ Fluid intake (8-10 glasses/d) ▪ Women: avoid breastfeeding ▪ Notify physician/dentist of sulfonamide use before general anesthesia ▪ Notify physician of fever, sore throat, difficult breathing, rash, bruising/bleeding.

NOTES:

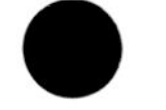

cromolyn sodium (sodium cromoglycate)/nedocromil sodium •

(kroe-moe-lin/ned-oh-kroe-mill)

CATEGORY: *Antiasthmatic (indirect)*

Rx; Preg Cat B

BRAND NAMES	DOSAGE FORMS
cromolyn	
Gastrocrom (Fisons)	PO capsule: 100mg
Intal (Fisons)	Aerosol: 800µg/spray Inhalation capsule: 20mg Nebulizer solution: 20mg/ampule
Nasalcrom (Fisons)	Nasal solution: 40mg/ml
nedocromil	
Tilade (Fisons)	Aerosol: 1.75mg/spray

USE: Prophylactic agent for management of bronchial asthma ▪ Prophylaxis & treatment of allergic rhinitis (nasal spray) ▪ Management of pts c̄ mastocytosis. **ACTION:** Indirect antiasthmatic activity due to inhibition of degranulation of sensitized mast cells. Exerts local effect on mucosa of lungs, prevents release of histamine, slow-reaction substance induced by inhalation of specific allergens. Has no antiinflammatory, antihistaminic, or bronchodilator activity.

PHARMACOKINETICS: cromolyn: after administration approximately 8% of dose is deposited in lungs, is absorbed & rapidly excreted unchanged in bile & urine. Remainder is exhaled or eventually swallowed & excreted in feces. nedocromil: after administration 8% is available after a single dose & 17% after multiple doses.

CONTRAINDICATIONS: Hypersensitivity. **CC:** Not indicated for status asthmaticus.

DOSAGE

cromolyn

Aerosol

Adult/Children ≥5y/o	2 sprays (1.6mg) qid at regular intervals. Prophylaxis of bronchospasms induced by exercise, cold air, etc. 2 sprays 10-60m before exposure

PO capsule

Children (2-12y/o)	100mg qid ½h ac/at hs

Inhalation capsule	
Adult/Children ≥2y/o	1 capsule (20mg) inhaled (Spinhaler) qid. Prophylaxis of bronchospasms induced by exercise, cold air, etc. 1 capsule inhaled before exposure
Nasal solution	
Adult/Children >6y/o	1 spray (5.2mg) 3-6 times/d
Nebulizer solution	
Adult/Children ≥2y/o	1 ampule (20mg) for nebulization qid
nedocromil	
Aerosol	
Adult/Children ≥12y/o	2 sprays (3.5mg) qid (14mg/d) at regular intervals

SIDE/ADVERSE EFFECTS: cromolyn: Aerosol/capsules: bronchospasm, cough, wheezing, dizziness, nasal congestion, rare laryngeal edema, lacrimation, dysuria, urinary frequency ▪ Nasal solution: nasal burning & irritation, headache, bad taste, epistaxis, postnasal drip ▪ Nebulizer solution: cough, nasal congestion, nausea, sneezing, wheezing. nedocromil: most common are unpleasant taste, coughing, pharyngitis, bronchospasm, headache.

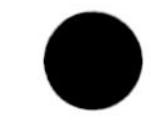

INTERACTIONS: Drug: Use $\bar{c}$ isoproterenol during pregnancy not recommended due to possible teratogenic effects.

NURSING MANAGEMENT PRIORITIES

ADMINISTRATION: Assess for hx of hypersensitivity ▪ Assess respiratory function, patency of nasal passages ▪ Avoid abrupt withdrawal ▪ Avoid exposure to heat/light in storage.

EVALUATION: Assess respiratory status, adequate inhalation ▪ Monitor frequency of asthmatic attacks.

EDUCATION: Take as directed by physician; do *not* abruptly D/C drug ▪ Notify physician/dentist of use before treatment ▪ Notify physician *immediately* of wheezing, respiratory distress ▪ Do *not* use for acute asthma attacks (prophylaxis only) ▪ Full drug effects may require several wks of therapy ▪ Proper use of aerosol/inhaler.

NOTES:

cyclophosphamide • (sye-klow-foss-fa-mide)

CATEGORY: *Alkylating agent:* antineoplastic

Rx; Preg Cat D

BRAND NAMES

Cytoxan (BM-ONC) (Bristol [Canada])
Neosar (Adria)
**Procytox (Horner)*

DOSAGE FORMS

Powder for injection (IV)
Tablet: 25, 50mg
Powder for injection (IV)
Powder for injection, tablet

USE: Treatment of malignant lymphomas incl Burkitt's lymphoma (drug of choice), follicular lymphoma, Hodgkin's disease, lymphoblastic lymphosarcoma, lymphocytic lymphosarcoma, reticulum cell sarcoma ▪ Treatment of leukemias incl acute pediatric lymphoblastic leukemias, acute myelogenous/monocytic leukemia, chronic granulocytic/lymphocytic leukemia ▪ Treatment of multiple myeloma, mycosis fungioides, solid malignancies, breast cancer. **ACTION:** Antineoplastic activity due to polyfunctional alkylating effects on DNA replication, RNA transcription; drug exhibits phosphorylating properties, immunosuppressive activity.

PHARMACOKINETICS: IV half-life about 4h; excretion via kidneys as metabolites, unchanged drug w/in 48h.

CONTRAINDICATIONS: Hypersensitivity, severe depression of bone marrow function. **CC:** Use ⬆ risk of oncogenesis, fertility impairment, mutagenic activity.

DOSAGE

Pediatric	*PO/IV*	Induction: loading dose 2-8mg/kg/d divided for ≥6d
	PO	Maintenance: 2-5mg/kg twice/wk
Adult	*PO/IV*	Induction: 1-5mg/kg/d or 40-50mg/kg divided for 2-5d. Loading dose may require $^1/_3$-$^1/_2$ ⬇ in presence of bone marrow dysfunction
	PO	Maintenance: 1-5mg/kg/d
	IV	10-15mg/kg q7-10d or 3-5mg/kg twice/wk

SIDE/ADVERSE EFFECTS: GI: *N/V/D,* oral ulcerations, ***hemorrhagic colitis*** ▪ GU: *hemorrhagic cystitis,* cystitis, fibrosis, amenorrhea, azoospermia ▪ HEM: *leukopenia,* ***thrombocytopenia,*** anemia ▪ INT: *alopecia,* skin/fingernail darkening, nonspecific dermatitis ▪ MET: hyperuricemia ▪ Other: ***secondary malignancies*** (incl bladder, myeloproliferative/lymphoproliferative), interstitial pulmonary fibrosis.

Note: Side/adverse effects: common in *italic;* serious in ***boldface italic.***

*Available in Canada only.

INTERACTIONS: Drug: Live vaccines contraindicated during therapy ▪ Radiation, other myelosuppressive drugs produce additive bone marrow depression ▪ Steroids produce additive immunosuppressant activity ▪ Barbiturates may ↑ cyclophosphamide metabolism ▪ Doxorubicin may ↑ cardiac toxicity ▪ Allopurinol may ↑ bone marrow suppression.

NURSING MANAGEMENT PRIORITIES

ADMINISTRATION: Check pt hx for recent course of radiation/antineoplastic therapy; report to physician ▪ Avoid exposure to moisture/light in storage ▪ Store between 36° & 90° F ▪ PO: administer 1h ac/2h pc ▪ Reconstitute powder for injection c̄ 5ml sterile/bacteriostatic H_2O (100mg/vial), 120ml (200mg/vial), 25ml (250mg/vial); may be administered IV, IM, intraperitoneally, intrapleurally, by infusion (added to 5% dextrose/normal saline solution) ▪ Force fluids (3000ml/d) ▪ Use reconstituted injection w/in 24h at room temperature or 6d refrigerated ▪ Administer antiemetic before therapy ▪ Provide emotional support.

EVALUATION: Monitor CBC throughout therapy ▪ Assess for infection, bleeding, anemia ▪ Assess for ↑ serum uric acid levels ▪ Monitor hepatic, renal function during therapy ▪ Assess hydration status (I&O, daily weight) ▪ False +: Pap test ▪ False −: skin tests (*Candida,* mumps, PPD, trichophyton) ▪ Monitor wound healing (delay) ▪ Check IV site closely; avoid extravasation.

EDUCATION: ↑ Fluid intake (10-12 glasses/d) PO: take on empty stomach ▪ Avoid exposure to infection ▪ Check c̄ physician before immunization (pt, family) ▪ Diet as tolerated; avoid spicy foods ▪ Maintain good oral hygiene; use soft-bristled toothbrush ▪ Notify physician of symptoms of bone marrow depression (fever, sore throat, bruising, bleeding, lethargy) ▪ Loss of hair may occur (reversible) ▪ Women: avoid breastfeeding ▪ Encourage ventilation of feelings ▪ Use contraception if sexually active.

NOTES:

cyclosporine • (sye-kloe-<u>spore</u>-een)

CATEGORY: *Immunosuppressive:* polypeptide antibiotic Rx; Preg Cat C

BRAND NAMES	DOSAGE FORMS
Neoral (Sandoz)	Microemulsion capsule: 25, 100mg Microemulsion oral solution: 100mg/ml
Sandimmune (Sandoz)	Capsules: 25,100mg IV injection: 50mg/ml Oral solution: 100mg/ml

USE: Suppression of rejection in liver, heart, kidney allogenic organ transplants ▪ Cyclosporine is always combined c̄ an adrenal corticosteroid for prophylaxis of organ rejection ▪ Treatment of chronic rejection in pts previously treated c̄ other immunosuppressive agents ▪ Microemulsion preparations have greater PO absorption, faster peak plasma levels. **ACTION:** Exact immunosuppressive mechanism not determined. Produces reversible inhibition of immunocompetent T-cell lymphocytes in the G_0 (resting) & G_1 (first growth) phase of cell cycle. This effect is most pronounced on T-helper cells. In addition, drug inhibits interleukin-1 & -2 release &/or synthesis of these lymphokines.

PHARMACOKINETICS

PO absorption	Peak	Half-life	Protein binding	Excretion
Incomplete	3.5h	10-27h	90%	About 94% primarily as metabolites via bile

CONTRAINDICATIONS: Hypersensitivity to drug or polyxyethylated castor oil. **CC:** Use ↑ risk of infection, lymphoma, other neoplasms ▪ Use requires experienced physicians ▪ Microemulsion preparation (*Neoral*) has ↑ bioavailability, cannot be used interchangeably c̄ nonmicroemulsion preparations (*Sandimmune*) w/out physician supervision.

DOSAGE

Children/Adult *PO* 15mg/kg as single dose 4-12h before transplant surgery. Continue initial daily postop dose for 1-2wks, then ↓ by 5%/wk to maintenance dose of 5-10mg/kg. Microemulsion preparations have same initial dose administered in 2 divided doses/d & subsequently adjusted to achieve specific therapeutic levels

IV Dosage is ⅓ PO dose: 5-6mg/kg as single dose 4-12h before surgery, continued daily (5-6mg/kg/d) postop until pt can be switched to PO forms

SIDE/ADVERSE EFFECTS: CNS: ***tremor convulsions***, headache, confusion ▪ CV: hypertension (50%), MI (rare) ▪ GI: N/V/D, upper GI bleeding (rare), abdominal discomfort ▪ GU: renal dysfunction, ***glomerular capillary thrombosis*** ▪ HEM: leukopenia, ***lymphoma, thrombocytopenia*** ▪ INT: hirsutism, acne ▪ Other: gum hyperplasia, sinusitis, gynecomastia.

INTERACTIONS: Drug: Use c̄ carbamazepine, phenobarbital, phenytoin will ⬇ cyclosporine levels ▪ Use c̄ bromocriptine, danazol, diltiazem, erythromycin, fluconazole, itraconazole, ketoconazole, metoclopramide, methylprednisolone, nicardipine, verapamil will ⬆ cyclosporine levels ▪ Use c̄ amphotericin B, cimetidine, diclofenac, gentamicin, ketoconazole, melphalan, ranitidine, TMP-SMZ, tobramycin, vancomycin will produce additive nephrotoxicity. **Food:** Taken c̄ meals ⬇ PO absorption esp high-fat content foods.

NURSING MANAGEMENT PRIORITIES

ADMINISTRATION: Assess for hx of hypersensitivity ▪ Assess renal function; notify physician if impaired ▪ PO: mix c̄ milk/juice in glass container ▪ IV: dilute immediately before administration according to manufacturer's directions; administer via slow infusion (2-6h); assess for allergic rx for up to 30m postinfusion ▪ Administer at same time qd to maintain optimum blood levels.

EVALUATION: Monitor VS, esp ⬆ BP ▪ Monitor I&O ▪ Monitor neurologic function (LOC, reflexes) ▪ Monitor AST, ALT (hepatotoxicity) ▪ Assess for abnormal electrophoresis, lipids (⬆) ▪ Assess for signs of rejection (⬆ temperature, graft tenderness, ⬆ creatinine).

EDUCATION: PO: take c̄ meals to ⬇ GI distress; take at same time qd; mix c̄ milk, fruit juice in glass container ▪ Take as directed by physician ▪ Keep scheduled appointments c̄ physician/for lab work ▪ Side effects are reversible after D/C drug ▪ Maintain good oral hygiene; notify dentist of use ▪ Report signs of infection/rejection *immediately* to physician ▪ Women: avoid breastfeeding.

NOTES:

cyproheptadine hcl • (si-proe-hep-ta-deen)

CATEGORY: *Antihistamine:* H1 blocker, antipruritic

Rx; Preg Cat B

BRAND NAMES
Periactin (Merck)
**Vimicon (Frosst)*

DOSAGE FORMS
Syrup: 2mg/5ml
Tablet: 4mg

USE: Symptomatic treatment of allergic disorders mediated by histamine. **ACTION:** H_1 antihistamine activity due to competitive inhibition of histamine at H_1 histamine receptors on effector cells; drug exhibits antiserotonin activity, is structurally related to azatadine maleate & has anticholinergic activity.

PHARMACOKINETICS: 40% of single dose excreted in urine, 2%-20% in feces.

CONTRAINDICATIONS: Hypersensitivity, neonates, nursing mothers, lower respiratory tract symptoms, angle-closure glaucoma, bladderneck obstruction, prostatic hypertrophy, pyloduodenal obstruction, stenosing peptic ulcer. **CC:** Use c̄ caution in children; pts c̄ bronchial asthma, cardiovascular disease, hypertension, hyperthyroidism, ↑ IOP due to atropinelike activity.

DOSAGE

Pediatric	*PO*	2-6y/o: 2mg 2-3 times/d. Do *not* exceed 12mg/d 7-14y/o: 4mg 2-3 times/d. Do *not* exceed 16mg/d
Adult	*PO*	4-20mg/d divided. Doses of 32mg/d may be required. Do *not* exceed 0.5mg/kg/d

SIDE/ADVERSE EFFECTS: CNS: *drowsiness*, dizziness, fatigue, euphoria, paresthesias ▪ CV: hypotension, palpitations, tachycardia, extrasystole ▪ EENT: blurred vision, nasal stuffiness ▪ GI: N/V, anorexia ▪ GU: early menses ▪ HEM: ***agranulocytosis, hemolytic anemia, thrombocytopenia*** ▪ INT: drug rash, photosensitivity ▪ RESP: thickening of bronchial secretions, wheezing ▪ Other: anticholinergic effects.

INTERACTIONS: Drug: Use c̄ anticholinergics, CNS depressants, TCAs produces additive effects ▪ MAO-I can intensify anticholinergic effects of antihistamines.

Note: Side/adverse effects: common in *italic;* serious in ***boldface italic.***

*Available in Canada only.

NURSING MANAGEMENT PRIORITIES

ADMINISTRATION: Assess for hx of antihistamine hypersensitivity ▪ Administer c̄ food ▪ Have support equipment available for anaphylaxis ▪ Avoid exposure to moisture/light in storage ▪ Maintain hydration.

EVALUATION: Monitor VS, esp BP ▪ Assess for excessive drowsiness, dizziness, weakness ▪ Monitor CBC c̄ prolonged therapy ▪ Monitor children for paradoxic rxs (CNS stimulation) ▪ Assess for tolerance to therapeutic dose; notify physician; another antihistamine may be substituted.

EDUCATION: Drowsiness, dizziness, lightheadedness may occur; use caution in potentially hazardous activities ▪ Avoid use c̄ alcohol, other CNS depressants ▪ Take c̄ meals ▪ Store in tightly closed, light-resistant container ▪ Use sugarless gum/hard candy to diminish dry mouth ▪ ↑ Fluid intake (8-10 glasses/d) ▪ Notify physician of symptoms of allergic rx (fever, difficult breathing, rash) ▪ Women: avoid breastfeeding ▪ Carry identification (MedicAlert) if antihistamine allergic ▪ Notify physician of antihistamine use before allergy testing.

NOTES:

cytarabine • (sye-tare-a-been)

CATEGORY: *Antineoplastic:* antimetabolite

Rx; Preg Cat D

BRAND NAME
Cytosar-U (Upjohn)

DOSAGE FORMS
Powder for injection (IV/SC): 100-, 500-mg; 1-, 2-g vials

USE: Treatment of acute myelocytic, lymphocytic leukemia, non-Hodgkin's lymphoma in children, intrathecal use in meningeal leukemia. Drug is not active PO. **ACTION:** Antimetabolic activity due to inhibition of DNA polymerase, resulting in cytotoxic effect in cells c̄ high rates of proliferation; exhibits immunosuppressive activity.

PHARMACOKINETICS: Route of administration determines peak, duration, half-life; protein binding about 13%; metabolized in liver, excreted via urine.

CONTRAINDICATIONS: Hypersensitivity/severe preexisting drug-induced bone marrow suppression. **CC:** Use requires experienced physicians ▪ Use c̄ caution c̄ preexisting drug-induced bone marrow depression due to potent bone marrow suppressant activity.

DOSAGE: *IV/SC* or *intrathecally*
Children/Adult

Nonlymphocytic leukemia	100mg/m²/d by continuous IV infusion days 1-7 or 100mg/m² IV q12h
Acute lymphocytic leukemia	Consult latest recommendations
Meningeal leukemia	Most frequent intrathecal dose 30mg/m² q4d until cerebrospinal fluid is normal. Usual dose range 5-75mg/m²

SIDE/ADVERSE EFFECTS: CNS: dizziness, neuritis, neural toxicity ▪ CV: chest pain ▪ EENT: conjunctivitis ▪ GI: *anorexia, V/D, oral/anal ulceration*, sore throat, esophageal ulcers, abdominal pain, bowel neurosis ▪ HEM: ***bone marrow suppression*** resulting in anemia, leukopenia, ***thrombocytopenia,*** megaloblastosis ▪ HEP: dysfunction, jaundice ▪ INT: rash, skin ulceration, freckling, alopecia, pruritus, urticaria ▪ Other: ***bleeding, thrombophlebitis.***

INTERACTIONS: Drug: Use of live vaccines contraindicated during therapy.

NURSING MANAGEMENT PRIORITIES

ADMINISTRATION: Check hx for recent course of radiation or antineoplastic agents; report to physician ▪ IV: reconstitute, dilute according to manufacturer's directions; stable for 48h at room temperature ▪ Do *not* administer discolored/precipitated solutions ▪ Avoid direct administration c̄ other antineoplastic agents (physical incompatibility) ▪ Administer antiemetic before therapy ▪ Provide emotional support.

EVALUATION: Monitor CBC throughout therapy ▪ Assess for infection, bleeding, anemia ▪ May produce ↑ serum uric acid level ▪ Monitor hepatic function ▪ Assess hydration status (I&O, daily weight) ▪ Check IV insertion site carefully (cellulitis).

EDUCATION: ↑ Fluid intake (8-10 glasses/d) ▪ Avoid exposure to infection ▪ Check c̄ physician before immunization (pt, family) ▪ Diet as tolerated; avoid spicy foods ▪ Avoid alcoholic beverages ▪ Maintain oral hygiene; use soft-bristled toothbrush ▪ Notify physician of symptoms of bone marrow depression (fever, sore throat, bruising, bleeding, lethargy) ▪ Loss of hair may occur (reversible after therapy is ended) ▪ Women: avoid breastfeeding ▪ Encourage ventilation of feelings ▪ Use contraception if sexually active.

NOTES:

danaparoid • (dah-nap-ah-roid)

CATEGORY: *Anticoagulant:* antithrombotic

Rx; Preg Cat B

BRAND NAME	DOSAGE FORM
Organ (Organon)	SC injection: 750 anti-Xa units/0.6 ml

USE: Prophylaxis of postop deep venous thrombosis in pts undergoing hip replacement surgery. **ACTION:** Antithrombotic activity due to inhibition of fibrin formation via thrombin coagulation pathway by activity of anti-Xa, which contains heparin sulfate, dermatan sulfate, chondroitin sulfate. Maximum activity usually occurs in 2-5h after SC administration. Drug has no appreciable effects on platelet function.

PHARMACOKINETICS: SC route provides almost 100% bioavailability & a half-life of 24h. Excretion is via urinary pathway.

CONTRAINDICATIONS: Hypersensitivity to drug or pork products ▪ Severe hemorrhagic diathesis (hemophilia, idiopathic thrombocytopenic purpura, active bleeding conditions). **CC:** Injection not intended for IM administration ▪ Use can result in hemorrhage from any body site ▪ Use in pts c̄ renal impairment requires caution, & careful monitoring is required ▪ Preparation cannot be dosed unit for unit c̄ any heparin preparation ▪ Safety & efficacy for pediatric pts not established ▪ Use can result in sodium sulfite allergies.

DOSAGE

Adult	750 anti-Xa units bid SC beginning 1-4h preop & not sooner than 2h postop for a usual range of 7-14d

SIDE/ADVERSE EFFECTS: CNS: headache, dizziness, insomnia ▪ GI: N/V, constipation ▪ INT: pruritus, rash ▪ Local: pain at injection site ▪ Other: edema, fever, UTI, anemia, urinary retention.

INTERACTIONS: Drug: None currently reported. **Lab:** Routine clotting tests PT, APTT, whole blood clotting time are not suitable for danaparoid monitoring ▪ CBC, platelet counts, occult stood blood tests are recommended.

NURSING MANAGEMENT PRIORITIES

ADMINISTRATION: Assess for hx of hypersenstiviity, incl sulfites ▪ Administer by deep SC injection; use lower abdomen; change needle after preparation, do *not* aspirate; rotate sites; check for hemorrhage; avoid massaging ▪ Avoid IM (danger of hematoma formation) ▪ Do *not* use discolored/precipitated solutions ▪ Avoid mixing c̄ other drugs in solution ▪ Have blood or platelets available for OD.

EVALUATION: Monitor hepatic, CV, renal status ▪ Observe for signs of hemorrhage, incl abdominal/lumbar pain; treat c̄ blood or platelet transfusion (w/in 30m of administration)

EDUCATION: Report any bleeding/bruising *immediately* ▪ Avoid smoking, use c̄ alcohol ▪ Use electric razor/depilatory for hair removal ▪ Avoid aspirin-containing products ▪ Check c̄ physician/pharmacist before taking OTC preparations ▪ Women: avoid breastfeeding.

NOTES:

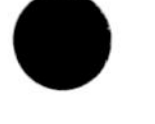

dexamethasone/dexamethasone acetate/ dexamethasone sodium phosphate • (dex-a-meth-a-sone)

CATEGORY: *Glucosteroid:* corticosteroid

Rx; Preg Cat NA

BRAND NAMES	**DOSAGE FORMS**
dexamethasone	
Decadron (Merck)	Elixir, tablet
**Dexasone (ICN)*	Elixir, tablet
Hexadrol (Organon)	Elixir, tablet
dexamethasone acetate	
Decadron-LA (Merck)	Injection suspension
dexamethasone sodium phosphate	
Decadron Phosphate (Merck)	Aerosol, injection
Hexadrol (Organon)	Injection

USE: Treatment of adrenocortical deficiency, allergic states, inflammatory/autoimmune disorders, cerebral edema, septic shock, TB meningitis ▪ Palliation of leukemia, lymphomas ▪ Remission of proteinuria in nephrotic states & acute multiple sclerosis. **ACTION:** Glucosteroids produce potent antiinflammatory effect, inhibit immune response.

PHARMACOKINETICS: PO administration usually produces peak effect in 1-2h, c̄ duration about 3d.

CONTRAINDICATIONS: Systemic fungal infections, hypersensitivity, administration of live viral vaccines c̄ immunosuppressive doses. **CC: Food:** Excessive consumption of licorice can ⬆ risk of hypokalemia.

DOSAGE

Pediatric	*Aerosol*	2 inhalations (0.3mg) 3-4 times/d. Do *not* exceed 8/d
Adult	*PO*	0.75-9mg/d
	IM/IV	0.5-9mg/d; intraarticular, intralesional, soft tissue, 0.2-6mg once q3-5d to once q2-3wks
	IM suspension	8-16mg q1-3wks prn. Intraarticular, 4-16mg q1-3wks prn. Intralesional, 0.8-1.6mg/injection site
	Aerosol	3 inhalations (0.3mg) 3-4 times/d. Do *not* exceed 12/d

SIDE/ADVERSE EFFECTS: CNS: ***convulsions***, headache, psychic impairment, mood swings, vertigo; ⬆ ICP c̄ papilledema may develop ▪ CV: CHF, hypertension ▪ EENT: ⬆ IOP, cataracts, exophthalmos ▪ END: cushingoid states, growth suppression in children, menstrual irregu-

Note: Side/adverse effects: common in *italic;* serious in ***boldface italic.***

*Available in Canada only.

larities, 2° adrenocortical/pituitary unresponsiveness, hyperglycemia, carbohydrate intolerance ▪ GI: peptic ulcer, ulcerative esophagitis ▪ INT: poor wound healing, fragile skin, petechiae/ecchymoses, facial erythema, ↑ sweating, urticaria, hirsutism ▪ MET: (−) nitrogen balance, hypokalemic alkalosis, edema ▪ MS: muscle weakness/loss of mass, pathologic fracture of long bones, osteoporosis, necrosis of femoral/humeral heads ▪ Other: ↑ susceptibility to infection.

INTERACTIONS: Drug: Severe hypokalemia can occur c̄ diuretics (nonpotassium sparing) ▪ Use c̄ ulcerogenic drugs (eg, aspirin, indomethacin) can produce additive effects ▪ Use c̄ antidiabetic agents may require higher doses of antidiabetic drugs.

NURSING MANAGEMENT PRIORITIES

ADMINISTRATION: Assess for hx of hypersensitivity ▪ PO: administer c̄ food, milk, antacids ▪ Do *not* administer acetate suspension IV ▪ IM: shake suspension well; do *not* freeze; inject *deep* into gluteal UOQ (avoid deltoid); rotate sites ▪ Avoid abrupt withdrawal ▪ Elderly may require ↓ dosage.

EVALUATION: Monitor VS, esp BP; mental status, blood glucose in diabetics (hyperglycemia), I&O, weight, serum K^+, Na^+; vision/IOP; stools for occult blood.

EDUCATION: Take c̄ food/milk (single daily dose *before* 9AM; multiple doses at equal intervals) ▪ Take as ordered by physician; do *not* ↑ dose, D/C ▪ Eat foods high in K^+, protein, calcium, vitamin D; avoid black licorice ▪ Follow low-Na^+ diet ▪ Check c̄ physician before immunization ▪ Avoid infection ▪ Report anorexia, difficult breathing, weakness, dizziness to physician *immediately* ▪ Notify physician of black/tarry stools, slow wound healing, blurred vision, bruising/bleeding, weight gain, emotional changes ▪ Avoid alcohol, caffeine ▪ Diabetics: closely monitor blood/urine glucose ▪ Safety precautions c̄ ↑ activity/exercise ▪ Notify physician/dentist of use before treatment ▪ Carry medical identification (MedicAlert) ▪ Keep appointment c̄ physician ▪ Women: avoid breastfeeding ▪ Body image changes may occur c̄ prolonged use.

NOTES:

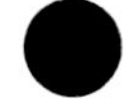

dextroamphetamine hcl • (dex-troe-am-fet-a-meen)

CATEGORY: *Anorexiant, CNS stimulant:* sympathomimetic

Rx C-II; Preg Cat C

BRAND NAME

Dexedrine (SKB)

DOSAGE FORMS

Elixir: 5mg/5ml
SR capsule (Spansules): 5, 10, 15mg
Tablet: 5mg

USE: Treatment of narcolepsy, behavioral syndrome (minimum brain dysfunction) in children ▪ Control of exogenous obesity. **ACTION:** Weak, indirect-acting sympathomimetic c̄ strong CNS-stimulant activity; peripheral effects incl respiratory-stimulant activity, ↑ in BP, weak bronchodilation; CNS effects incl alerting rxs.

PHARMACOKINETICS: Good PO absorption; hepatic metabolism c̄ 10-12h half-life in adults, 7h in children.

CONTRAINDICATIONS: Hypersensitivity, advanced arterial sclerosis, symptomatic CV disease, significant hypertension, hypothyroidism, glaucoma. **CC:** Use can produce dependence, withdrawal symptoms ▪ D/C use when anorexic effect ceases.

DOSAGE

Pediatric

Behavioral: 3-5y/o: Initial dose 2.5mg/d, raised in 2.5-mg increments weekly until desired effect is reached
≥6y/o: Initial dose 5-mg 1-2 times/d, raised in 5-mg increments weekly until desired effect is reached. Some cases may require ≥40mg/d
Narcolepsy: 6-12y/o: 5mg/d, raised in 5-mg increments weekly until desired effect is reached

Adult *PO*

Obesity: 10-30mg/d divided
Narcolepsy: 5-60mg/d depending on response

SIDE/ADVERSE EFFECTS: CNS: dizziness, insomnia, euphoria, dyskinesia, headache, exacerbation of tics, rare psychotic episodes, *restlessness* ▪ CV: ↑ in BP, palpitations, tachycardia ▪ GI: anorexia, dry mouth, diarrhea, constipation, unpleasant taste ▪ GU: impotence ▪ INT: urticaria.

INTERACTIONS: Drug: Use c̄ MAO-I can produce hypertensive crisis ▪ Use can antagonize effects of guanethidinelike drugs ▪ Diabetic pts may require insulin adjustments ▪ Urinary alkalizers will ↓ urinary excretion, prolong activity.

NURSING MANAGEMENT PRIORITIES

ADMINISTRATION: Assess for hx of catecholamine hypersensitivity ▪ Do *not* administer w/in 6h of hs or w/in 14d after MAO-I therapy ▪ Administer tablets ac for obesity ▪ Do *not* crush Spansule; administer whole ▪ Avoid abrupt withdrawal; D/C gradually.

EVALUATION: Monitor VS, esp BP/pulse ▪ Assess for tolerance to therapeutic effect ▪ Diabetics: closely monitor blood glucose ▪ Check for signs of dependence.

EDUCATION: Dizziness, restlessness may occur; use caution when engaging in potentially hazardous activities ▪ Take as directed by physician; do *not* ↑ dose ▪ Swallow Spansule whole ▪ Do *not* take w/in 6h of hs; may cause insomnia ▪ Avoid caffeine-containing products ▪ Weight-reduction diet ▪ Diabetics: monitor blood/urine glucose carefully ▪ Physical dependence may occur ▪ Use sugarless gum/hard candy to diminish dry mouth ▪ Notify physician of nervousness, dizziness, insomnia ▪ Women: avoid breastfeeding ▪ Check c̄ physician/pharmacist before taking OTC cough/cold preparations.

NOTES:

diazepam • (dye-<u>az</u>-e-pam)

CATEGORY: *Benzodiazepine:* antianxiety agent, anxiolytic, anticonvulsant Rx C-IV; Preg Cat NA

BRAND NAMES

**E-Pam (ICN)*
**Meval (Medic)*
**Rival (Riva)*
Valium (Roche)
**Vivol (Horner)*

DOSAGE FORMS: Capsule, injection (IM/IV), rectal gel, tablet.

USE: Treatment of anxiety, tension, alcohol withdrawal symptoms ▪ Convulsive disorders ▪ Preop/instrumental exam anxiety ▪ Adjunct for relief of skeletal muscle spasm.

ACTION: Benzodiazepines appear to potentiate the inhibitory effects of gamma aminobutyric acid (GABA) in central-mediated neurotransmission. Anxiolytic activity due to depression of CNS at brainstem reticular formation, limbic, thalamic areas. Drug exhibits muscle relaxant & moderate anticonvulsant properties.

CONTRAINDICATIONS: Hypersensitivity, narrow-angle glaucoma. **CC:** Not indicated for psychotic disorders ▪ Extended use can result in dependence, withdrawal symptoms ▪ Do not mix diazepam injection c̄ other drugs or solutions.

DOSAGE

PO: anxiety, alcoholism, spasm, convulsive disorders

Pediatric >6mo	1.25mg 3-4 times/d
Adult	2-10mg 2-4 times/d
Geriatric	2-2.5mg 1-2 times/d

PHARMACOKINETICS

	Onset	Peak	Duration	Half-life	Protein binding	Excretion
PO	30-60m	1-2h	3h	20-50h	80%-98%	As conjugates in urine
IM	15-30m	Erratic	1-3h	20-50h	80%-98%	
IV	1-5m	—	15m-1h	20-50h	80%-98%	

Note: Side/adverse effects: common in *italic;* serious in ***boldface italic.***

*Available in Canada only.

Parenteral *(IM/IV)*
Pediatric

Tetanus	>30d: 1-2mg, repeat in 3-4h prn ≥5y/o: 5-10mg, repeat in 3-4h prn
S. epilepticus	>30d: 0.2-0.5mg q2-5m to a maximum of 5mg ≥5y/o: 1mg q2-5m to a maximum of 10mg

Adult

Anxiety	2-10mg, repeat in 3-4h prn
Alcoholism	10mg, then 5-10mg in 3-4h prn
Cardioversion	5-10mg IV w/in 5-10m before procedure
Endoscopy	10-20mg IV before procedure
Preop	10mg IM before surgery
Spasm	5-10mg, repeat in 3-4h prn
S. epilepticus	5-10mg, repeat at 10-15m intervals to a maximum of 30mg. Repeat in 3-4h prn

SIDE/ADVERSE EFFECTS: CNS: *drowsiness, fatigue,* ataxia ▪ CV: hypotension ▪ HEM: neutropenia (rare) ▪ PSYCH: paradoxic anxiety, hallucinations, hyperexcited states.

INTERACTIONS: Drug: Use c̄ other CNS depressants produces additive effects ▪ Use c̄ MAO-I can produce toxic effects.

NURSING MANAGEMENT PRIORITIES

ADMINISTRATION: Assess for hx of benzodiazepine hypersensitivity ▪ Do *not* mix/dilute parenteral preparations (incompatibility) ▪ IM: inject *deep, slowly* into large muscle mass ▪ IV: assess respirations before each dose; administer *slowly* (5mg/m) as close to venipuncture site as possible; keep pt recumbent for 3h ▪ Avoid abrupt withdrawal.

EVALUATION: Assess for symptoms of abrupt withdrawal (tremors, abdominal/muscle cramps, convulsions) c̄ prolonged use ▪ Check for signs of dependence (↑ drug request)/tolerance ▪ Monitor activity status (safety precautions) ▪ Assess for paradoxic rxs (CNS stimulation), esp in elderly ▪ Check for depression; suicide precautions prn.

EDUCATION: Use caution in potentially hazardous activities ▪ Avoid use c̄ alcohol, other CNS depressants ▪ Indiscriminate use may lead to dependence ▪ Do *not* keep at bedside ▪ Take as ordered by physician; do *not* ↑ dose ▪ Women: avoid breastfeeding.

OVERDOSE MANAGEMENT: *See* Benzodiazepines.

NOTES:

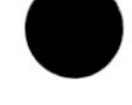

diazoxide • (dye-az-ox-ide)

CATEGORY: *Antihypertensive:* antihypoglycemic Rx; Preg Cat C

BRAND NAMES
Hyperstat IV (Schering)
Proglycem (Baker Norton)
(Schering [Canada])

DOSAGE FORMS
Injection (IV): 300mg/20m
Capsule: 50mg
PO Suspension: 50mg/ml

USE: IV: management of hypertensive emergencies ▪ PO: management of hypoglycemia due to hyperinsulinism associated c̄ extrapancreatic malignancy, inoperable islet cell adenoma/carcinoma, leucine sensitivity/nesidioblastosis. **ACTION:** Antihypertensive effect (IV administration) due to direct relaxing of smooth muscle in peripheral vascular beds; PO use produces antihypoglycemic effect due to inhibition of insulin release from pancreas & by ↑ hepatic glucose release.

CONTRAINDICATIONS: Hypersensitivity (incl other sulfonamidelike drug allergies), compensatory hypertension associated c̄ coarctation/arteriovenous shunt; functional hypoglycemia. **CC:** Use c̄ caution when treating severely elevated BP.

DOSAGE

Adult	*IV*	Bolus dose 300mg or a mini bolus dose 1-3mg/kg repeated at 5-15m intervals. Mini bolus dosage has become the most recommended schedule because it produces a more controlled reduction of BP. Maintenance doses can be given at 4-24h intervals if needed. Pediatric dose: mini bolus schedule

PHARMACOKINETICS

	Onset	Duration	Half-life	Protein binding	Excretion
PO	1h	Up to 8h	20-36h	>90%	Slowly via urine as unchanged drug, metabolites
IV	5m	Up to 12h	20-36h	>90%	

Adult/ Pediatric	*PO*	3-8mg/kg in 2-3 equal doses q8-12h
Neonates/ Infants	*PO*	8-15mg/kg in 2-3 equal doses q8-12h

SIDE/ADVERSE EFFECTS: CNS: cerebral ischemia, *dizziness*, lightheadedness, drowsiness, anxiety, headache ▪ CV: sodium/H_2O retention, *orthostatic hypotension*, ***arrhythmias***, bradycardia ▪ GI: N/V, anorexia, abdominal discomfort, ***acute pancreatitis*** (rare) ▪ INT: hirsutism in women (PO) ▪ MET: hyperglycemia in diabetic pts (IV).

INTERACTIONS: Drug: Use c̄ PO anticoagulants may require dosage ↓ due to displacement of anticoagulant from protein storage sites ▪ Use c̄ thiazides can produce additive hyperglycemic/antihypertensive activity ▪ Use c̄ hydralazine may cause severe hypotension ▪ Avoid IV use for 6h after administration of antihypertensives, papaverine-like drugs, nitrites. **Lab:** False – insulin response to glucagon.

NURSING MANAGEMENT PRIORITIES

ADMINISTRATION: Assess for hx of hypersensitivity (incl sulfonamides) ▪ Assess BP, pulse; notify physician of extremes ▪ Assess renal function; may require ↓ dosage if impaired ▪ Assess serum electrolytes, blood glucose, CBC ▪ IV: place pt in supine position, maintain for 1h after injection; inject over 10-30s ▪ Do *not* administer IM or SC ▪ PO suspension: shake well before pouring ▪ Do *not* administer discolored/precipitated solutions ▪ Administer c̄ diuretic to ↓ Na^+/H_2O retention, esp c̄ multiple doses.

EVALUATION: Monitor BP q5m, then qh when stable ▪ Monitor I&O, daily weight ▪ Assess for CHF (dyspnea, peripheral edema, ↑ weight); notify physician ▪ Diabetics: closely monitor blood glucose (hyperglycemia) ▪ Check IV insertion site carefully; avoid extravasation ▪ May produce ↑ serum uric acid.

EDUCATION: Dizziness may occur; use caution in potentially hazardous activities ▪ Avoid changing positions (lying/sitting/standing) rapidly ▪ Notify physician of abnormal rxs (difficulty breathing, chest pain, irregular heartbeat) ▪ Diabetics: monitor blood/urine glucose carefully ▪ Excessive hair growth may occur c̄ prolonged PO therapy (reversible after therapy).

NOTES:

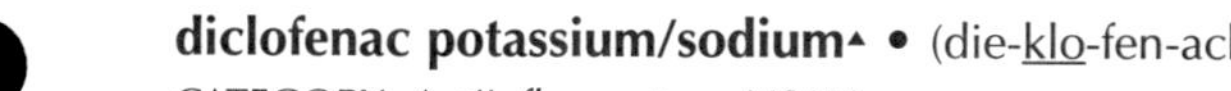

diclofenac potassium/sodium▲ • (die-klo-fen-ack)

CATEGORY: *Antiinflammatory:* NSAIA

Rx; Preg Cat B

BRAND NAMES
Cataflam (C-G)
Voltaren▲ (C-G)

DOSAGE FORMS
Tablet: 50mg
Enteric-coated tablet: 25, 50, 75mg
0.1% ophthalmic solution

COMBINATION PRODUCT

Arthrotec (Searle) 50mg; 75mg diclofenac/200µg misoprostal/tablet

USE: Treatment of rheumatoid/osteoarthritis & ankylosing spondylitis ▪ Management of pain, 1° dysmenorrhea (tablet) ▪ Treatment of postop inflammation following cataract surgery (ophthalmic). **ACTION:** Antiinflammatory activity appears related to inhibition of prostaglandin synthesis.

PHARMACOKINETICS

PO absorption	Peak	Protein binding	Excretion
Complete	2-3h	99%	Via urine, bile as conjugates

CONTRAINDICATIONS: Hypersensitivity, aspirin/other antiinflammatory agent hypersensitivity. **CC:** Use ↑ risk of GI bleeding, ulcers, perforation.

DOSAGE: Adult *PO*

Osteoarthritis	100-150mg/d divided 2-3 times/d. Daily dose >150mg not currently evaluated
Rheumatoid arthritis	150-200mg/d divided 3-4 times/d. Daily dose >200mg not currently evaluated
Ankylosing spondylitis	100-125mg/d given as 25mg qid & 25mg at hs if needed. Daily dose >125mg not currently evaluated
Ophthalmic solution	1gtt qid starting 24h after surgery for 2wks
Pain/dysmenorrhea	50mg tid. Do *not* exceed 200mg/d
Arthrotec	1 tablet 3-4 times/d

SIDE/ADVERSE EFFECTS: CNS: *headache, dizziness,* depression, anxiety ▪ CV: palpitations, chest pain, tachycardia, PVC, possible & rare ***MI*** ▪ EENT: amblyopia, night blindness, vitreous floaters, blurred vision, tinnitus, reversible hearing loss ▪ GI: *pain, cramps, constipation,* *nausea*, stomatitis, ***GI bleeding***, colitis, V/D, flatulence ▪ GU: oliguria, proteinuria, ***acute renal failure, interstitial nephritis, nephrotic syndrome, papillary necrosis*** ▪ HEM: leukopenia, ***thrombocytopenia, agranulocytosis, aplastic anemia*** ▪ INT: rash, urticaria, photosensitivity, ***Stevens-Johnson syndrome, erythema multiforme*** ▪ Other: asthma, excessive perspiration.

INTERACTIONS: Drug: Use c̄ ulcerogenic drugs produces additive effects ▪ Use c̄ PO anticoagulants may ↑ their activity ▪ Use c̄ aspirin will ↓ diclofenac plasma levels ▪ Use c̄ methotrexate, digoxin, cyclosporin may ↑ their toxicity ▪ Use c̄ lithium requires monitoring of lithium levels.

NURSING MANAGEMENT PRIORITIES

ADMINISTRATION: Assess for hx of NSAIA, salicylate hypersensitivity ▪ Avoid administration to pts c̄ hx of asthma, bleeding disorders, salicylate hypersensitivity ▪ Assess GI, renal, hepatic function; use caution if impaired ▪ May be administered c̄ food; *best* on empty stomach (1h ac/2h pc); do *not* crush tablets (enteric coated) ▪ Administer c̄ full glass of liquid; encourage upright position for 15-30m ▪ Avoid exposure to moisture during storage ▪ *Not* recommended for pts c̄ restricted Na^+ intake ▪ Elderly may require ↓ dosage.

EVALUATION: Monitor hepatic, renal status c̄ prolonged use ▪ Monitor pt receiving anticoagulant therapy; may potentiate bleeding ▪ Monitor I&O, daily weight ▪ Monitor AST, ALT ▪ Assess for edema in extremities ▪ Assess for visual/hearing disturbances; D/C drug, notify physician.

EDUCATION: Dizziness/drowsiness may occur; use caution in potentially hazardous activities ▪ Take on empty stomach (1h ac/2h pc), c̄ food if GI distress occurs; swallow tablet whole; take c̄ full glass of liquid; maintain upright position for 15-30m ▪ Take as ordered by physician; do *not* ↑ dose ▪ Notify physician *immediately* of bleeding, ↓ urine output, swelling of feet/legs, lethargy, GI distress, jaundice, visual/hearing disturbances ▪ Avoid taking c̄ aspirin, other NSAIAs ▪ Avoid use c̄ alcohol ▪ Check c̄ physician/pharmacist before taking OTC preparations ▪ Notify physician/dentist of use before treatment ▪ Store in tightly closed container ▪ Women: avoid breastfeeding ▪ Full drug effects may require several wks of therapy.

NOTES:

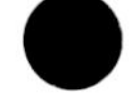

didanosine (ddl) • (dye-dan-o-seen)

CATEGORY: *Antiviral*

Rx; Preg Cat B

BRAND NAME
Videx (BM-ONC)

DOSAGE FORMS
Powder for PO solution: 100-, 167-, 250-, 375-mg foil packets
Ped powder for PO solution: 2-g (4-oz), 4-g (8-oz) bottles
Chewable tablet: 25, 50, 100, 150mg

USE: Management of advanced HIV infection in adults & children >6mo of age who have significant immunologic deterioration or are intolerant to zidovudine therapy.
ACTION: Antiviral activity due to inhibition of viral replication in HIV; drug is a nucleoside analog of deoxyadenosine that is converted by cellular enzymes into the active antiviral metabolite dideoxyadenosine triphosphate (dd ATP), which, when incorporated into viral DNA, leads to chain termination & subsequent inhibition of viral replication. In addition, dd ATP inhibits HIV reverse transcriptase enzymes required for viral DNA synthesis.

PHARMACOKINETICS

PO absorption (ac)	Half-life	Excretion
33%-37%	8-24h	Via urine as metabolites

CONTRAINDICATIONS: Hypersensitivity. **CC:** Use ↑ risk of pancreatitis (sometimes fatal), peripheral neuropathy, liver failure ▪ Current pediatric use requires dilated retinal exam q6mo to preclude retinal depigmentation.

DOSAGE

Pediatric *PO*		
Body surface area (m²)	Tablets	Pediatric solution
1.1-1.4	100mg bid	125mg/12.5ml bid
0.8-1.0	75mg bid	94mg/9.5ml bid
0.5-0.7	50mg bid	62mg/6ml bid
≤0.5	25mg bid	31mg/3ml bid
Adult *PO*		
Weight	Tablets	Solution (packet)
≤75kg	300mg bid	375mg bid
50-74kg	200mg big	250mg bid
35-49kg	125mg bid	167mg bid

SIDE/ADVERSE EFFECTS: CNS: headache, peripheral neuropathy, insomnia, depression, dizziness ▪ CV: hypertension, vasodilation ▪ GI: anorexia, N/V/D, abdominal pain, constipation, stomatitis, taste changes, dry mouth, ***pancreatitis*** ▪ HEM: ***leukopenia***, granulocytopenia, ***thrombocytopenia*** ▪ HEP: ***liver failure*** ▪ INT: alopecia, rash, pruritus, eczema ▪ MS: arthritis, myalgia, asthenia ▪ RESP: asthma, cough, rhinitis, rhinorrhea ▪ Other: otic pain, malaise, photophobia.

INTERACTIONS: Drug: Use c̄ tetracycline best avoided ▪ Administer drugs such as dapsone, ketoconazole, whose absorption is affected by stomach acidity, 2h before didanosine administration ▪ Use c̄ drugs that cause peripheral neuropathy, pancreatitis requires close monitoring. **Food:** Meals ⬇ PO absorption (administer ac).

NURSING MANAGEMENT PRIORITIES

ADMINISTRATION: Assess for hx of hypersensitivity ▪ Administer on empty stomach (1h ac/2h pc) ▪ Chewable tablets: chew thoroughly or mix in 1oz H_2O to form dispersion; drink immediately ▪ PO solution: reconstitute & dilute c̄ antacid according to manufacturer's directions; shake admixture well before use; refrigerate, store in tightly closed container.

EVALUATION: Monitor VS, esp temperature ▪ Assess for development of neuropathy (numbness, tingling, pain in distal extremities) ▪ Monitor hepatic, renal status.

EDUCATION: Take as ordered by physician at equal intervals around clock to maintain blood levels; do *not* ⬆ dose ▪ Do *not* share drug ▪ Women: avoid breastfeeding ▪ Used to control, *not* cure, HIV infections ▪ Notify physician of any change in health status ▪ Check c̄ physician/pharmacist before taking OTC preparations ▪ Avoid sexual contact, blood donation (risk of HIV transmission) ▪ Keep scheduled appointments c̄ physician/for blood work.

NOTES:

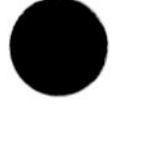

diethylstilbestrol/diethylstilbestrol diphosphate • (dye-eth-ul-stil-bess-trole)

CATEGORY: *Estrogenic agent*

Rx; Preg Cat X

AVAILABLE PREPARATIONS	DOSAGE FORMS
Diethylstilbestrol (various)	Tablet: 0.1, 0.25, 0.5, 1, 5mg
Diethylstilbestrol Diphosphate *Stilphostrol (Miles)*	Injection (IV): 0.25g/ampule Tablet: 50mg

USE: Palliation of breast/prostatic cancer. Diphosphate salt is currently limited to prostatic cancer palliation. **ACTION:** Drug appears to have same mechanism as natural estrogens: development, maintenance of female reproductive system, 2° sex characteristics.

PHARMACOKINETICS: Drug exhibits good PO absorption, slow metabolism, & is excreted as metabolites via urine, feces.

CONTRAINDICATIONS: Known/suspected pregnancy, estrogen-dependent neoplasms, breast cancer except in appropriately selected pts; abnormal genital bleeding, active or in pts c̄ a hx of thrombophlebitis/thrombophlebitic disorders (except breast/prostate cancer treatment). **CC:** Estrogenic agents have been reported to ⬆ risk of endometrial cancer, gallbladder disease ▪ Not indicated for postcoital contraception.

DOSAGE

Adult *PO* Usual palliation dose for prostate cancer 1-3mg/d, which can be ⬇ to 1mg/d. Usual dose for breast cancer 15mg/d. Dose of diphosphate salt 50mg tid & ⬆ depending on pt tolerance. Do *not* exceed 1g/d. Usual IV dose 0.5g/d & ⬆ to 1g on subsequent days for ≥5d followed by 0.25-0.5g maintenance dose 1-2 times/wk

SIDE/ADVERSE EFFECTS: CNS: headache, migraine, dizziness, mental depression ▪ EENT: intolerance to contact lenses, steepening of corneal curvature ▪ GI: N/V, abdominal cramps, bloating ▪ GU: amenorrhea, breakthrough bleeding, dysmenorrhea, candidiasis, change in menstrual flow, spotting, ⬆ size of uterine fibromyomas ▪ INT: melasma, ***erythema multiforme***/nodosum, alopecia, hirsutism, urticaria ▪ MET: ⬇ carbohydrate tolerance ▪ Other: weight changes, edema, porphyria exacerbation.

INTERACTIONS: Drug: Use c̄ TCAs may result in toxic rxs.

NURSING MANAGEMENT PRIORITIES

ADMINISTRATION: Assess for hx of hypersensitivity ▪ Administer cyclically (3wks on, 1wk off) c̄ meals ▪ Do *not* crush enteric-coated tablets; administer whole ▪ Schedule pregnancy test for sexually active women before administration ▪ Avoid abrupt withdrawal; D/C gradually.

EVALUATION: Monitor hepatic, renal status ▪ Monitor BP ▪ Assess PT; may ⬇ anticoagulant effect ▪ Diabetics: careful blood/urine testing; may ⬇ antidiabetic drug effect ▪ Assess for behavioral changes, depression ▪ Monitor pt weight; observe for edema.

EDUCATION: Review package insert c̄ pt ▪ Nausea may occur during first 2wks of therapy ▪ Women: avoid pregnancy, breastfeeding ▪ Breast self-exam (incl men) ▪ Avoid smoking (⬆ CV complications) ▪ Take c̄ food ▪ Notify physician/dentist of use before treatment ▪ Keep scheduled appointments c̄ physician ▪ Avoid exposure to direct sunlight, UV light (sunlamps); use sunscreen, protective clothing ▪ D/C drug, notify physician if pregnancy is suspected ▪ Notify physician *immediately* of chest/leg pain, unusual vaginal bleeding, difficult breathing, slurred speech ▪ Men: enlarged breasts, impotence reversible after therapy ▪ Check weight, swelling in feet/legs daily.

NOTES:

digitoxin • (di-ji-tox-in)

CATEGORY: *Cardiac glycoside*

Rx; Preg Cat C

BRAND NAME
Crystodigin (Lilly)

DOSAGE FORMS
Tablet: 0.05, 0.1mg

USE: Treatment of CHF, supraventricular arrhythmias. **ACTION:** Dig glycosides ⬆ force of myocardial contractions; ⬆ refractory period of AV, SA nodes; ⬇ conductivity of AV node, bundle of His, heart rate.

DOSAGE: Dig doses usually administered w/in 24h divided.

Pediatric	*PO*	Dig dose usually divided, ≥6h between doses Premature: 0.022mg/kg Newborn: 0.025mg/kg 2wks-1yr: 0.040-0.045mg/kg 1-2y/o: 0.040mg/kg 2-12y/o: 0.020-0.030mg/kg
Adult	*PO*	Dig dose usually 0.6mg followed by 0.4mg & 0.2mg at 4-6h intervals. Usual maintenance dose 0.05-0.3mg/d

PHARMACOKINETICS

Route	Absorption	Onset	Peak	Half-life	Protein binding	Excretion
PO	Complete	30m-2h	4-12h	120-168h	97%	Up to 14-21d for complete renal excretion; also in feces
IM/IV	——	24m-2h	4-12h	120-168h	97%	

CONTRAINDICATIONS: Hypersensitivity, ventricular tachycardia, presence of toxic effects. **CC:** Use for management of idiopathic hypertrophic subaortic stenosis is doubtful in absence of severe cardiac failure.

SIDE/ADVERSE EFFECTS: CNS: apathy, headache, psychosis (rare) ▪ CV: conduction disturbances, PVCs ▪ EENT: blurred, yellow/red/green vision ▪ GI: N/V/D, anorexia ▪ Other: diaphoresis, gynecomastia, fatigue.

INTERACTIONS: Drug: Acetazolamide, amphotericin B, chlorthalidone, ethacrynic acid, furosemide, laxatives, thiazides, other K^+-reducing agents ↑ dig toxicity by inducing hypokalemia ▪ Parenteral Ca administration can produce serious arrhythmias ▪ Antacids, antidiarrheals, ion-exchange resins ↓ PO dig absorption ▪ Barbiturates, hydantoins, phenylbutazone ↓ dig activity by enzyme induction ▪ Use cautiously c̄ adrenergics, β blockers, quinidine, procainamide. **Food:** Excessive consumption of licorice can ↑ dig toxicity.

NURSING MANAGEMENT PRIORITIES

ADMINISTRATION: Loading dose must be administered to achieve therapeutic blood levels; assess for dig ingestion w/in past 2wks ▪ Assess for toxicity before administering each dose (N/V, bradycardia, arrhythmias) ▪ Check apical pulse for 1m before administration; if <60/>120 hold dose, notify physician ▪ Administer single PO dose in AM c̄ food ▪ Elderly may require ↓ dosage.

EVALUATION: Monitor serum electrolytes (hypokalemia, hypercalcemia, hypomagnesemia ↑ dig toxicity) ▪ Check cardiac monitor for arrhythmias ▪ Assess cardiopulmonary, renal status; monitor I&O ▪ Therapeutic serum dig level: 25-35ng/ml.

EDUCATION: Take as ordered by physician; do *not* skip dose w/out notifying physician ▪ Notify physician of symptoms of toxicity (loss of appetite, N/D, visual problems, irregular heartbeat) ▪ Eat foods high in K^+, esp if taking diuretics; avoid black licorice ▪ Procedure for radial pulse determination ▪ Check radial pulse each AM for 1m; notify physician if slow (<60)/irregular ▪ Maintain optimum weight; avoid high-Na^+ substances ▪ Check c̄ physician before taking other medications ▪ Store in cool, dry, light-resistant container.

OVERDOSE MANAGEMENT: *See* Cardiac Glycosides.

NOTES:

digoxin • (di-jox-in)

CATEGORY: *Cardiac glycoside*

Rx; Preg Cat C

BRAND NAMES

Lanoxicaps (G-W)
Lanoxin (G-W)

DOSAGE FORMS

Capsule: 0.05, 0.1, 0.2mg
Pediatric elixir: 0.05mg/ml
Pediatric injection: 0.1mg/ml
Injection: 0.25mg/ml
Tablet: 0.125, 0.25, 0.5mg

USE: Treatment of CHF, supraventricular arrhythmias. **ACTION:** Dig glycosides ↑ force of myocardial contraction; ↑ refractory period of AV, SA nodes; ↓ conductivity of AV node, bundle of His, heart rate.

CONTRAINDICATIONS: Hypersensitivity, ventricular tachycardia, presence of toxic effects. **CC:** Use c̄ active glomerulonephritis requires extreme caution esp during digitalization.

DOSAGE: Dig doses usually given w/in 24h; first dose 50% of total dose, followed by two 25% doses given at 48-h intervals.

Pediatric *IV*
Premature: 0.015-0.025mg/kg
Newborn: 0.020-0.030mg/kg
1mo-2y/o: 0.030-0.050mg/kg
2-5y/o: 0.025-0.035mg/kg
5-10y/o: 0.015-0.030mg/kg
>10y/o: 0.008-0.012mg/kg

PO
Premature: 0.020-0.030mg/kg
Newborn: 0.025-0.035mg/kg
1mo-2y/o: 0.035-0.060mg/kg
2-5y/o: 0.030-0.040mg/kg
5-10y/o: 0.020-0.035mg/kg
>10y/o: 0.010-0.015mg/kg

PHARMACOKINETICS

	PO absorption	Onset	Peak	Duration	Half-life	Protein binding	Excretion
PO	50%-90%	50m-2h	2-6h	2-4d	36h	20%-25%	Renal, feces
IV	—	5-30m	1-4h	2-4d	36h	20%-25%	Renal, feces

	Usual pediatric maintenance dose is 20%-35% of dig dose
Adult *PO/IV*	Usual dig dose 1-1.5mg/d, c̄ usual maintenance dose 0.125-0.5mg/d

SIDE/ADVERSE EFFECTS: CNS: apathy, headache, psychosis (rare) ▪ CV: conduction disturbances, PVCs, bradycardia ▪ EENT: blurred, yellow/red/green vision ▪ GI: N/V/D, anorexia ▪ Other: diaphoresis, gynecomastia, fatigue.

INTERACTIONS: Drug: Acetazolamide, amphotericin B, chlorthalidone, ethacrynic acid, furosemide, laxatives, thiazides, other K^+-reducing agents ↑ dig toxicity by inducing hypokalemia ▪ Parenteral Ca administration can produce serious arrhythmias ▪ Antacids, antidiarrheals, ion-exchange resins ↓ PO dig absorption ▪ Barbiturates, hydantoins, phenylbutazone ↓ dig activity by enzyme induction ▪ Use cautiously c̄ adrenergics, β blockers, quinidine, procainamide. **Food:** Excessive consumption of licorice can ↑ dig toxicity.

NURSING MANAGEMENT PRIORITIES

ADMINISTRATION: Loading dose must be administered to achieve therapeutic blood levels; assess for dig ingestion w/in past 2wks ▪ Assess renal function; may require ↓ dosage ▪ Assess for toxicity before administering each dose (N/V, bradycardia, arrhythmias) ▪ Check apical pulse for 1m before administration; if <60/>120 hold dose, notify physician ▪ Administer single PO dose in AM c̄ food ▪ IV: preferred parenteral route; administer *slowly* ▪ Elderly may require ↓ dosage.

EVALUATION: Monitor serum electrolytes (K^+, Ca^{++}, Mg^{++}) ▪ Monitor I&O ▪ Therapeutic serum digoxin level: 0.5-2.0ng/ml.

EDUCATION: Take as ordered by physician; do *not* skip dose w/out notifying physician ▪ Notify physician of symptoms of toxicity (loss of appetite, N/D, visual problems, irregular heartbeat) ▪ Eat foods high in K^+, esp if taking diuretics; avoid black licorice ▪ Check radial pulse each AM for 1m; notify physician if slow (<60)/irregular ▪ Maintain optimum weight; avoid high-Na^+ substances ▪ Check c̄ physician before taking other medications ▪ Store in cool, dry, light-resistant container.

OVERDOSE MANAGEMENT: *See* Cardiac Glycosides.

NOTES:

diltiazem hcl • (dil-tye-a-zem)

CATEGORY: *Calcium blocker:* antianginal, slow channel blocker Rx; Preg Cat C

BRAND NAMES	DOSAGE FORMS
Cardizem (MMD) *(Nordic [Canada])*	SR capsule: 60, 90, 120mg CD capsule: 120, 180, 240, 300mg Tablet: 30, 60, 90, 120mg IV injection: 5mg/ml
Dilacor XR (RPR)	Capsule: 180, 240mg

USE: Treatment of chronic stable angina (CD, XR capsules) ▪ Treatment of vasospastic angina (tablet) ▪ Treatment of hypertension as a sole agent (CD, SR, XR, capsules)/in combination c̄ other antihypertensives ▪ Treatment of atrial fibrillation/flutter, paroxysmal supraventricular tachycardia (IV). **ACTION:** Antianginal effect due to inhibition of extracellular Ca^{+}-ion transmembrane migration in cardiac, vascular smooth muscle via slow channel passageway, resulting in coronary vasodilation; ↑ myocardial oxygen supply, ↓ oxygen consumption.

CONTRAINDICATIONS: Hypersensitivity, sick sinus syndrome or 2nd/3rd° AV block (except in presence of pacemaker), hypotension (<90 systolic), acute MI, & pulmonary congestion (documented by x-ray film). **CC:** ↑ CHF is possible in pts c̄ preexisting ventricular function impairment.

DOSAGE

Adult *PO*

Chronic angina	120-180mg once/d c̄ doses up to 480mg
Vasospastic angina	Initial dose 30mg qid (ac, at hs). Usual range 180-240mg divided 3-4 doses/d
Hypertension	180-540mg once/d

PHARMACOKINETICS

	PO absorption	Onset	Peak	Half-life	Protein binding	Excretion
Tablet	>95%	30m	2-4h	3-4.5h	70%-80%	Via urine, feces primarily as metabolites

Adult	*IV*	
Arrhythmias		Bolus dose 0.25mg/kg over 2m. Second dose 0.35mg/kg over 2m after 15m prn. Then 5-15mg/h by continuous infusion for 24h

SIDE/ADVERSE EFFECTS: CNS: *headache, dizziness,* nervousness, sleep disturbances ▪ CV: *peripheral edema,* ***arrhythmias***, palpitations, CHF, *bradycardia* ▪ GI: *nausea,* diarrhea, constipation ▪ INT: rash, pruritus, photosensitivity.

INTERACTIONS: Drug: Use c̄ dig may ↑ dig serum level ▪ Use c̄ β blockers may prolong cardiac conduction time. **Lab:** Transient ↑ in ALT, AST, LDH.

NURSING MANAGEMENT PRIORITIES

ADMINISTRATION: Assess for hx of hypersensitivity ▪ Assess for hx of heart failure; use c̄ caution ▪ Assess BP, heart rate; if apical pulse <60, hold dose, notify physician ▪ Administer ac, at hs; may crush tablets ▪ Elderly may require ↓ dosage.

EVALUATION: Monitor VS, esp BP, pulse ▪ Monitor I&O ▪ Monitor hepatic, renal status ▪ Assess for CHF (dyspnea, peripheral edema, ↑ weight); notify physician ▪ Monitor PR interval (may ↑) ▪ Digitalized pts: assess for dig toxicity (bradycardia, anorexia, palpitations).

EDUCATION: Dizziness may occur; use caution in potentially hazardous activities ▪ Avoid changing positions (lying/sitting/standing) rapidly ▪ Procedure for checking radial pulse ▪ If pulse slow (<60)/irregular, do *not* take dose, notify physician ▪ Avoid caffeine ▪ Check c̄ physician/pharmacist before taking OTC preparations ▪ Take as ordered by physician; do *not* change dosage ▪ Notify physician of difficult breathing, chest pain, swelling of hands/legs; D/C drug ▪ Keep scheduled appointments c̄ physician ▪ Continue SL nitroglycerin (if ordered) to relieve sudden chest pain or for prophylaxis before exertion ▪ Avoid use c̄ alcohol.

NOTES:

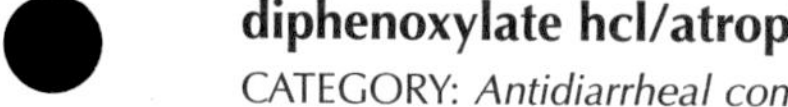

diphenoxylate hcl/atropine sulfate • (dye-fen-ox-i-late/a-troe-peen)

CATEGORY: *Antidiarrheal combination*

Rx C-V; Preg Cat C

BRAND NAME
Lomotil (Searle)

DOSAGE FORMS
Diphenoxylate/atropine per 5ml liquid/tablet: 2.5mg/0.025mg

USE: Adjunct in management of diarrhea. **ACTION:** Antidiarrheal effect due to slowing of intestinal motility.

PHARMACOKINETICS: Combination has good PO absorption, rapid metabolism, & is excreted primarily as metabolites via urine, feces.

CONTRAINDICATIONS: Hypersensitivity, diarrhea associated c̄ pseudomembranous enterocolitis or enterotoxin-producing bacteria, obstructive jaundice. **CC:** Complete management of diarrhea requires appropriate electrolyte, fluid replacement ▪ Use c̄ caution in young children c̄ strict dosage compliance due to possible delayed toxicity; greater response variables in this age group.

DOSAGE

Pediatric *PO*	2y/o: 1.5-3ml qid
	3y/o: 2-3ml qid
	4y/o: 2-4ml qid
	5y/o: 2.5-4.5ml qid
	6-8y/o: 2.5-5ml qid
	9-12y/o: 3.5-5ml qid
Adult *PO*	2 tablets/10ml liquid qid. Control usually maintained c̄ 2 tablets/10ml/d

SIDE/ADVERSE EFFECTS: CNS: sedation, dizziness, depression, numbness of extremities, euphoria, lethargy ▪ GI: N/V, abdominal discomfort, paralytic ileus, ***toxic megacolon,*** anorexia ▪ INT: pruritus ▪ Other: anticholinergic: normal effects due to atropine (eg, dry mouth, blurred vision), respiratory depression, angioneurotic edema, swollen gums.

INTERACTIONS: Drug: Use c̄ CNS depressants produces additive effects ▪ Use c̄ anticholinergics produces additive effects ▪ Use c̄ MAO-I not recommended.

NURSING MANAGEMENT PRIORITIES

ADMINISTRATION: Assess for hx of hypersensitivity to either compounds ▪ Assess F/E balance; do *not* administer if severely impaired ▪ Assess hepatic function; ↓ dosage if impaired ▪ Avoid exposure to moisture/light in storage; do *not* freeze liquid form ▪ May crush tablet, administer c̄ food.

EVALUATION: Monitor bowel function; ⬇ dose as diarrhea is controlled ▪ Assess for atropinism (dry mouth, blurred vision, tachycardia) ▪ Assess hydration status (I&O, daily weight) ▪ Check for signs of dependence c̄ prolonged use ▪ Assess for abdominal distention; D/C drug ▪ Monitor children, elderly closely (⬆ susceptibility to adverse effects).

EDUCATION: Follow clear liquid/bland diet until diarrhea subsides ▪ Take as directed by physician; do *not* ⬆ dose ▪ Avoid use c̄ alcohol, caffeine ▪ Do *not* take c̄ CNS depressants ▪ May cause drowsiness/dizziness; use caution in potentially hazardous activities ▪ Indiscriminate use may lead to dependence ▪ Use sugarless gum/hard candy to diminish dry mouth ▪ Maintain fluid intake (6-8 glasses/d) ▪ Store in tightly closed, light-resistant container ▪ Women: avoid breastfeeding ▪ Notify physician if diarrhea persists (>48h), fever occurs.

NOTES:

dipyridamole • (dye-peer-id-a-mole)

CATEGORY: *Platelet inhibitor:* anticoagulant

Rx; Preg Cat B

BRAND NAMES	DOSAGE FORMS
**Apo-Dipyridamole (Apotex)*	Tablet: 25, 50, 75mg
Persantine (B-I)	Tablet: 25, 50, 75mg

USE: Adjunct to coumarin anticoagulants in preventing postoperative thromboembolic rxs in prosthetic heart valve replacement. **ACTION:** Anticoagulant activity due to a dose-dependent lengthening of abnormally shortened platelet survival time that occurs c̄ prosthetic heart valve replacement.

PHARMACOKINETICS: Exhibits slow absorption c̄ a peak in about 75m; high protein binding; fecal (biliary) excretion as glucuronide conjugates.

CONTRAINDICATIONS: Hypersensitivity. **CC:** Use c̄ caution in pts c̄ hypotension due to possible peripheral vasodilation ▪ Drug is excreted in breast milk. Use c̄ caution in nursing mothers ▪ Safety & efficacy in children ≤12y/o not established.

DOSAGE

Adult *PO* — Usual adjunct dose 75-100mg qid

SIDE/ADVERSE EFFECTS: CNS: headache, dizziness, syncope ▪ GI: nausea, distress ▪ INT: skin rash ▪ Other: flushing, weakness.

INTERACTIONS: Drug: Use c̄ heparin requires caution ▪ Use c̄ aspirin produces additive antiplatelet activity.

NURSING MANAGEMENT PRIORITIES

ADMINISTRATION: Assess for hx of hypersensitivity ▪ Administer 1h ac/2h pc c̄ full glass H_2O; may crush, mix c̄ food; may administer c̄ meals if GI distress occurs.

EVALUATION: Monitor VS, esp BP ▪ Assess for bleeding, esp c̄ anticoagulants, aspirin.

EDUCATION: Dizziness may occur; use caution in potentially hazardous activities ▪ Avoid changing positions (lying/sitting/standing) rapidly ▪ Take as ordered by physician; do *not* change frequency ▪ May take c̄ meals; *best* on empty stomach (1h ac/2h pc) ▪ Avoid changing brand-name preparations ▪ Avoid use c̄ alcohol ▪ Avoid smoking ▪ Check c̄ physician/pharmacist before taking OTC preparations ▪ Notify physician of unusual bleeding/bruising ▪ Full drug effects may require several wks of therapy.

NOTES:

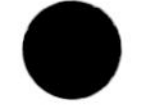

dirithromycin • (di-rith-row-mye-sin)

CATEGORY: *Antibiotic:* macrolide antibiotic (semisynthetic) Rx; Preg Cat C

BRAND NAME
Dynabac (Sanofi)

DOSAGE FORM
Enteric tablet: 250mg

USE: Treatment of infections caused by susceptible strains of *Legionella pneumophilia, Moraxella catarrhalis, Mycoplasma pneumoniae, Staphylococcus aureus* (methicillin-resistant), *Streptococcus pyogenes* (pharyngitis/tonsillitis).
ACTION: Bacteriostatic activity due to inhibition of ribosomal protein synthesis. Drug is inactive (pro-drug) & is converted into active metabolite erythromycylamine by hydrolysis during PO absorption.

PHARMACOKINETICS

PO absorption	Peak	Half-life	Protein binding	Excretion
Adequate	3.9-4.1h	8h	15%-30%	Via bile, feces primarily as unchanged metabolites

CONTRAINDICATIONS: Hypersensitivity to drug or other macrolide antibiotics. **CC:** Use can result in pseudomembranous colitis ▪ Not indicated for *Streptococcus pyogenes* skin/skin structure infections, *Haemophilus* spp. respiratory infections, bacteremias ▪ Safety & efficacy in <12y/o not established.

DOSAGE

Adult/Children >12y/o	*PO*	500mg once/d for 7-14d, depending on infection

SIDE/ADVERSE EFFECTS: CNS: dizziness, headache, insomnia ▪ GI: abdominal pain, N/V/D, flatulence, ***pseudomembranous colitis***, dyspepsia ▪ HEM: ↑ in eosinophilia, neutrophilia platelet count ▪ Other: asthenia, dyspnea, nonspecific pain, rash.

INTERACTIONS: Drug: Bacteriostatic antibiotics can antagonize effects of bactericidal antibiotics ▪ Use c̄ H_2-blockers, antacids (c̄ immediate administration) can ↑ PO absorption of dirithromycin (erythromycylamine). ▪ Use c̄ triazolam can ↑ its effects ▪ Macrolides can ↑ toxicity of ergotamine, dihyroergotamine, oral anticoagulants

Food: Administration c̄ food after eating or w/in 1h will ↑ PO absorption.

NURSING MANAGEMENT PRIORITIES

ADMINISTRATION: Assess for erythromycin/macrolide sensitivity ▪ Obtain C&S before therapy ▪ Administer w/out regard to meals c̄ full glass H_2O (avoid citrus juice); do *not* crush ▪ Avoid antacids w/in 2h of administration.

EVALUATION: Monitor VS, esp temperature ▪ Monitor GI status ▪ Observe for signs of superinfection (diarrhea, perineal itching, oral ulcers).

EDUCATION: Dizziness may occur; use caution in potentially hazardous activities ▪ Complete full course of therapy ▪ Can be taken c̄ meals (avoid citrus juice); swallow whole ▪ Take at equal intervals around clock to maintain blood levels ▪ Diarrhea may occur; notify physician ▪ Notify physician of symptoms of allergic rx (fever, difficult breathing, rash).

NOTES:

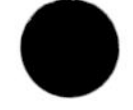

disopyramide phosphate • (dye-soe-peer-a-mide)

CATEGORY: *Antiarrhythmic*

Rx; Preg Cat C

BRAND NAMES

Norpace (Searle)

**Rythmodan (Rouscel)*

DOSAGE FORMS

Capsule: 100, 150mg
CR Capsule: 100, 150mg
Capsule: 100,150mg

USE: Treatment of cardiac arrhythmias incl unifocal, multifocal premature (ectopic) ventricular contractions, paired premature ventricular contractions, episodes of ventricular tachycardia. **ACTION:** Antiarrhythmic effect similar to procainamide, quinidine (type 1 antiarrhythmics); ↓ rate of diastolic depolarization in cells c̄ augmented automaticity, upstroke velocity, while ↑ action potential duration of normal cardiac cells.

PHARMACOKINETICS

PO absorption	Peak	Half-life	Protein binding	Excretion
Complete	2h	6.7h	50%-65%	Via urine as unchanged drug, metabolites

CONTRAINDICATIONS: Hypersensitivity, cardiogenic shock, preexisting 2nd, 3rd° AV block (if no pacemaker present), congenital Q-T prolongation. **CC:** Use in CHF can exacerbate condition ▪ D/C use c̄ QRS widening ▪ >25% Q-T prolongation c̄ continued ectopy requires consideration for D/C ▪ Use c̄ type 1a antiarrhythmics should be limited to life-threatening arrhythmias ▪ ↓ Dosage if 1° heart block develops.

DOSAGE

Adult *PO* — Usual dose 150mg q6h, 300mg (CR) q12h, c̄ daily range 400-800mg divided

SIDE/ADVERSE EFFECTS: CNS: dizziness, headache, nervousness, depression, insomnia ▪ CV: ***hypotension***, ↑ CHF, conduction disturbances, esp ***QRS widening*** ▪ EENT: blurred vision; dry nose, throat, eyes ▪ GI: *dry mouth, gas bloating* c̄ pain, constipation, anorexia, N/V/D ▪ GU: *urinary hesitancy*, impotence, dysuria ▪ INT: rash, dermatoses, pruritus ▪ MET: hypokalemia ▪ MS: muscle aches, pains.

Note: Side/adverse effects: common in *italic;* serious in ***boldface italic.***

*Available in Canada only.

INTERACTIONS: Drug: Use c̄ anticholinergics produces additive effects ▪ Use c̄ phenytoin (enzyme inducer) produces ↓ blood levels.

NURSING MANAGEMENT PRIORITIES

ADMINISTRATION: Assess for hx of hypersensitivity ▪ Assess for hx of heart failure; use c̄ caution ▪ Assess apical pulse; if <60/>120, hold dose, notify physician ▪ Monitor ECG; D/C if widened QRS/↑ arrhythmias ▪ Assess hepatic, renal function, IOP in glaucoma; notify physician if abnormal, hold drug ▪ Assess serum K^+ (normal: 3.5-5mEq/L); correct imbalances ▪ Administer 1h ac/2h pc ▪ Administer SR capsules whole; do *not* crush ▪ Avoid abrupt withdrawal; D/C gradually ▪ Elderly may require ↓ dosage.

EVALUATION: Monitor hepatic, renal status ▪ Monitor VS, esp BP, heart rate ▪ Monitor I&O, daily weight ▪ Assess for CHF (dyspnea, peripheral edema, ↑ weight); notify physician ▪ Monitor serum K^+, glucose levels (hypoglycemia) ▪ Therapeutic blood levels: 2-4μg/ml.

EDUCATION: Take on empty stomach (1h ac/2h pc); swallow SR capsules whole ▪ Take as ordered by physician; do *not* change dose or time intervals ▪ Check c̄ physician/pharmacist before taking any OTC preparations ▪ Use sugarless gum/hard candy to diminish dry mouth ▪ Avoid exposure to direct sunlight/UV light (sunlamps); use sunscreen, protective clothing ▪ Dizziness, blurred vision may occur; use caution in potentially hazardous activities ▪ Avoid use c̄ alcohol ▪ Constipation may occur; ↑ fluid, roughage in diet ▪ Notify physician of eye pain, swelling in hands/legs ▪ Avoid ↑ exercise, temperature extremes ▪ Diabetics: hypoglycemia may occur; take sugar, notify physician.

NOTES:

dobutamine hcl • (doe-byoo-ta-meen)

CATEGORY: *Sympathomimetic:* β_1-adrenergic

Rx; Preg Cat B

BRAND NAME	DOSAGE FORM	DOSAGE	
Dobutrex (Lilly)	Powder for injection (IV): 250mg/vial	Adult *IV infusion*	Usual dose 2.5-10μg/kg/m. Doses up to 40μg/kg/m may be required

USE: Short-term treatment of cardiac decompensation due to depressed contractility associated c̄ organic heart disease or cardiac surgical procedures. **ACTION:** β_1-Receptor activity produces cardiac stimulation, positive inotropic effect, ↑ cardiac output, ↑ stroke volume; ↓ peripheral resistance; does not cause release of norepinephrine.

PHARMACOKINETICS

Onset	Peak	Half-life	Excretion
1-2m	Up to 10m	2m	Primarily via urine as metabolites

CONTRAINDICATIONS: Hypersensitivity, idiopathic hypertrophic subaortic stenosis. **CC:** Use may cause significant ↑ in heart rate or BP ▪ Powder for injection contains sodium bisulfite, which can cause rare bronchospasm, other hypersensitivities.

SIDE/ADVERSE EFFECTS: CNS: headache ▪ CV: *dose-related ↑ heart rate,* BP, ***ventricular ectopic activity;*** palpitation, anginal pain ▪ GI: nausea ▪ RESP: shortness of breath.

INTERACTIONS: Drug: Use c̄ nitroprusside may result in ↑ cardiac output, ↓ pulmonary wedge pressure ▪ Use c̄ β blockers antagonizes therapeutic effects ▪ Use c̄ halogenated general anesthetics may cause serious arrhythmias ▪ Use c̄ MAO-I will ↑ pressor effects; ↓ doses are needed.

NURSING MANAGEMENT PRIORITIES

ADMINISTRATION: Assess for hx of catecholamine hypersensitivity ▪ Assess fluid balance; correct hypovolemia ▪ Do *not* mix c̄ sodium bicarbonate, other alkaline solutions ▪ Reconstitute c̄ 10ml sterile H_2O for injection/5% dextrose injection; if not completely dissolved, add 10ml diluent; further dilute to 50ml, administer c̄ 5% dextrose/0.9% NaCl/sodium lactate injection, use w/in 24h;

administer via infusion pump ▪ Reconstituted solution stable 6h at room temperature, 48h refrigerated ▪ Do *not* freeze (crystallizes) ▪ Pink discoloration does *not* affect potency ▪ Do *not* mix in same IV line c̄ heparin, hydrocortisone, cefazolin, cefamandole, cephalothin, penicillin, sodium ethacrynate.

EVALUATION: Monitor VS, esp BP, heart rate q2-5m ▪ Monitor ECG, hemodynamic status q15m ▪ Monitor I&O q15-30m ▪ Check IV infusion site carefully; avoid extravasation.

EDUCATION: Notify nurse/physician of abnormal rxs (difficult breathing, chest pain, irregular heartbeat).

NOTES:

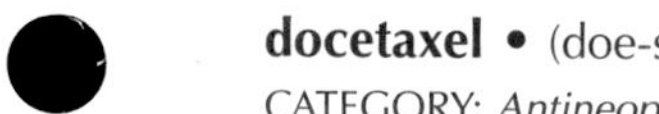

docetaxel • (doe-seh-tax-el)

CATEGORY: *Antineoplastic:* antimicrotubule agent — Rx; Preg Cat D

BRAND NAME	**DOSAGE FORMS**
Taxotere (RPR)	IV injection: 20, 80mg/vial

USE: Treatment of advanced metastatic breast cancer in pts who have progressed or relapsed c̄ anthracycline-based therapy. **ACTION:** Semisynthetic antineoplastic obtained from the yew shrub. Antineoplastic activity related to antimicrotubule activity resulting in inhibition of cell replication. Docetaxel promotes synthesis of stable & nonfunctional microtubule that cannot be reorganized into a functional microtubule network, which is an essential part of the mitotic spindle during cell replication.

PHARMACOKINETICS: Following IV injection there is an initial rapid ↓ in plasma concentrations, which is followed by a second & slow influx of the drug from peripheral body compartments into plasma. Drug exhibits a three-phase half-life of 4m, 36m, 11.1h. Protein binding is 94%, excretion is primarily via feces as metabolites.

CONTRAINDICATIONS: Hypersensitivity to drug or polysorbate 80 formulated drugs, <1500mm^3 baseline neutrophil counts. **CC:** Use requires qualified physicians & baseline neutrophil counts >1500/mm^3 ▪ Toxic deaths have occurred at doses of 100mg/m^2 in pts c̄ normal & abnormal liver function. ▪ Use can produce severe fluid retention (6% of pts) even c̄ a premedication regimen ▪ Use in pts c̄ > normal bilirubin, AST, ALT levels is not usually recommended due to ↑ risk of grade 4 neutropenia.

DOSAGE

Adult	*IV*	60-100mg/m^2 administered over 1h q3wks

SIDE/ADVERSE EFFECTS: CNS: peripheral neuropathy (paresthesia most frequent) ▪ CV: ***atrial fibrillation, pulmonary edema/embolism, thrombophlebitis,*** tachycardia ▪ GI: N/V/D, stomatitis ▪ HEM: anemia, ***neutropenia, leukopenia, thrombocytopenia*** ▪ HEP ↑ levels of ALT, AST ▪ Other: asthenia, alopecia, arthralgia.

INTERACTIONS: Drug: Use c̄ other bone marrow depressants will produce additive effects ▪ Use c̄ erythromycin, ketoconazole, terfenadine requires caution due to alteration of their metabolism. **Lab:** ↑ Levels of ALT, AST.

NURSING MANAGEMENT PRIORITIES

ADMINISTRATION: Check pt hx for recent course of radiation/antineoplastic agents ▪ May premedicate c̄ PO corticosteroids (hypersensitivity) ▪ Administer antiemetic before therapy ▪ Dilute c̄ NSS or 5% dextrose according to manufacturer's directions before administration ▪ Diluted solution stable for 8h at room temperature or store refrigerated; stand at room temperature for 5m before using ▪ Administer by IV infusion over 1h ▪ Avoid exposure to heat/light in storage ▪ Provide emotional support.

EVALUATION: Monitor neurologic, hepatic, renal function ▪ Check IV site closely; avoid extravasation ▪ Monitor CBC throughout therapy, esp WBCs ▪ Assess for anaphylactic rxs; have support equipment available ▪ Assess for infection, bleeding, anemia ▪ Assess hydration status (I&O, daily weight).

EDUCATION: ↑ Fluid intake (8-10 glasses/d) ▪ Avoid exposure to infection ▪ Check c̄ physician before immunization (pt, family) ▪ Diet as tolerated, avoid spicy foods ▪ Maintain good oral hygiene; use soft-bristled toothbrush ▪ Loss of hair may occur (reversible) ▪ Notify physician of symptoms of bone marrow depression (fever, sore throat, bruising, bleeding, lethargy) ▪ Women: avoid breastfeeding ▪ Encourage ventilation of feelings ▪ Use contraception if sexually active.

NOTES:

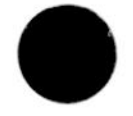

donepezil hcl • (don-eh-peh-zil)

CATEGORY: *Centrally acting cholinesterase inhibitor:* antidementia agent Rx; Preg Cat C

BRAND NAME	DOSAGE FORMS
Aricept (Pfizer)	Tablet: 5, 10mg

USE: Palliative treatment of mild to moderate symptoms of dementia of Alzheimer's disease. **ACTION:** Alzheimer's disease is associated c̄ ⬇ in cholinergic neurons in the brain, resulting in a deficiency of acetylcholine. Anticholinesterase activity of donepezil in the brain results in ⬆ acetylcholine levels, which help ⬇ early symptoms of dementia associated c̄ Alzheimer's disease.

PHARMACOKINETICS

PO absorption	Peak	Half-life	Protein binding	Excretion
Excellent	3-4h	70h	96%	Via feces, urine primarily as metabolites

CONTRAINDICATIONS: Hypersensitivity to drug or piperidine-derived drugs. **CC:** Use c̄ caution in pts c̄ conduction dysfunction caused by possible vagotonic activity, hx of ulcer diseases caused by ⬆ acid secretion, asthma ▪ Presence in breast milk not determined ▪ Safety, efficacy in children not established.

DOSAGE

Adult	*PO*	5 or 10mg once/d at hs. Do *not* ⬆ to 10mg/d until pt has been on 5mg/d for 4-6wks

SIDE/ADVERSE EFFECTS: CNS: headache, insomnia, dizziness, depression, abnormal dreams ▪ CV: hypertension, ECG abnormalities (eg, fibrillation, AV block), peripheral vascular disease ▪ EENT: blurred vision, ***glaucoma, cataract,*** tinnitus ▪ GI: N/V/D, anorexia, ***bleeding,*** ⬆ appetite ▪ GU: urinary irregularities ▪ RESP: bronchitis, sore throat, pulmonary congestion ▪ Other: bone fracture, ***thrombocytopenia.***

INTERACTIONS: Drug: Use c̄ anticholinergics can produce mutual antagonism ▪ Use c̄ succinylcholine-type muscle relaxants will produce ⬆ muscular relaxation ▪ Use c̄ other parasympathomimetics (cholinergics) can produce additive results ▪ Use c̄ NSAIAs may result in GI bleeding.

NURSING MANAGEMENT PRIORITIES

ADMINISTRATION: Assess for hx of hypersensitivity ▪ Administer at hs before sleep ▪ Institute safety precautions ▪ Avoid abrupt withdrawal; D/C gradually (cognitive deterioration).

EVALUATION: Monitor VS, IOP ▪ Monitor I&O, fluid retention, CHF ▪ Monitor for active or occult GI bleeding in high-risk pts (ulcer development).

EDUCATION: Dizziness/drowsiness may occur; use caution in potentially hazardous activities ▪ Take at hs ▪ Notify physician of clinical improvement (↑ mental function); abnormal rxs (diarrhea, rash, jaundice) ▪ Used to control, *not* cure, symptoms of Alzheimer's disease ▪ Keep scheduled appointments c̄ physician ▪ Full drug effects may require several wks of therapy.

NOTES:

dopamine hcl • (doe-pa-meen)

CATEGORY: *Sympathomimetic:* β_1-adrenergic

Rx; Preg Cat C

BRAND NAMES

Generic

***Revimine (USV)**

DOSAGE FORMS

Injection (IV): 40, 80, 160mg/ml

Injection (IV): 40mg/ml

USE: Treatment of shock syndrome due to chronic cardiac decompensation, endotoxic septicemia, MI, open heart surgery, renal failure, trauma. **ACTION:** Direct stimulation of β_1 receptors, dopaminergic receptors; in high doses, affects α receptors; sum total of adrenergic, dopaminergic activity results in positive inotropic effect, ↑ renal & mesenteric blood flow; α-adrenergic effects more pronounced c̄ higher doses, produces vasoconstriction, ↑ BP.

PHARMACOKINETICS

Onset	Half-life	Excretion
3-5m	2m	Via urine as metabolites in 24h

CONTRAINDICATIONS: Pheochromocytoma. **CC:** Do not use in presence of uncorrected tachyarrhythmias or ventricular fibrillation ▪ Do not mix injection c̄ any alkaline dilution solution due to chemical inactivation.

DOSAGE

Adult *IV infusion*	Start c̄ 1-5µg/kg/m. May be ↑ if needed. In severe cases, start c̄ 5µg/kg/m, gradually ↑ in 5-10µg/kg/m increments to 20-50µg/kg/m if needed

SIDE/ADVERSE EFFECTS: CNS: headache ▪ CV: anginal pain, ***ectopic beats,*** hypotension, tachycardia, vasoconstriction ▪ GI: N/V ▪ RESP: dyspnea ▪ Other: necrosis, tissue sloughing c̄ extravasation.

INTERACTIONS: Drug: Use c̄ cyclopropane/halogenated general anesthetics may cause serious arrhythmias ▪ Use c̄ MAO-I will ↑ pressor effects, ↓ doses are needed.

NURSING MANAGEMENT PRIORITIES

ADMINISTRATION: Assess for hx of catecholamine hypersensitivity ▪ Assess fluid balance; correct hypovolemia ▪ Monitor ABG; correct acidosis ▪ Dilute (stable for 24h); infuse into large vein, titrate rate according to findings following physician guidelines; use infusion pump ▪ Do *not* mix c̄ sodium bicarbonate, other alkaline solutions ▪ Do *not* mix alkaline drugs in same IV line ▪ Do *not* use discolored/precipitated solutions ▪ Have phentolamine available for extravasation ▪ Avoid exposure to light.

EVALUATION: Monitor VS, esp BP, heart rate (assess for ↓ BP when infusion is stopped) ▪ Monitor ECG, hemodynamic status q5-15m ▪ Monitor I&O q5-15m ▪ Check IV insertion site carefully; avoid extravasation ▪ Observe pts c̄ hx of peripheral vascular disease for change in color/temperature of extremities; assess peripheral pulses; notify physician of abnormalities.

EDUCATION: Notify nurse/physician of abnormal rxs (difficult breathing, chest pain, irregular heartbeat, pain at IV insertion site).

NOTES:

doxazosin mesylate/prazosin • (dox-ay-zoe-sin/pra-zoe-sin)

CATEGORY: *Antihypertensive:* α_1-blocker

Rx; Preg Cat B/C

BRAND NAMES	DOSAGE FORMS
doxazosin	
Cardura (Pfizer)	Tablet: 1, 2, 4, 8mg
prazosin	
Minipress (Pfizer)	Capsule: 1, 2, 5mg

COMBINATION PRODUCTS

Minizide 1, 2, 5 (Pfizer)	prazosin hcl/polythiazide per capsule: 1mg/0.5mg, 2mg/0.5mg, 5mg/0.5mg

PHARMACOKINETICS

PO absorption	Peak	Half-life	Protein binding	Excretion
doxazosin				
Good	2-3h	22h	98%	Via feces, urine as metabolites
prazosin				
Good	2-3h	2-4h	95%-97%	Via feces, urine as metabolites

USE: Treatment of hypertension as sole agent/in combination c̄ other antihypertensives, esp thiazides or β-adrenergic blockers ▪ Treatment of benign prostatic hyperplasia (BPH) (doxazosin). **ACTION:** Antihypertensive effect due to α_1-adrenergic blockage, resulting in ⬇ peripheral vascular resistance. Can exhibit first-dose syncope effect.

CONTRAINDICATIONS: Hypersensitivity. **CC:** To ⬇ first dose effect, initiate treatment c̄ 1mg/d & adjust ⬆ slowly.

DOSAGE: Adult *PO*

doxazosin	
Hypertension	Initial dose 1mg once/d; adjust if necessary to achieve desired effect. Doses of 16mg/d may be required.
BPH	4-8mg/d
prazosin	
Hypertension	Initial dose 1mg 2-3 times/d, may ⬆ to total 20mg/d. Usual maintenance range 6-15mg/d
Minizide	Usual dosage 1 capsule (1,2,5) 2-3 times/d

SIDE/ADVERSE EFFECTS: CNS: *dizziness, headache,* drowsiness, syncope, paresthesia, nervousness, depression ▪ CV: edema, palpitations, ***arrhythmia***, postural hypotension ▪ EENT: blurred vision, tinnitus, eye pain, rhinitis ▪ GI: N/D, dyspepsia, flatulence, dry mouth ▪ GU: polyuria ▪ INT: pruritus, rash ▪ RESP: dyspnea, chest pain ▪ Other: *fatigue, malaise,* pain, asthenia.

INTERACTIONS: Drug: Use c̄ other high protein-bound drugs can result in displacement from inactive protein binding sites ▪ Use c̄ β-blockers, thiazides produces additive hypotensive effects. **Lab:** Prazosin can produce false + screening test for pheochromocytoma.

NURSING MANAGEMENT PRIORITIES

ADMINISTRATION: Assess for hx of hypersensitivity ▪ Assess BP before administration ▪ Assess renal function; may require ↓ dose if impaired ▪ Administer c̄ food ▪ Elderly may require ↓ dosage.

EVALUATION: Monitor VS, esp BP ▪ Monitor for first-dose phenomenon (syncope); maintain recumbent position for 4h ▪ Monitor I&O, daily weight ▪ Assess peripheral circulation ▪ Assess for edema in extremities ▪ Monitor CV, renal status.

EDUCATION: Dizziness may occur; use caution in potentially hazardous activities ▪ Avoid changing positions (lying/sitting/standing) rapidly ▪ Take as directed by physician; do *not* change dose ▪ Used to control, *not* cure, hypertension ▪ Avoid use c̄ alcohol ▪ Use sugarless gum/hard candy to diminish dry mouth ▪ Avoid ↑ exercise, temperature extremes, smoking ▪ Maintain optimum weight ▪ Avoid high-Na^+ foods (canned soups, lunch meats, cheese) ▪ Check c̄ physician/pharmacist before taking OTC preparations ▪ Notify physician/dentist of use before treatment ▪ Do *not* D/C w/out checking c̄ physician ▪ Keep scheduled appointments c̄ physician; have BP checked regularly ▪ Carry identification (MedicAlert) if hypertensive ▪ Full drug effects may require several wks of therapy.

NOTES:

doxepin hcl • (dox-e-pin)

CATEGORY: *Tricyclic antidepressant:* mood elevator Rx; Preg Cat C

BRAND NAME

Sinequan (Roerig)
(Pfizer [Canada])

DOSAGE FORMS

Capsule: 10, 25, 50, 75, 100, 150mg
PO concentrate: 10mg/ml

USE: Treatment of endogenous depression ▪ Treatment of depression/anxiety c̄ alcoholism or organic disease ▪ Treatment of psychotic depressive disorders c̄ anxiety & manic-depressive conditions. **ACTION:** Antidepressant activity appears related to inhibition of norepinephrine re-uptake in central adrenergic neurons.

PHARMACOKINETICS

PO absorption	Peak	Half-life	Excretion
Rapid	2h	6-8h	Via urine as metabolites

CONTRAINDICATIONS: Hypersensitivity, MAO-I therapy, MI (acute recovery period), glaucoma, urinary retention. **CC:** Caution is required c̄ once-a-day dosage schedule for pts c̄ intercurrent illness or c̄ concurrent drug administration, esp c̄ drugs that have anticholinergic effect.

DOSAGE

Adult *PO* 75-150mg/d. Do *not* exceed 300mg/d

SIDE/ADVERSE EFFECTS: CNS: *drowsiness,* dizziness, headache, incoordination, tremors, extrapyramidal symptoms, paresthesia (extremities), insomnia ▪ CV: ***arrhythmias, MI*** (rare), stroke (rare), ***heart block*** (rare), orthostatic hypotension ▪ EENT: tinnitus ▪ GI: anorexia, N/V/D, stomatitis, cramps, black tongue, dry mouth, constipation ▪ GU: gynecomastia, testicular swelling, galactorrhea, breast enlargement, urinary hesitancy, urinary retention ▪ HEM: ***agranulocytosis,*** eosinophilia, ***thrombocytopenia*** ▪ HEP: cholestatic jaundice ▪ INT: skin rash, photosensitivity, alopecia ▪ PSYCH: disorientation, delusions, hallucinations, exacerbation of psychosis, confusion ▪ Other: parotid swelling.

INTERACTIONS: Drug: Significant depressant effects c̄ alcohol ▪ Anticholinergics, chlorpromazine produce ↑ atropinelike effects; paralytic ileus could occur ▪ Significant ↑ in activity c̄ epinephrine, levarterenol, other adrenergic agents ▪ Significant antagonism to effects of reserpine, clonidine, guanethidine-type antihypertensives ▪ Use c̄ MAO-I best avoided.

NURSING MANAGEMENT PRIORITIES

ADMINISTRATION: Assess for hx of TCA hypersensitivity ▪ Assess for impaired hepatic, renal function; hx of glaucoma, prostatic hypertrophy; may require ⬇ dosage ▪ PO: administer as single dose/d at hs c̄ food ▪ PO concentrate: use calibrated dropper; dilute in 120ml H_2O, milk, fruit, or tomato juice before administering; do *not* mix c̄ carbonated beverages ▪ Institute safety precautions ▪ Institute suicide precautions ▪ ⬆ Dosage *slowly*; maintenance dose lowest dose that will maintain remission of depression ▪ Avoid abrupt withdrawal; D/C gradually ▪ Heavy smokers may require ⬆ dosage ▪ Elderly may require ⬇ dosage.

EVALUATION: Monitor CV, hepatic, renal status ▪ Monitor VS, esp BP ▪ Monitor CBC, esp long-term ▪ Monitor fluid retention (I&O, daily weight), constipation ▪ Assess for symptoms of abrupt withdrawal (nausea, headache, malaise) ▪ Assess for actual swallowing of PO forms.

EDUCATION: Dizziness/drowsiness may occur; use caution in potentially hazardous activities ▪ Avoid changing positions (lying/sitting/standing) rapidly ▪ Avoid use of alcohol, other CNS depressants up to 1 wk after ending therapy ▪ Take PO forms c̄ food to ⬇ GI irritation ▪ Take as directed by physician ▪ Use sugarless gum/hard candy to diminish dry mouth ▪ Constipation may occur; ⬆ fluids, bulk-containing foods ▪ Check c̄ physician before taking OTC/Rx preparations ▪ May produce peculiar taste ▪ Notify physician/dentist of use before treatment ▪ Store in tightly closed container ▪ Avoid exposure to direct sunlight, UV light (sunlamps); use sunscreen, protective clothing ▪ Encourage recreational/diversional interests ▪ Notify physician of fever, sore throat, malaise ▪ Keep scheduled appointments c̄ physician ▪ Full drug effects may require several wks of therapy.

NOTES:

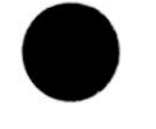

doxycycline hyclate/minocycline hcl •

(dox-i-sye-kleen/mi-noe-sye-kleen)

CATEGORY: *Tetracycline:* broad-spectrum antibiotic Rx; Preg Cat D

BRAND NAMES	**DOSAGE FORMS**
doxycycline	
Doryx (P-D)	Capsule, injection (IV), PO suspension, syrup, tablet
Doxychel Hyclate (Rachelle)	
Vibramycin (Pfizer)	
Vibra-Tabs (Pfizer)	
minocycline	
Minocin (Lederle)	Capsule, injection (IV), syrup

USE: Drug(s) of choice for chlamydial, mycoplasmal, rickettsial infections; acne control, balantidiasis, brucellosis, chancroid, cholera, granuloma inguinale, shigellosis, spirochetal relapsing fever ▪ Alternative in penicillin allergy, infections in which bacteriologic testing indicates good activity ▪ Infections due to susceptible strains of *Escherichia coli, Enterobacter aerogenes, Francisella tularensis,* gonococcal (male) urethritis, *Haemophilus influenzae, Klebsiella* spp, *Yersinia pestis* ▪ Malaria prophylaxis (doxycycline) starting 1-2d before travel & continue for 4wks after completion of travel. **ACTION:** Bacteriostatic effect due to inhibition of ribosomal protein synthesis.

CONTRAINDICATIONS: Hypersensitivity, pregnancy, nursing mothers, children <8y/o. **CC:** Use in children ≤8y/o or during the last half of pregnancy may cause yellow-gray-brown teeth discoloration.

DOSAGE

doxycycline *PO/IV*

Pediatric	>8y/o: 2mg/lb d1, then 1-2mg/lb/d
Children >8y/o	Malaria prophylaxis: 2mg/kg/d

PHARMACOKINETICS

	PO absorption: No food	PO absorption: Food	PO peak	Half-life	Protein binding	Excretion
doxycycline	90%-100%	70%-80%	2-12h	14-24h	30%-90%	Via feces, urine
minocycline	90%-100%	70%-80%	2-12h	11-26h	55%-80%	Via feces, urine

Note: Side/adverse effects: common in *italic;* serious in ***boldface italic.*** *Available in Canada only.

Adult	200mg d1, then 100-200mg/d Malaria prophylaxis: 100mg/d
minocycline *PO/IV*	
Pediatric	>8y/o: 4mg/kg followed by 2mg/kg q12h
Adult	200mg followed by 100mg q12h. Do *not* exceed 400mg/d IV

SIDE/ADVERSE EFFECTS: GI: gastric upset, diarrhea, bleeding, enterocolitis ▪ GU: dose-related ↑ BUN ▪ HEM: ***hemolytic anemia, thrombocytopenia***, ▪ INT: monilial overgrowth, maculopapular rash, ***exacerbation of SLE***, photosensitivity ▪ MS: reversible bulging fontanel in neonates, fetal skeletal retardation, discoloration of teeth ▪ Other: phlebitis at infusion site.

INTERACTIONS: Drug: Do *not* use c̄ antacids, antidiarrheals, bactericidal antibiotics, dairy products, methoxyflurane ▪ PO anticoagulants may require ↓ doses, esp during extended antibiotic therapy.

NURSING MANAGEMENT PRIORITIES

ADMINISTRATION: Assess for hx of tetracycline hypersensitivity ▪ Obtain C&S before therapy ▪ Avoid PO administration c̄ milk, dairy products, antacids/antidiarrheal suspensions, iron salts ▪ Shake PO suspensions well before pouring ▪ Administer PO dose c̄ full glass H_2O ▪ IV: dilute; administer *slowly* (over 1h) ▪ Use reconstituted IV solution immediately ▪ Avoid exposure to heat/moisture/light in storage ▪ Do *not* administer to pregnant women, neonates, children <8y/o (permanent discoloration of teeth, ↓ bone growth).

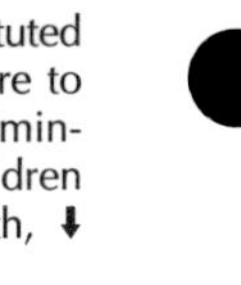

EVALUATION: Monitor pt receiving anticoagulant therapy; may potentiate bleeding ▪ Assess renal, hepatic status ▪ Monitor VS, esp temperature ▪ Observe for signs of superinfection (diarrhea, itching, coated tongue) ▪ Assess for ↑ BUN, AST, creatinine.

EDUCATION: Complete full course of therapy (usually 10d), even if symptoms subside ▪ Avoid prolonged exposure to direct sunlight, UV light ▪ Take c̄ full glass H_2O; do *not* take w/in 1h of hs ▪ Take at equal intervals around clock to maintain blood levels ▪ Diarrhea may occur ▪ Store in dry, tightly closed, light-resistant container ▪ Avoid taking products containing Al^{+++}, Mg^{++}, Ca^{++}, Fe^{++}, Zn^{++} concurrently ▪ Discard outdated preparations ▪ Can be taken c̄ meals; avoid dairy products ▪ Women: avoid breastfeeding.

NOTES:

edrophonium chloride • (ed-roe-foe-nee-um)

CATEGORY: *Parasympathomimetic:* anticholinesterase — Rx; Preg Cat NA

BRAND NAME
Tensilon (ICN)

DOSAGE FORM
Injection (IM/IV): 10mg/ml

USE: Differential diagnosis of myasthenia gravis; adjunct in evaluating treatment ▪ To reverse neuromuscular blockage of curarelike drugs. **ACTION:** Anticholinesterase activity results in higher levels of acetylcholine, which produce indirect parasympathomimetic activity; ↑ acetylcholine levels at somatic myoneural nicotinic receptors alleviate symptoms of myasthenia gravis.

PHARMACOKINETICS

IV onset	Duration	Excretion
30-60s	10m	Route, metabolism not determined

CONTRAINDICATIONS: Hypersensitivity, mechanical urinary obstructions. **CC:** Use c̄ caution c̄ bronchial asthma, cardiac arrhythmias ▪ Injection contains sodium sulfite, which can cause allergic rxs.

DOSAGE

Pediatric	*IV*	1mg for children ≤75lbs, 2mg for children ≥75lbs. If no response after 45s, dose may be titrated up to 5mg in children <75lbs, up to 10mg in bigger children, given at increments of 1mg q30-45s 0.5mg for infants
	IM	2mg for children ≤75lbs, 5mg for children ≥75lbs. Rx time delayed 2-10m
Adult	*IV*	Start c̄ 10-mg dose, c̄ 2mg administered in 15-30s. If no response after 45s, remaining 8mg injected. If muscarinic rx c̄ 2-mg dose, test stopped, atropine 0.4-0.5mg given. As antagonist to curare-like drugs, 10mg IV over 30-40s. Repeat if needed. Do *not* exceed maximum dose 40mg
	IM	10mg; repeat in 30m c̄ 2mg to rule out false negative

SIDE/ADVERSE EFFECTS: CNS: ***convulsions***, dysarthria, dysphonia ▪ CV: bradycardia, hypotension ▪ EENT: miosis, ↑ lacrimation ▪ GI: ↑ secretions, N/V, abdominal cramps, dysphagia ▪ GU: urinary frequency.

INTERACTIONS: Drug: Use c̄ caution in pts already receiving anticholinesterase therapy.

NURSING MANAGEMENT PRIORITIES

ADMINISTRATION: Assess for hx of hypersensitivity ▪ Assess for hx of cardiac problems; test dose administered ▪ Administered by physician; assist as necessary ▪ Do *not* administer c̄ other cholinergics ▪ Monitor BP, pulse, respirations throughout administration ▪ Have atropine injection available for OD ▪ Have emergency support equipment available ▪ Test for myasthenia gravis; assess muscle strength before, after administration ▪ Use protective measures (bedrails) to prevent injury from possible restlessness.

EVALUATION: Monitor VS, esp respirations ▪ Myasthenic crisis (↑ respiratory status); cholinergic crisis (↓ respiratory status).

EDUCATION: Notify nurse/physician *immediately* of sweating, abdominal cramps, salivation ▪ Effects of drug will last approximately 30m.

NOTES:

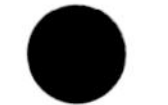

enalapril maleate/enalaprilat* • (e-nal-a-pril)

CATEGORY: *Antihypertensive:* angiotensin inhibitor Rx; Preg Cat C/D†

BRAND NAME	DOSAGE FORMS
Vasotec (Merck)	IV injection*: 1.25mg/ml Tablet: 2.5, 5, 10, 20mg

USE: Treatment of hypertension as sole agent/in combination c̄ other antihypertensives ▪ Treatment of heart failure usually in combination c̄ a diuretic & digitalis ▪ Treatment of asymptomatic left ventricular dysfunction (ejection fraction ≤35%). **ACTION:** Antihypertensive activity appears related to suppression of renin-angiotensin-aldosterone system by competitive inhibition of ACE, which produces angiotensin II from angiotensin I; this results in reduction of peripheral arterial resistance, aldosterone secretion.

CONTRAINDICATIONS: Hypersensitivity; hx of angioedema c̄ other ACE-1. D/C during pregnancy as soon as possible. **CC:** Risk of anaphylactoid rxs, angioedema, agranulocytosis, & neutropenia c̄ use.

DOSAGE: Adult

Hypertension	*PO*	Start c̄ 5mg/d. ↑ Slowly to 10-40mg/d as single dose or in 2 equal doses.
	IV	1.25mg q6h over a 5-m period
Heart failure		Initial dose of 2.5mg/d c̄ range of 2.5-20mg/d bid. Do *not* exceed 40mg/d
Left ventricular dysfunction		Initial dose of 2.5mg bid c̄ slow ↑ to optimum dose of 20mg/d divided

SIDE/ADVERSE EFFECTS: CNS: *headache, dizziness* ▪ CV: hypotension, tachycardia, chest pain, palpitations, ***MI*** (rare), CHF, Raynaud's syndrome ▪ GI: V/D, pain, dyspep-

PHARMACOKINETICS

PO absorption	Onset	Peak	Half-life	Duration	Excretion
60%	1h	4-6h	1-1.5h	Up to 24h	95% via urine in 24h

Note: Side/adverse effects: common in *italic;* serious in ***boldface italic.***

*Available in Canada only.
†1st trimester, C; 2nd & 3rd trimesters, D.

sia ▪ HEM: ***agranulocytosis***, neutropenia, anemia, ***thrombocytopenia*** ▪ INT: rash, pruritus, ***angioedema*** ▪ Other: loss of taste (reversible), *fatigue*.

INTERACTIONS: Drug: Aspirin, indomethacin, other NSAIAs may antagonize therapeutic response ▪ Use K^+-sparing diuretics c̄ caution (hyperkalemia) ▪ Use c̄ lithium requires caution. **Lab:** ↑ In liver enzyme, serum bilirubin.

NURSING MANAGEMENT PRIORITIES

ADMINISTRATION: Assess for hx of hypersensitivity ▪ Assess BP; notify physician of extremes ▪ Assess renal function; may require ↓ dosage if impaired ▪ Diuretics may be D/C for 2-3d before beginning drug to avoid hypotension ▪ PO: may crush, administer c̄ liquid; *best* on empty stomach (1h ac) ▪ IV: administer slowly (over 5m); may be diluted c̄ up to 50ml compatible diluent ▪ Assess serum Na^+ (normal: 135-145mEq/L) ▪ Assess for rapid ↓ in BP w/in 3h after administration of 1st dose (c̄ hyponatremia) ▪ SLE, elderly may require ↓ dosage ▪ Avoid abrupt withdrawal; D/C gradually.

EVALUATION: Monitor VS, esp BP ▪ Monitor CBC (esp WBC, differential) throughout therapy ▪ Monitor electrolyte status (↑K^+, ↓Na^+) ▪ Monitor I&O, daily weight ▪ Monitor renal function (proteinuria); notify physician ▪ Assess for loss of taste ▪ Assess for edema in extremities.

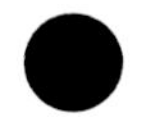

EDUCATION: Dizziness may occur; use caution in potentially hazardous activities ▪ Avoid changing positions (lying/sitting/standing) rapidly ▪ Notify physician of fever, sore throat, bruising/bleeding, swelling of feet/legs ▪ Take as ordered by physician even if symptom free; do *not* skip doses ▪ Take 1h ac ▪ Do *not* D/C w/out notifying physician ▪ Check c̄ physician/pharmacist before taking OTC/Rx preparations ▪ Avoid high-Na^+ foods (canned soups, lunch meats, cheese) ▪ Avoid high-K^+ foods (bananas, citrus juices, raisins) ▪ Check c̄ physician/pharmacist before using salt substitutes ▪ Avoid ↑ exercise, temperature extremes, ↑ smoking ▪ Loss of taste may occur, which may result in loss of appetite ▪ Tablets may smell like sulfur ▪ Used to control, *not* cure, hypertension ▪ Maintain optimum weight ▪ Keep scheduled appointments c̄ physician; have BP checked regularly ▪ Women: avoid breastfeeding ▪ Full drug effects may require several wks of therapy.

NOTES:

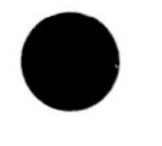

ephedrine sulfate • (e-fed-rin)

CATEGORY: *Sympathomimetic:* adrenergic, bronchodilator, decongestant

Rx/OTC; Preg Cat C

AVAILABLE PREPARATIONS
Capsule (OTC): 15, 25, 30, 50mg
Injection (IM/IV/SC) (Rx): 5, 25, 50mg/ml
Nose drops (OTC): 0.5%, 1%, 3%
Syrup (OTC): 11, 20mg/5ml

USE: Symptomatic treatment of asthma ▪ Topical, systemic decongestant ▪ Pressor agent for hypotension, shock ▪ Treatment of enuresis. **ACTION:** Sympathomimetic effect due to activity on α-, β-adrenergic receptors, resulting in vasoconstriction, ↑ BP, stimulation of heart, dilation of bronchioles; drug exhibits strong CNS stimulation.

PHARMACOKINETICS: Complete PO, parenteral absorption; bronchodilation onset 15-60m PO, c̄ duration 2-4h; cardiac, pressor duration IV about 1h; drug extensively metabolized, excreted via urine.

CONTRAINDICATIONS: Hypersensitivity, narrow-angle glaucoma, psychoneurosis. **CC:** Use may cause hypertension ▪ Extensive use for bronchospastic disease may result in ↓ therapeutic effect ▪ Topical use as nasal decongestant can result in ↓ effectiveness due to "rebound phenomenon."

DOSAGE

Pediatric	*PO*	2-3mg/kg/d in 4-6 divided doses
	IM/IV/SC	3mg/kg/d divided in 4-6 doses
	Topical	1-3gtt q3-4h for nasal decongestion
Adult	*PO*	12.5-50mg 3-4 times/d
	IM/IV/SC	25-50mg. Do *not* exceed daily maximum dose of 150mg
	Topical	1-3gtt q3-4h for nasal decongestion

SIDE/ADVERSE EFFECTS: CNS: *nervousness*, insomnia, ***restlessness***, headache ▪ CV: ***arrhythmias***, precordial pain, palpitations ▪ EENT: rebound nasal congestion c̄ long-term/excessive local application ▪ GU: vesicle sphincter spasm, possible urinary retention ▪ PSYCH: mood changes, hallucinations.

INTERACTIONS: Drug: Use c̄ MAO-I can produce hypertensive crisis ▪ Use c̄ dig, anesthetics may cause arrhythmias ▪ Use c̄ other sympathomimetics, TCAs best avoided ▪ Use c̄ guanethidine, reserpine, hydralazine can antagonize antihypertensive effects ▪ Use c̄ β-adrenergic blocking agents can antagonize their effects.

NURSING MANAGEMENT PRIORITIES

ADMINISTRATION: Assess for hx of catecholamine hypersensitivity ▪ Assess BP, hx of cardiac problems; do *not* administer ▪ Do *not* crush timed-release preparations ▪ Do *not* administer discolored/precipitated solutions; discard unused portions ▪ PO: do *not* administer just before hs ▪ IV: inject *slowly* ▪ Protect from light; do *not* freeze ▪ Elderly may require ⬇ dosage.

EVALUATION: Monitor VS, esp BP, heart rate ▪ Monitor I&O ▪ Assess for tolerance to therapeutic effect; D/C for few days, then resume.

EDUCATION: Avoid taking before hs; insomnia may occur ▪ Notify physician of pressure sensation in eyes, heart/bladder problems; D/C drug ▪ Take as ordered by physician; do *not* ⬆ dosage ▪ Check c̄ physician/pharmacist before using OTC cough/cold preparations ▪ Procedure for intranasal administration.

NOTES:

epinephrine • (ep-i-nef-rin)

CATEGORY: *Sympathomimetic:* bronchodilator, vasopressor

Rx/OTC; Preg Cat C

BRAND NAMES

Adrenalin (P-D)
AsthmaHaler Mist (Norcliff Thayer)
Bronitin Mist (Whitehall)
Bronkald Mist (Winthrop)
**Dysne-Inhal (Rougier)*
**Epifrin (Allergan)*
**Glaucon (Alcon)*
Medihaler-Epi (3M)
Primatene Mist (Whitehall)

DOSAGE FORMS

Aerosol (OTC); injection (Rx); nasal solution (OTC), ophthalmic solution (Rx)

USE: To relieve respiratory distress due to bronchospasm ▪ Treatment of mucosal congestion, hypersensitivity rxs, esp anaphylaxis ▪ To prolong activity of infiltration local anesthetics ▪ To restore cardiac rhythm in cardiac arrest ▪ Hemostatic agent ▪ Management of open-angle glaucoma, ophthalmic/nasal congestion. **ACTION:** Sympathomimetic effect due to direct activity on both α-, β-adrenergic receptors, resulting in vasoconstriction, ↑ BP, stimulation of heart, dilation of bronchioles.

PHARMACOKINETICS: Onset in asthma attacks instant via inhalation, about 5-10m SC; excretion via urine primarily as metabolites.

CONTRAINDICATIONS: Hypersensitivity, narrow angle glaucoma, organic brain damage; shock due to trauma, cyclopropane, halogenated general anesthetics, c̄ local anesthetics for use in toes/fingers, labor, coronary insufficiency. **CC:** Use may cause severe hypertension c̄ accidental IV administration c̄ SC doses or OD ▪ Use c̄ caution c̄ cardiac arrhythmias, organic heart disease, or hypertension.

DOSAGE

Pediatric	*Parenteral*	10µg/kg/dose SC
Adult	*Parenteral*	100µg-1mg SC/IM, 25-400µg IV
Adult/Pediatric	*Inhalation*	Proper dose automatically dispensed by nebulizer/aerosol dosage unit
	Ophthalmic	1-2gtt in eye prn

Note: Side/adverse effects: common in *italic;* serious in ***boldface italic.***

*Available in Canada only.

SIDE/ADVERSE EFFECTS: CNS: headache, *restlessness*, tremor, insomnia ▪ CV: *palpitations*, chest pain ▪ EENT: dry mouth, sore throat c̄ aerosol ▪ PSYCH: transient anxiety ▪ Other: tissue necrosis from repeated injections.

INTERACTIONS: Drug: Use c̄ MAO-I produces significant hypertension ▪ Use c̄ adrenergic blockers antagonizes their effects ▪ Use c̄ other sympathomimetics may cause additive effects, ↑ toxicity.

NURSING MANAGEMENT PRIORITIES

ADMINISTRATION: Assess for hx of catecholamine hypersensitivity ▪ Administer while awake (except in cardiac arrest) ▪ Auscultate breath sounds; notify physician if abnormal ▪ Check preparation, dosage calculations c̄ another RN for accuracy ▪ Do *not* expose to light ▪ SC: refrigerate suspension; shake well before administration, use TB syringe; massage injection site (↓ vasoconstriction); rotate sites ▪ IV: use cardiac monitoring; check compatibility chart for mixing; dilute 1mg (1:1000 solution) c̄ 10ml NaCl injection to produce 1:10,000 solution, inject *slowly* (1mg/m); may dilute further c̄ 5% dextrose solution; discard unused portion ▪ IM: do *not* inject intragluteally; use deltoid ▪ Do *not* use discolored/precipitated solution ▪ Ophthalmic: put pressure on lacrimal sac for 1m after instillation.

EVALUATION: Monitor VS, esp BP, heart rate ▪ Monitor respiratory status ▪ Assess I&O, urinary retention ▪ Assess for signs of excessive CNS stimulation; hold drug, notify physician ▪ Diabetics: closely monitor blood glucose (hyperglycemia).

EDUCATION: Take as ordered by physician; do *not* ↑ dose ▪ Diabetics: check blood/urine glucose carefully ▪ Notify physician of irritability, difficult breathing, chest pain, insomnia ▪ Check c̄ physician/pharmacist before taking OTC preparations ▪ Women: avoid breastfeeding ▪ Procedure for ophthalmic, intranasal, inhalation, SC (Autoinjector) administration.

NOTES:

ergonovine maleate/methylergonovine maleate •

(er-gone-oh-veen/meth-ill-er-gone-oh-veen)

CATEGORY: *Oxytoxic*

Rx; Preg Cat NA/C

BRAND NAMES	DOSAGE FORMS
ergonovine	
Generic	Injection (IM/IV): 0.2mg/ml
methylergonovine	
Methergine (Sandoz)	Injection (IM/IV): 0.2mg/ml Tablet: 0.2mg

USE: Treatment/prevention of postpartum/postabortal hemorrhage due to uterine atony ▪ With full supervision, may be given in second stage of labor following delivery of anterior shoulder (methylergonovine). **ACTION:** Oxytoxic effect due to direct stimulation of uterine smooth muscle, resulting in intense contractions followed by periods of relaxation; accordingly, ↑ uterine tone, ↓ postpartum uterine bleeding; drug can occasionally produce severe hypertensive episodes, esp in toxemic pts.

CONTRAINDICATIONS: Hypersensitivity, threatened spontaneous abortion. **CC:** Hyperstimulation of uterus during labor can induce uterine tetany, ↓ uteroplacental blood flow.

PHARMACOKINETICS

Onset of contractions				
PO	IM	IV	Duration	Excretion
10m	2-5m	Immediate	≥3h	Primarily via feces

DOSAGE

ergonovine

Adult	*IM*	0.2mg; may be repeated for severe hemorrhage
	IV	Route should be restricted to lifesaving situations because of higher rate of side effects

methylergonovine

Adult	*PO*	0.2mg; 3-4 times/d in puerperium for a maximum of 1wk
	IM	0.2mg after delivery of anterior shoulder, placenta, or during puerperium prn q2-4h
	IV	Route limited to life-saving situations because of ↑ rate of adverse effects

SIDE/ADVERSE EFFECTS: CNS: headache ▪ CV: hypertension, particularly when administered IV ▪ GI: N/V ▪ Other: possible symptoms of ergot poisoning.

INTERACTIONS: Drug: Concurrent/sequential use c̄ vasoconstrictors/regional anesthesia may affect BP.

NURSING MANAGEMENT PRIORITIES

ADMINISTRATION: *Not* routinely used before delivery ▪ Assess BP ▪ Assess serum calcium; IV calcium gluconate if hypocalcemic ▪ PO: avoid excessive moisture in storage ▪ Injection: store in cold place (<46° F); do *not* exceed 60d at room termperature ▪ Do *not* administer discolored/precipitated solutions ▪ IV: use infusion control device; administer *slowly* ▪ Have emergency support equipment available ▪ Provide emotional support.

EVALUATION: Monitor BP, pulse ▪ Monitor serum calcium ▪ Observe for signs of ergotism (N/V, dizziness, cramps, headache, confusion) ▪ Postpartum: monitor fundal height/tone; assess amount/character of lochia.

EDUCATION: Explain procedure, rationale to pt, family ▪ Occurrence of contractions ▪ Relaxation techniques ▪ Comfort measures ▪ Store in tightly closed container ▪ Avoid smoking ▪ Notify physician of infection, signs of ergotism (cramps, vomiting, thirst, weakness, tingling in extremities).

NOTES:

ergotamine tartrate • (er-got-a-meen)

CATEGORY: α-*adrenergic blocker:* antimigraine, sympatholytic Rx; Preg Cat X

BRAND NAMES
Ergostat (P-D)
Medihaler Ergotamine (3M)

DOSAGE FORMS
Sublingual tablets: 2mg
0.36mg metered/dose

COMBINATION PRODUCTS

Cafergot (Sandoz)	Ergotamine/caffeine
Wigraine (Organon)	1mg/100mg/tablet
	2mg/100mg/suppository

USE: Treatment of vascular headache. **ACTION:** Produces direct vasoconstriction on cranial blood vessels to relieve vascular pulsations probably responsible for vascular headache; exhibits oxytoxic activity.

PHARMACOKINETICS

Peak	Half-life	Excretion
0.5-3h	2.7h, then 27h	90% in bile as metabolites; unmetabolized in saliva

CONTRAINDICATIONS: Coronary heart disease, hypersensitivity, hypertension, impaired hepatic/renal function, peripheral vascular disease, pregnancy, sepsis. **CC:** Extended use c̄ ↑ doses can result in ergotism.

DOSAGE

Adult	*SL*	2mg, repeat at ½-h intervals. Do *not* exceed 6mg/d, 10mg/wk
	Aerosol	One inhalation (0.36mg), repeat at ≥5-m intervals. Do *not* exceed 6 inhalations/d, 15/wk
Cafergot/Wigraine	*PO*	2 tablets, then 1 q½h to a maximum of 6 tablets/attack, or 10/wk
	Rectal	1 suppository, then 1 in 1h (maximum of 2/attack or 5/wk)

SIDE/ADVERSE EFFECTS: CNS: headache, tremors, convulsions ▪ CV: blood vessel contraction (↓ circulation esp limbs; ***gangrene*** possible) ▪ GI: N/V.

Note: Side/adverse effects: common in *italic;* serious in ***boldface italic.***

*Available in Canada only.

INTERACTIONS: Drug: Propranolol, other β blockers may interfere c̄ activity of ergotamine.

NOTES:

NURSING MANAGEMENT PRIORITIES

ADMINISTRATION: Used to abort *acute* vascular headache; administer at onset of pain/during prodromal stage ▪ Assess characteristics of pain ▪ Assess psychosocial factors associated c̄ pain ▪ Aerosol: shake well before use ▪ Provide pt comfort during headache attacks ▪ Provide ↓ environmental stimuli ▪ Avoid exposure to moisture/light in storage; use original container.

EVALUATION: Observe for signs of ergotism (N/V/D, drowsiness, dizziness, headache, mental confusion) ▪ Monitor hepatic status ▪ Monitor VS, esp heart rate ▪ Assess peripheral pulses c̄ prolonged therapy.

EDUCATION: Take drug when pain starts (used to stop *acute* attacks) ▪ Lie down in darkened, quiet room for several hrs after taking drug ▪ Compliance c̄ prescribed dosage regimen; do *not* exceed recommended dose/wk allowable ▪ Notify physician immediately of signs of ergotism (N/V/D, drowsiness, dizziness, headache, mental confusion) ▪ Store in tightly closed, light-resistant container ▪ Women: avoid breastfeeding ▪ Procedure for inhalation/SL administration.

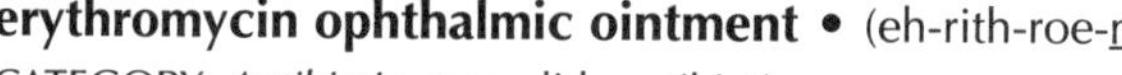

erythromycin ophthalmic ointment • (eh-rith-roe-mye-sin)

CATEGORY: *Antibiotic:* macrolide antibiotic   Rx; Preg Cat B

BRAND NAMES	DOSAGE FORMS
Generic	Ophthalmic ointment: 0.5% (5mg/g)
Ilotycin (Dista) (Lilly [Canada])	Ophthalmic ointment: 0.5% (5mg/g)

USE: Treatment of ophthalmic infections due to susceptible organisms ▪ Prophylaxis of gonococcal/chlamydial ophthalmia neonatorum. **ACTION:** Bacteriostatic activity due to inhibition of ribosomal protein synthesis in susceptible microorganisms; topical ophthalmic application has limited tissue penetration, may fail to protect against gonococcal penicillinase-producing strains of *Neisseria gonorrhoeae.*

CONTRAINDICATIONS: Hypersensitivity. **CC:** Use may result in overgrowth of nonsusceptible organisms.

DOSAGE

Ophthalmic infection	Apply ribbon (approximately 1cm) of ointment to infected eye(s), usually in conjunctival sac, ≥1 time/d
Ophthalmia neonatorum	Use new tube for each infant. Apply ribbon (0.5-1cm) of ointment in each conjunctival sac *not* later than 1h after delivery

SIDE/ADVERSE EFFECTS: EENT: local ophthalmic irritation ▪ Other: possible overgrowth of nonsusceptible organisms.

NURSING MANAGEMENT PRIORITIES

ADMINISTRATION: Assess for hx of hypersensitivity ▪ Avoid contamination of ointment tube tip ▪ Use new tube of ointment for each neonate ▪ Apply thin strip into lower conjunctival sac after delivery ▪ Do *not* flush from eye after administration ▪ Avoid excessive heat/light in storage; do *not* freeze.

EVALUATION: Observe for signs of local hypersensitivity; notify physician.

EDUCATION: Explain procedure, rationale to family ▪ Report signs of local hypersensitivity (redness, tearing, irritation) immediately ▪ Avoid using common towels/washcloths among family members ▪ Procedure for ophthalmic administration.

NOTES:

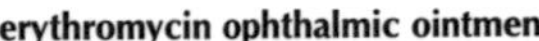

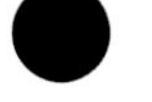

erythromycin salts • (eh-rith-roe-mye-sin)

CATEGORY: *Antibiotic:* macrolide antibiotic Rx; Preg Cat B

BRAND NAMES

erythromycin base
E-Mycin (Boots), Ery-Tab (Abbott), ERYC (P-D)
erythromycin estolate
Ilosone (Dista) (Lilly [Canada])
erythromycin ethylsuccinate
*E.E.S. (various), *Erythrocin (Abbott), EryPed (Abbott)*
erythromycin gluceptate
Ilotycin Gluceptate IV (Dista) (Lilly [Canada])
erythromycin lactobionate
Erythrocin Lactobionate IV (Abbott)
erythromycin stearate
Erythrocin Stearate (Abbott), Wyamycin S (W-A)

DOSAGE FORMS

Capsule, chewable tablet, injection (IV), suspension, tablet

USE: Treatment of systemic infections caused by susceptible strains of α-hemolytic streptococci, *Bordetella pertussis, Chlamydia trachomatis, C. urethritis, Entamoeba histolytica* (intestinal amebiasis only), group A β-hemolytic streptococci, *Haemophilus influenzae, Legionella pneumophila, Listeria monocytogenes, Mycoplasma pneumoniae, Neisseria gonorrhoeae,* staphylococci, *Streptococcus pneumoniae, Treponema pallidum, Ureaplasma* urethritis ▪ Treatment of erythrasma (*Corynebacterium minutissimum)* ▪ Adjunct to antitoxin therapy in treating *Corynebacterium* diphtheria infections ▪ Treatment of diphtheria carriers. **ACTION:** Bacteriostatic activity due to inhibition of ribosomal protein synthesis in susceptible organisms.

PHARMACOKINETICS

PO absorption	Peak	Half-life	Protein binding	Excretion
Good	1-4h	1.5-2h	73%-96%	Primarily via feces as unchanged drug

CONTRAINDICATIONS: Hypersensitivity. **CC:** Use may produce hepatic impairment, esp estolate salt.

Note: Side/adverse effects: common in *italic;* serious in ***boldface italic.***

*Available in Canada only.

DOSAGE

Base, estolate, stearate

Pediatric	*PO*	30-50mg/kg/d divided. Severe infection, up to 60-100mg/kg/d
Adult	*PO*	250mg qid. Severe infection: ≤4g/d. Primary syphilis: 30-50g divided for 10-15d. Urethritis: 500mg qid for 7d

Ethylsuccinate

Adult	*PO*	400mg qid. Primary syphilis: 48-64g divided for 10-15d. Urethritis: 800mg tid for 7d

Gluceptate, lactobionate

Pediatric/Adult	*IV*	15-20mg/kg/d. Severe infection, higher doses

SIDE/ADVERSE EFFECTS: EENT: hearing loss (reversible) ▪ GI: *abdominal cramps*, N/V/D ▪ HEP: hepatotoxicity ▪ INT: urticaria, rash ▪ Other: ***anaphylaxis***, thrombophlebitis (IV).

INTERACTIONS: Drug: Bacteriostatic antibiotics can antagonize effects of bacterial antibiotics ▪ Use c̄ carbamazepine, PO anticoagulants, theophylline can ↑ their toxicity ▪ Use c̄ astemizole not recommended ▪ Use c̄ cisapride can produce fatal cardiac arrhythmias.

NURSING MANAGEMENT PRIORITIES

ADMINISTRATION: Assess for erythromycin sensitivity ▪ Obtain C&S before therapy ▪ PO: administer 1h ac/2h pc c̄ full glass H_2O (avoid citrus juice); do *not* crush delayed-release/enteric-coated preparations; estolate, ethylsuccinate, enteric-coated preparations can be taken w/out regard to meals ▪ IV: dilute c̄ 10ml (250-, 500-mg vial), 20ml (1-g vial) sterile H_2O for injection; further dilute to 1g/L normal saline, lactated Ringer, 5% dextrose solution according to manufacturer's directions; administer via *slow*, continuous infusion (20-60m).

EVALUATION: Monitor VS, esp temperature; hepatic status ▪ Observe for signs of superinfection (diarrhea, perineal itching, oral ulcers).

EDUCATION: Complete full course of therapy ▪ Take on empty stomach; estolate, ethylsuccinate, enteric-coated preparations can be taken c̄ meals (avoid citrus juice); swallow delayed-release, enteric-coated preparations whole; shake suspension well before pouring; keep refrigerated; chewable tablet should *not* be swallowed whole, chew thoroughly ▪ Take at equal intervals around clock to maintain blood levels ▪ Diarrhea may occur.

NOTES:

estazolam/quazepam • (ess-taz-oh-lam/kway-ze-pam)

CATEGORY: *Benzodiazepine:* hypnotic

Rx C-IV; Preg Cat X

BRAND NAMES	**DOSAGE FORMS**
estazolam	
ProSom (Abbott)	Tablet: 1, 2mg
quazepam	
Doral (Wallace)	Tablet: 7.5, 15mg

USE: Short-term treatment of insomnia associated c̄ difficulty in falling asleep, frequent awakenings, or early morning awakening. **ACTION:** Hypnotic activity extends to all stages (0-4) of sleep; improves total sleep time, ⬇ number of nocturnal awakenings; REM sleep not affected.

CONTRAINDICATIONS: Hypersensitivity. **CC:** Use can produce dependence; abrupt D/C can result in withdrawal symptoms.

DOSAGE: *PO*

estazolam	
Adult	1-2mg at hs
Geriatric	0.5mg or higher at hs
quazepam	
Adult	7.5 or 15mg at hs
Geriatric	Adult dosage ⬇ after 1-2d

PHARMACOKINETICS

	PO absorption	Peak	Half-life	Protein binding	Excretion
estazolam	Readily	2h	18.4h	93%	96% via urine, 4% via feces as metabolites
quazepam	Rapid	2h	39h	95%	23% via urine, 31% via feces as metabolites over 5-d period

SIDE/ADVERSE EFFECTS: CNS: *drowsiness,* headache, hypokinesia, nervousness, dizziness, hangover ▪ CV: infrequent flushing, palpitation ▪ GI: dry mouth, N/V ▪ HEM: leukopenia (rare) ▪ Other: asthenia, abnormal vision, malaise.

INTERACTIONS: Drug: Use c̄ other CNS depressants produces additive effects ▪ Use c̄ MAO-I can produce serious toxic effects.

NURSING MANAGEMENT PRIORITIES

ADMINISTRATION: Assess for hx of benzodiazepine hypersensitivity ▪ Avoid exposure to heat/moisture/light in storage ▪ Avoid abrupt withdrawal ▪ Elderly may require ↓ dosage ▪ ↓ Environmental stimuli.

EVALUATION: Monitor renal, hepatic status ▪ Assess for symptoms of abrupt withdrawal (tremors, abdominal/muscle cramps, convulsions) c̄ prolonged use ▪ Check for signs of dependence (↑ drug request)/tolerance ▪ Monitor activity status (safety precautions) ▪ Assess for paradoxic rxs (CNS stimulation), esp in elderly ▪ Check for depression; suicide precautions prn ▪ Assess pt sleep patterns.

EDUCATION: Drowsiness may occur; use caution in potentially hazardous activities ▪ Avoid use c̄ alcohol, other CNS depressants ▪ Indiscriminate use may lead to dependence ▪ Do *not* smoke after taking drug ▪ Do *not* keep at bedside ▪ Take as ordered by physician; do *not* ↑ dose ▪ Women: avoid breast-feeding ▪ Check c̄ physician/pharmacist before taking OTC preparations ▪ Practice relaxation exercises, ventilation of feelings ▪ Utilize sleep producers (reading, warm milk, soft music).

NOTES:

estradiol/estrogens, conjugated • (ess-tra-dye-ole/ess-troe-jenz)

CATEGORY: *Estrogenic agent* Rx; Preg Cat X

BRAND NAMES	**DOSAGE FORMS**
Estrace (MJP)	Tablets: Vaginal cream
Estraderm (Ciba)	Transdermal patch
Premarin (W-A)	Injection, tablets, vaginal cream

USE: Treatment of moderate/severe symptoms associated c̄ menopause, atrophic vaginitis, kraurosis vulvae, female hypogonadism, female castration, breast/prostate cancer palliation, osteoporosis prevention, primary ovarian failure ▪ Prevention of postpartum breast enlargement conjugated estrogens (Premarin). **ACTION:** Estrogens required for development, maintenance of female reproductive system, 2° sex characteristics.

PHARMACOKINETICS: Rapid PO absorption, extensive protein binding & metabolism, excretion via urine.

CONTRAINDICATIONS: Known/suspected pregnancy, estrogen-dependent neoplasia, breast cancer except in appropriately selected pts; abnormal genital bleeding, active or hx of estrogen-associated thrombophlebitis/thromboembolic disorders (except for breast/prostate cancer treatment). **CC:** Use can ⬆ risk of endometrial cancer in postmenopausal women ▪ Sustained ⬆ dose therapy can ⬆ risk of breast cancer.

DOSAGE: Drug should be given cyclically for short-term use; lowest dose that will control symptoms should be chosen, D/C as soon as possible

estradiol

PO	Usual initial dose 1-2mg/d administered cyclically For cancer palliation, usual starting dose 1-2mg tid
Vaginal	2-4g cream (marked on applicator)/d for 1-2wks. Gradually ⬇ to half initial dose for similar period. Usual maintenance dose 1g 1-3 times/wk
Transdermal	Initiate c̄ 0.5mg/d patch 2 times/wk, adjust for control of symptoms.

conjugated estrogens

Adult *PO*

Menopause	1.25mg/d. If pt is menstruating, start on day 5 of bleeding for cyclic administration
Atrophic vaginitis, kraurosis vulvae	≥0.3mg/d, depending on response Administer cyclically
Hypogonadism	2.5-7.5mg/d divided for 20d followed by rest period of 10d

Castration, ovarian failure	1.25mg/d, cyclically
Postpartum breast enlargement	3.75mg q4h for 5 doses or 1.25mg q4h for 5d
Prostatic cancer	1.25-2.5mg tid
Breast cancer	10mg tid for at least 3mo
IM/IV	
Abnormal uterine bleeding	25mg, repeat in 6-12h prn. Start PO doses as soon as possible
Vaginal	2-4g intravaginally/topical

SIDE/ADVERSE EFFECTS: CNS: headache, migraine, dizziness, mental depression ▪ CV: edema ▪ EENT: intolerance to contact lenses, steepening of corneal curvature ▪ GI: *nausea*, vomiting, abdominal cramps, bloating ▪ GU: amenorrhea, breakthrough bleeding, dysmenorrhea, candidiasis, change in menstrual flow, spotting, ⬆ size of uterine fibromyomas ▪ INT: melasma, ***erythema multiforme***/nodosum, alopecia, hirsutism, urticaria ▪ MET: ⬇ carbohydrate tolerance ▪ Other: weight changes, porphyria exacerbation ▪ Use c̄ PO anticoagulants may ⬇ their activity.

INTERACTIONS: Drug: Use c̄ TCAs may result in toxic rxs.

NURSING MANAGEMENT PRIORITIES

ADMINISTRATION: Assess for hx of hypersensitivity ▪ PO: administer cyclically (3wks on, 1wk off) c̄ meals ▪ Avoid abrupt withdrawal; D/C gradually ▪ Vaginal: apply c̄ plastic dose applicator; maintain in recumbent position 30m after application.

EVALUATION: Monitor BP ▪ Monitor hepatic, renal status ▪ Assess for endometrial cancer (Pap test, physical exam) ▪ Monitor PT; may ⬇ anticoagulant effect ▪ Diabetics: careful blood/urine testing; may ⬇ antidiabetic drug effect ▪ Assess for behavioral changes, depression ▪ Monitor weight; observe for edema.

EDUCATION: Review package insert c̄ pt ▪ Take PO dosage form c̄ food ▪ Nausea may occur during first 2wks of therapy ▪ Women: avoid pregnancy, breastfeeding ▪ Breast self-exam (incl men) ▪ Avoid smoking (⬆ CV complications) ▪ Notify physician/dentist of use before treatment ▪ Avoid exposure to direct sunlight, UV light (sunlamps); use sunscreen, protective clothing ▪ D/C drug, notify physician if pregnancy is suspected ▪ Vaginal: apply at hs; use sanitary napkin (avoid tampons) to protect clothing; procedure for using plastic dose applicator ▪ Notify physician *immediately* of chest/leg pain, unusual vaginal bleeding, difficult breathing, slurred speech ▪ Men: enlarged breasts, drug-related impotence reversible after therapy ▪ Check weight, swelling in feet/legs daily ▪ Keep scheduled appointments c̄ physician (Pap test, physical exam).

NOTES:

ethambutol hcl • (e-tham-byoo-tole)

CATEGORY: *Antitubercular*

Rx; Preg Cat NA

BRAND NAMES	**DOSAGE FORMS**
**Etibi (ICN)*	
Myambutol (Lederle)	Tablet: 100, 400mg

USE: Combined treatment of pulmonary TB c̄ isoniazid, streptomycin, both, or other agents. **ACTION:** Tuberculostatic activity due to interference of protein synthesis by inhibition of RNA synthesis in actively growing susceptible tubercular bacilli; use c̄ isoniazid ↓ mycobacterial resistance to isoniazid.

PHARMACOKINETICS

PO absorption	Peak	Half-life	Protein binding	Excretion
75%-80%	2-4h	3.3h	22%	50% via urine as unchanged drug in 24h, 8%-15% as metabolites

CONTRAINDICATIONS: Hypersensitivity, known optical neuritis (unless clinically required). **CC:** Use c̄ caution & ↓ dosage in pts c̄ renal impairment ▪ Safety in children <13y/o not established ▪ Use can result in unilateral or bilateral loss of vision acuity. Testing before & during therapy of vision is required ▪ Periodic hepatic, hematologic, renal assessment is required esp for long-term therapy.

DOSAGE

Adult *PO*	Initial dose 15mg/kg as single daily dose. Retreatment dose 25mg/kg as single daily dose

SIDE/ADVERSE EFFECTS: CNS: optic/peripheral neuritis, headache, dizziness, mental confusion, possible hallucinations ▪ EENT: dose-related loss of visual acuity (optic neuritis) ▪ GI: gastric distress, anorexia, N/V, abdominal pain ▪ INT: dermatitis, pruritus ▪ MS: joint pain, exacerbation of gout ▪ Other: fever.

INTERACTIONS: Drug: Aluminum-containing products (antacids) may ↓ PO absorption of ethambutol.

NURSING MANAGEMENT PRIORITIES

ADMINISTRATION: Assess for hx of hypersensitivity ▪ Obtain sputum C&S before therapy ▪ May administer c̄ food ▪ Avoid exposure to heat/moisture/light in storage ▪ Assess renal function; ↓ dose if impaired.

Note: Side/adverse effects: common in *italic;* serious in ***boldface italic.***

*Available in Canada only.

EVALUATION: Monitor hepatic, renal status ▪ Assess for visual disturbances (ocular toxicity) ▪ Monitor serum for ↑ uric acid, AST, ALT.

EDUCATION: Take as directed by physician; do *not* skip doses ▪ May take c̄ food ▪ Keep scheduled appointments for eye exams ▪ Notify physician *immediately* of visual problems ▪ Women: avoid pregnancy, breastfeeding ▪ May produce gouty symptoms ▪ Emotional support during long-term therapy.

NOTES:

ethosuximide • (eth-oh-sux-i-mide)

CATEGORY: Anticonvulsant

Rx; Preg Cat NA

BRAND NAME
Zarontin (P-D)

DOSAGE FORMS
Capsule: 250mg
Syrup: 250mg/5ml

USE: Drug of choice for petit mal. **ACTION:** Anticonvulsant activity due to motor cortex depression, ↑ in convulsive threshold; drug ↓ paroxysmal spike/wave patterns of petit mal seizure.

PHARMACOKINETICS

PO absorption	Peak	Half-life	Excretion
Good	4h	30-60h	Primarily via urine as metabolites

CONTRAINDICATIONS: Hypersensitivity. **CC:** Use may produce blood dyscrasias.

DOSAGE

Pediatric	*PO*	3-6y/o: Start c̄ 250mg/d, adjust to achieve control ≥6y/o: Start c̄ 500mg/d, adjust to achieve control. 20mg/kg/d is optimum dose in most children
Adult	*PO*	Start c̄ 500mg/d, ↑ by 250mg q4-7d to achieve control. Doses >1.5g require close supervision. Usual maintenance dose 500mg-1.5g/d

SIDE/ADVERSE EFFECTS: CNS: *drowsiness*, headache, dizziness, euphoria, sleep disturbances, hiccoughs, ataxia, agitation, aggressiveness ▪ GI: N/V/D, anorexia, cramps, pain ▪ GU: vaginal bleeding ▪ HEM: ***agranulocytosis, aplastic anemia,*** leukopenia, pancytopenia, eosinophilia ▪ INT: urticaria, erythematous rash, ***Stevens-Johnson syndrome, SLE*** ▪ Other: gum hypertrophy, swollen tongue.

INTERACTIONS: Drug: Use c̄ chloramphenicol, other bone marrow depressants results in significant blood dyscrasia.

NURSING MANAGEMENT PRIORITIES

ADMINISTRATION: Assess for hx of anticonvulsant hypersensitivity ▪ Assess hepatic, hematologic, renal function ▪ Administer c̄ food/milk ▪ Avoid abrupt withdrawal; institute strict seizure precautions if drug abruptly withdrawn ▪ Avoid exposure to light (syrup)/moisture in storage; do *not* freeze syrup.

EVALUATION: Monitor occurrence/characteristics of seizures ▪ Monitor hepatic, hematologic, renal status ▪ Assess for behavioral changes ▪ Assess for skin rash; notify physician, D/C drug ▪ Monitor activity status (safety precautions) ▪ Assess for symptoms of abrupt withdrawal (tremors, abdominal/muscle cramps, convulsions) ▪ Therapeutic blood level: 40-100mg/ml.

EDUCATION: Do *not* omit doses ▪ Drowsiness/dizziness may occur; use caution in potentially hazardous activities ▪ Do *not* smoke after taking drug ▪ Take c̄ food/milk ▪ Carry medical identification (MedicAlert) ▪ Take at equal intervals ▪ Keep scheduled appointments c̄ physician ▪ Store in tightly closed container ▪ Syrup: do *not* freeze; protect from light/moisture ▪ Check c̄ physician/pharmacist before taking OTC/Rx preparations.

NOTES:

etodolac/sulindac • (eh-toe-doe-lack/sul-in-dak)

CATEGORY: *Antiinflammatory:* analgesic, NSAIA

Rx; Preg Cat C

BRAND NAMES	DOSAGE FORMS
etodolac	
Lodine (W-A)	Capsules: 200, 300mg
sulindac	
Clinoril (Merck)	Tablet: 150, 200mg

USE: Treatment of acute & long-term arthritis ▪ Relief of mild/moderate pain ▪ Gout, painful shoulder, spondylitis (sulindac). **ACTION:** Antiinflammatory, analgesic activity appears related to inhibition of prostaglandin synthesis.

CONTRAINDICATIONS: Hypersensitivity, pts c̄ aspirin- or other NSAIA-induced allergies (asthma, rhinitis, etc.) **CC:** Risk of GI ulceration, bleeding, & perforation c̄ use.

DOSAGE: Adult *PO*

etodolac

Osteoarthritis	Initial dose of 800-1200mg/d divided. Then adjust between 600-1200mg/d. Do *not* exceed 1200mg/d or 20mg/kg for pts ≤60kg
Pain	200-400mg q6-8h prn. Do *not* exceed 1200mg/d or 20mg/kg for pts ≤60kg

sulindac

Arthritis, spondylitis	150mg bid then adjust. Do *not* exceed 400mg/d
Painful shoulder, gout	200mg bid. ⬇ Dosage after improvement, usually 7-14d for painful shoulder, 7d for gout

SIDE/ADVERSE EFFECTS: CNS: confusion, headache, paresthesia, dizziness, depression ▪ CV: fluid retention, edema, hypertension, palpitation, CHF ▪ EENT: blurred vision, tinnitus, taste changes ▪ GI: dyspepsia, abdominal pain, bleeding, N/V/D, flatulence, constipation ▪ GU: dysuria, urinary frequency, renal impairment ▪ HEM: anemia, ***thrombocytopenia*** (rare) ▪ INT: pruritus, rash, urticaria ▪ Other: asthenia, asthma, tinnitus.

INTERACTIONS: Drug: Use c̄ ulcerogenic drugs produces additive effects ▪ Phenylbutazone will ⬆ plasma levels due to protein displacement ▪ Use c̄ cyclosporine, digoxin, lithium methotrexate can ⬆ their activity.

NURSING MANAGEMENT PRIORITIES

ADMINISTRATION: Assess for hx of NSAIA hypersensitivity ▪ Avoid administration to pts c̄ hx of asthma, bleeding disorders, salicylate hypersensitivity ▪ Assess for hx of peptic ulcer; use c̄ caution if impaired ▪ Administer c̄ food/milk to ↓ GI irritation; encourage upright position for 15-30m ▪ Avoid exposure to moisture in storage ▪ Elderly may require ↓ dosage.

EVALUATION: Monitor hepatic, renal status c̄ prolonged use ▪ Monitor pts receiving anticoagulant therapy; may potentiate bleeding ▪ Monitor I&O, daily weight ▪ Assess for edema in extremities ▪ Assess for visual/hearing disturbances; D/C drug, notify physician.

EDUCATION: Dizziness/drowsiness may occur; use caution in potentially hazardous activities ▪ Take c̄ food/milk to ↓ GI distress; maintain upright position for 15-30m ▪ Take as ordered by physician; do *not* ↑ dose ▪ Notify physician *immediately* of bleeding, ↓ urine output, swelling of feet/legs, lethargy, GI distress, jaundice, visual disturbance ▪ Avoid taking c̄ aspirin, other NSAIAs ▪ Avoid use c̄ alcohol ▪ Check c̄ physician/pharmacist before taking OTC preparations ▪ Notify physician/dentist of use before treatment ▪ Store in tightly closed container ▪ Schedule eye exams c̄ prolonged use ▪ Women: avoid breastfeeding ▪ Full drug effects may require several wks of therapy.

NOTES:

fenoprofen calcium/oxaprozin • (fen-oh-proe-fen/ox-ah-proe-zin)

CATEGORY: *Antiinflammatory:* analgesic, NSAIA Rx; Preg Cat NA/C

BRAND NAMES	DOSAGE FORMS
fenoprofen	
Nalfon (Distal) (Lilly [Canada])	Capsule (Pulvule): 200, 300mg Tablet: 600mg
oxaprozin	
Daypro (Searle)	Caplet: 600mg

USE: Treatment of rheumatoid arthritis/osteoarthritis ▪ Relief of mild/moderate pain. **ACTION:** Antiinflammatory, analgesic activity appears related to inhibition of prostaglandin synthesis.

PHARMACOKINETICS

PO absorption	Peak	Half-life	Protein binding	Excretion
fenoprofen				
Rapid	2h	2-4h	99%	90% via urine primarily as metabolities in 24h
oxaprozin				
High	3-5h	42-50h	99.9%	Via urine, bile as conjugates

CONTRAINDICATIONS: Hypersensitivity, aspirin hypersensitivity, impaired renal function. **CC:** Risk of GI ulceration, bleeding, perforation c̄ use.

DOSAGE

fenoprofen

Adult *PO*

Pain	200mg q4-6h prn
Arthritis	Starting dose 300-600mg qid. Do *not* exceed 3200mg/d

oxaprozin

Adult *PO*

Pain	1200mg once/d. Do *not* exceed 1800mg or 26mg/kg/d

SIDE/ADVERSE EFFECTS: CNS: *headache, somnolence,* dizziness, nervousness, tremor, confusion ▪ CV: palpitations, tachycardia ▪ EENT: tinnitus, ↓ hearing, blurred vision ▪ GI: abdominal pain, *dyspepsia*, constipation, N/V, pain, anorexia, flatulence, dry mouth, ***hemorrhage*** ▪ GU: rare acute interstitial nephritis ▪ HEM: anemia, leukopenia, ***thrombocytopenia*** ▪ INT: pruritus, rash, urticaria.

Note: Side/adverse effects: common in *italic;* serious in ***boldface italic.***

*Available in Canada only.

INTERACTIONS: Drug: Use c̄ ulcerogenic drugs produces additive effects ▪ Use c̄ PO anticoagulants, thrombolytic agents may ↑ their activity ▪ Use c̄ aspirin will ↓ fenoprofen plasma levels ▪ Use c̄ other ↑ protein-bound drugs can produce displacement from inactive binding sites ▪ Use c̄ H_2 blockers will ↓ oxaprozin body clearance. **Lab:** Fenoprofen can produce false ↑ in triiodothyroxine c̄ Amerlex-M kit.

NURSING MANAGEMENT PRIORITIES

ADMINISTRATION: Assess for hx of NSAIA, salicylate hypersensitivity ▪ Avoid administration to pts c̄ hx of asthma, bleeding disorders, salicylate hypersensitivity ▪ Assess GI, renal, hepatic function; use caution if impaired ▪ May be administered c̄ food, milk, antacid; *best* on empty stomach (1h ac/2h pc); tablets may be crushed, capsules opened; encourage upright position for 15-30m ▪ Avoid exposure to moisture in storage ▪ Elderly may require ↓ dosage.

EVALUATION: Monitor hepatic, renal status c̄ prolonged use ▪ Monitor pt receiving anticoagulant therapy; may potentiate bleeding ▪ Monitor I&O, daily weight ▪ Assess for edema in extremities ▪ Assess for visual/hearing disturbances; D/C drug, notify physician.

EDUCATION: Dizziness/drowsiness may occur; use caution in potentially hazardous activities ▪ Take on empty stomach (1h ac/2h pc), c̄ food/milk if GI distress occurs; maintain upright position for 15-30m ▪ Take as ordered by physician; do *not* ↑ dose ▪ Notify physician *immediately* of bleeding, urine output, swelling of feet/legs, lethargy, GI distress, jaundice, visual/hearing disturbances ▪ Avoid taking c̄ aspirin, other NSAIAs ▪ Avoid use c̄ alcohol ▪ Check c̄ physician/pharmacist before taking OTC preparations ▪ Notify physician/dentist of use before treatment ▪ Store in tightly closed container ▪ Full drug effects may require several wks of therapy.

NOTES:

fentanyl citrate • (fen-ta-nil)

CATEGORY: *Narcotic:* synthetic opiate

Rx C-II; Preg Cat C

BRAND NAMES	DOSAGE FORMS
Duragesic (Janssen)	Transdermal 25, 50, 75, 100μg/h
Sublimaze (Janssen)	Injection (IM/IV): 0.05mg/ml

USE: Relief of moderate/severe pain ▪ Preop sedation; operative, preop analgesia ▪ Relief of chronic pain requiring opioids (transdermal). **ACTION:** Narcotics produce analgesia, euphoria, sedation; 0.1-mg dose approximately equivalent to 10mg morphine, 75-g meperidine.

PHARMACOKINETICS

	Onset	Duration	Excretion
IM	7-8m	1-2h	Via urine as unchanged drug, metabolites
IV	1-3m	30-60m	

Transdermal provides a dose of 25, 50, 75, or 100μg/h for 72h

CONTRAINDICATIONS: Hypersensitivity; use c̄ extreme caution in head injuries. **CC:** Use should be restricted to qualified physicians ▪ Opioid antagonists & oxygen-resuscitative, intubation equipment should be readily available ▪ Caution is required when used in pts c̄ head injuries, ↑ ICP, impaired respiration ▪ Use can produce dependence, abrupt D/C can result in withdrawal symptoms.

DOSAGE

Pediatric (2-12y/o)	*IM/IV*	Induction, maintenance: 0.02-0.03mg/kg
Adult	*IM/IV*	
Preop		0.05-0.1mg IV before surgery
Adjunct to general anesthesia		Induction: low dose 0.002mg/kg; moderate dose 0.002-0.02mg/kg; high dose 0.02-0.05mg/kg Maintenance: low dose 0.002mg/kg; moderate dose 0.002-0.02mg/kg; high dose 0.02-0.5mg/kg
Adjunct to regional anesthesia		0.05-0.1mg. May be repeated
Postop		0.05-0.1mg. May be repeated in 1-2h prn
Adult	*Transdermal*	Start c̄ 25μg/h & adjust

SIDE/ADVERSE EFFECTS: CNS: *sedation, lightheadedness*, euphoria, dysphoria, tremor, disorientation, ↓ convulsive threshold ▪ CV: hypotension, palpitations, flushing of face, phlebitis at IV site ▪ EENT: miosis ▪ GI: N/V, dry mouth, constipation, biliary tract spasm ▪ GU: urinary retention ▪ INT: pruritus, urticaria ▪ RESP: ***respiratory depression***.

INTERACTIONS: Drug: Use c̄ alcohol, antihistamines, barbiturates, benzodiazepines, methotrimeprazine, phenothiazines, other CNS depressants produces additive CNS depression; ↓ dosage may be required ▪ Use c̄ TCAs may produce additive respiratory depression.

NURSING MANAGEMENT PRIORITIES

ADMININISTRATION: Assess for hx of hypersensitivity ▪ Store under double lock/key; document use accurately ▪ Check compatibility for mixing c̄ other drugs in solution ▪ Do *not* administer if respirations are <12/m ▪ IM: inject *deep* into muscle ▪ IV: dilute; administer *slowly* (1-2m) ▪ Have narcotic antagonist, support measures available ▪ Elderly may require ↓ dosage ▪ Administer subsequent initial narcotic analgesic at ↓ dosage ($^1/_4$ - $^1/_3$ usual dose).

EVALUATION: Monitor VS, esp BP, respirations ▪ Assess renal function, urinary retention ▪ Assess for potentiation of CNS depressant effect ▪ Assess for signs of OD (coma, pinpoint pupils, respiratory depression).

EDUCATION: Avoid excessive sensory stimulation ▪ Keep bedrails up ▪ Turn, cough, deep breathe after surgery ▪ Avoid changing positions (lying/sitting/standing) rapidly ▪ Avoid smoking.

NOTES:

finasteride • (fin-as-teh-ride)

CATEGORY: *Testosterone inhibitor:* antiprostatitis agent Rx; Preg Cat X

BRAND NAMES	DOSAGE FORMS
Proscar (MSD)	Tablet: 5mg
Propecia (Merck)	Tablet: 1mg

USE: Treatment of symptomatic benign prostatic hyperplasia (BPH). A 6-mo treatment period may be required to determine if therapy is successful. Treatment usually produces 20%-30% ⬇ in prostate size ▪ Treatment of male hair loss (Propecia). **ACTION:** Antiprostatitis activity (BHP) due to competitive inhibition of enzyme 5 α-reductase, which metabolizes testosterone into 5 α-dihydrotestosterone (DHT), a potent androgen that stimulates prostate gland. Accordingly, ⬇ DHT levels alleviate symptoms of BPH.

PHARMACOKINETICS

PO absorption	Half-life	Protein binding	Excretion
Good	3-16h	90%	Via urine, feces as metabolites

CONTRAINDICATIONS: Hypersensitivity, pregnancy (abnormal fetal male genitalia). Pregnant women should avoid coitus c̄ males taking the drug. Pregnant women should avoid contact c̄ broken tablets. **CC:** Not indicated for use in children ▪ Treatment may require a minimum of 6mo to determine a positive clinical response ▪ Before therapy all disease conditions that can mimic BPH must be ruled out. Examples include cancer, infection, hypotonic bladder, structural abnormalities ▪ Use c̄ caution in pts c̄ liver impairment.

DOSAGE

BPH Adult males *PO*	5mg once/d
Hair Loss	1mg once/d

SIDE/ADVERSE EFFECTS: CNS: ⬇ libido ▪ GU: impotence, ⬇ ejaculate volume ▪ Other: breast tenderness, enlargement.

INTERACTIONS: Drug: No significant rxs currently reported.

NURSING MANAGEMENT PRIORITIES

ADMINISTRATION: Assess for hx of hypersensitivity ▪ Assess GU function (incl digital rectal exam) ▪ Assess hepatic function; use caution if impaired ▪ Take c̄ or w/out food ▪ Not indicated for use in women or children.

EVALUATION: Monitor GU, hepatic status.

EDUCATION: May be taken w/out regard to food ▪ Changes in sexual activity/performance may occur ▪ Pregnant women should avoid contact c̄ crushed drug or pt's semen ▪ Full drug effects may require several mos of therapy.

NOTES:

flecainide acetate • (flek-a-nide)

CATEGORY: *Antiarrhythmic* Rx; Preg Cat C

BRAND NAME	DOSAGE FORMS
Tambocor (3M)	Tablet: 50, 100, 150mg

USE: Treatment of documented ventricular arrhythmias ▪ Treatment of paroxysmal atrial flutter/fibrillation (PAF) ▪ Treatment of paroxysmal supraventricular tachycardia (PSVT). **ACTION:** Antiarrhythmic effect due to dose-related depression of cardiac conduction, esp in His-Purkinje system; drug has no appreciable effect on atrial arrhythmias, produces effects similar to group 1C antiarrhythmics, is reserved for documented serious ventricular arrhythmias.

PHARMACOKINETICS

PO absorption	Peak	Half-life	Protein binding	Excretion
Almost complete	3h	20h	40%	Via urine as unchanged drug, metabolites

CONTRAINDICATIONS: Hypersensitivity, cardiogenic shock, 2°/3° AV block, right bundle branch block when associated c̄ left hemiblock w/out pacemaker. **CC:** Not recommended for use c̄ chronic atrial fibrillation due to drug's proarrhythmic effect.

DOSAGE

Adult *PO*

Sustained ventricular tachycardia	Initial dose 100mg q12h c̄ 50-mg increments if needed. ↑ 50mg bid q4d until satisfactory response. Usual dose 150mg q12h c̄ daily maximum 400mg
Nonsustained tachycardia, ventricular complexes	Initial dose 100mg q12h c̄ 50-mg increments if needed bid q4d until satisfactory response. Usual range 200-400mg/d c̄ maximum 600mg/d
PAF/PSVT	Initial dose of 50mg q12h. ↑ 50mg bid q4d if needed. Do *not* exceed 300mg/d

SIDE/ADVERSE EFFECTS: CNS: *dizziness, headache, tremor*, convulsions, confusion, paresthesia, depression, drowsiness ▪ CV: CHF, ***proarrhythmic effect,*** palpitations, ***heart block***, bradycardia, angina, hypotension, hypertension, chest pain ▪ EENT: *blurred vision*, visual spots, tinnitus, photophobia ▪ GI: N/V, anorexia, constipation, abdominal pain ▪ GU: impotence ▪ HEM: leukopenia, ***thrombocytopenia*** ▪ INT: rash, urticaria, pruritus, ***exfoliative dermatitis*** ▪ MS: arthralgia ▪ RESP: *dyspnea*.

INTERACTIONS: Drug: Use c̄ propranolol will ↑ plasma levels of both drugs, possible summation of negative inotropic effects ▪ Use c̄ disopyramide or verapamil requires extreme caution.

NURSING MANAGEMENT PRIORITIES

ADMINISTRATION: Assess for hx of hypersensitivity ▪ Assess hepatic, renal function; may require ↓ dosage if impaired ▪ May be administered w/out regard to meals ▪ Assess serum K^+ levels (normal: 3.5-5mEq/L); correct imbalances before administration ▪ Maintain blood levels; administer at equal intervals around clock ▪ Avoid exposure to moisture in storage ▪ Elderly may require ↓ dosage.

EVALUATION: Monitor VS, esp heart rate, BP ▪ Assess for CHF (dyspnea, peripheral edema, ↑ weight); notify physician ▪ Monitor serum for ↑ alkaline phosphatase c̄ prolonged use ▪ Monitor ECG, CBC, blood levels throughout therapy ▪ Assess for tremors (signifies maximum dose) ▪ Therapeutic blood levels: 0.4-1.0µg/ml.

EDUCATION: Dizziness may occur; use caution in potentially hazardous activities ▪ Avoid changing positions (lying/sitting/standing) rapidly, esp elderly ▪ Take as ordered by physician even if symptom free; do *not* skip doses ▪ Take at equal intervals around clock ▪ Procedure for checking radial pulse ▪ Notify physician *immediately* of irregular pulse, fever, sore throat, bruising/bleeding ▪ Keep scheduled appointments c̄ physician ▪ Notify physician/dentist of use before treatment ▪ Full drug effect may require several days of therapy.

NOTES:

fluconazole • (floo-koe-na-zole)

CATEGORY: *Broad-spectrum antifungal* Rx; Preg Cat C

BRAND NAME
Diflucan (Pfizer)

DOSAGE FORMS
IV infusion: 2mg/ml in 100-, 200-ml units
Tablet: 50, 100, 200mg

USE: Treatment of oropharyngeal, esophageal, & serious systemic UTI, pneumonia, peritonitis & vaginal infections caused by susceptible strains of *Candida* spp ▪ Treatment of cryptococcal meningitis ▪ Prophylaxis of *Candida* infection in bone marrow transplantation (BMT) associated c̄ cytotoxic drugs or radiation therapy. **ACTION:** Antifungal activity may be related to selective inhibition of fungal sterol demethylation (cytochrome P-450 sterol C-14 α-demethylation) resulting in the accumulation of 14 α-methyl sterols, which are fungistatic.

PHARMACOKINETICS

PO absorption	Peak	Half-life	Protein binding	Excretion
Almost complete	1-2h	30h	11%-20%	Primarily as unchanged drug via urine

CONTRAINDICATIONS: Hypersensitivity. **CC:** Use can cause significant hepatotoxicity incl fatalities ▪ Dosage for neonates ≤ 2wks old must be administered q72h.

DOSAGE: For pts c̄ normal renal function. The PO & IV doses are the same. The IV dose should be administered at a maximum rate of about 200mg/h as a continuous infusion.

Candidiasis

Oropharyngeal	Adult PO suspension: 50, 200mg/5ml. Initial dose 200mg/d followed by 100mg once/d for at least 2wks. Doses up to 400mg/d may be required. Children: 6mg/kg on day 1 then 3mg/kg/d
Esophageal	Initial dose 200mg/d followed by 100mg once/d. Doses up to 400mg/d may be used. Minimum treatment time is at least 3wks & 2 or more wks following resolution of symptoms. Children: 6mg/kg on day 1 then 3mg/kg/d
Systemic	Adult: initial dose 400mg/d followed by 200mg once/d for at least 4wks &

	at least 2wks following resolution of symptoms. Children: 6-12mg/kg/d
Vaginal	Adult: 150mg as a single dose
Meningitis	Adult: initial dose 400mg/d followed by 200mg once/d for 10-12wks after negative CSF cultures. Prophylactic dose of 200mg/d required in AIDS pts. Children: 12mg/kg on day 1 then 6mg/kg/d
BMT	400mg/d. Start several days before BMT in pts c̄ severe granulocytopenia & continue for 7d after satisfactory neutrophil levels have been reached

SIDE/ADVERSE EFFECTS: Substantially higher c̄ HIV-infected pts ▪ CNS: *headache* ▪ GI: N/V/D, abdominal pain ▪ HEP: ↑ in serum transaminase ▪ INT: ***Stevens-Johnson syndrome.***

INTERACTIONS: Drug: Use c̄ PO anticoagulants can ↑ PT & requires careful monitoring ▪ Use c̄ phenytoin & cyclosporine can ↑ their plasma concentrations ▪ Use c̄ PO hypoglycemic agents will ↓ their metabolism & ↑ their plasma concentrations, & dosage adjustments may be required ▪ Use c̄ astemizole not recommended ▪ Use c̄ cisapride can produce fatal cardiac arrhythmias.

NURSING MANAGEMENT PRIORITIES

ADMINISTRATION: Assess for hx of hypersensitivity to azole antifungal agent ▪ Obtain C&S before therapy ▪ Assess hepatic, renal function; ↓ dosage if impaired ▪ IV: Administer via continuous infusion at a maximum rate of 200mg/h; do *not* use if solution is cloudy or precipitated; do *not* add other medication to the IV solution; do *not* administer IM or SC ▪ Avoid exposure to moisture in storage.

EVALUATION: Monitor VS, esp temperature ▪ Monitor hepatic function ▪ Assess for occurrence of rash; D/C drug, notify physician.

EDUCATION: Take as ordered by physician at same time qd; do *not* change dose ▪ Take c̄ food to avoid GI upset ▪ Report skin rash to physician *immediately*; D/C drug ▪ Check c̄ physician/pharmacist before taking OTC preparations ▪ Store in tightly closed container.

NOTES:

flucytosine • (floo-sye-toe-seen)

CATEGORY: *Antifungal:* antimonilial, fluorinated pyrimidine Rx; Preg Cat D

BRAND NAME
Ancobon (Roche)

DOSAGE FORMS
Capsule: 250, 500mg

USE: Treatment of infections caused by susceptible strains of *Cryptococcus* (meningitis, pulmonary, urinary tract, septicemia) & *Candida* (endocarditis, septicemia, urinary tract). **ACTION:** Antifungal activity appears related to ⬇ purine, pyrimidine uptake via competitive inhibition. In addition, drug is converted into antimetabolite 5-fluorouracil after absorption into susceptible fungi. Thus fungal RNA & DNA synthesis is inhibited. Constant sensitivity tests required during therapy because resistant strains can emerge quickly.

PHARMACOKINETICS

PO absorption	Peak	Half-life	Protein binding	Excretion
Almost complete	2h	2.4-4.8h	2.9%-4%	Via urine primarily as unchanged drug

CONTRAINDICATIONS: Hypersensitivity. **CC:** Use c̄ caution c̄ bone marrow depression, impaired renal function ▪ Electrolyte, hematologic, & renal assessment should be determined before & monitored during treatment.

DOSAGE

Pediatric/Adult	*PO*	50-250mg/kg/d equally divided into 4 doses
Children	*PO*	<50kg:1.5-4.5g/m² is suggested

SIDE/ADVERSE EFFECTS: CNS: headache, ataxia, sedation, paresthesia, peripheral neuropathy, parkinsonism, vertigo, confusion, hallucinations ▪ CV: ***cardiac arrest*** ▪ GI: N/V/D, anorexia, dry mouth, duodenal ulcer, ***hemorrhage, ulcerative colitis,*** abdominal pain ▪ GU: ***azotemia, crystalluria, renal failure,*** ⬆ in BUN, creatinine ▪ HEM: ***agranulocytosis,*** anemia, ***aplastic anemia, thrombocytopenia,*** eosinophilia, leukopenia ▪ HEP: jaundice, *hepatic dysfunction* ▪ INT: photosensitivity, rash, pruritus, urticaria ▪ RESP: chest pain, dyspnea, ***respiratory arrest*** ▪ Other: hypoglycemia, hypokalemia, weakness, psychosis.

INTERACTIONS: Drug: Use c̄ other bone marrow–depressing drugs or during radiation therapy can produce significant toxicity ▪ Use c̄ hepatotoxic drugs is best avoided ▪ Use c̄ amphotericin B can produce ↑ therapeutic effects. **Lab:** Serum creatinine levels should be determined by Jaffé method.

NURSING MANAGEMENT PRIORITIES

ADMINISTRATION: Assess for hx of hypersensitivity ▪ Obtain C&S before therapy ▪ Administer in early AM ▪ Assess hepatic function; ↓ dosage if impaired ▪ Administer c̄ food.

EVALUATION: Monitor VS, esp temperature ▪ Monitor hepatic function ▪ Diabetics: monitor blood glucose (hypoglycemia).

EDUCATION: Dizziness/drowsiness may occur; use caution in potentially hazardous activities ▪ Take as directed by physician at same time qd, do *not* change dose ▪ Take c̄ food ▪ Take antacids at least 2h after taking drug ▪ Avoid exposure to bright light; wear sunglasses to ↓ discomfort ▪ May require several wks/mos of treatment; take until lab tests are normal ▪ Check c̄ physician/pharmacist before taking OTC preparations ▪ Store in tightly closed container ▪ Women: avoid breastfeeding ▪ Avoid use c̄ alcohol.

NOTES:

flumazenil • (floo-maz-eh-nil)

CATEGORY: *Benzodiazepine* antagonist: antidote

Rx; Preg Cat C

BRAND NAME
Romazicon (Roche)

DOSAGE FORM
IV injection: 0.1mg/ml

USE: Complete or partial reversal of sedative effects of benzodiazepine (therapeutic or diagnostic procedures) ▪ Treatment of benzodiazepine OD. **ACTION:** Benzodiazepine antagonism due to competitive inhibition c̄ benzodiazepines for CNS receptor sites (GABA/benzodiazepine receptor complex).

PHARMACOKINETICS: Initial half-life of 7-15m c̄ a terminal half-life of 41-79m; protein binding 50%; excreted via urine (90%-95%), feces (5%-10%) primarily as metabolites. Moderate liver dysfunction ↓ renal clearance by 40%-60% & severe liver dysfunction to 25% of normal.

CONTRAINDICATIONS: Hypersensitivity to drug or benzodiazepines, serious cyclic antidepressant OD, benzodiazepine control of potentially life-threatening conditions (ICP, status epilepticus). **CC:** Use in pts c̄ extended benzodiazepine use or c̄ high seizure potential can result in seizures ▪ Not recommended for serious cyclic antidepressant OD.

DOSAGE
Adult *IV*

Sedation reversal	0.2mg over 15s. If unsatisfactory after 45s, repeat dose of 0.2mg at 60-s intervals to a maximum total dose of 1mg
Overdose	0.2mg over 30s. If unsatisfactory after 30s, give 0.3mg over 30s. If required, 0.5mg over 30-60s to a maximum total dose of 3mg

SIDE/ADVERSE EFFECTS: CNS: ***convulsions***, headache, confusion, stupor, dizziness, agitation ▪ CV: cutaneous vasodilation, *arrhythmia,* hypertension ▪ EENT: blurred vision, transient hearing impairment, tinnitus ▪ GI: N/V ▪ Other: injection site pain and/or ***thrombophlebitis***, rash, speech disorders, shivering, hyperventilation.

INTERACTIONS: Drug: Use caution in cases of mixed drug OD because of possible convulsions & cardiac arrhythmias (esp c̄ cyclic antidepressants).

Note: Side/adverse effects: common in *italic;* serious in ***boldface italic.***

*Available in Canada only.

NURSING MANAGEMENT PRIORITIES

ADMINISTRATION: Assess for hx of benzodiazepine hypersensitivity ▪ Assess hepatic status; use caution if impaired ▪ Administer via IV infusion site into large vein ▪ Compatible c̄ D_5W, lactated Ringer, normal saline solutions; discard after 24h; keep in vial until just before use ▪ Avoid use in cyclic antidepressant toxicity ▪ Avoid use in children.

EVALUATION: Monitor VS, esp BP, heart rate ▪ Monitor activity status (safety precautions) ▪ Check IV insertion site carefully; avoid extravasation ▪ Assess for visual/hearing disturbances; notify physician.

EDUCATION: Notify nurse/physician of rx (abnormal heartbeat, confusion, pain at injection site) ▪ Use caution in potentially hazardous activities for up to 24h after taking drug ▪ Avoid use c̄ alcohol, OTC preparations for up to 24h after taking drug.

NOTES:

fluorouracil • (flure-oh-yoor-a-sill)

CATEGORY: *Antineoplastic:* antimetabolite — Rx; Preg Cat D

BRAND NAMES	DOSAGE FORMS
Adrucil (Adria)	Injection (IV): 50mg/ml
Efudex (Roche)	Topical cream: 5%
	Solution: 2%, 5%
Fluoroplex (Herbert)	Topical cream: 1% (5% in Canada)
	Solution: 1%

USE: Palliative treatment of colon, rectum, breast, stomach, pancreatic cancer ▪ Topical treatment of superficial basal cell carcinomas when conventional treatment is impractical ▪ Topical treatment of actinic or solar keratosis. **ACTION:** Antimetabolite activity due to competitive inhibition of enzyme thymidylate synthetase, resulting in deficiency of thymidine, which inhibits DNA synthesis.

PHARMACOKINETICS: After IV administration, drug is distributed into bone marrow, intestinal mucosa, liver, tumors; no intact drug can be detected in blood after 3h; excretion via urine primarily as metabolites.

CONTRAINDICATIONS: Depressed bone marrow function, poor nutritional state, serious infections; topical: local hypersensitivity. **CC:** Hospitalization is recommended for first course of treatment ▪ Use c̄ caution in pts c̄ hx of high-dose pelvic radiation, alkylating agents, widespread metastatic tumors involving bone marrow.

DOSAGE

Adult *IV*	Start c̄ 12mg/kg/d for 4 successive days. Do *not* exceed total daily dose 800mg. If no toxicity, give 6mg/kg on days 6, 8, 10, 12; do not give on days 5, 7, 9, 11; D/C on day 12 For poor-risk pts, start c̄ 6mg/kg/d for 3 successive days. If no toxicity, give 3mg/kg on days 5, 7, 9; do not give on days 4, 6, 8. Do *not* exceed total daily dose 400mg. Usual maintenance dose 10-15mg/kg/wk c̄ ⬇ doses for poor-risk pts. Do *not* exceed 1g/wk
Topical Actinic/solar keratosis	Apply cream/solution bid to lesions. Continue until inflammatory response reaches erosion, necrosis, ulceration stage. Usually requires 2-4wks; complete healing may require up to 2mos

Superficial basal cell carcinoma	Apply 5% cream/solution bid to lesions for at least 3-6wks. Therapy may require 10-12wks

SIDE/ADVERSE EFFECTS: GI: esophagopharyngitis, stomatitis, anorexia, N/V/D ▪ HEM: ***myelosuppression, thrombocytopenia*** ▪ INT: alopecia, dermatitis, dry skin, loss of nails ▪ Other: photophobia, lacrimation, ***acute cerebellar syndrome*** ▪ Topical: local pain, burning, pruritus, hyperpigmentation, scarring, suppuration, scaling, swelling.

INTERACTIONS: Drug: Radiation therapy, other myelosuppressive drugs produce additive bone marrow depression.

NURSING MANAGEMENT PRIORITIES

ADMINISTRATION: Check hx for radiation/antineoplastic therapy ▪ IV: dilute according to manufacturer's directions; administer antiemetic before therapy; administer via direct injection (1-2m) or slow IV infusion (2-24h); precipitate may form when exposed to cold temperatures; heat to 60°C to redissolve, shake vigorously; cool to body temperature before using ▪ Topical: cleanse area, apply c̄ applicator/fingers; wash hands before, after application ▪ Provide emotional support ▪ Assess oral cavity for ulceration; notify physician ▪ Avoid exposure to heat/moisture/light in storage ▪ Contact dermatitis may occur.

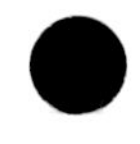

EVALUATION: Monitor hepatic, renal function; CBC, esp WBC, platelets throughout therapy; notify physician if ↓ ▪ Assess for infection, bleeding, anemia ▪ May produce ↑ serum uric acid level ▪ Assess hydration status (I&O, daily weight) ▪ Check IV insertion site carefully (cellulitis).

EDUCATION: ↑ Fluid intake (8-10 glasses/d) ▪ Avoid exposure to infection ▪ Check c̄ physician before immunization ▪ Diet as tolerated; avoid spicy foods ▪ Maintain oral hygiene; use soft-bristled toothbrush ▪ Notify physician of symptoms of bone marrow depression ▪ Loss of hair may occur (reversible) ▪ Women: avoid breastfeeding ▪ Use contraception if sexually active ▪ Topical: avoid exposure to direct sunlight, UV light (sunlamps); use sunscreen; avoid application near eyes, nose, mouth; local discomfort may occur; apply as ordered; store in tightly closed, light-resistant container; wash hands before, after application.

NOTES:

fluoxetine hcl • (floo-ox-uh-teen)

CATEGORY: *Antidepressant:* selective serotonin reuptake inhibitor (SSRI) Rx; Preg Cat B

BRAND NAME
Prozac (Dista)

DOSAGE FORMS
Pulvule (capsule): 10, 20mg
PO liquid: 20mg/5ml

USE: Treatment of depression that closely resembles DSM-IV category 296 of major depressive disorder. Long-term use requires reevaluation of clinical effectiveness ▪ Treatment of obsessive compulsive disorder (DSM-IV category 301.4) ▪ Treatment of bulimia nervosa. **ACTION:** Antidepressant activity appears related to inhibition of serotonin (5-hydroxytryptamine) reuptake at presynaptic membrane in the CNS resulting in subsequent serotonergic activity.

PHARMACOKINETICS

PO absorption	Peak	Half-life	Protein binding	Excretion
Good ac/pc	6-8h	7-9d	94.5%	Mainly as inactive metabolites via urine

CONTRAINDICATIONS: Hypersensitivity. **CC:** Use can result in rash, other allergic rxs.

DOSAGE: Adult *PO*

Depression	Usual dose 20mg/d in AM. If no clinical improvement is obtained after several wks, ⬆ may be required. Doses >20mg/d require bid administration, in the AM & at noontime. Do *not* exceed 80mg/d
Bulimia	60mg/d

SIDE/ADVERSE EFFECTS: CNS: *anxiety, nervousness, insomnia, drowsiness, tremor, headache,* dizziness, abnormal dreams ▪ CV: angina, hot flashes, palpitations, rare conduction disturbances, lymphadenopathy ▪ GI: *anorexia* c̄ significant weight loss, N/D, dry mouth, dyspepsia, constipation, abdominal pain ▪ GU: frequent urination, painful menstruation, sexual dysfunction ▪ INT: *rash, pruritus, excessive sweating, erythema multiforme* ▪ RESP: flulike symptoms, pharyngitis, bronchitis ▪ Other: *fatigue,* visual disturbances, tinnitus, anemia.

INTERACTIONS: Drug: Use c̄ MAO-I & tryptophan is best avoided ▪ Use c̄ diazepam may ⬆ its half-life ▪ Use c̄ highly protein-bound drugs (digitoxin, warfarin, etc.) can result in adverse effects of these drugs and/or fluoxetine because of protein displacement. **Lab:** Mild ↑ in proteinuria, transaminase levels.

NURSING MANAGEMENT PRIORITIES

ADMINISTRATION: Assess for hx of hypersensitivity ▪ Assess for hx of seizures; use caution ▪ Assess hepatic, renal status; ↓ dosage if impaired ▪ Administer consistently c̄ or w/out food; single dose in AM, divided dose in AM & noon ▪ Institute safety, seizure precautions ▪ Institute suicide precautions ▪ Avoid abrupt withdrawal; D/C gradually ▪ Avoid moisture/heat/direct light in storage ▪ Elderly may require ↓ dosage.

EVALUATION: Monitor CV, hepatic, renal status ▪ Monitor fluid retention (I&O, daily weight), constipation ▪ Assess for weight loss (anorectic effect) ▪ Assess for symptoms of abrupt withdrawal (nausea, headache, malaise) ▪ Assess for actual swallowing of PO forms ▪ Assess for skin rash, hives; notify physician, D/C drug.

EDUCATION: Dizziness/drowsiness may occur; use caution in potentially hazardous activities ▪ Avoid changing positions (lying/sitting/standing) rapidly ▪ Avoid use of alcohol, other CNS depressants for up to 1wk after end of therapy ▪ Take consistently c̄ or w/out food ▪ Take as directed by physician ▪ Use sugarless gum/hard candy to diminish dry mouth ▪ Constipation may occur; ↑ fluids, bulk-containing foods ▪ Notify physician of skin rash, hives; D/C drug ▪ Check c̄ physician/pharmacist before taking OTC/Rx preparations ▪ Notify physician/dentist of use before treatment ▪ Store in tightly closed, light-resistant container ▪ Encourage recreational/diversional interests ▪ Notify physician of weight loss, fever, sore throat, malaise ▪ Keep scheduled appointments c̄ physician ▪ Women: notify physician of pregnancy possibility; avoid breastfeeding ▪ Full drug effects may require several wks of therapy.

NOTES:

fluphenazine decanoate/enanthate/hcl • (floo-fen-a-zeen)

CATEGORY: *Phenothiazine:* antipsychotic, neuroleptic Rx; Preg Cat NA

BRAND NAMES	DOSAGE FORMS
**Modecate (Squibb)*	Injection (SC/IM): 5mg/ml, 25mg/5ml
**Moditen (Squibb)*	Injection (SC/IM): 5mg/ml, 25mg/5ml
Permitil (Schering)	PO concentrate: 5mg/ml Tablet: 2.5, 5, 10mg
Prolixin (Apothecon)	Elixir: 2.5mg/5ml Injection (IM): 2.5mg/ml PO concentrate: 5mg/ml Tablet: 1, 2.5, 5, 10mg
Prolixin Decanoate (Apothecon)	Injection (SC/IM): 25mg/ml
Prolixin Enanthate (Apothecon)	Injection (SC/IM): 25mg/ml

USE: Treatment of psychoses. **ACTION:** Antipsychotic activity appears associated c̄ ⬇ in neural transmission in central dopamine-dependent pathways, resulting in tranquilizing effect; decanoate/enanthate injection effects have onset between 24-72h; psychotic symptoms controlled w/in 48-96h.

PHARMACOKINETICS

PO absorption	Onset	Peak	Duration	Excretion
Rapid	1h	2h	6-8h	Via urine, feces

CONTRAINDICATIONS: Hypersensitivity, comatose states, bone marrow depression, presence of large amounts of CNS depressants, liver impairment, renal damage. **CC:** Extended use may produce extrapyramidal symptoms, tardive dyskinesia, neuroleptic malignant syndrome.

DOSAGE

decanoate/enanthate		
Adult	*SC/IM*	12.5-25mg usually adequate. Do *not* exceed 100mg/dose
hcl		
Adult	*PO*	0.5-20mg/d
	IM	2.5-10mg/d
Geriatric	*PO*	1-2.5mg/d

SIDE/ADVERSE EFFECTS: CNS: drowsiness, extrapyramidal rxs, tardive dyskinesia, seizures, depression,

Note: Side/adverse effects: common in *italic;* serious in ***boldface italic.*** *Available in Canada only.

catatonialike states ▪ CV: postural hypotension, tachycardia, ECG changes ▪ EENT: blurred vision; corneal, lenticular changes; nasal congestion ▪ END: menstrual irregularities, galactorrhea ▪ HEM: ***agranulocytosis***, eosinophilia, ***hemolytic anemia***, thrombocytopenic purpura ▪ HEP: cholestatic jaundice ▪ INT: urticaria, photosensitivity, ***exfoliative dermatitis*** ▪ Other: fever, hyperpyrexia, hypothermia.

INTERACTIONS: Drug: Al^{+++}/Mg^{++} antacid preparations ↓ absorption ▪ Use c̄ narcotics, barbiturates, other CNS depressants ↑ CNS depression ▪ Guanethidine, related antihypertensive effects antagonized.

NURSING MANAGEMENT PRIORITIES

ADMINISTRATION: Assess for hx of phenothiazine hypersensitivity ▪ Assess VS, esp BP ▪ PO: administer c̄ food ▪ PO concentrate: dilute before administration c̄ >60ml fluid ▪ IM/SC: keep pt lying down for 30m after injection ▪ Discard markedly discolored/precipitated solution ▪ Avoid skin contact c̄ liquid forms (contact dermatitis) ▪ Avoid abrupt withdrawal; D/C gradually ▪ Heavy smokers may require ↑ dosage.

EVALUATION: Monitor hepatic, ophthalmic, renal status; BP, CBC; fluid retention; constipation; seizures ▪ Assess for extrapyramidal symptoms (tics/spasms, trembling, shuffling gait); jaundice, agranulocytosis ▪ Assess for symptoms of abrupt withdrawal (nausea, dyskinesia, trembling, dizziness).

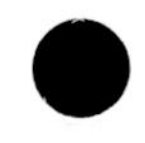

EDUCATION: Dizziness/drowsiness may occur; use caution in potentially hazardous activities ▪ Avoid changing positions (lying/sitting/standing) rapidly ▪ Avoid use c̄ alcohol, other CNS depressants ▪ Take PO forms c̄ meals ▪ Store in tightly closed, light-resistant container ▪ Use sugarless gum/hard candy to diminish dry mouth ▪ Constipation may occur; ↑ fluids, bulk-containing foods ▪ May turn urine pink/red/brown ▪ Avoid contact c̄ liquid forms ▪ Women: avoid breastfeeding ▪ Avoid exposure to temperature extremes; direct sunlight, UV light (sunlamps); use sunscreen, protective clothing ▪ Notify physician of fever, sore throat, bruising/bleeding, extrapyramidal symptoms (tics/spasms, trembling, shuffling gait) ▪ Take as directed by physician ▪ Check c̄ physician before taking OTC preparations ▪ Extended-action injectable effects may last up to 6wks ▪ Do *not* take antacids/antidiarrheals w/in 2h of drug ▪ Full drug effects may require several wks of therapy.

OVERDOSE MANAGEMENT: *See* Phenothiazines.

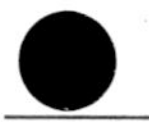

flurazepam hcl • (flure-az-e-pam)

CATEGORY: *Benzodiazepine:* hypnotic — Rx C-IV; Preg Cat X

BRAND NAMES	DOSAGE FORMS
**Apo-Flurazepam (Apotex)*	
Dalmane (Roche)	Capsule: 15, 30mg
**Somnol (Horner)*	
**Som-Pam (ICN)*	

USE: Short-term treatment of insomnia associated c̄ difficulty in falling asleep, frequent awakenings, early-morning awakening. **ACTION:** Hypnotic activity extends to all stages (0-4) of sleep; improves total sleep time; ⬇ number of nocturnal awakenings, REM sleep not affected.

PHARMACOKINETICS

PO absorption	Peak	Half-life	Excretion
Rapid	30-60m	2-3h	Via urine primarily as metabolites, which have long half-life

CONTRAINDICATIONS: Hypersensitivity, pregnancy. **CC:** Use can produce dependence; abrupt D/C can result in withdrawal symptoms.

DOSAGE

Adult *PO*	15-30mg at hs
Geriatric/debilitated	15mg at hs

SIDE/ADVERSE EFFECTS: CNS: *drowsiness, fatigue, ataxia* ▪ CV: hypotension ▪ EENT: dry mouth ▪ HEM: neutropenia (rare) ▪ INT: skin rash ▪ PSYCH: paradoxic anxiety, hallucinations, hyperexcited states.

INTERACTIONS: Drug: Use c̄ other CNS depressants produces additive effects ▪ Use c̄ MAO-I can produce serious toxic effects.

NURSING MANAGEMENT PRIORITIES

ADMINISTRATION: Assess for hx of benzodiazepine hypersensitivity ▪ Avoid exposure to heat/moisture/light in storage ▪ Avoid abrupt withdrawal ▪ Elderly may require ⬇ dosage ▪ ⬇ Environmental stimuli.

EVALUATION: Monitor renal, hepatic status ▪ Assess for symptoms of abrupt withdrawal (tremors, abdominal/muscle cramps, convulsions) c̄ prolonged use ▪ Check for signs of dependence (⬆ drug request) ▪ Monitor activity sta-

Note: Side/adverse effects: common in *italic;* serious in ***boldface italic.*** — *Available in Canada only.

tus (safety precautions) ▪ Assess for tolerance to therapeutic dose ▪ Assess for paradoxic rxs (CNS stimulation), esp in elderly ▪ Check for depression, suicide precautions prn ▪ Assess pt sleep patterns.

EDUCATION: Drowsiness may occur; use caution in potentially hazardous activities ▪ Avoid use c̄ alcohol, other CNS depressants ▪ Indiscriminate use may lead to dependence ▪ Do *not* smoke after taking drug ▪ Do *not* keep at bedside ▪ Take as ordered by physician; do *not* ↑ dose ▪ Women: avoid breastfeeding ▪ Check c̄ physician/pharmacist before taking OTC preparations ▪ Practice relaxation exercises, ventilation of feelings ▪ Utilize sleep producers (reading, warm milk, soft music).

NOTES:

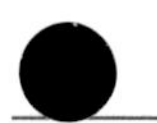

CATEGORY: *Antiinflammatory:* analgesic, NSAIA Rx; Preg Cat B

BRAND NAMES	**DOSAGE FORMS**
flurbiprofen	
Ansaid (Upjohn)	Tablet: 50, 100mg
*Ocufen (Allergan)**	Ophthalmic solution: 0.03%
ketoprofen	
Orudis (W-A)	Capsules: 25, 50, 75mg
Oruvail (W-A)	ER capsules: 100, 150, 200mg

USE: Treatment of rheumatoid arthritis/osteoarthritis ▪ Inhibition of intraoperative miosis (flurbiprofen/ophthalmic) ▪ Relief of mild/moderate pain, primary dysmenorrhea (ketoprofen). **ACTION:** Antiinflammatory, analgesic activity appears related to inhibition of prostaglandin synthesis.

PHARMACOKINETICS

PO absorption	Peak	Half-life	Protein binding	Excretion
flurbiprofen				
Good	1.5h	5.7h	99%	Via urine as conjugates
ketoprofen				
Complete	0.5-2h	2-4h	99%	Via urine as conjugates

CONTRAINDICATIONS: Hypersensitivity, aspirin/other antiinflammatory agent hypersensitivity. **CC:** Risk of GI ulcerations, bleeding, perforation c̄ use.

DOSAGE

flurbiprofen

Adult *PO*

Arthritis	200-300mg/d divided 2, 3, or 4 times/d. Do *not* exceed a single dose of 100mg. Total daily dose above 300mg not currently recommended
Ophthalmic solution	1gtt q½h starting 2h before surgery

ketoprofen

Adult *PO*

Arthritis	150-300mg/d divided in 3 or 4 doses. Do *not* exceed 300mg/d
Pain	25-50mg q6-8h
Dysmenorrhea	25-50mg q6-8h

SIDE/ADVERSE EFFECTS: CNS: *headache*, nervousness, dizziness, drowsiness ▪ CV: hypertension, heart failure, edema ▪ EENT: tinnitus, conjunctivitis, visual disturbance ▪ GI: *abdominal pain, N/D, **GI bleeding**,* vomiting, flatulence ▪ GU: symptoms of renal infection, rare ***interstitial nephritis***, hematuria ▪ HEM: rare ***hemolytic anemia, thrombocytopenia,*** leukopenia ▪ INT: rash, urticaria, pruritus, photosensitivity, rare ***toxic epidermal necrolysis,*** rhinitis ▪ Other: asthma.

INTERACTIONS: Drug: Use c̄ ulcerogenic drugs produces additive effects ▪ Use c̄ PO anticoagulants may ↑ their activity ▪ Use c̄ aspirin not recommended ▪ Use c̄ furosemide requires monitoring ▪ Use c̄ other protein-bound drugs can produce displacement from inactive protein sites ▪ Use c̄ methotrexate will ↑ its toxicity ▪ Ketoprofen will ↓ urinary excretion of K^+ and Cl^- of hydrochlorothiazide.

NURSING MANAGEMENT PRIORITIES

ADMINISTRATION: Assess for hx of NSAIA, salicylate hypersensitivity ▪ Avoid administration to pts c̄ hx of asthma, bleeding disorders, salicylate hypersensitivity ▪ Assess GI, renal, hepatic function; use caution if impaired ▪ May be administered c̄ food, milk, antacid; *best* on empty stomach (1h ac/2h pc); tablets may be crushed (except SR form); administer c̄ full glass of liquid; encourage upright position for 15-30m ▪ Avoid exposure to moisture during storage ▪ Elderly may require ↓ dosage.

EVALUATION: Monitor VS, esp BP ▪ Monitor hepatic, renal status c̄ prolonged use ▪ Monitor pt receiving anticoagulant therapy; may potentiate bleeding ▪ Monitor stool for occult blood ▪ Monitor I&O, daily weight ▪ Assess for edema in extremities ▪ Assess for visual disturbances; D/C drug, notify physician.

EDUCATION: Dizziness/drowsiness may occur; use caution in potentially hazardous activities ▪ Take on empty stomach (1h ac/2h pc) c̄ food/milk if GI distress occurs; take c̄ full glass liquid; maintain upright position for 15-30m ▪ Take as ordered by physician; do *not* ↑ dose ▪ Notify physician *immediately* of bleeding, ↓ urine output, swelling of feet/legs, lethargy, GI distress, jaundice, visual disturbances ▪ Avoid taking c̄ aspirin, other NSAIAs ▪ Avoid use c̄ alcohol ▪ Check c̄ physician/pharmacist before taking OTC preparations ▪ Notify physician/dentist of use before treatment ▪ Women: avoid breastfeeding ▪ Store in tightly closed container ▪ Full drug effects may require several wks of therapy.

NOTES:

fluvoxamine maleate • (flew-vox-ah-mean)

CATEGORY: *Antidepressant:* selective serotonin reuptake inhibitor (SSRI) Rx; Preg Cat C

BRAND NAME
Luvox (Solvay)

DOSAGE FORMS
Tablet: 25, 50, 100mg

USE: Treatment of obsessive-compulsive disorder as defined in DSM-IV. Treatment requires at least 2-3wks for therapeutic activity. **ACTION:** Antidepressant activity appears related to inhibition of serotonin (5-hydroxytryptamine) reuptake at presynaptic membrane in the CNS & subsequent serotonergic activity.

PHARMACOKINETICS

PO absorption	Peak	Half-life	Protein binding	Excretion
Good	3-8h	13-16h	77%-80%	Via urine

CONTRAINDICATIONS: Hypersensitivity, use c̄ astemizole, MAO-I, terfenadine. **CC:** Use c̄ caution c̄ severe liver dysfunction, ⬇ renal clearance in elderly pts.

DOSAGE

Adult	*PO*	Start c̄ 50mg at hs. Thereafter dosage may be ⬆ by 50mg q3-7d to a maximum of 300mg/d.
Geriatric	*PO*	Initiate c̄ 25mg at hs & adjust

SIDE/ADVERSE EFFECTS: CNS: *headache*, somnolence, insomnia, nervousness, dizziness ▪ CV: palpitations, vasodilation ▪ GI: N/V/D, dry mouth, anorexia, constipation, dyspepsia, taste changes ▪ Other: *asthenia*, respiratory infections, excessive sweating.

INTERACTIONS: Drug: Use c̄ astemizole, MAO-I, terfenadine contraindicated ▪ Use c̄ alcohol, tryptophan best avoided ▪ Smoking will ⬆ fluvoxamine metabolism. **Food:** Meals will not ⬇ PO absorption.

NURSING MANAGEMENT PRIORITIES

ADMINISTRATION: Assess for hx of hypersensitivity ▪ Assess for hx of seizures; use caution ▪ Assess hepatic, renal status; ⬇ dosage if impaired ▪ Administer consistently c̄ or w/out food in PM (single dose) or in AM & PM (divided doses) ▪ Institute safety, seizure precautions ▪ Avoid abrupt withdrawal; D/C gradually ▪ Avoid moisture/heat/direct light in storage ▪ Elderly may require ⬇ dosage.

EVALUATION: Monitor CV, hepatic, renal status ▪ Monitor fluid retention (I&O, daily weight), constipation ▪ Assess for weight loss (anorectic effect) ▪ Assess for symptoms of abrupt withdrawal (nausea, headache, malaise) ▪

Note: Side/adverse effects: common in *italic;* serious in ***boldface italic.***

*Available in Canada only.

Assess for skin rash, hives; notify physician, D/C drug ▪ Diabetics: monitor blood glucose (hypoglycemia).

EDUCATION: Dizziness/drowsiness may occur; use caution in potentially hazardous activities ▪ Avoid changing positions (lying/sitting/standing) rapidly ▪ Diarrhea may occur ▪ Avoid use c̄ alcohol, other CNS depressants for up to 1wk after end of therapy ▪ Take consistently c̄ or w/out food ▪ Take as directed by physician ▪ Use sugarless gum/hard candy to diminish dry mouth ▪ Constipation may occur; ↑ fluids, bulk-containing foods ▪ Notify physician of skin rash, hives; D/C drug ▪ Avoid exposure to direct sunlight, UV light (sun lamps); use sunscreen, protective clothing ▪ Check c̄ physician/pharmacist before taking OTC/Rx preparations ▪ Notify physician/dentist of use before treatment ▪ Store in tightly closed, light-resistant container ▪ Encourage recreational/diversional interests ▪ Notify physician of weight loss, fever, sore throat, malaise ▪ Keep scheduled appointments c̄ physician ▪ Women: notify physician of possibility of pregnancy; avoid breastfeeding ▪ Full drug effects may require several wks of therapy.

NOTES:

foscarnet sodium (phosphonoformic acid trisodium) • (foss-car-net)

CATEGORY: *Antiviral* Rx; Preg Cat C

BRAND NAME	DOSAGE FORM
Foscavir (Astra)	IV injection 24mg/ml

USE: Treatment of cytomegalovirus (CMV) retinitis in AIDS pts ▪ Treatment of acyclovir-resistant mucocutaneous herpes simplex virus (HSV) in immunocompromised pts.
ACTION: Antiviral activity due to inhibition of viral replication of herpes viruses including CMV, herpes HS-1, herpes HS-2, human herpes HHV-6, Epstein-Barr, & varicella-zoster virus; drug is an organic analog of inorganic pyrophosphate that inhibits virus-specific DNA polymerase & reverse transcriptase enzymes required for DNA synthesis.

PHARMACOKINETICS

Protein binding	Half-life	Excretion
14%-17%	3h	80%-90% via urine as unchanged drug

CONTRAINDICATIONS: Hypersensitivity. **CC:** Most common adverse effect that occurs in most pts to some degree is renal toxicity ▪ Alteration in electrolytes can produce seizures.

DOSAGE: For normal renal function

Adult *IV*	Initial dose 60mg/kg (adjusted for renal function) given over a minimum of 1h q8h for 2-3wks. Usual maintenance range 90-120mg/kg/d over 2h
HSV	40mg/kg q8 or 12h for 2-3wks

SIDE/ADVERSE EFFECTS: CNS: seizures (10%), headache (26%), dizziness, neuropathy (both central & peripheral), cerebral edema, ***encephalopathy,*** tremor, paresthesia, extrapyramidal symptoms, neuralgia, ataxia, EEG abnormalities, aphasia, paraplegia, tetany, dementia, confusion, anxiety, hallucinations ▪ CV: ***ECG abnormalities, cardiomyopathy, cardiac failure & arrest,*** palpitations, arrhythmias ▪ EENT: vision abnormalities, eye pain, conjunctivitis, photophobia blindness, retinal detachment, tinnitus, otitis ▪ GI: diarrhea (30%), nausea (47%), vomiting, anorexia, rectal hemorrhage, ***pseudomembranous colitis,*** abdominal pain, flatulence, dry mouth, ulcers (duodenal & esophageal), ulcerative proctitis & stomatitis, constipation, pancreatitis ▪ HEM: anemia (33%), granulocytopenia, leukopenia, ***pulmonary embolism, thrombosis, thrombocytopenia*** ▪ INT: pruritus, rash, ulceration, acne, alopecia, urticaria ▪ MET: hypocalcemia (15%), hypomagnesemia (15%), hypokalemia (16%), hypophosphatemia (8%), hyperphosphatemia (6%) ■ REN: albuminuria, dysuria, ***acute renal failure,*** hematuria, ***glomerulonephritis,*** UTIs, nocturia ■ RESP: coughing, dyspnea, pneumonia, sinusitis, pulmonary infiltration ■ Other: neoplasms, ↑ AST, ↑ ALT, fever (65%), arthralgia, myalgia, inflammation/pain at local injection site.

INTERACTIONS: Drug: Use c̄ nephrotic drugs produces additive effects ■ Use c̄ pentamidine can ↑ hypocalcemia ■ Use c̄ zidovudine can produce additive anemia. **Lab:** ↓ In serum Ca, K, Mg, P electrolytes.

NURSING MANAGEMENT PRIORITIES

ADMINISTRATION: Assess for hx of hypersensitivity ■ Assess for renal impairment; requires ↓ dosage ■ Administer via infusion-control device at rate <1mg/kg/m ■ Administer c̄ normal saline solution or 5% dextrose solution; do *not* add another drug/supplement to IV line ■ Maintain hydration.

EVALUATION: Monitor VS, esp temperature ■ Monitor hepatic, renal status ■ Monitor electrolyte balance; notify physician of abnormalities ■ Assess for paresthesias; notify physician ■ May ↑ serum creatinine ■ Seizure precautions, esp in pts c̄ hx of convulsive disorders ■ Assess for visual disturbances.

EDUCATION: Used to control, *not* cure, HIV-related infections ■ Notify physician of any change in health status ■ Avoid sexual contact, blood donation (risk of HIV transmission) ■ Keep scheduled appointments c̄ physician/for blood work ■ Notify physician of numbness, tingling in extremities ■ ↑ Fluid intake (8-10 glasses/d) ■ Women: avoid breastfeeding ■ IV injection site may be painful ■ Loss of taste may occur ■ Keep appointments c̄ physician/for eye exams.

NOTES:

fosfomycin tromethamine • (foss-foe-mye-sin)

CATEGORY: *Urinary tract bactericidal antibiotic* Rx; Preg Cat C

BRAND NAME
Monurol (Forest)

DOSAGE FORM
Granule packet: 3g

USE: Treatment of uncomplicated UTI in females caused by susceptible strains of *Escherichia coli, Enterococcus faecalis.* **ACTION:** Bactericidal activity due to inactivation of bacterial enzymes required for proper cell wall synthesis in susceptible organisms.

PHARMACOKINETICS

PO absorption	Peak	Half-life	Protein binding	Excretion
Rapid	2-4h	5.7h	0%	Unchanged via urine/feces

CONTRAINDICATIONS: Hypersensitivity. *CC:* Not indicated for pyelonephritis, perinephric abscess ▪ Safety & efficacy in children ≤12y/o not established ▪ Drug crosses placental barrier ▪ Inform physician if symptoms of infection do not improve in 2-3d ▪ Drug must be mixed c̄ H_2O for proper PO administration ▪ Do *not* exceed a single treatment for a sole episode of acute cystitits.

DOSAGE
Females ≥18y/o *PO* Single dose (1 packet) of 3g in H_2O

SIDE/ADVERSE EFFECTS: CNS: headache, dizziness ▪ GI: abdominal pain, diarrhea (most frequent), dyspepsia, nausea ▪ GU: dysmenorrhea, vaginitis ▪ RESP: pharyngitis, rhinitis ▪ Other: asthenia, back pain, rash.

INTERACTIONS: Drug: Use c̄ metoclopramide may ↓ fosfomycin serum levels & renal excretion. **Lab:** Transient ↑ in ALT, AST, bilirubin, eosinophil count. **Food:** May be taken c̄ or w/out meals.

NURSING MANAGEMENT PRIORITIES
ADMINISTRATION: Assess for hx of hypersensitivity ▪ Obtain C&S before therapy ▪ Administer in 4oz cold H_2O, take *immediately* after mixing ▪ Maintain hydration ▪ Avoid exposure to mositure/light in storage.

EVALUATION: Monitor VS, esp temperature, CBC, UA; I&O, hepatic/renal status.

EDUCATION: Procedure for dissolving drug; do *not* take dry ▪ Maintain good personal hygiene (esp perineal, oral) ▪ Maintain fluid intake (6-8 glasses/d) ▪ Women: avoid breastfeeding ▪ Notify physician of fever, sore throat, difficult breathing, rash.

NOTES:

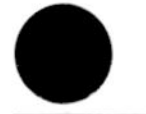

furosemide • (fur-oh-se-mide)

CATEGORY: *Loop diuretic:* antihypertensive

Rx; Preg Cat C

BRAND NAMES
**Furoside (ICN)*
Lasix (H-M-R)
(Hoechst [Canada])
**Neo-Renal (Neolab)*
**Novosemide*
(Novopharm)
**Uritol (Horner)*

DOSAGE FORMS
Injection (IM/IV): 10mg/ml; PO solution: 10mg/ml; tablet: 20, 40, 80mg

USE: Treatment of edema due to renal dysfunction ▪ Treatment of hypertension as sole agent/in combination c̄ other antihypertensives ▪ Adjunct in treating edema due to CHF, hepatic cirrhosis, acute pulmonary edema. **ACTION:** Diuretic activity due to excretion of H_2O, Na^+, Cl^-, other electrolytes by inhibiting tubular reabsorption, esp in medullary, cortical portions of ascending limb of loop of Henle; antihypertensive effect due to ⬇ in peripheral vascular resistance.

CONTRAINDICATIONS: Hypersensitivity, anuria, severe electrolyte imbalance. **CC:** Hospitalization is recommended for initiation of treatment in pts c̄ hepatic cirrhosis, ascites ▪ Use in premature neonates can ⬆ risk of persistent PDA.

DOSAGE

Pediatric	*PO*	2mg/kg as single dose. Do *not* exceed 6mg/kg/d
	IM/IV	1mg/kg
Adult	*PO*	
Edema		20-80mg/d as single dose. Refractory pts may require 600mg/d as single dose or divided
Hypertension		40mg bid. Adjust dosage according to response

PHARMACOKINETICS

PO absorption	Onset	Peak	Duration	Half-life	Protein binding	Excretion
60%	1h	1-2h	6-8h	30-50m	95%	50% via urine in 24h

Note: Side/adverse effects: common in *italic;* serious in ***boldface italic.***

*Available in Canada only

Adult	*IM/IV*
Edema	20-40mg. May be repeated in 2h
Acute pulmonary edema	40mg IV, repeat 1-1.5h later prn

SIDE/ADVERSE EFFECTS: CNS: dizziness, paresthesia, headache ▪ CV: orthostatic hypotension ▪ EENT: blurred vision, hearing loss, tinnitus ▪ GI: anorexia, N/V, cramping, jaundice, ***pancreatitis*** ▪ HEM: anemia, leukopenia, ***thrombocytopenia, aplastic anemia*** ▪ INT: purpura, rash, urticaria, ***exfoliative dermatitis, erythema multiforme***, photosensitivity.

INTERACTIONS: Drug: Use c̄ neurotoxic drugs incl aminoglycosides, capreomycin, chloroquine, vancomycin can result in significant toxicity ▪ Induced hypokalemia ⬆ dig toxicity ▪ Avoid use c̄ lithium, clofibrate ▪ Use c̄ corticosteroid can produce severe hypokalemia ▪ Use c̄ tubocurarine can ⬆ its activity. **Food:** Excessive consumption of licorice can ⬆ hypokalemia.

NURSING MANAGEMENT PRIORITIES

ADMINISTRATION: Assess for hx of hypersensitivity (incl sulfonamides) ▪ PO: administer c̄ food/milk on arising ▪ IV: use infusion w/in 24h after preparation; administer *slowly* (2m), hearing loss may occur c̄ rapid bolus ▪ Slight discoloration of tablets does *not* affect potency ▪ Assess serum K^+ (normal level: 3.5-5mEq/L) ▪ Elderly may require ⬇ dosage ▪ IM: inject *deep, slowly* into gluteal UOQ.

EVALUATION: Monitor VS, esp BP, pulse; fluid retention (I&O, daily weight) ▪ Monitor serum for ⬆ BUN, creatinine, uric acid; ⬇ K^+ ▪ Assess for ⬇ hearing (ototoxicity).

EDUCATION: Expect ⬆ urine output ▪ May cause weakness, lethargy ▪ Take PO forms c̄ food ▪ Take on waking up, at same time qd ▪ Take even if symptom free ▪ Notify physician of signs of hypokalemia (muscle cramps, lethargy, nausea)/hyponatremia (thirst, dry mouth, drowsiness) ▪ Avoid changing positions (lying/sitting/standing) rapidly ▪ Take as directed; do *not* skip doses ▪ Eat foods high in K^+; avoid black licorice ▪ Avoid high-Na^+ foods ▪ Check c̄ physician/pharmacist before taking OTC/Rx preparations ▪ Diabetics: check blood/urine glucose carefully ▪ Women: avoid breastfeeding ▪ Avoid exposure to direct sunlight, UV light ▪ May produce sweet taste.

NOTES:

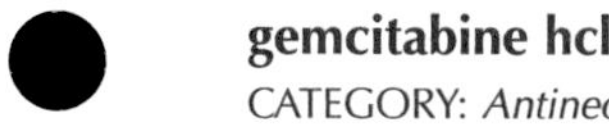

gemcitabine hcl • (gem-sit-ah-bean)

CATEGORY: *Antineoplastic:* antimetabolite

Rx; Preg Cat D

BRAND NAME	**DOSAGE FORMS**
Gemzar (Lilly)	Powder for IV injection: 200-mg, 1-g vial

USE: Treatment of locally advanced (nonresectable Stage II or III) or metastatic (Stage IV) adenocarcinoma of the pancreas ▪ Treatment of inoperable & locally advanced Stage IIIA/IIIB or metastatic (Stage IV) non-small cell lung cancer in combination with cisplatin. **ACTION:** Gemcitabine is a synthetic pyrimidine nucleoside antimetabolite that produces a dual cytotoxic antineoplastic effect on DNA synthesis by (1) inhibition of ribonucleotide enzyme that catalyzes rxs required for DNA synthesis & (2) incorporation of the drug into the DNA chain, resulting in termination of DNA synthesis.

PHARMACOKINETICS: Pharmacokinetic values for the drug are variable due to the influence of age, gender, & time length of the IV infusion. Short infusion administration time (<70m) produced a half-life of 32-94m, depending on age & gender whereas a long infusion time (70-285m) produced a half-life of 245-638m. Protein binding is negligible. Excretion is almost 95%-98% via urine.

CONTRAINDICATIONS: Hypersensitivity. **CC:** Use requires experienced physicians ▪ Pt should be monitored for blood values, hepatic & renal function before/during treatment ▪ ⬆ Toxicity c̄ infusion >60m or more frequently than weekly dosing ▪ Use can ⬇ bone marrow function, incl anemia, leukopenia, thrombocytopenia ▪ Safety & efficacy not established for children.

DOSAGE

Adult *IV*

Pancreatic cancer	1000mg/m² over 30m once/wk for 7wks and/or toxic manifestations occur. Rest for 1 wk followed by treatment cycles of 1 weekly infusion for 3 consecutive wks out of q4wks
Non-small lung cancer	3-wk schedule: 1250mg/m² over 30m on d1, 8 of each 21-d cycle 4-wk schedule: 1000mg/m² over 30m on d1, 8, 15 of each 28-d cycle Cisplatin, 100mg/m² on d1 after administration of gemcitabine for both schedules

SIDE/ADVERSE EFFECTS: CV: ***MI, CVA,*** arrhythmias, hypertension, edema ▪ GI: N/V/D ▪ GU: ***rare hemolytic uremic syndrome*** ▪ HEM: anemia, leukopenia, ***thrombocytopenia*** ▪ RESP: dyspnea, bronchospasm, ***rare parenchymal lung toxicity,*** flulike symptoms ▪ Other: mild alopecia, fever, infection, paresthesias.

INTERACTIONS: Drug: None currently reported. **Lab:** Transient ↑ in alkaline phosphatase, ALT, AST.

NURSING MANAGEMENT PRIORITIES

ADMINISTRATION: Check pt hx for recent course of radiation/antineoplastic agents ▪ Administer antiemetic before therapy ▪ Provide emotional support ▪ Reconstitute according to manufacturer's directions, shake to dissolve, use w/in 24h of reconstitution; avoid excessive agitation.

EVALUATION: Monitor hepatic, neurologic, renal function: CBC, esp WBC, platelets throughout therapy; notify physician if ↓ ▪ Assess for infection, bleeding, anemia ▪ Assess hydration status (I&O, daily weight) ▪ Monitor for hepatic toxicity (jaundice, clay-colored stools) ▪ Assess for anaphylactic rxs; have support equipment available.

EDUCATION: ↑ Fluid intake (8-10 glasses/d) ▪ Avoid expoure to infection ▪ Check $\bar{c}$ physician before immunization ▪ Diet as tolerated; avoid spicy foods ▪ Maintain good oral hygiene; use soft-bristled toothbrush ▪ Notify physician of symptoms of bone marrow depression (fever, sore throat, bruising, bleeding, lethargy) ▪ Dizziness/drowsiness may occur; use caution in potentially hazardous activities ▪ Notify physician of symptoms of allergic rx (fever, difficult breathing, rash) ▪ Women: avoid pregnancy, breastfeeding; use contraception if sexually active.

NOTES:

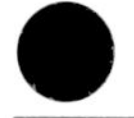

gentamicin sulfate • (jen-ta-mye-sin)

CATEGORY: *Aminoglycoside:* antibiotic — Rx; Preg Cat C

BRAND NAMES	DOSAGE FORMS
**Alcomicin (Alcon)*	Injection, ophthalmic
**Cidomycin (Roussel)*	gtt/ointment, pediatric injection,
Garamycin (Schering)	topical cream/ointment

USE: Treatment of infections caused by susceptible strains of *Enterobacter aerogenes, Escherichia coli, Klebsiella pneumoniae, Proteus* spp, *Pseudomonas aeruginosa, Salmonella* spp, *Serratia* (nonpigmented), *Shigella* spp ▪ Alternative for penicillin-resistant staphylococcal infections ▪ In combination c̄ carbenicillin for treating stubborn *Pseudomonas* infection ▪ With penicillin for treating sepsis, staphylococcal pneumonia in neonates. **ACTION:** Bactericidal activity due to inhibition of ribosomal protein synthesis in susceptible organisms.

PHARMACOKINETICS

IM peak	Half-life	Protein binding	Excretion
0.5-1h	2-2.5h	0%-30% in 24h	70% unchanged in urine

CONTRAINDICATIONS: Hypersensitivity, hx of serious aminoglycoside toxicity. **CC:** Use of aminoglycosides during pregnancy can result in bilateral congenital deafness ▪ Use can produce significant ototoxicity, nephrotoxicity ▪ Injection contains sodium bisulfite, which can cause allergic rxs.

DOSAGE: For pts c̄ normal renal function; treatment usually 7-10d; dosage for pts c̄ impaired renal function must be adjusted according to manufacturer's recommendation.

Pediatric	*IM/IV*	Neonates (<1wk old): 5mg/kg/d or 2.5mg/kg q12h Neonates/infants: 7.5mg/kg/d or 2.5mg/kg q8h Children: 6-7mg/kg/d q8h in equal doses
Adult	*IM/IV*	3mg/kg/d q8h in equal doses Serious infection: 5mg/kg/d in 3-4 doses. ⬇ To 3mg/kg/d when clinically indicated
	Topical/ Ophthalmic	Apply to affected area as directed by physician

SIDE/ADVERSE EFFECTS: CNS: headache, paresthesia ▪ EENT: ***ototoxicity*** (auditory/vestibular damage: dizziness, vertigo, tinnitus, roaring in ears, hearing loss) ▪ INT: rash ▪ REN: ***nephrotoxicity*** (casts, proteinuria, ↑ BUN, NPN, serum creatinine) ▪ Other: fever.

INTERACTIONS: Drug: Avoid use c̄ neurotoxic/nephrotoxic drugs (eg, other aminoglycosides, colistin, ethacrynic acid, furosemide, polymyxin B, vancomycin) ▪ Dimenhydrinate can mask aminoglycoside ototoxicity ▪ ↑ Activity of succinylcholine/tubocurarine; Ca salts can reverse blockade ▪ PO anticoagulant activity may ↑ due to ↓ intestinal vitamin K synthesis.

NURSING MANAGEMENT PRIORITIES

ADMINISTRATION: Assess for hx of aminoglycoside hypersensitivity ▪ Obtain C&S before therapy ▪ Obtain pt weight for dose calculation ▪ Determine creatinine clearance before administration ▪ IV: single dose may be diluted in 50-250ml sterile normal saline/5% dextrose solution; infuse over ½-1h; use less diluent for pediatric IV; may mix c̄ dextrose, lactated Ringer, Ringer injection, normal saline solution ▪ Do *not* mix c̄ other drugs, incl carbenicillin, other extended-spectrum penicillins ▪ IM: administer by *deep, slow* injection; rotate sites; avoid inflamed areas ▪ Do *not* administer SC ▪ Maintain hydration ▪ Elderly may require ↓ dosage ▪ Therapeutic blood levels: 4-10µg/ml.

EVALUATION: Assess for hearing dysfunction ▪ Monitor VS, esp temperature ▪ Assess for edema in extremities ▪ Assess for neuromuscular blockade, respiratory paralysis, nephrotoxicity ▪ Observe for signs of superinfection (diarrhea, URI, coated tongue) ▪ Assess peak (<12µg/ml), trough (<2µg/ml) serum concentrations.

EDUCATION: Report hearing, balance difficulties to physician at once ▪ ↑ Fluid intake (10-12 glasses/d) ▪ Notify physician of symptoms of allergic rxs (fever, difficult breathing, rash, burning/stinging in eyes).

NOTES:

glipizide/glyburide/glimepiride • (<u>glip</u>-i-zide/<u>glye</u>-byoo-ride/<u>glih</u>-meh-per-ide) 154

CATEGORY: *Oral hypoglycemic:* second-generation sulfonylurea Rx; Preg Cat C/B/C

BRAND NAMES	DOSAGE FORMS
glipizide	
Glucotrol (Roerig)	Tablet: 5, 10mg
glyburide	
DiaBeta (H-M-R)	Tablet: 1.25, 2.5, 5mg
**Euglucon (USV)*	Tablet: 5mg
Glynase PresTab (Upjohn)	Tablet: 1.5, 3mg
Micronase (Upjohn)	Tablet: 1.25, 2.5, 5mg
glimepiride	
Amaryl (H-M-R)	Tablet: 1, 2, 4mg

USE: Management of type II (non-insulin-dependent) diabetes that cannot be controlled by diet alone. **ACTION:** Antidiabetic activity due to stimulation of insulin release from functioning β cells of pancreas; drug appears to ↑ action of insulin at peripheral postreceptor sites.

CONTRAINDICATIONS: Hypersensitivity, diabetic ketoacidosis c̄, w/out coma. **CC:** Use may be associated c̄ ↑ rate of cardiovascular mortality, secondary failure, stress.

DOSAGE: Adult PO

glipizide	Must be individualized. Usual maintenance range 2.5-40mg/d
glyburide	Must be individualized. Usual maintenance range 1.25-20mg/d
glimepiride	Must be individualized. Usual maintenance range 1-8mg/d

SIDE/ADVERSE EFFECTS: GI: *nausea,* epigastric fullness, heartburn ▪ HEM: ***aplastic anemia, agranulocytosis,*** leukopenia, ***hemolytic anemia***, pancytopenia, ***thrombocytopenia*** ▪ INT: erythema, morbilliform/maculopapular eruptions, photosensitivity ▪ MET: ***hypoglycemia***.

PHARMACOKINETICS

	PO absorption	Onset	Peak	Duration	Half-life	Binding	Excretion
glipizide	Complete	1h	1-3h	Up to 24h	2-4h	98%-99%	90% via urine as metabolites
glyburide	Complete	1-2h	3-4h	Up to 24h	10h	NA	50% via bile, 50% via urine
glimepiride	Complete	1-2h	2-3h	Up to 24h	NA	99.5%	60% via urine as metabolites

Note: Side/adverse effects: common in *italic;* serious in ***boldface italic.*** *Available in Canada only.

INTERACTIONS: Drug: Use c̄ alcohol, MAO-I, β blockers can significantly ↑ hypoglycemic effects ▪ Use c̄ anabolic steroids, chloramphenicol, guanethidine, PO anticoagulants, probenecid, salicylates, sulfinpyrazone, sulfonamides ↑ hypoglycemic effects ▪ Use c̄ adrenergics, corticosteroids, phenytoin, thiazides, thyroid preparations ↓ hypoglycemic effects.

NURSING MANAGEMENT PRIORITIES

ADMINISTRATION: Assess for hx of hypersensitivity (incl sulfonamides) ▪ Administer ½h ac in single AM dose/divided doses ▪ Avoid exposure to moisture/light in storage ▪ Elderly may require ↓ dosage.

EVALUATION: Monitor hepatic, renal, hematologic status ▪ Monitor FBS ▪ Evaluate pt closely during first wk to assess effectiveness ▪ Monitor for signs of hypoglycemia/hyperglycemia.

EDUCATION: Compliance c̄ special diet therapy ▪ Blood/urine glucose/ketone testing procedures ▪ Symptoms of hypoglycemia (anxiety, headache, fatigue, nausea, sweating); notify physician *immediately* ▪ Always carry lump of sugar/candy for quick use in hypoglycemia ▪ Avoid alcohol ▪ Check c̄ physician before taking OTC preparations ▪ Symptoms of hyperglycemia (excessive hunger, thirst, urination, rapid pulse, sweet-smelling breath, weight loss); notify physician *immediately* ▪ Maintain good personal hygiene ▪ Carry medical identification (MedicAlert) ▪ Store in tightly closed container ▪ Keep scheduled appointments c̄ physician/for blood glucose determinations ▪ Schedule periodic eye exams ▪ Maintain optimum body weight ▪ Avoid prolonged exposure to sunlight; use sunscreen, protective clothing ▪ Women: avoid breastfeeding ▪ PO hypoglycemic needs may change c̄ ↑ stress, ↑ exercise, ↓ appetite; notify physician ▪ Report skin rash, itching to physician.

NOTES:

granisetron hcl/ondansetron hcl • (gran-iss-e-tron/on-dan-se-tron)

CATEGORY: *Antiemetic:* antiserotonergic, 5-HT_3 receptor antagonist   Rx; Preg Cat B

BRAND NAMES
granisetron hcl
Kytril (SKB)
ondansetron hcl
Zofran (Cerenex)

DOSAGE FORMS
IV injection: 1.12mg/ml vial
Tablet: 1mg
IV injection: 2mg/ml
Tablet: 4, 8mg

USE: Prevention of N/V c̄ emetogenic antineoplastic therapy incl high-dose cisplatin treatment ▪ Prevention of postop nausea (ondansetron) ▪ Prevention of N/V c̄ radiotherapy. **ACTION:** Antiemetic activity due to selective antagonism of 5-hydroxytryptamine$_3$ receptors (5-HT_3-receptors). Receptors are located on peripheral vagus nerve terminals & in the chemoreceptor trigger zone in the CNS. Drugs block access of 5-hydroxytryptamine (serotonin) to 5-HT_3 receptors, resulting in an antiemetic effect. The main site of antagonism appears related to peripheral receptors on vagal nerve terminals.

CONTRAINDICATIONS: Hypersensitivity. **CC:** Dosage adjustments (⬇) are suggested for elderly pts.

PHARMACOKINETICS

PO absorption	Half-life	Protein binding	Excretion
granisetron			
Well	0.9-31h (mean-8.95h)	65%	Via urine, feces primarily as metabolites
ondansetron			
Well	2.4-6.2h (mean-4h)	70%-75%	Via urine, feces primarily as metabolites

DOSAGE

granisetron		
Children (2-16y/o)/ Adult	*IV*	10µg/kg given over 5m given 30m before chemotherapy
Adult	*PO*	1mg bid given 1h before chemotherapy & 12h after first dose only on day(s) of chemotherapy
ondansetron		
Children (4-18y/o)	*IV*	Three doses of 0.15mg/kg c̄ first dose infused over 15m & administered 30m before chemotherapy, repeated 4 & 8h after first dose

(4-12y/o) *PO* 4mg tid c̄ first dose administered 30m before chemotherapy, repeated 4 & 8h after first dose

Adult *IV* Three doses of 0.15mg/kg c̄ first dose infused over 15m & administered 30m before chemotherapy, repeated 4 & 8h after first dose; 32mg infused over 15m & administered 30m before chemotherapy. For postop nausea, 4mg over 2-5m

PO 8mg tid c̄ first dose administered 30m before chemotherapy, repeated 4 & 8h after first dose, followed by 8mg q8h for 1-2d after completion of chemotherapy. For radiotherapy 8mg 1-2h before treatment, then 8mg q1-2d after completion of treatment. For postop nausea prevention, 16mg as a single dose 1h before anesthesia

SIDE/ADVERSE EFFECTS: CNS: headache, dizziness, insomnia, rare extrapyramidal symptoms, ***grand mal seizures*** ▪ CV: angina, EKG changes, hypotension, ***rare cases of heart block*** ▪ GI: constipation, diarrhea ▪ EENT: blurred vision, taste disorders ▪ HEP: ↑ AST, ALT ▪ Other: rash, hypokalemia, fever.

INTERACTIONS: Drug: None currently reported, however, ondansetron administered c̄ food ↑ PO absorption.

NURSING MANAGEMENT PRIORITIES

ADMINISTRATION: Assess for hx of hypersensitivity ▪ Assess hepatic function; use caution if impaired ▪ PO: administer 30m before chemotherapy ▪ IV: dilute according to manufacturer's directions in D_5W or normal saline solution; infuse over 15m ▪ Store at room temperature.

EVALUATION: Monitor VS, esp BP ▪ Monitor F/E imbalance ▪ Monitor CV status (tachycardia, angina) ▪ Monitor bowel function; constipation may occur ▪ Observe for potentiation of CNS depressant effect ▪ Assess for absence of N/V.

EDUCATION: Dizziness may occur, use caution in potentially hazardous activities ▪ Constipation may occur: ↑ fluids, bulk-containing foods ▪ Notify physician if headache occurs, analgesic will be prescribed ▪ Use sugarless gum/hard candy to diminish dry mouth ▪ Notify physician *immediately* of rash, difficulty breathing.

guanabenz acetate/guanfacine hcl • (gwahn-a-benz/gwahn-fa-seen)

CATEGORY: *Antihypertensive:* α_2-adrenergic

Rx; Preg Cat C/B

BRAND NAMES	DOSAGE FORMS
guanabenz	
Wytensin (W-A)	Tablet: 4, 8mg
guanfacine	
Tenex (Robins)	Tablet: 1, 2mg

USE: Treatment of hypertension as sole agent/in combination c̄ thiazide diuretic. **ACTION:** Antihypertensive effect due to agonist activity c̄ central α_2 receptors, resulting in ⬇ sympathetic outflows from bulbar level of brain to circulatory system.

PHARMACOKINETICS

PO absorption	Peak	Half-life	Protein binding	Excretion
guanabenz				
75%	2-5h	4-14h	90%	Via urine primarily as metabolites
guanfacine				
Good	1-4h	10-36h	70%	Via urine as unchanged drug & metabolites

CONTRAINDICATIONS: Hypersensitivity. **CC:** Abrupt D/C can result in a rebound ⬆ in BP ▪ Use c̄ caution in pts c̄ severe coronary/cerebrovascular disease, recent MI, chronic hepatic/renal failure ▪ guanabenz: Not indicated for children <12y/o ▪ Use during pregnancy can result in fetal harm.

DOSAGE

guanabenz

Adult *PO*	Starting dose 4mg bid. May be ⬆ in 4-8mg increments/d q1-2wks. Doses >32mg bid may be required in rare cases

guanfacine

Adult *PO*	Usual dose is 1mg at hs. May be ⬆ to 2-3mg/d at hs after 3-4wks

SIDE/ADVERSE EFFECTS: CNS: *drowsiness, dizziness, headache,* anxiety, depression, sleep disturbances ▪ CV: ***arrhythmias***, palpitations, edema, chest pain ▪ EENT: conjunctivitis, rhinitis, blurred vision, nasal congestion ▪ END: gynecomastia ▪ GI: dry mouth, N/V/D, pain, constipation, taste disorders ▪ GU: urinary frequency, sex function disturbances ▪ INT: rash, pruritus ▪ MS: muscle aches ▪ Other: asthenia, dyspnea, hypokinesia, impotence.

INTERACTIONS: Drug: Use c̄ CNS depressants produces additive sedation.

NOTES:

NURSING MANAGEMENT PRIORITIES

ADMINISTRATION: Assess for hx of hypersensitivity ▪ Assess BP; notify physician of extremes ▪ Administer last dose at hs ▪ Elderly may require ⬇ dosage ▪ Avoid abrupt withdrawal; D/C gradually.

EVALUATION: Monitor VS, esp BP ▪ Monitor electrolyte status ▪ Monitor I&O, daily weight ▪ Assess for edema in extremities.

EDUCATION: Dizziness/drowsiness may occur; use caution in potentially hazardous activities ▪ Avoid changing positions (lying/sitting/standing) rapidly ▪ Take last dose at hs ▪ Take as ordered by physician even if symptom free; do *not* skip doses ▪ Use sugarless gum/hard candy to diminish dry mouth ▪ Used to control, *not* cure, hypertension ▪ Do *not* D/C w/out notifying physician ▪ Check c̄ physician/pharmacist before taking OTC/Rx preparations ▪ Do *not* use c̄ alcohol, other CNS depressants ▪ Avoid high-Na^+ foods (canned soups, lunch meats, cheese) ▪ Avoid ⬆ exercise, cold, smoking ▪ Maintain optimum weight ▪ Check for swelling in feet/legs daily; notify physician if present.

guanethidine monosulfate • (gwahn-eth-i-deen)

CATEGORY: *Antihypertensive:* norepinephrine depletor Rx; Preg Cat C

BRAND NAMES	DOSAGE FORMS
**Apo-Guanethidine (Apotex); Ismelin (C-G)*	Tablet: 10, 25mg

COMBINATION PRODUCT

Esimil (C-G)	Guanethidine 10mg/ hydrochlorothiazide 25mg/tablet

USE: Treatment of hypertension as sole agent/in combination c̄ other antihypertensives ▪ Treatment of renal hypertension. **ACTION:** Antihypertensive effect due to slow depletion, inhibition of norepinephrine release at sympathetic fibers.

PHARMACOKINETICS: PO absorption is incomplete, up to 50% of single dose reaches circulatory system; at least 2wks required for full therapeutic effect; excretion via urine as unchanged drug, metabolites.

CONTRAINDICATIONS: Hypersensitivity, pheochromocytoma, use c̄ MAO-I, frank CHF not due to hypertension. **CC:** Use can cause orthostatic hypotension esp in AM, hot weather during exercise ▪ Use c̄ caution in pts c̄ bronchial asthma, renal disease, or severe cardiac failure ▪ ↑ Any dosage adjustment slowly due to cumulative effects of drug.

DOSAGE

Pediatric	*PO*	Initial dose 0.2mg/kg/d, ↑ by same amount if needed q7-10d to maximum dose 3mg/kg/d
Adult	*PO*	Initial dose 10mg/d, ↑ gradually if needed. For hospitalized pts, initial dose 25-50mg, ↑ by 25-50mg/d qod if needed
Esimil		Usual adult starting dose 2 tablets/d

SIDE/ADVERSE EFFECTS: CNS: dizziness, syncope, mental depression, weakness ▪ CV: bradycardia, edema, CHF, postural/exertional hypotension ▪ EENT: blurred vision, parotid tenderness, nasal congestion ▪ GI: ↑ bowel movement/diarrhea, dry mouth ▪ GU: inhibition of ejaculation, urinary incontinence ▪ HEM: anemia, leukopenia ▪ INT: alopecia ▪ MS: myalgia ▪ RESP: asthma ▪ Other: weight gain.

INTERACTIONS: Drug: Use c̄ amphetamines, MAO-I, TCAs, phenothiazines, PO contraceptives may antagonize effects of guanethidine ▪ Use c̄ epinephrine, other direct-acting adrenergics may ↑ their vasopressor effect ▪ Use c̄ *Rauwolfia* derivatives may cause significant hypotension, bradycardia, mental depression ▪ Use c̄ alcohol can ↑ orthostatic hypotension.

NURSING MANAGEMENT PRIORITIES

ADMINISTRATION: Assess for hx of hypersensitivity ▪ Assess BP, apical pulse; if <60/m, hold drug, notify physician ▪ May crush tablet ▪ Avoid abrupt withdrawal; D/C gradually ▪ Elderly may require ↓ dosage.

EVALUATION: Monitor VS, esp BP ▪ Monitor electrolyte status ▪ Monitor I&O, daily weight ▪ Assess for edema in extremities.

EDUCATION: Dizziness/drowsiness may occur, use caution in potentially hazardous activities ▪ Avoid changing positions (lying/sitting/standing) rapidly ▪ Avoid ↑ exercise, temperature extremes, smoking ▪ Procedure for checking radial pulse ▪ Check pulse before taking; if <60/m, do *not* take drug, notify physician ▪ Take as ordered by physician even if symptom free; do *not* skip doses ▪ Used to control, *not* cure, hypertension ▪ Do *not* D/C w/out notifying physician ▪ Check c̄ physician/pharmacist before taking OTC/Rx preparations ▪ Do *not* use c̄ alcohol, other CNS depressants ▪ Avoid high-Na^+ foods (canned soups, lunch meats, cheese) ▪ Maintain optimum weight ▪ Check for swelling in feet/legs daily; notify physician if present ▪ Men: impotence may occur; inform physician ▪ Notify physician/dentist of use before treatment ▪ Notify physician of diarrhea, frequent dizziness/fainting.

NOTES:

haloperidol/haloperidol decanoate▲ • (ha-loe-per-i-dole)

CATEGORY: *Antipsychotic:* butyrophenone neuroleptic   Rx; Preg Cat C

BRAND NAMES	DOSAGE FORMS
Haldol (McNeil)	Injection (IM): 5mg/ml PO concentrate: 2mg/ml Tablet: 0.5, 1, 2, 5, 10, 20mg
Haldol Decanoate (McNeil)▲	Injection (IM): 50mg/ml, 100mg/ml

USE: Treatment of psychotic states (decanoate salt is intended for chronic psychotic pts) ▪ Treatment of Gilles de la Tourette syndrome ▪ Treatment of severe behavior problems in children ▪ Short-term treatment in hyperactive children. **ACTION:** Antipsychotic activity may be due to brainstem depression; drug inhibits ascending reticular activating system of brainstem; exhibits anti-α-adrenergic, anticholinergic, antiemetic, antidopaminergic, hypotensive, hypothermic, sedative properties.

PHARMACOKINETICS

PO absorption	Peak	Protein binding	Excretion
Good (70%)	2-6h	92%	Via urine, feces

CONTRAINDICATIONS: Hypersensitivity, comatose states, presence of large amount of CNS depressants, Parkinson's disease. **CC:** Extended use can produce extrapyramidal symptoms, tardive dyskinesia, neuroleptic malignant syndrome.

DOSAGE

Pediatric	*PO*	
Psychosis		0.05-0.15 mg/kg/d
Tourette syndrome & nonpsychotic behavior		0.05-0.075mg/kg/d
Adult	*PO*	
Moderate psychosis		0.5-2mg 2-3 times/d or more
Severe psychosis		3-5mg 2-5 times/d or up to 100mg/d
	IM	2-5mg q4-8h. Initial dose of decanoate salt is calculated to be 10-15 times previous daily PO dose, should *not* exceed 100mg. Doses >300mg/mo not well studied. Dosing intervals usually 4wks
Geriatric/ Debilitated	*PO*	0.5-2mg 2-3 times/d or more

SIDE/ADVERSE EFFECTS: CNS: *drowsiness*, extrapyramidal rxs, tardive dyskinesia ▪ CV: hypotension, tachycardia, ECG changes ▪ END: lactation, breast enlargement, menstrual irregularities, gynecomastia, impotence ▪ GI: anorexia, N/V, dry mouth ▪ GU: urinary retention ▪ HEM: anemia, lymphomonocytosis, ***agranulocytosis*** ▪ INT: acneiform maculopapular rash, photosensitivity, alopecia ▪ RESP: bronchospasm, laryngospasm ▪ Other: ***neuroleptic malignant syndrome.***

INTERACTIONS: Drug: Use c̄ lithium can produce significant encephalopathic syndrome ▪ Use c̄ alcohol, narcotics, barbiturates, other CNS depressants will ↑ CNS depression.

NURSING MANAGEMENT PRIORITIES

ADMINISTRATION: Assess VS, esp BP ▪ PO concentrate: dilute before administration c̄ >60ml H_2O; do *not* use coffee, tea, lithium citrate syrup ▪ PO: administer c̄ food/full glass of H_2O or milk ▪ IM: inject *slowly, deep* into UOQ of buttock; keep pt lying down for ½h after injection ▪ Avoid exposure to moisture/light in storage ▪ Avoid abrupt withdrawal; D/C gradually ▪ Maintain hydration ▪ Elderly/debilitated may require ↓ dosage ▪ Avoid administration c̄ lithium.

EVALUATION: Monitor hepatic, ophthalmic, renal status ▪ Monitor BP, CBC ▪ Monitor fluid retention (I&O, daily weight) ▪ Assess for extrapyramidal symptoms (tics/spasms, trembling, shuffling gait) ▪ Seizure precautions in pts c̄ hx of convulsive disorders ▪ Long-term therapy: assess for jaundice, agranulocytosis ▪ Assess for symptoms of abrupt withdrawal (nausea, dyskinesia, trembling, dizziness) ▪ Assess IOP.

EDUCATION: Dizziness/drowsiness may occur; use caution in potentially hazardous activities ▪ Avoid changing positions (lying/sitting/standing) rapidly ▪ Avoid use c̄ alcohol, CNS depressants ▪ Take as ordered by physician ▪ Take PO forms c̄ meals ▪ Store in tightly closed, light-resistant container ▪ Use sugarless gum/hard candy to diminish dry mouth ▪ Maintain fluid intake (6-8 glasses/d) ▪ Avoid exposure to direct sunlight, UV light (sunlamps); use sunscreen, protective clothing ▪ Notify physician of fever, sore throat, bruising/bleeding ▪ Notify physician of extrapyramidal symptoms (tics/spasms, trembling, shuffling gait) ▪ Avoid ↑ exercise, temperature extremes ▪ Avoid smoking ▪ Check c̄ physician/pharmacist before taking OTC preparations ▪ Schedule periodic eye exams ▪ Full drug effects may require several wks of therapy ▪ Procedure for PO concentrate administration.

NOTES:

heparin sodium • (hep-a-rin)

CATEGORY: *Anticoagulant* Rx; Preg Cat C

BRAND NAMES
**Calilean (Harris)*
Hep-Lock (Elkins-Sinn)
**Hepalean (Harris)*
Liquaemin Sodium (Organon)

DOSAGE FORM
Injection (IV/SC)

USE: Prophylaxis, treatment of arterial embolism, pulmonary embolism, venous thrombosis & extensions ▪ Atrial fibrillation c̄ embolization ▪ Prevention of clotting during arterial/heart surgery ▪ Diagnosis, treatment of acute/chronic consumption coagulopathies (disseminated intravascular coagulation) ▪ Anticoagulant for use in blood transfusion, extracorporeal circulation, dialysis, laboratory blood samples ▪ Controversial adjunct in treating coronary occlusion c̄ acute MI. **ACTION:** Anticoagulant activity due to inhibition of conversion of prothrombin to thrombin; heparin also appears to have antithrombin action, ⬇ agglutination of platelets; has no effect on existing clots; does not cross placental barrier.

PHARMACOKINETICS

Onset SC	Onset IV	Half-life	Excretion
20-60m	Immediate	1-2h	Reticular endothelial system; small amount excreted via urine

CONTRAINDICATIONS: Hypersensitivity, any uncontrolled bleeding. **CC:** Use can produce hemorrhage from any site in the body ▪ Not intended for IM use.

DOSAGE

Pediatric	*IV*	Usual dose 50U/kg followed by 100U/kg q4h
Adult	*SC*	Usual dose 10,000-20,000U followed by 8000-10,000U tid
	IV	Usual dose 10,000U followed by 5000-10,000U 4-6 times/d Usual infusion dose 20,000-40,000U/d

Note: Side/adverse effects: common in *italic*; serious in ***boldface italic***

*Available in Canada only.

SIDE/ADVERSE EFFECTS: CV: hemorrhage (10%), vasospastic rx may develop ▪ HEM: acute reversible ***thrombocytopenia,*** rebound hyperlipemia ▪ Other: ↓ renal function, osteoporosis c̄ long-term therapy; local irritation at SC site.

INTERACTIONS: Drug: Aspirin, other drugs that affect platelet function (esp cefamandole, cefoperazone) ↑ anticoagulant effect ▪ PO anticoagulants ↑ anticoagulant effect ▪ Use c̄ streptokinase, urokinase is best avoided.

NURSING MANAGEMENT PRIORITIES

ADMINISTRATION: Assess for hx of hypersensitivity ▪ Administer by deep SC injection, intermittent IV injection, continuous IV infusion ▪ Avoid IM (danger of hematoma formation) ▪ Can be mixed c̄ dextrose, dextrose/NaCl, normal saline, invert sugar, protein hydrolysate, Ringer solution; lactated Ringer injection ▪ Prepare fresh solutions; avoid storage for >24h ▪ Do *not* use discolored/precipitated solutions ▪ SC: use lower abdomen; change needle after preparation; do *not* aspirate; rotate sites; check for hemorrhage; avoid massaging ▪ IV: use infusion pump ▪ Regulate dosage according to APTT, coagulation studies ▪ Avoid mixing c̄ other drugs in solution ▪ Have protamine sulfate available for OD ▪ Elderly may require ↓ dosage.

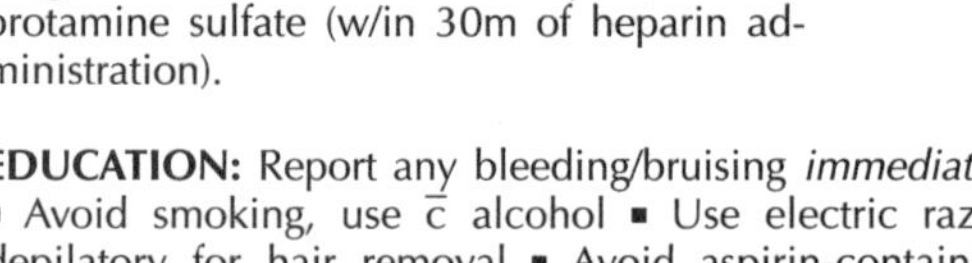

EVALUATION: Monitor hepatic, CV, renal status ▪ Monitor APTT; maintain at 1.5-2.5 times control value ▪ Observe for signs of hemorrhage, incl abdominal/lumbar pain; treat c̄ protamine sulfate (w/in 30m of heparin administration).

EDUCATION: Report any bleeding/bruising *immediately* ▪ Avoid smoking, use c̄ alcohol ▪ Use electric razor/depilatory for hair removal ▪ Avoid aspirin-containing products ▪ Check c̄ physician/pharmacist before taking OTC preparations ▪ Women: avoid breastfeeding.

OVERDOSE MANAGEMENT: *See* protamine sulfate.

NOTES:

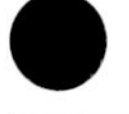

hydralazine hcl • (hye-<u>dral</u>-a-zeen)

CATEGORY: *Antihypertensive*

Rx; Preg Cat C

BRAND NAME

Apresoline HCl (Novartis)

DOSAGE FORMS

Injection (IM/IV): 20mg/ml
Tablet: 10, 25, 50, 100mg

COMBINATION PRODUCTS

Apresazide 25/25 (Novartis)	hydralazine hcl/hydrochlorothiazide per capsule: 25mg/25mg
Apresazide 50/50 (Novartis)	hydralazine hcl/hydrochlorothiazide per capsule: 50mg/50mg
Apresazide 100/50 (Novartis)	hydralazine hcl/hydrochlorothiazide per capsule: 100mg/50mg
Ser-Ap-Es (Novartis)	reserpine/hydralazine hcl/hydrochlorothiazide per tablet: 0.1mg/25mg/15mg

USE: Treatment of hypertension as sole agent/in combination c̄ other antihypertensives. **ACTION:** Antihypertensive effect due to direct relaxing, vasodilation of arteriolar smooth muscle.

PHARMACOKINETICS

PO absorption	Peak	Half-life	Protein binding	Excretion
Rapid	1-2h	3-7h	87%	Via urine primarily as metabolites

CONTRAINDICATIONS: Hypersensitivity, coronary artery disease, mitral valvular/rheumatic heart disease. **CC:** Use can produce rare episodes of simulated SLE.

DOSAGE

Pediatric	*PO*	0.75mg/kg divided, ↑ slowly for 2-3wks to daily maximum 7.5mg/kg prn
Adult	*PO*	Initial dose 10mg qid for 2-4d, ↑ to 25mg qid for balance of wk, 50mg qid wk 2. Adjust to lowest effective dose for maintenance
	IM/IV	20-40mg, repeat prn. Switch to PO as soon as possible
Combination products		Dosage must be adjusted for each pt, in general 1-2U (capsules/tablets) 1-3 times/d

SIDE/ADVERSE EFFECTS: CNS: *headache,* peripheral neuritis, dizziness, tremors, anxiety, psychotic rxs ▪ CV: *palpitations, tachycardia, angina pectoris,* edema, paradoxic hypertension ▪ EENT: nasal congestion, conjunctivitis ▪ GI: *anorexia, N/V/D,* constipation, paralytic ileus ▪ GU: difficult urination ▪ HEM: anemia, leukopenia, ***agranulocytosis,*** lymphadenopathy ▪ HEP: hepatitis ▪ INT: rash, urticaria, pruritus ▪ RESP: dyspnea.

INTERACTIONS: Drug: Use c̄ adrenergic drugs may antagonize hypotensive effect ▪ Use c̄ other antihypertensives, MAO-I produces additive hypotensive effects.

NURSING MANAGEMENT PRIORITIES

ADMINISTRATION: Assess for hx of hypersensitivity ▪ Assess renal function; ⬇ dosage if impaired ▪ PO: administer c̄ meals; switch from parenteral form w/in 48h ▪ IV: administer *slowly* (10mg/m); monitor BP, heart rate ▪ Elderly may require ⬇ dosage ▪ Avoid abrupt withdrawal ▪ Have pyridoxine (vitamin B_6) available for neurotoxicity.

EVALUATION: Monitor VS, esp BP, electrolyte status, I&O, daily weight ▪ Assess for edema in extremities; mental status (depression, disorientation, anxiety).

EDUCATION: Dizziness/drowsiness may occur; use caution in potentially hazardous activities ▪ Avoid changing positions (lying/sitting/standing) rapidly ▪ Take as ordered by physician, even if symptom free; do *not* skip doses ▪ Take c̄ meals ▪ Do *not* D/C w/out notifying physician ▪ Check c̄ physician/pharmacist before taking OTC/Rx preparations ▪ Notify physician *immediately* of tingling/numbness of hands/feet; D/C drug ▪ Physician may order vitamin B_6 supplements to alleviate neurotoxic effects ▪ Avoid high-Na^+ foods ▪ Avoid ⬆ exercise, temperature extremes, smoking ▪ Used to control, *not* cure, hypertension ▪ Maintain optimum weight ▪ Avoid use c̄ alcohol, CNS depressants ▪ Keep scheduled appointments c̄ physician; have BP checked regularly ▪ Check for swelling in feet/legs daily ▪ Men: impotence may occur.

NOTES:

hydroxyzine hcl/hydroxyzine pamoate▲ • (hye-drox-i-zeen)

CATEGORY: *Antianxiety:* antihistamine   Rx; Preg Cat NA

BRAND NAMES
Atarax (Pfizer)
**Multipax (U.S.U.)*
Vistaril (Pfizer)

DOSAGE FORMS: Capsule▲, injection, PO suspension▲, syrup, tablet

USE: Treatment of anxiety, tension ▪ Preop/postop sedative ▪ Management of N/V, allergic pruritus. **ACTION:** Anxiolytic activity appears related to depression of CNS at brainstem reticular formation, hypothalamus; drug also exhibits antiemetic, antihistamine properties.

PHARMACOKINETICS: Rapid PO absorption c̄ 4-6h sedation; excretion via feces primarily as metabolites.

CONTRAINDICATIONS: Hypersensitivity. **CC:** Not recommended for use in nursing mothers.

DOSAGE

Pediatric		
Anxiety/pruritus	*PO*	<6y/o: 50mg/d divided ≥6y/o: 50-100mg/d divided
Sedation	*PO*	Preop/postop: 0.6mg/kg
Nausea/vomiting	*IM*	0.5mg/lb
Adult		
Anxiety	*PO*	50-100mg qid
	IM	50-100mg q4-6h prn
Pruritus	*PO*	25mg 3-4 times/d
Sedation	*PO*	Preop/postop: 50-100mg
	IM	Preop/postop, prepartum/ postpartum: 25-100mg
Nausea/vomiting	*IM*	25-100mg

SIDE/ADVERSE EFFECTS: Drowsiness, dry mouth, involuntary motor activity (rare).

INTERACTIONS: Drug: Use c̄ CNS depressant ↑ depression, may require dosage adjustments ▪ Use c̄ anticholinergics, TCAs may produce ↑ anticholinergic effects.

Note: Side/adverse effects: common in *italic*; serious in ***boldface italic***.

*Available in Canada only.

NURSING MANAGEMENT PRIORITIES

ADMINISTRATION: Assess for hx of hypersensitivity ▪ PO: may crush tablets/open capsules ▪ PO suspension: shake well before administering ▪ IM: inject *deep, slowly* into large muscle mass; rotate sites; do *not* administer IV/SC ▪ Avoid abrupt withdrawal; D/C gradually ▪ Avoid exposure to heat/moisture/light in storage ▪ Elderly may require ↓ dosage ▪ Problem discussion, sympathetic listening contribute to relief of anxiety.

EVALUATION: Monitor renal, hepatic status ▪ Assess for symptoms of abrupt withdrawal (tremors, abdominal/muscle cramps, convulsions) c̄ prolonged use ▪ Check for signs of dependence (↑ drug request) ▪ Monitor activity status (safety precautions) ▪ Assess for tolerance to therapeutic dose ▪ Check for depression; suicide precautions prn.

EDUCATION: Dizziness/drowsiness may occur; use caution in potentially hazardous activities ▪ Avoid use c̄ alcohol, other CNS depressants ▪ Indiscriminate use may lead to dependence ▪ Do *not* keep at bedside ▪ Take as ordered by physician; do *not* ↑ dose ▪ Use sugarless gum/hard candy to diminish dry mouth ▪ Maintain good oral hygiene; use soft-bristled toothbrush ▪ Check c̄ physician/pharmacist before taking OTC/Rx preparations ▪ Women: avoid breastfeeding ▪ Store in tightly closed, light-resistant container ▪ Practice relaxation exercises, ventilation of feelings, stress management techniques.

NOTES:

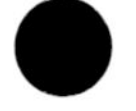

ibuprofen • (eye-byoo-proe-fen)

CATEGORY: *Antiinflammatory:* analgesic, antipyretic, NSAIA — Rx/OTC▲; Preg Cat NA

BRAND NAMES	DOSAGE FORMS
Advil▲ (Whitehall)	Caplet: 200mg Tablet: 200mg
**Amersol (Horner)*	Capsule: 200, 300, 400mg
Children's Advil (Whitehall)	Suspension: 100mg/5ml
Motrin (Upjohn)	Tablet: 300, 400, 600, 800mg
Motrin IB▲ (Upjohn)	Caplet: 200mg Tablet: 200mg
**Novoprofen (Novopharm)*	Tablet: 400, 600, 800mg
Nuprin▲ (B-M)	Caplet: 200mg Tablet: 200mg
Children's Motrin (McNeil)	Suspension: 100mg/5ml

USE: Treatment of rheumatoid arthritis/osteoarthritis ▪ Relief of mild/moderate pain, primary dysmenorrhea ▪ Antipyretic. **ACTION:** Antiinflammatory, analgesic, antipyretic activity appears related to inhibition of prostaglandin synthesis.

PHARMACOKINETICS

PO absorption	Peak	Half-life	Protein binding	Excretion
80%	1-2h	1.8-2h	90%-99%	Via urine primarily as metabolites in 24h

CONTRAINDICATIONS: Hypersensitivity, aspirin/other antiinflammatory agent hypersensitivity. **CC:** Use can ↑ risk of GI bleeding, ulcers, perforation.

DOSAGE

Adult *PO*	
Arthritis	400-800mg 3-4 times/d. Do *not* exceed 3.2g/d
Pain	200-400mg q4-6h
Dysmenorrhea	200-400mg q4-6h
Fever	200-400mg q4-6h
Children *PO*	
Fever	6mo-12y/o: 5mg/kg if <102.5° F; 10mg/kg if >102.5° F. Do *not* exceed maximum dose 40mg/kg/d

*Available in Canada only

SIDE/ADVERSE EFFECTS: CNS: *dizziness,* headache, drowsiness ▪ CV: edema, palpitations, CHF ▪ EENT: tinnitus, ↓ hearing, blurred vision ▪ GI: *abdominal pain, N/V,* constipation, stomatitis ▪ GU: ***glomerular nephritis,*** hematuria, ***interstitial nephritis,*** nephrotic syndrome ▪ HEM: ***agranulocytosis, aplastic anemia, hemolytic anemia*** ▪ INT: *rash,* alopecia, pruritus, purpura, urticaria ▪ Other: thirst, eosinophilic pneumonia.

INTERACTIONS: Drug: Use c̄ ulcerogenic drugs produces additive effects ▪ Use c̄ PO anticoagulants may ↑ their activity ▪ Aspirin will ↓ ibuprofen plasma levels.

NURSING MANAGEMENT PRIORITIES

ADMINISTRATION: Assess for hx of NSAIA hypersensitivity ▪ Avoid administration to individuals c̄ hx of asthma, bleeding disorders, salicylate hypersensitivity ▪ May be administered c̄ food/milk; *best* on empty stomach (1h ac/2h pc); encourage upright position for 15-30m ▪ Avoid exposure to moisture/light in storage ▪ Elderly may require ↓ dosage.

EVALUATION: Monitor hematologic, hepatic, renal status c̄ prolonged use ▪ Monitor pts receiving anticoagulant therapy; may potentiate bleeding ▪ Monitor I&O, daily weight c̄ prolonged use ▪ Assess for edema in extremities ▪ Assess for visual disturbances, skin rash; D/C drug, notify physician.

EDUCATION: Dizziness/drowsiness may occur; use caution in potentially hazardous activities ▪ Take on empty stomach (1h ac/2h pc), c̄ food/milk if GI distress occurs; maintain upright position for 15-30m ▪ Take as ordered by physician; do *not* ↑ dose ▪ Notify physician *immediately* of bleeding, ↑ urine output, swelling of feet/legs, lethargy, GI distress, jaundice, visual disturbance ▪ Avoid taking c̄ aspirin, other NSAIAs ▪ Avoid use c̄ alcohol ▪ Check c̄ physician/pharmacist before taking OTC preparations ▪ Notify physician/dentist of use before treatment ▪ Store in tightly closed container ▪ Full drug effects may require several wks of therapy.

NOTES:

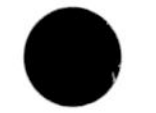

imipenem/cilastatin sodium • (i-mi-pen-em/sye-la-stat-in)

CATEGORY: *Antibiotic combination*

Rx; Preg Cat C

BRAND NAME
Primaxin (Merck)

DOSAGE FORMS
IM powder: 50mg/vial
IV powder: 250-, 500-mg vials, infusion bottles

USE: Treatment of bone, joint, gynecologic, lower respiratory, skin, urinary tract infections caused by susceptible strains of *Acinetobacter* spp, *Bacteroides* spp, *Bifidobacterium* spp, *Citrobacter* spp, *Clostridium* spp, *Enterobacter* spp, *Escherichia coli, Fusobacterium* spp, *Gardnerella vaginalis,* groups A, B, D streptococci, *Haemophilus* spp, *Klebsiella* spp, *Peptococcus* spp, *Peptostreptococcus* spp, *Propionibacterium* spp, *Proteus* spp, *Providencia* spp, *Pseudomonas aeruginosa, Serratia marcescens, Staphylococcus* spp ▪ Penicillinase-producing *Staphylococcus* endocarditis. **ACTION:** Imipenem is a β-lactam antibiotic. Bactericidal activity due to inhibition of cell wall synthesis in susceptible organisms. Cilastatin sodium inhibits the renal enzyme dipeptidase, which inactivates imipenem, resulting in higher urinary levels of imipenem. Both drugs are present in the IV powder for injection in equivalent amounts (250mg/250mg or 500mg/500mg).

PHARMACOKINETICS

	Half-life	Protein binding	Excretion
imipenem	1h	20%	Up to 70% of both recovered in urine within 10h
cilastatin	1h	40%	

CONTRAINDICATIONS: Hypersensitivity. **CC:** β-lactam antibiotics can produce serious/fatal (anaphylaxis) hypersensitivity rxs ▪ Possible cross allergenicity c̄ other β-lactam antibiotics.

DOSAGE: For normal renal function

Adult *IV*	
Mild infections	250-500mg q6h
Moderate/severe infections	500mg-1g q6h or q8h
UTIs	250mg q6h; 500mg q6h for complicated infections
Adult *IM*	
Mild/moderate infections	500-750mg q12h

SIDE/ADVERSE EFFECTS: CNS: dizziness, headache, ***encephalopathy***, paresthesia, psychic disturbances ▪ CV: palpitations, tachycardia, hypotension ▪ EENT: transient hearing loss, tinnitus ▪ GI: *N/V/D*, ***pseudomembranous & hemorrhagic colitis***, pain, glossitis, ↑ salivation ▪ HEP: ↑ alkaline phosphatase, AST, ALT, LDH ▪ HEM: ***agranulocytosis***, ↓ WBC count ▪ INT: rash, pruritus, urticaria, erythema multiforme ▪ RESP: dyspnea, hyperventilation ▪ Other: ↑ BUN & *local phlebitis*, thrombophlebitis, pain, erythema, asthenia, fever, candidiasis.

INTERACTIONS: Drug: Use c̄ bacteriostatic antibiotics can lead to antibiotic antagonism.

NURSING MANAGEMENT PRIORITIES

ADMINISTRATION: Assess for hx of β-lactam hypersensitivity ▪ Obtain C&S before therapy ▪ Assess renal function; ↓ dosage if impaired ▪ Reconstitute, dilute according to manufacturer's directions ▪ Administer via IV infusion only, over 20-30m period; avoid aminoglycoside administration at same site ▪ Do *not* administer cloudy solutions; yellow-amber color does *not* indicate ↓ potency ▪ Have support equipment available for anaphylaxis ▪ Na^+ content: 0.8mEq (18.8mg)/250mg; calculate in Na^+-restricted diets.

EVALUATION: Monitor VS, esp temperature ▪ Monitor renal, hepatic status ▪ Observe for signs of superinfection (diarrhea, itching, oral ulcers) ▪ May ↑ serum ALT, AST, LDH, alkaline phosphatase, bilirubin, creatinine, BUN; ↓ H&H; + Coombs test ▪ Assess for tremors, seizures; notify physician (may ↓ dose or D/C).

EDUCATION: ↑ Fluid intake (8-10 glasses/d) ▪ Maintain good personal hygiene (esp perineal, oral) ▪ Diarrhea may occur; check c̄ physician before taking any antidiarrheal agents ▪ Notify nurse/physician of symptoms of allergic rx (difficult breathing, rash) ▪ Carry identification (Medic-Alert) if β-lactam allergic.

NOTES:

imipramine hcl/imipramine pamoate/desipramine hcl •

(im-ip-ra-meen/dess-ip-ra-meen)

CATEGORY: *Tricyclic antidepressant*: mood elevator — Rx; Preg Cat C

BRAND NAMES	DOSAGE FORMS
imipramine hcl	
**Impril (ICN)*	Tablet: 10, 25, 50, 75mg
**Novopramine (Novopharm)*	
Tofranil (Novartis)	Injection (IM): 25mg/2m Tablet: 10, 25, 50mg
imipramine pamoate	
Tofranil-PM (Novartis)	Capsule: 75, 100, 125, 150mg
desipramine hcl	
Norpramin (H-M-R)	Tablet: 10, 25, 50, 75, 100, 150mg

USE: Treatment of endogenous depression ▪ Childhood enuresis (imipramine hcl). **ACTION:** Antidepressant activity appears related to inhibition of norepinephrine reuptake in central adrenergic neurons; imipramine converted to desipramine in body.

PHARMACOKINETICS

PO absorption	Peak	Half-life	Excretion
Complete	1-2h	8-16h	40% via urine as metabolites in 24h

CONTRAINDICATIONS: Hypersensitivity, MAO-I therapy, MI (acute recovery period). **CC:** Do not exceed 2.5mg/d during childhood ▪ Injection contains sodium bisulfite, which can cause allergic rxs.

DOSAGE

imipramine hcl

Enuresis	*PO*	≥6y/o: 25mg/d 1h before hs >12y/o: up to 75mg/d 1h before hs Do *not* exceed 75mg/d
Depression		
Adolescent	*PO*	30-40mg divided. Do *not* exceed 100mg/d
Adult	*PO*	75-200mg/d divided
	IM	Up to 100mg/d divided

Note: Side/adverse effects: common in *italic*; serious in ***boldface italic***.

*Available in Canada only.

Geriatric	*PO*	30-40mg divided. Do *not* exceed 100mg/d
imipramine pamoate		
Adult	*PO*	75-200mg/d divided
desipramine hcl		
Adolescent	*PO*	25-100mg/d divided
Adult	*PO*	75-300mg/d divided
Geriatric	*PO*	25-100mg/d divided

SIDE/ADVERSE EFFECTS: CNS: *drowsiness,* extrapyramidal symptoms, paresthesia (extremities) ▪ CV: ***arrhythmias,*** postural hypotension ▪ EENT: tinnitus ▪ GI: anorexia, N/V, dry mouth, constipation ▪ GU: gynecomastia, urinary hesitancy ▪ HEM: ***agranulocytosis,*** eosinophilia, ***thrombocytopenia*** ▪ HEP: cholestatic jaundice ▪ INT: skin rash, photosensitivity, alopecia ▪ PSYCH: delusions, hallucinations, exacerbation of psychosis, confusion.

INTERACTIONS: Drug: Significant depressant effects c̄ alcohol, other CNS depressants ▪ Use c̄ anticholinergics, chlorpromazine may produce ↑ atropinelike effects; paralytic ileus could occur ▪ Significant ↑ in activities c̄ epinephrine, levarterenol, other adrenergic agents ▪ Significant antagonism to effects of reserpine, clonidine, guanethidine-type antihypertensives.

NURSING MANAGEMENT PRIORITIES

ADMINISTRATION: Assess for hx of TCA hypersensitivity; glaucoma; prostatic hypertrophy; renal, hepatic disease ▪ PO: administer c̄ food ▪ Parenteral: do *not* administer IV ▪ Institute suicide/safety precautions ▪ ↑ Dosage *slowly* ▪ Avoid abrupt withdrawal.

EVALUATION: Monitor hepatic, renal status; BP, CBC, I&O, daily weight, constipation ▪ Assess for symptoms of abrupt withdrawal (nausea, headache, malaise) ▪ Assess for actual swallowing of PO forms.

EDUCATION: Dizziness/drowsiness may occur; use caution in potentially hazardous activities ▪ Avoid changing positions (lying/sitting/standing) rapidly ▪ Avoid use c̄ alcohol, CNS depressants for up to 1wk after end of therapy ▪ Take PO forms c̄ food to ↓ GI irritation ▪ Use sugarless gum/hard candy to diminish dry mouth ▪ Constipation may occur; ↑ fluids, bulk-containing foods ▪ Check c̄ physician/pharmacist before taking OTC/Rx preparations ▪ Use sunscreen, protective clothing ▪ Notify physician/dentist of use before treatment ▪ Notify physician of fever, sore throat, malaise ▪ Full drug effects may require several wks of therapy.

NOTES:

imiquimod • (im-ick-weh-mod)

CATEGORY: *Topical antiviral:* immune response modifier Rx; Preg Cat B

BRAND NAME	DOSAGE FORM
Aldara (3M)	Cream: 5%

USE: Treatment of external genital & perianal warts (condyloma acuminata) in adults. **ACTION:** Precise antiviral mechanism is unknown for treating human papillomavirus, the etiologic agent causing condyloma, which is usually transmitted sexually. The drug may induce a local immune response modulation involving interferon-alpha & cytokines, resulting in antiviral activity.

PHARMACOKINETICS: Topical absorption is minimal. Less than 1% following application is excreted in the feces & urine.

CONTRAINDICATIONS: Hypersensitivity. **CC:** Not indicated for other human papillomavirus diseases of the genital area (urethral, cervical, intravaginal, interanal, rectal) ▪ Safety & efficacy in pts <18y/o not established ▪ Avoid contact c̄ eyes & sexual activity while medication is on the skin.

DOSAGE

Adult	Apply to affected areas 3 times/wk (skipping 1d between treatment) before hs & leave on skin for 6-10h

SIDE/ADVERSE EFFECTS: Systemic: headache, flulike symptoms ▪ Local: burning, edema, erosion, erythema, fungal infection, induration, pain, scabbing, ulceration.

INTERACTIONS: None currently reported.

NURSING MANAGEMENT PRIORITIES

ADMINISTRATION: Assess for hx of hypersensitivity ▪ Use glove for application to prevent microbial transmission; apply thin layer, rub in until cream is no longer visible; use nonocclusive dressings ▪ Avoid temperature extremes in storage.

EVALUATION: Monitor skin for abnormal rxs (erythema, erosion, edema); notify physician.

EDUCATION: Take exactly as directed by physician ▪ Procedure for topical application ▪ Wash treatment area c̄ mild soap & H_2O 6-10h following application ▪ Avoid contact c̄ eyes ▪ Avoid sexual contact when applied ▪ Notify physician *immediately* of severe skin rxs (burning, bleeding, excoriation) ▪ Used to control, *not* cure, genital warts.

NOTES:

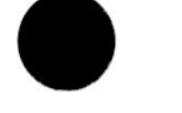

indomethacin/indomethacin sodium trihydrate▲ •

(in-doe-meth-a-sin)

CATEGORY: *Antiinflammatory* Rx; Preg Cat NA

BRAND NAME
Indocin (Merck)
(Indocid [Canada])

DOSAGE FORMS
Capsule: 25, 50, 75mg (SR)
PO suspension: 25mg/5ml
Powder for injection▲ (IV): 1mg/vial
Suppository: 50mg

USE: Treatment of rheumatoid arthritis/osteoarthritis, ankylosing spondylitis, acute gout, acute painful shoulder ▪ PDA closure in premature infants (IV). **ACTION:** Antiinflammatory activity appears related to inhibition of prostaglandin synthesis.

PHARMACOKINETICS

PO absorption	Peak	Half-life	Protein binding	Excretion
90%	2-4h	4.5h	90%	Via urine (60%), feces (33%) as unchanged drug, metabolites

CONTRAINDICATIONS: Hypersensitivity, aspirin/other antiinflammatory hypersensitivity, proctitis/rectal bleeding (suppositories); IV: infants c̄ infection, hemorrhage, thrombocytopenia, necrotizing enterocolitis, impaired renal function, or congenital heart disease in whom PDA is necessary for adequate pulmonary/systemic blood flow. **CC:** Use lowest possible effective dose ▪ Use can ↑ risk of GI bleeding, ulcers, perforation.

DOSAGE

Adults/Children

>14y/o	*PO*	
Arthritis, spondylitis		Start 25mg 2-3 times/d & adjust. Usual range 150-200mg/d divided. Do *not* exceed 200mg/d
Gout		50mg tid. ↓ To cessation as soon as possible
Painful shoulder		75-150mg/d in 3-4 divided doses. Usual treatment 7-14d
Infants	*IV*	Doses at 12-24h intervals based on age: <48h: dose 1, 0.2mg/kg; doses 2 & 3, 0.1mg/kg

2-7d: all 3 doses 0.2mg/kg
>7d: dose 1, 0.2mg/kg; doses 2 & 3, 0.25mg/kg
Second course of 3 doses may be given, c̄ each dose separated 12-24h as described

SIDE/ADVERSE EFFECTS: CNS: *headache, somnolence,* dizziness, tremor, confusion ▪ CV: palpitations, tachycardia, edema ▪ EENT: tinnitus, ↓ hearing, blurred vision, corneal deposits ▪ GI: *dyspepsia*, constipation, N/V, pain, anorexia, flatulence, dry mouth, ***hemorrhage*** ▪ GU: vaginal bleeding ▪ INT: pruritus, rash, urticaria.

INTERACTIONS: Drug: Use c̄ ulcerogenic drugs produces additive effects ▪ Use c̄ PO anticoagulants, thrombolytic agents may ↑ their activity ▪ Use c̄ triamterene will ↓ kidney function.

NURSING MANAGEMENT PRIORITIES

ADMINISTRATION: Assess for hx of NSAIA hypersensitivity (incl aspirin) ▪ Avoid administration to pts c̄ hx of asthma, bleeding disorders, salicylate hypersensitivity ▪ Assess renal, hepatic function; use c̄ caution if impaired ▪ PO: administer c̄ food/milk, encourage upright position for 15-30m; shake suspension well before pouring ▪ Administer SR capsules whole ▪ IV: reconstitute c̄ 1-2ml 0.9% NaCl, sterile H_2O for injection (w/out preservatives); use *immediately*; administer direct IV (5-10s), avoid extravasation; discard unused portion ▪ Avoid exposure to moisture/light in storage ▪ Store suppositories in refrigerator; do *not* freeze ▪ Elderly may require ↓ dosage.

EVALUATION: Monitor pt receiving anticoagulant therapy; may potentiate bleeding ▪ Monitor I&O, daily weight ▪ Assess for edema in extremities, visual disturbances; D/C drug, notify physician.

EDUCATION: Dizziness/blurred vision may occur; use caution in potentially hazardous activities ▪ Take c̄ food/milk to ↓ GI distress; maintain upright position for 15-30m ▪ Swallow SR capsules whole ▪ Take as ordered by physician; do *not* ↑ dose ▪ Store in tightly closed, light-resistant container ▪ Notify physician *immediately* of bleeding, rash, flulike symptoms, swelling of feet/legs, GI distress, jaundice, visual disturbances ▪ Avoid use c̄ alcohol, aspirin, other NSAIAs ▪ Check c̄ physician/pharmacist before taking OTC preparations ▪ Keep appointments for blood work/eye exams ▪ Women: avoid breastfeeding.

NOTES:

ipecac syrup • (ip-e-kak)

CATEGORY: *Emetic*

OTC; Preg Cat C

AVAILABLE PREPARATION
Syrup; available from various manufacturers/distributors in 1-, 2-oz bottles

USE: Emetic, expectorant. **ACTION:** Emetic activity due to central stimulation of chemoreceptor trigger zone, local irritation of gastric mucosa.

PHARMACOKINETICS: Normally effective 90% of time w/in 15-20m.

CONTRAINDICATIONS: Semiconsciousness; pregnancy; ingestion of convulsants, corrosive substances, kerosene, strychnine, caustic substances. **CC:** Consider gastric lavage if vomiting does not occur w/in 30-45m after second dose.

DOSAGE

Emetic		
Pediatric	*PO*	≤1y/o: usually 5ml. Repeat in 20m if no emesis 1-12y/o: 10-15ml. Repeat in 20m if no emesis
Adult	*PO*	15-30ml. Repeat in 20m if no emesis
Expectorant		
Adult/Children	*PO*	0.5-1ml

SIDE/ADVERSE EFFECTS: No emesis: absorbed alkaloid (emetine) can cause cardiac conduction disturbances ▪ After emesis: GI upset, diarrhea.

INTERACTIONS: Drug: Use c̄ activated charcoal will ↓ chances of emesis; may give activated charcoal after vomiting has occurred.

NURSING MANAGEMENT PRIORITIES
ADMINISTRATION: Administer only to conscious pts ▪ Follow administration c̄ H_2O: 1-2 glasses, adult; ½-1 glass, child ▪ Avoid concurrent administration c̄ milk, activated charcoal, carbonated beverages ▪ Do *not* administer in cases of corrosive poisoning ▪ Avoid exposure to heat/direct light in storage.

EVALUATION: Monitor VS, esp heart rate (cardiotoxic) ▪ Assess for vomiting; repeat dose in 20-30m if emesis does *not* occur.

EDUCATION: Telephone number for poison control center/emergency room/physician; call before taking drug ▪ Give only to alert/conscious pts ▪ Procedure for home use: take exactly as prescribed on label, follow c̄ H_2O; do *not* use c̄ milk/carbonated beverages; do not take more than 2 doses ▪ *Not* recommended at home for children <1y/o; physician supervision necessary ▪ Store in tightly closed, light-resistant container out of reach of children; check expiration date routinely, replace before expiration.

NOTES:

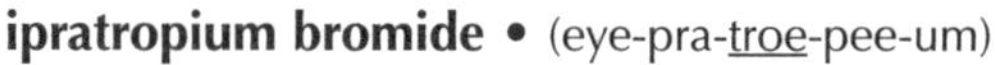

ipratropium bromide • (eye-pra-troe-pee-um)

CATEGORY: *Anticholinergic:* bronchodilator — Rx; Preg Cat B

BRAND NAME

Atrovent (B-I)

DOSAGE FORMS

Aerosol: 18mg/dose
Inhalation solution: 0.02%
Nasal spray: 0.03% (21µg/spray), 0.06% (42µg/spray)

USE: Treatment of bronchospasm associated c̄ COPD ▪ Treatment of rhinorrhea associated c̄ common cold (0.06% spray) & allergic & nonallergic perennial rhinitis (0.03% spray). **ACTION:** Bronchodilation due to local specific site anticholinergic antagonism of muscarinic receptor in bronchial smooth muscle. Drug does not produce systemic anticholinergic effect.

PHARMACOKINETICS: After inhalation: onset of 15m, peak 1-2h, duration 3-6h, & half-life 2h.

CONTRAINDICATIONS: Hypersensitivity to drug, atropine, soya lecithin, soybean, peanuts. **CC:** Not indicated for acute bronchospasm requiring rapid therapeutic response ▪ Use c̄ caution in pts c̄ bladder neck obstruction, narrow-angle glaucoma, prostatic hypertrophy ▪ Nasal spray limited to ≥12y/o.

DOSAGE

Children (≥12y/o)/Adult

Aerosol	2 inhalations (36mg) qid. Do *not* exceed 12 doses in 24h
Solution	2.5ml (500mg) PO nebulization q6-8h
Spray	2 sprays (0.03 or 0.06%) 2-4 times/d

SIDE/ADVERSE EFFECTS: CNS: nervousness, dizziness, headache ▪ CV: palpitations ▪ GI: nausea, *dry mouth* (solution) ▪ RESP: cough, ↑ in symptoms, bronchitis & URI (solution) ▪ Other: blurred vision (aerosol), chest & back pain (solution).

INTERACTIONS: Drug: No significant rxs reported esp c̄ other bronchodilators & steroids.

NURSING MANAGEMENT PRIORITIES

ADMINISTRATION: Assess for hx of hypersensitivity, incl soy products ▪ Assess respiratory function, patency of nasal passages ▪ Avoid abrupt withdrawal ▪ Avoid exposure to heat/light in storage.

EVALUATION: Monitor VS, esp heart rate; I&O ▪ Observe for anticholinergic effects ▪ Assess respiratory status, adequate inhalation.

EDUCATION: Advise pt of expected anticholinergic side effects (dry mouth, photophobia, constipation) ▪ Notify physician *immediately* of skin rash, flushing of skin, eye pain; D/C drug ▪ Avoid strenuous work/exercise during hot, humid weather ▪ Use sugarless gum/hard candy to diminish dry mouth ▪ Avoid OTC cough/hay fever preparations ▪ Avoid potentially hazardous activities ▪ ↑ Fluid intake (10-12 glasses/d) ▪ Take as directed by physician; do *not* abruptly D/C drug ▪ Notify physician/dentist of use before treatment ▪ Proper use of aerosol/inhaler (do *not* puncture/incinerate aerosol container) ▪ Avoid contact of solution c̄ eyes (temporary blurred vision may occur).

NOTES:

isoniazid • (eye-soe-nye-a-zid)

CATEGORY: *Antitubercular*

Rx; Preg Cat NA

BRAND NAMES
INH (Ciba)
**Isotamine (ICN)*
Laniazid (Lannett)
Nydrazid (Apothecon)

DOSAGE FORMS
Injection (IM): 100mg/ml
Tablet: 50, 100, 300mg

PHARMACOKINETICS

PO absorption	Peak	Half-life	Excretion
Good	1-2h	1-4h	Via urine primarily as unchanged drug

USE: Treatment of all forms of tuberculosis (TB) as sole agent/in combination c̄ other antitubercular agents ▪ Prophylactic therapy for (listed by priority): (a) household members, other close associates of persons c̄ recently diagnosed TB; (b) positive tuberculin skin test reactors c̄ chest x-ray films consistent c̄ nonprogressive TB, & c̄ neither positive bacteriologic findings nor hx of adequate chemotherapy; (c) newly infected persons; (d) positive tuberculin skin test reactors c̄ prolonged therapy c̄ corticosteroids, immunosuppressive therapy, leukemia, Hodgkin's disease, diabetes, silicosis, recent gastrectomy; (e) other positive tuberculin reactors ≤35y/o. **ACTION:** Antitubercular activity appears due to inhibition of transaminase activity, other pyridoxine-linked enzymes in actively growing susceptible tubercle bacilli; emergence of mycobacterial strains resistant to isoniazid can be significantly ⬇ by combination c̄ other antimycobacterial agents.

CONTRAINDICATIONS: Hypersensitivity, hepatic dysfunction. **CC:** Use can result in serious/fatal age-related hepatitis, which can develop after mos of treatment ▪ Preventive treatment should be delayed in pts c̄ acute hepatic diseases.

DOSAGE

Tuberculosis

Pediatric	*PO/Parenteral*	10-20mg/kg/d as single dose
Adult	*PO/Parenteral*	5mg/kg/d as single dose

Prophylaxis

Pediatric	*PO/Parenteral*	10mg/kg/d as single dose
Adult	*PO/Parenteral*	300mg/d as single dose

SIDE/ADVERSE EFFECTS: CNS: peripheral neuropathy, ***toxic encephalopathy, convulsions***, memory impairment, toxic psychosis ▪ EENT: optic neuritis ▪ END: gynecomastia ▪ GI: N/V, epigastric distress, anorexia ▪ EM: ***agranulocytosis; hemolytic, sideroblastic, aplastic anemia; thrombocytopenia*** ▪ HEP: age-related hepatitis (usually elderly); ↑ in AST, ALT; ***jaundice***, bilirubinemia ▪ INT: maculopapular or morbilliform rashes, ***exfoliative dermatitis*** ▪ Other: vitamin B_6 deficiency, pellagra, gynecomastia.

INTERACTIONS: Drug: Use c̄ rifampin, cycloserine, ethionamide may produce ↑ CNS toxicity ▪ Use c̄ antacid suspensions may ↓ isoniazid absorption ▪ Use c̄ phenytoin may require dosage adjustments for phenytoin.

NURSING MANAGEMENT PRIORITIES

ADMINISTRATION: Assess for hx of hypersensitivity (incl ethionamide, pyrazinamide, niacin) ▪ Obtain C&S before therapy ▪ PO: may administer on empty stomach, or c̄ meals to ↓ GI irritation; administer 1h before antacids ▪ IM: massage site after injection; rotate sites ▪ Avoid exposure to heat/moisture/light in storage ▪ Assess hepatic function; ↓ dose if impaired ▪ Have IV pyridoxine (vitamin B_6) available for OD.

EVALUATION: Monitor VS, esp temperature, BP; hepatic, renal status; serum for ↑ uric acid, AST, ALT ▪ Assess for visual disturbances (ocular toxicity) ▪ Use Clinistix/Diastix for urine testing.

EDUCATION: Take as ordered by physician, even if symptom free; do *not* skip doses ▪ May take on empty stomach or c̄ meals to ↓ GI irritation ▪ Do *not* take antacids for at least 1h after drug ▪ Avoid changing positions rapidly ▪ Keep appointments for eye exams/c̄ physician ▪ Notify physician *immediately* of visual problems, tingling/numbness of hands/feet, jaundice, lethargy, dark urine; D/C drug ▪ Women: avoid pregnancy, breastfeeding ▪ Safety precautions c̄ ↑ activity ▪ Emotional support during long-term therapy ▪ Avoid use of alcohol, tyramine-containing (aged, fermented) foods ▪ Store in tightly closed, light-resistant container ▪ Physician may order vitamin B_6 supplements to alleviate neurotoxic effects ▪ Diabetics: use Clinistix/Diastix to check urine glucose ▪ Full drug effects may require several wks of therapy.

NOTES:

isoproterenol hcl • (eye-soe-proe-ter-e-nole)

CATEGORY: *Sympathomimetic:* β adrenergic, bronchodilator — Rx; Preg Cat C

BRAND NAMES	**DOSAGE FORMS**
Isuprel (Winthrop)	Injection (IV): 0.2mg/ml Mistometer: 131μg/spray Solution: 0.5%, 1% SL tablet (Glossets): 10, 15mg
Medihaler-Iso (3M)	Aerosol: 80μg/spray

USE: Treatment of bronchospasm associated c̄ acute/chronic asthma, pulmonary emphysema, bronchitis, bronchiectasis ▪ Adjunct in treatment of shock ▪ Treatment of cardiac arrest, carotid sinus hypersensitivity, Adams-Stokes syndrome, ventricular arrhythmias due to AV block. **ACTION:** Sympathomimetic activity selective for β receptors, c̄ no appreciable α-receptor activity; β_1-adrenergic activity results in positive inotropic, chronotropic cardiac effect, c̄ ⬆ output, stroke volume, oxygen consumption; β_2-adrenergic activity produces bronchial, GI, uterine smooth muscle relaxation.

PHARMACOKINETICS: Bronchodilation after inhalation immediate; duration about 1h, 1-2h c̄ SC/SL administration; excretion via urine.

CONTRAINDICATIONS: Hypersensitivity, digitalis tachycardia, preexisting cardiac arrhythmias. **CC:** Excessive PO inhalation use can result in ⬇ effectiveness. Use in pts c̄ a failing or injured heart can result in harmful effect.

DOSAGE

Bronchospasm	*SL*	
Pediatric		5-10mg. Do *not* exceed 30mg/d
Adult		10-20mg. Do *not* exceed 60mg/d
Heart block		
Pediatric		½ initial adult dose
Adult		10-15mg 4-6 times/d
Asthma/bronchospasm		
	Inhalation	1-5 treatments prn
Shock	*IV*	0.5-5μg/m. Dosage adjusted to heart rate, BP, urine flow. Doses up to 30μg/m may be required for advanced shock

Heart block/arrhythmias

Intracardiac	0.02mg
IM	Initial dose 0.2mg, subsequent range 0.02-1mg
IV	Initial dose 0.02-0.06mg, subsequent range 0.01-0.2mg
IV infusion	0.5-5μg/m
SC	Initial dose 0.2mg, subsequent range 0.15-0.2mg

SIDE/ADVERSE EFFECTS: CNS: mild tremors, headache, nervousness, dizziness ▪ CV: tachycardia, pulmonary edema, paradoxic Adams-Stokes seizures ▪ Other: flushing of face, sweating.

INTERACTIONS: Drug: Use c̄ MAO-I can produce significant hypertensive crisis ▪ Use c̄ TCAs, epinephrine best avoided ▪ Use c̄ propranolol antagonizes isoproterenol effects.

NURSING MANAGEMENT PRIORITIES

ADMINISTRATION: Assess for hx of catecholamine hypersensitivity (incl sulfites) ▪ Avoid concurrent epinephrine administration ▪ SL: have pt dissolve under tongue; do *not* swallow; rinse mouth c̄ H_2O after absorption ▪ Inhalation: consult manufacturer's directions (do *not* inject); excessive use may ⬇ effectiveness; rinse mouth c̄ H_2O after administration ▪ Do *not* use discolored/precipitated solution ▪ IV: cardiac monitoring; use infusion pump; have emergency support equipment available ▪ Intracardiac: administer chest compressions to perfuse drug into myocardium ▪ Avoid exposure to heat/direct sunlight in storage ▪ Elderly may require ⬇ dosage.

EVALUATION: Monitor VS, esp BP, heart rate (D/C drug if >120) ▪ Monitor hemodynamic status, ABGs (parenteral) ▪ Monitor I&O.

EDUCATION: Take as ordered by physician; do *not* ⬆ dose ▪ Take on arising ▪ Notify physician *immediately* of rapid/"skipped" heartbeats, chest pain, tremors; D/C drug ▪ May turn saliva pink/red (SL, inhalation) ▪ Procedure for inhalation/SL administration.

NOTES:

isosorbide dinitrate • (eye-soe-sor-bide)

CATEGORY: *Antianginal:* coronary vasodilator — Rx; Preg Cat C

BRAND NAMES	**DOSAGE FORMS**
Dilatrate (Schwarz)	SR capsule: 40mg
Isordil (W-A)	SL tablet: 2.5, 5mg
	Titradose tablet: 5, 10, 20, 30, 40mg
	Tembids (SR) tablet: 40mg
Sorbitrate (Zeneca)	Chewable tablet: 5mg
	Tablet: 5, 10, 20, 30, 40mg

USE: Treatment/prophylaxis of angina pectoris. **ACTION:** Vasodilation due to direct relaxation of smooth muscle blood vessels, esp in coronary circulation; ↑ blood supply to myocardium helps relieve ischemia, thereby ↓ anginal pain.

PHARMACOKINETICS

	Onset	Duration	Excretion
SL chewable tablet	1-3m	1-2h	Via urine primarily as metabolites
PO tablet	1h	4-6h	
Extended action forms	0.5-1h	Up to 12h	

CONTRAINDICATIONS: Hypersensitivity to drug, nitrates/nitrites. **CC:** Use in pts c̄ CHF or MI not established.

DOSAGE

Adult	*Chewable/SL*	2.5-10mg prn
	PO	5-30mg 3-4 times/d or more

SIDE/ADVERSE EFFECTS: CNS: headache, dizziness, restlessness ▪ CV: postural hypotension, cutaneous vasodilation, flushing ▪ GI: N/V ▪ INT: rash, exfoliative dermatitis.

INTERACTIONS: Drug: Use c̄ calcium blockers, alcohol, β blockers, phenothiazines results in additive hypotensive effects.

NURSING MANAGEMENT PRIORITIES

ADMINISTRATION: Assess for hx of nitrate hypersensitivity ▪ Administer 1h ac/2h pc ▪ Chewable tablet: have pt chew well, hold in mouth for 2m before swallowing ▪ SR: have pt swallow whole ▪ SL: administer c̄ pt sitting/lying; avoid talking, drinking, eating, smoking until absorbed ▪ Avoid exposure to heat/moisture in storage.

EVALUATION: Monitor VS, esp BP ▪ Assess for headache; notify physician ▪ Assess for tolerance c̄ prolonged use.

EDUCATION: Dizziness may occur; use caution in potentially hazardous activities ▪ Avoid changing positions (lying/sitting/standing) rapidly ▪ Avoid use c̄ alcohol ▪ Take 1h ac/2h pc ▪ Swallow SR capsules/tablets whole ▪ Store in cool, dry area ▪ Chewable tablet: chew well, hold in mouth for 2m before swallowing ▪ SL: dissolve under tongue; do *not* eat, drink, talk, smoke during use; notify physician/go to emergency room if not relieved w/in 15m ▪ Take prescribed analgesic for headache ▪ Notify physician of any ↓ in drug effect (persistent chest pain) ▪ Avoid ↑ exercise, exposure to temperature extremes ▪ Carry medical identification (MedicAlert).

NOTES:

itraconazole • (it-rah-koe-na-zol)

CATEGORY: *Broad-spectrum antifungal*

Rx; Preg Cat C

BRAND NAME
Sporanox (Jannsen)

DOSAGE FORM
Capsule: 100mg
Oral solution: 10mg/ml

USE: Treatment of oropharyngeal/esophageal candidiasis (oral solution) ▪ Treatment of blastomycosis, histoplasmosis fungal infections. In addition, exhibits antifungal activity against wide array of other systemic & topical fungal infections ▪ Treatment of aspergillosis in pts c̄ intolerance of, refractory to amphotericin B ▪ Treatment of onychomycosis due to susceptible dermatophytes. **ACTION:** Antifungal activity appears related to ↓ synthesis of ergosterol, which is an essential component of the cell membrane. ↓ Cytochrome P-450–dependent synthesis of ergosterol.

PHARMACOKINETICS

PO absorption	Half-life	Protein binding	Excretion
Moderate	64h	19.8%	Via urine, feces primarily as metabolites

CONTRAINDICATIONS: Hypersensitivity, concurrent use c̄ astemizole, cisapride, terfenadine. **CC:** Use associated c̄ extremely rare cases of reversible idiosyncratic hepatitis ▪ Hepatic enzyme values before/during treatment must be monitored ▪ Drug is excreted in breast milk; use in nursing mothers is not recommended.

DOSAGE

Adult *PO*	200mg once/d c̄ food. May ↑ to maximum 400mg/d divided if required. For life-threatening infections loading dose 200mg tid may be given for first 3d of treatment.
Onychomycosis	200mg/d for 12wks. For fingernails (only) 100mg bid for 1wk c̄ 3wks rest & repeated for 1 or more cycles
Candidiasis	
Oropharyngeal	10ml PO solution swished in mouth for several seconds & then swallowed. Usual daily dose range 20ml (200 mg) for 1-2wks
Esophageal	10 ml (100 mg)/d for 5wks

SIDE/ADVERSE EFFECTS: CNS: headache, dizziness, somnolence, depression, insomnia ▪ CV: hypertension, edema ▪ EENT: tinnitus ▪ GI: *N/V/D,* anorexia, abdominal pain, flatulence ▪ INT: *rash,* pruritus ▪ Other: fatigue, fever, malaise, hepatic dysfunction, hypokalemia, impotence.

INTERACTIONS: Drug: Use c̄ cisapride can produce fatal cardiac arrhythmias ▪ Use c̄ cyclosporine, digoxin, PO hypoglycemics, PO anticoagulants, tacrolimus will ↑ their respective activities ▪ ↓ Itraconazole levels can result c̄ H_2 blockers, isoniazid, rifampin ▪ Use c̄ triazolam is best avoided ▪ Use c̄ other hepatotoxic drugs can produce additive toxicity. **Food:** Administer c̄ food to ↑ PO absorption.

NURSING MANAGEMENT PRIORITIES

ADMINISTRATION: Assess for hx of hypersensitivity ▪ Obtain C&S before therapy ▪ Administer in early AM ▪ Assess hepatic function; ↓ dosage if impaired ▪ Administer c̄ food.

EVALUATION: Monitor VS, esp temperature, BP ▪ Monitor hepatic function ▪ Diabetics: monitor blood glucose (hypoglycemia).

EDUCATION: Dizziness/drowsiness may occur; use caution in potentially hazardous activities ▪ Take as directed by physician at same time qd; do *not* change dose ▪ Take c̄ food ▪ Take antacids at least 2h after taking drug ▪ Avoid exposure to bright light; wear sunglasses to ↓ discomfort ▪ May require several wks/mos of treatment; take until lab tests are normal ▪ Check c̄ physician/pharmacist before taking OTC preparations ▪ Store in tightly closed container ▪ Women: avoid breastfeeding ▪ Avoid use c̄ alcohol.

NOTES:

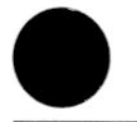

kanamycin sulfate • (kan-a-mye-sin)

CATEGORY: *Aminoglycoside:* antibiotic

Rx; Preg Cat D

BRAND NAMES

**Anamid*

Kantrex (Apothecon)

DOSAGE FORMS

Capsule: 500mg
Injection (IM/IV): 500mg/2ml, 1g/3ml
Pediatric injection: (IM/IV): 75mg/2ml

USE: Treatment (parenteral) of infections caused by susceptible strains of *Enterobacter aerogenes, Escherichia coli, Klebsiella pneumoniae, Mima-Herellea (Acinetobacter), Proteus* spp, *Serratia marcescens* ▪ Alternative for penicillin-resistant staphylococcal infection (parenteral) ▪ Treatment of cirrhotic pts c̄ hepatic coma caused by nitrogen-producing bacteria (PO) ▪ Intestinal antisepsis (PO). **ACTION:** Bactericidal activity due to inhibition of ribosomal protein synthesis in susceptible organisms; toxicity usually limits systemic use to serious gram-negative infection; dosage must be adjusted to pts c̄ impaired renal function.

PHARMACOKINETICS

IM peak	Half-life	Excretion
1h	2-2.5h	50% via urine in 4h, complete w/in 24-48h

CONTRAINDICATIONS: Hypersensitivity, hx of serious aminoglycoside toxicity. **CC:** Use c̄ renal impairment will ↑ toxicity ▪ Use can result in nephrotoxicity; ototoxicity may produce irreversible bilateral deafness ▪ Neuromuscular blockade c̄ respiratory paralysis has been reported c̄ aminoglycoside use.

DOSAGE

Pediatric/Adult	*IM/IV*	Usual dose 15mg/kg/d in 2 doses. Do *not* exceed 1.5g/d
Adult	*PO*	
Hepatic encephalopathy		8-12g/d divided
Intestinal antisepsis		1g q4h for 4 doses, followed by 1g q6h for 36-72h

SIDE/ADVERSE EFFECTS: CNS: headache, paresthesia ▪ EENT: ***ototoxicity*** (auditory, vestibular damage: dizziness, vertigo, tinnitus, roaring in ears, hearing loss) ▪ GU: ***nephrotoxicity*** (casts, proteinuria; ↑ BUN, NPN, serum creatinine) ▪ INT: rash ▪ Other: fever.

INTERACTIONS: Drug: Avoid use c̄ neurotoxic/nephrotoxic drugs (eg, other aminoglycosides, colistin, ethacrynic acid, furosemide, polymyxin B, vancomycin) ▪ Dimenhydrinate can mask aminoglycoside ototoxicity ▪ Use c̄ succinylcholine/tubocurarine ↑ their activity; Ca^{++} salts can reverse blockade ▪ PO anticoagulant activity may ↑ due to ↓ intestinal vitamin K synthesis.

NURSING MANAGEMENT PRIORITIES

ADMINISTRATION: Assess for hx of aminoglycoside hypersensitivity ▪ Obtain C&S before therapy ▪ Obtain pt weight for dosage calculation ▪ Determine creatinine clearance before administration ▪ IM: administer by *deep, slow* injection into gluteal UOQ ▪ IV: dilute 500mg/vial in 200ml normal saline/5% dextrose (1-g vial in 400ml) solution; administer 60-80gtt/m; may mix c̄ dextrose, Ringer injection, normal saline solution ▪ Inhalation: dilute 250mg in 3ml normal saline solution, nebulize ▪ Intraperitoneal: instill 500mg in 20ml sterile distilled H_2O ▪ Do *not* mix c̄ other drugs ▪ Avoid exposure to moisture in storage; store in original container ▪ Darkened color does *not* indicate ↓ potency ▪ Maintain hydration ▪ Elderly may require ↓ dosage.

EVALUATION: Assess for hearing dysfunction ▪ Monitor hepatic, renal, VIII CN function ▪ Monitor VS, esp temperature ▪ Assess for edema in extremities ▪ Assess for neuromuscular blockade, respiratory paralysis, nephrotoxicity ▪ Observe for signs of superinfection (diarrhea, URI, coated tongue) ▪ Assess for hypersensitivity (fever, difficult breathing, rash) ▪ Assess peak (<35µg/ml), trough (<5µg/ml) serum concentrations.

EDUCATION: Report hearing, balance difficulties to physician at once ▪ ↑ Fluid intake (10-12 glasses/d).

NOTES:

ketoconazole • (key-toe-koe-na-zol)

CATEGORY: *Antifungal*

Rx; Preg Cat C

BRAND NAME
Nizoral (Janssen)

DOSAGE FORMS
Cream: 2%
Tablet: 200mg
Shampoo: 2%

USE: Treatment of fungal infection (blastomycosis, candidiasis, chromomycosis, coccidioidomycosis, histoplasmosis, paracoccidioidomycosis) caused by susceptible strains ▪ Treatment of cutaneous dermatophyte infections not responsive to topical therapy ▪ Cream used in the topical treatment of candidiasis, dermatophytes, & tinea versicolor. **ACTION:** Antifungal activity, usually fungistatic, due to inhibition of ergosterol synthesis, a vital fungal cell membrane component; this results in cell membrane permeability changes, inhibition of purine transport; drug not suitable for fungal meningitis.

PHARMACOKINETICS

PO absorption	Peak	Half-life	Protein binding	Excretion
Variable	1-2h	2h	99%	Via feces primarily as metabolites c̄ some urinary excretion

CONTRAINDICATIONS: Hypersensitivity, concurrent use c̄ astemizole, cisapride, terfenadine. **CC:** Systemic use may cause hepatic (hepatocellular) toxicity incl rare cases of fatalities.

DOSAGE

Pediatric	*PO*	>2y/o: 3.3-6.6mg/kg/d as single dose
Adult	*PO*	200mg/d as single dose. Serious infections may require 400mg once/d
Cream		Once/d over area of infection
Shampoo		Use twice/wk for 4wks c̄ at least 3d between each shampooing followed by occasional use to maintain control

SIDE/ADVERSE EFFECTS: CNS: headache, dizziness, somnolence, photophobia ▪ END: gynecomastia ▪ GI: N/V/D, pain ▪ GU: impotence ▪ HEM: ***thrombocytopenia*** ▪ HEP: ***hepatocellular toxicity.***

INTERACTIONS: Drug: Use c̄ cisapride can produce fatal cardiac arrhythmias ▪ Use c̄ cyclosporine, digoxin, PO hypoglycemics, PO anticoagulants, tacrolimus will ↑ their respective activities ▪ ↓ Ketoconazole levels can result c̄ H_2 blockers, isoniazid, rifampin ▪ Use c̄ triazolam is best avoided ■ Use c̄ other hepatotoxic drugs can produce additive toxicity. **Food:** Administer c̄ food to ↑ PO absorption.

NURSING MANAGEMENT PRIORITIES

ADMINISTRATION: Assess for hx of hypersensitivity ■ Obtain C&S before therapy ■ Administer in early AM ■ Assess hepatic function; ↓ dosage if impaired ■ Do *not* administer w/in 2h of alkaline substances (requires acid media to dissolve); may be ordered c̄ dilute HCl, sip through glass/plastic straw placed behind teeth, follow c̄ glass of H_2O.

EVALUATION: Monitor VS, esp temperature ■ Monitor hepatic function.

EDUCATION: Dizziness/drowsiness may occur; use caution in potentially hazardous activities ■ Take as ordered by physician at same time qd; do *not* change dose ■ Take c̄ food ■ Avoid exposure to bright light; wear sunglasses to ↓ discomfort ■ May require several wks/mos of treatment; take until lab tests normal ■ Check c̄ physician/pharmacist before taking OTC preparations ■ Store in tightly closed container ■ Women: avoid breastfeeding ■ Avoid use c̄ alcohol.

NOTES:

ketorolac tromethamine • (key-<u>toe</u>-roe-lack)

CATEGORY: *Analgesic:* antiinflammatory, NSAIA — Rx; Preg Cat C

BRAND NAMES	DOSAGE FORMS
Acular (Allergan)	Ophthalmic solution: 0.5%
Toradol (Roche)	IM/IV: 15, 30mg/ml
	Tablets: 10mg

USE: Short-term relief of pain (up to 5d) ▪ Produces maximum IM/IV effect in 1-2h c̄ a duration of 4-6h ▪ Treatment of seasonal allergic conjunctivitis (ophthalmics). **ACTION:** Analgesic activity appears related to inhibition of prostaglandin synthesis.

CONTRAINDICATIONS: Hypersensitivity, c̄ nasal polyps or aspirin & other NSAIA-induced allergies, peptic ulcer/bleeding/perforation, advanced renal impairment or pts at high risk for renal failure, labor/delivery, nursing mothers, epidural/intrathecal administration, confirmed cerebral bleeding, & other hemorrhaging conditions. **CC:** For short-term use of 1-5d that requires opiate level analgesia ▪ Use c̄ caution c̄ coagulation disorders.

DOSAGE: Do *not* exceed 5d

Adult <65y/o	*PO*	20mg as a first dose for pts who received 60mg IM or 30mg IV single dose followed by 10mg q4-6h. Do *not* exceed 40mg/d
>65y/o		10mg as a first dose for pts who received 30mg IM or 15mg IV single dose followed by 10mg q4-6h. Do *not* exceed 40mg/d
<65y/o	*IM/IV*	30mg q6h. Do *not* exceed 120mg/d
>65y/o		15mg q6h. Do *not* exceed 60mg/d
	Ophthalmic	1gtt qid

SIDE/ADVERSE EFFECTS: CNS: headache (17%), drowsiness, dizziness, paresthesia, nervousness, convulsions, tre-

Note: Side/adverse effects: common in *italic;* serious in ***boldface italic.***

*Available in Canada only.

mors ▪ CV: hypertension, palpitations, edema ▪ EENT: abnormal taste & vision, tinnitus, hearing loss ▪ GI: nausea (12%), dyspepsia (12%), pain (13%), ulcers, bleeding, stomatitis, V/D, pancreatitis ▪ HEM: purpura, leukopenia, eosinophilia ▪ INT: rash, pruritus, exfoliative dermatitis, urticaria, maculopapular rash, Lyell's syndrome, ***Stevens-Johnson syndrome*** ▪ REN: ***acute renal failure,*** azotemia, nephritis, hematuria ▪ RESP: asthma, dyspnea, rhinitis, cough ▪ Other: asthenia, anaphylaxis, fever.

INTERACTIONS: Drug: Use c̄ ulcerogenic drug produces additive effects ▪ Use c̄ warfarin, other high protein-binding drugs can ↑ their activity due to protein displacement ▪ Use c̄ lithium, methotrexate, nondepolarizing muscle relaxants may ↑ their activity ▪ Use c̄ furosemide may ↓ diuretic effect.

NURSING MANAGEMENT PRIORITIES

ADMINISTRATION: Assess for hx of NSAIA hypersensitivity ▪ Avoid administration to individuals c̄ hx of asthma, bleeding disorders, salicylate hypersensitivity ▪ PO: may be administered c̄ food/milk; *best* on empty stomach (1h ac/2h pc); encourage upright position for 15-30m ▪ Avoid exposure to moisture/light in storage ▪ Elderly may require ↓ dosage.

EVALUATION: Monitor hematologic, hepatic, renal status c̄ prolonged use ▪ Monitor pt receiving anticoagulant therapy; may potentiate bleeding ▪ Monitor I&O, daily weight c̄ prolonged use ▪ Assess for edema in extremities ▪ Assess for visual disturbances, skin rash; D/C drug, notify physician.

EDUCATION: Dizziness/drowsiness may occur; use caution in potentially hazardous activities ▪ Take on empty stomach (1h ac/2h pc), c̄ food/milk if GI distress occurs; maintain upright position of 15-30m ▪ Take as ordered by physician; do *not* ↑ dose ▪ Notify physician *immediately* of bleeding, ↓ urine output, swelling of feet/legs, lethargy, GI distress, jaundice, visual disturbance ▪ Avoid taking c̄ aspirin, other NSAIAs ▪ Avoid use c̄ alcohol ▪ Check c̄ physician/pharmacist before taking OTC preparations ▪ Notify physician/dentist of use before treatment ▪ Store in tightly closed container.

NOTES:

labetalol hcl • (la-bet-a-lole)

CATEGORY: *α–β blocker:* antihypertensive Rx; Preg Cat C

BRAND NAMES
Normodyne (Schering)
Trandate (G-W)

DOSAGE FORMS
Normodyne: Injection (IV): 5mg/ml; Tablet: 100, 200, 300mg
Trandate: Injection (IV): 5mg/ml; Tablet: 100, 200, 300mg

USE: Treatment of hypertension as sole agent/in combination c̄ other antihypertensives, esp thiazide or loop diuretic; severe hypertensive states treated IV. **ACTION:** Selective α_1, nonselective β blockage produces enhanced hypotensive effects.

PHARMACOKINETICS

PO absorption	Peak	Half-life	Protein binding	Excretion
Complete	1-2h	6-8h	55%-60%	Via urine, bile primarily as metabolites

CONTRAINDICATIONS: Hypersensitivity, bronchial asthma, cardiac failure, cardiogenic shock, greater than 1° heart block, severe bradycardia. **CC:** Use can produce severe hepatocellular toxicity c̄ possible hepatic necrosis & death ▪ Extended use in pts c̄ cardiac failure requires caution ▪ Use can mask signs of hypoglycemia.

DOSAGE

Adult	*PO*	Usual starting dose 100mg bid. Usual maintenance dose 200-400mg bid
	IV	Repeated injection: 20mg by slow injection. Additional doses 40-80mg may be given at 10-m intervals until desired results or total 300mg injected. Usual infusion rate 2mg/m

SIDE/ADVERSE EFFECTS: CNS: *dizziness,* drowsiness, paresthesias, headache ▪ CV: edema, *bradycardia,* postural hypotension ▪ EENT: nasal stuffiness, vision disturbance ▪ GI: *N/V/D,* dyspepsia, pain, taste distortion ▪ GU: impotence, ejaculation inhibition, ***acute urinary bladder retention*** ▪ HEP: ***hepatic necrosis*** ▪ INT: rash ▪ RESP: dyspnea, ***bronchospasm*** ▪ Other: *fatigue.*

INTERACTIONS: Drug: Use c̄ β adrenergics will antagonize therapeutic effects ▪ Use c̄ halothane ↑ hypotensive effects of IV labetalol ▪ Use c̄ cimetidine will ↑ hypotensive effects due to greater labetalol bioavailability ▪ Use c̄

TCAs ↑ incidence of tremors ▪ Dosage adjustments may be required c̄ antidiabetic drugs.

NURSING MANAGEMENT PRIORITIES

ADMINISTRATION: Assess for hx of hypersensitivity ▪ Assess apical pulse; if <60/m hold drug, notify physician ▪ Assess respiratory function; do *not* administer if impaired ▪ PO: administer c̄ food ▪ IV: place pt in supine position, maintain for 3h; assess BP; prepare according to manufacturer's directions; administer direct (over 2m), use infusion-control device for continuous infusion ▪ Elderly may require ↓ dosage ▪ Avoid abrupt withdrawal; D/C gradually.

EVALUATION: Monitor VS, esp BP (lying/standing), heart rate (parenteral: q5-15m) ▪ Monitor I&O, daily weight ▪ Assess peripheral circulation ▪ Diabetics: closely monitor blood glucose (hypoglycemia) ▪ Assess for edema in extremities ▪ Monitor hepatic, CV, renal, hemopoietic status c̄ long-term use.

EDUCATION: Dizziness may occur; use caution in potentially hazardous activities ▪ Avoid changing positions (lying/sitting/standing) rapidly ▪ Procedure for checking radial pulse ▪ Check pulse before taking; if <60/m do *not* take drug, notify physician ▪ Take as ordered by physician, even if symptom free; do *not* change dose ▪ Take c̄ food to ↓ GI irritation ▪ Used to control, *not* cure hypertension ▪ Avoid use c̄ alcohol ▪ Avoid ↑ exercise, temperature extremes, smoking ▪ Notify physician of muscle cramps, difficult breathing, cold extremities, leg edema ▪ Keep scheduled appointments c̄ physician; have BP checked regularly ▪ Maintain optimum weight ▪ Avoid high-Na^+ foods (canned soups, lunch meats, cheese) ▪ Check c̄ physician/pharmacist before taking OTC preparations ▪ Notify physician/dentist of use before treatment ▪ Do *not* D/C drug w/out checking c̄ physician ▪ Carry medical identification (MedicAlert) if hypertensive.

NOTES:

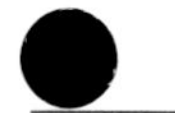

lansoprazole/omeprazole • (lan-so-prae-zol/oh-mep-ra-zol)

CATEGORY: *Antisecretory:* gastric acid pump inhibitor — Rx; Preg Cat B/C

BRAND NAMES	DOSAGE FORMS
lansoprazole	
Prevacid (TAP)	Delayed capsule: 15, 30mg
omeprazole	
Prilosec (Astra/Merck)	Delayed capsule: 20mg

USE: Short-term treatment of active duodenal ulcer ▪ Short-term treatment of active benign gastric ulcer ▪ Maintenance of healed duodenal ulcer ▪ Short-term treatment of severe erosive esophagitis (grade 2 or above) diagnosed by endoscopy ▪ Short-term treatment of esophagitis that does not respond well to H_2 blocker therapy ▪ Long-term treatment of Zollinger-Ellison syndrome, multiple endocrine adenomas, systemic mastocytosis (pathologic hypersecretory conditions) ▪ Treatment of gastroesophageal reflux disease (GERD) (omeprazole).

ACTION: Antisecretory activity due to blockage of final metabolic step of gastric acid synthesis (gastric acid pump inhibitor) by specific inhibition of the H^+, K^+ adenosine triphosphatase enzyme system w/in the gastric mucosa (secretory surface of gastric parietal cells). Drug exhibits no anticholinergic or H_2 blocking activity.

PHARMACOKINETICS

PO absorption	Peak	Half-life	Protein binding	Excretion
lansoprazole				
Rapid	1.7h	0.5-7.5h	97%	Via urine, feces as metabolites
omeprazole				
Rapid	0.5-3.5h	0.5-1h	95%	

CONTRAINDICATIONS: Hypersensitivity. **CC:** Long-term use may cause atrophic gastritis (omeprazole) ▪ Adequate response to treatment does not preclude gastric malignancy ▪ Not recommended for maintenance therapy in pts c̄ duodenal ulcers ▪ Efficacy for GERD >8wks of treatment not established (omeprazole) ▪ Use can produce dose-related gastric enterochromaffinlike (ECL) hyperplasia cell carcinoids in rats.

DOSAGE: Adult *PO*

lansoprazole

Active duodenal ulcer	15mg/d for 4-8wks
Active gastric ulcer	40mg/d for 4-8wks
Healed duodenal ulcer	15mg/d
Esophagilis	30mg/d up to 8wks

Hypersecretory conditions	60mg/d. Doses 120mg/d should be divided
omeprazole	
Active duodenal ulcer	20mg/d for 4-8wks
Esophagitis	20mg/d for 4-8wks
Hypersecretory condition	Individualized dosage starting 60mg once/d Doses of >80mg/d should be given in divided doses. Doses up to 120mg tid may be required
GERD	20mg/d for 4-8wks

SIDE/ADVERSE EFFECTS: CNS: anxiety, dream disorders, apathy, vertigo, insomnia, paresthesia ▪ CV: bradycardia, chest pain, tachycardia, peripheral edema ▪ EENT: taste perversion, tinnitus ▪ GI: anorexia, dry mouth, fecal discoloration, tongue mucosal atrophy ▪ GU: proteinuria, hematuria, glycosuria, testicular pain ▪ HEM: anemia, neutropenia, pancytopenia, ***thrombocytopenia*** ▪ INT: alopecia, dry skin, hyperhidrosis, pruritus, urticaria ▪ RESP: epistaxis, pharyngeal pain ▪ Other: fever, pain, abdominal swelling, weight gain.

INTERACTIONS: Drug: Use c̄ diazepam, phenytoin, warfarin may ↑ their effects ▪ Use c̄ sucralfate can ↓ lansoprazole absorption. **Lab:** ↑ In serum alkaline phosphatase, ALT, AST, creatinine.

NURSING MANAGEMENT PRIORITIES

ADMINISTRATION: Assess for hx of hypersensitivity ▪ Avoid exposure to moisture/light in storage ▪ Take in AM ac; swallow capsule whole, do *not* open ▪ May administer w/out regard to antacids.

EVALUATION: Monitor GI, hepatic, neurologic, renal status ▪ Monitor serum for ↑ creatinine, AST, ALT, alkaline phosphatase, total bilirubin ▪ Assess for reversible confusion in elderly/debilitated pts.

EDUCATION: Take in AM ac; swallow capsule whole ▪ Dizziness may occur; use caution in potentially hazardous activities ▪ Women: avoid breastfeeding ▪ Men: breast enlargement may occur ▪ Avoid smoking ▪ Avoid GI-irritating foods ▪ Check c̄ physician/pharmacist before taking OTC preparations ▪ Avoid anxiety-producing situations ▪ Take as ordered by physician ▪ Store in tightly closed, light-resistant container ▪ Notify physician *immediately* if experiencing diarrhea, black tarry stools, abdominal pain.

NOTES:

latanoprost • (lah-tan-oh-prost)

CATEGORY: *Antiglaucoma agent:* prostaglandin agonist Rx; Preg Cat C

BRAND NAME	**DOSAGE FORM**
Xalatan (Pharmacia)	Ophthalmic solution: 0.005%

USE: Treatment of open-angle glaucoma, ocular hypertension as a sole agent/in combination c̄ other antiglaucoma agents in pts c insufficient response &/or intolerance to other antiglaucoma agents. **ACTION:** ⬇ Of IOP due to ⬆ in aqueous humor outflow.

PHARMACOKINETICS

Onset	Duration	Half-life (serum)	Excretion
3-4h	8-12h	17m	Via urine primarily as metabolites

CONTRAINDICATIONS: Hypersensitivity. **CC:** Use can cause a slow iris color change to brown ▪ Remove contact lens before administration & 15m after administration to avoid absorption of benzalkonium chloride, which is present in the ophthalmic solution by the contact lenses ▪ Safety & efficacy not established for children.

DOSAGE

Adult	1 gtt (1.5µg) once daily in PM to affected eye(s)

SIDE/ADVERSE EFFECTS: Local: blurred vision, burning, conjunctival hyperemia ⬆ iris pigmentation, photophobia, tearing punctate, epithelial keratopathy, diplopia ▪ Other: systemic ocular absorption, URI infection, body pain, skin rash.

INTERACTIONS: Drug: Concurrent use c̄ ophthalmic solutions that contain the preservative, thimerosal, will cause precipitation c̄ latanoprost solution. To avoid rx, wait at least 5m between administration of the solutions.

NURSING MANAGEMENT PRIORITIES

ADMINISTRATION: Assess for hx of hypersenstiviity ▪ Wash hands thoroughly before administration ▪ Avoid contamination of solution, dropper tip ▪ Apply pressure to lacrimal sac 1-2m after instillation; instruct pt to keep eyes closed for 3-5m after insertion of gtt ▪ Avoid exposure to moisture/heat in storage ▪ Administer topical ophthalmic drugs at least 5m apart.

EVALUATION: Monitor IOP ▪ Monitor hepatic, CV, renal function; use caution if impaired ▪ Assess for signs of contact allergy (burning, itching), ocular dryness; D/C drug; notify physician.

EDUCATION: Dizziness, drowsiness, blurred vision may occur; avoid potentially hazardous activities ▪ Take as ordered by physician; do *not* ↑ dose ▪ Notify physician *immediately* of eye irritation; D/C drug ▪ Keep scheduled appointments $\bar{c}$ ophthalmologist ▪ Procedure for ophthalmic administration ▪ Women: avoid breastfeeding ▪ Iris color change may occur ▪ Avoid use $\bar{c}$ contact lenses.

NOTES:

letrozole • (let-roe-zol)

CATEGORY: *Antineoplastic:* nonsteroidal antiestrogenic agent Rx; Preg Cat D

BRAND NAME	DOSAGE FORM
Femara (Novarin)	Tablet: 2.5mg

USE: Treatment of advanced breast cancer c̄ progression following antiestrogen therapy in postmenopausal females. **ACTION:** Antineoplastic effect due to competitive inhibition of aromatase enzyme resulting in ↓ biosynthesis of adrenal androgens (androstenedione, testosterone) into estrogens (estradiol, estrone) in all body tissue, incl cancer tissue. ↓ Estrogen levels are obtained in 2-3d c̄ a subsequent regression in estrogen-dependent tumors. Drug has no effect on adrenal glucosteroid/mineralosteroid synthesis.

PHARMACOKINETICS

PO absorption	Half-life	Protein binding	Excretion
Complete	2d	Low	Via urine primarily as glucuronide conugates

CONTRAINDICATIONS: Hypersensitivity. **CC:** Use can result in transient ↓ in lymphocyte count ▪ Abnormalities occurred in liver function (about 3%).

DOSAGE

Adult	*PO*	2.5mg once/d until tumor regression is observed

SIDE/ADVERSE EFFECTS: CNS: dizziness, headache, somnolence ▪ CV: hypertension, peripheral edema ▪ GI: N/V/D, anorexia, dyspepsia, abdominal pain, constipation ▪ INT: pruritus, rash ▪ RESP: cough, dyspnea ▪ Other: fatigue, arthralgia, chest pain, hypercholesterolemia.

INTERACTIONS: None currently reported.

NURSING MANAGEMENT PRIORITIES

ADMINISTRATION: Check pt hx for recent course of radiation/antineoplastic agents ▪ Assess renal function; may require ↓ dosage if impaired ▪ Administer antiemetic before therapy ▪ Provide emotional support ▪ Avoid exposure to moisture/light in storage.

EVALUATION: Monitor hepatic, renal function; CBC, esp WBCs, platelets throughout therapy; notify physician if ↓ ▪ Assess for infection, bleeding, anemia ▪ Assess hydration status (I&O, daily weight).

EDUCATION: Store in dry, tightly closed, light-resistant container ▪ ↑ Fluid intake (8-10 glasses/d) ▪ Avoid exposure to infection ▪ Check c̄ physician before immunization (pt, family) ▪ Diet as tolerated; avoid spicy foods ▪ Maintain good oral hygiene; use soft-bristled toothbrush ▪ Notify physician of symptoms of bone marrow depression (fever, sore throat, bruising, bleeding, lethargy) ▪ Compliance c̄ prescribed dosage regimen ▪ Women: avoid breastfeeding ▪ Check c̄ physician/pharmacist before taking OTC preparations ▪ Use contraception if sexually active.

NOTES:

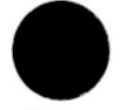

levodopa • (lee-voe-doe-pa)

CATEGORY: *Antiparkinsonian agent:* dopaminergic agonist Rx; Preg Cat NA

BRAND NAME
Larodopa (Roche)

DOSAGE FORMS
Capsule, tablet: 0.1, 0.5g

COMBINATION PRODUCTS

Sinemet 10/100, 25/100, 25/250, 50/200 (Du Pont)	Carbidopa/levodopa: 10mg/100mg, 25mg/100mg, 25mg/250mg, CR 25mg/100mg, 50mg/200mg

USE: Treatment of idiopathic, postencephalitic Parkinson's disease ▪ Treatment of symptomatic parkinsonism due to carbon monoxide poisoning, cerebral arteriosclerosis.
ACTION: Parkinson's disease related to ↓ levels of dopamine in corpus striatum. Levodopa enters CNS, is converted into dopamine in basal ganglia; concentration of dopamine ↑, symptoms of Parkinson's disease ↓. Carbidopa combined c̄ levodopa inhibits decarboxylation of levodopa; thus ↑ levels of levodopa available for transport to brain.

PHARMACOKINETICS

PO absorption	CNS transport	Half-life	Excretion
Good	1%	1h	80%-85% via urine w/in 24h

CONTRAINDICATIONS: Hypersensitivity, narrow-angle glaucoma, hx of melanoma/undiagnosed skin lesions, pt receiving MAO-I. **CC:** Use c̄ caution in presence of bronchial asthma & cardiovascular, endocrine, hepatic, pulmonary, renal disease ▪ Use can ↑ risk of bleeding in pts c̄ hx of peptic ulcers.

DOSAGE

Adult *PO*	Initial dose: 0.5-1g/d in ≥2 doses. ↑ Dose to 0.75g q3-7d as tolerated. Usual optimum dose should *not* exceed 8g
Sinemet 10/100	1 tablet 3-4 times/d. May ↑ to 8 tablets/d prn
Sinemet 25/100	1 tablet tid. May ↑ to 6 tablets/d prn
Sinemet 25/250	1 tablet 3-4 times/d if pt requires 1500mg/d of levodopa

SIDE/ADVERSE EFFECTS: CNS: *choreiform, dystonic, other involuntary movements;* headache, dizziness ▪ CV: cardiac irregularities, palpitations, orthostatic hypotension, phlebitis ▪ EENT: blurred vision ▪ HEM: ***hemolytic anemia, agranulocytosis*** ▪ PSYCH: delusions, agitation, anxiety, suicidal/psychotic episodes ▪ Other: dark urine/ sweat, hot flashes.

INTERACTIONS: Drug: Use c̄ MAO-I can produce hypertensive crisis ▪ Vitamin B_6 (pyridoxine), phenothiazine will antagonize effects of levodopa ▪ Use c̄ antihypertensives can produce additive hypotensive effects. **Food:** Consumption of liver, pork, wheat germ can ⬇ therapeutic effect.

NURSING MANAGEMENT PRIORITIES

ADMINISTRATION: Assess for hx of hypersensitivity ▪ Administer c̄ food ▪ Avoid exposure to moisture/light in storage ▪ Avoid abrupt withdrawal ▪ Elderly may require ⬇ dosage.

EVALUATION: Monitor CV, pulmonary, hepatic, renal status ▪ Monitor serum for ⬆ AST, ALT, BUN, LDH, bilirubin, alkaline phosphatase ▪ False + Coombs' test ▪ Urine glucose determinations inaccurate ▪ Assess for depression/ suicidal tendencies ▪ Monitor VS, esp BP.

EDUCATION: Take exactly as ordered by physician ▪ Full drug effects may require several mos ▪ Dizziness may occur on arising; change positions slowly ▪ Avoid preparations containing vitamin B_6 ▪ May darken urine/ sweat ▪ Maintain good personal hygiene (daily bath) ▪ Store in tightly closed, light-resistant container ▪ Take c̄ food ▪ Women: avoid breastfeeding ▪ Safety precautions c̄ ⬆ activity.

NOTES:

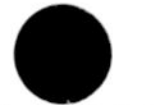

levothyroxine sodium (T_4) • (lee-voe-thye-rox-een)

CATEGORY: *Thyroid hormone*

Rx; Preg Cat A

BRAND NAMES	DOSAGE FORMS
**Eltroxin (Glaxo)*	Tablet: 50, 100, 150, 200, 300μg
Levothroid (Forest)	Injection (IM/IV): 200, 500 μg/vial Tablet: 25, 50, 75, 88, 100, 112, 125, 137, 150, 175, 200, 300μg
Synthroid (Knoll)	Injection (IM/IV): 200, 500μg/vial Tablet: 25, 50, 75, 88, 100, 112, 125, 150, 175, 200, 300μg

USE: Treatment of hypothyroidism ▪ Suppression of pituitary TSH in prevention/treatment of various types of goiters. **ACTION:** Thyroid hormones regulate general body metabolism by controlling cellular oxidative process; influence growth, tissue differentiation, maturation.

PHARMACOKINETICS

PO absorption	Half-life	Protein binding	Excretion
Up to 80%	6-7d	99%	Via urine, feces as metabolites

CONTRAINDICATIONS: Thyrotoxicosis, uncorrected adrenocortical deficiency, acute MI. **CC:** Not indicated for obesity; use as sole agent/in combination c̄ an anorexiant adrenergic can produce serious toxicity, which can be life threatening.

DOSAGE: Must be individualized. IM/IV can be substituted for PO if necessary.

Pediatric	*PO*	Suggested starting doses: 0-6mo: 8-10μg/kg/d 6-12mo: 6-8μg/kg/d 1-5y/o: 5-6μg/kg/d 6-12y/o: 4-5μg/kg/d >12y/o: 2-3μg/kg/d 11-20y/o: 3μg/kg/d
Adult	*PO*	Usual maintenance dose 50-200μg/d. For geriatric myxedematous infiltration c̄ cardiovascular dysfunction, starting dose 25μg/d suggested c̄ subsequent ⬆ at 3-4wks until desired effect is obtained

Note: Side/adverse effects: common in *italic;* serious in ***boldface italic.***

*Available in Canada only.

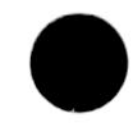

SIDE/ADVERSE EFFECTS: Usually limited to overdosage ▪ CNS: headache, insomnia, nervousness, tremors ▪ CV: angina, ***cardiac arrhythmias,*** palpitations, tachycardia ▪ GI: diarrhea ▪ Other: intolerance to heat; sweating, weight loss.

INTERACTIONS: Drug: Use c̄ epinephrine in pts c̄ coronary disease may induce coronary insufficiency ▪ Use c̄ PO anticoagulants will ↑ their activity, requires lower anticoagulant doses ▪ Use c̄ cholestyramine ↓ PO absorption of thyroid preparations ▪ Use in diabetic pts may require ↑ dosage of hypoglycemic agents.

NURSING MANAGEMENT PRIORITIES

ADMINISTRATION: Assess for hx of hypersensitivity ▪ Administer daily dose before breakfast ▪ Parenteral: reconstitute c̄ 5ml 0.9% NaCl injection (w/out preservative); shake well to dissolve; do *not* add to other IV fluids; discard unused portion ▪ Avoid exposure to moisture/ light in storage ▪ Elderly may require ↓ dosage.

EVALUATION: Monitor VS, esp heart rate ▪ Observe for signs of OD (chest pain, fever, nervousness, rapid/irregular heartbeat) ▪ Monitor thyroid function tests (T_3, T_4, TSH); evaluate pt use of iodine-containing substances before exam ▪ Diabetics: closely monitor blood glucose (hyperglycemia) ▪ May potentiate anticoagulant effect; assess for bleeding/bruising.

EDUCATION: Take as ordered by physician; do *not* change dose ▪ Avoid high-iodine foods (soybeans, cabbage, shellfish) ▪ Procedure for checking radial pulse ▪ Take pulse on arising qd; notify physician if ↑ /irregular; D/C drug ▪ Keep scheduled appointments for lab work/c̄ physician ▪ Do *not* change brand-name preparations ▪ Notify physician *immediately* of difficult breathing, chest pain, rapid/irregular heartbeat; D/C drug ▪ Check c̄ physician/pharmacist before taking OTC preparations ▪ Notify physician/dentist of use before treatment ▪ Store in dry, tightly closed, light-resistant container.

NOTES:

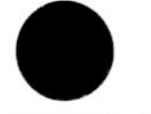

lidocaine hcl • (lye-doe-kane)

CATEGORY: *Antiarrhythmic:* local anesthetic

Rx; Preg Cat B

BRAND NAMES
LidoPen (Survival)
Xylocaine HCl (Astra)

DOSAGE FORMS
Injection (IM): 100mg/ml
Injection (IV): 10, 20, 40, 200mg/ml

Available in a wide array of preparations intended for local anesthesia.

USE: Treatment of acute ventricular arrhythmias occurring during MI/cardiac surgical procedures ▪ Local anesthetic.
ACTION: Antiarrhythmic effect due to depression of ventricular automaticity, depolarization; drug has no effect on atrial arrhythmias; local anesthetic effect due to reversible blocking of nerve conduction by undetermined mechanism.

CONTRAINDICATIONS: Hypersensitivity to amide-type local anesthetics, Stokes-Adams syndrome, Wolff-Parkinson-White syndrome, severe SA/AV intraventricular block. **CC:** Use requires constant ECG monitoring ▪ Use c̄ caution in presence of CHF, ⬇ cardiac output, elderly pts, digitalis toxicity c̄ AV blockage ▪ ⬇ Dosage or D/C c̄ exacerbation of arrhythmias.

DOSAGE

Pediatric	*IV*	Suggested bolus dose 0.5-1mg/kg. Usual maintenance infusion rate 10-50µg/kg/m
Adult	*IM*	4.3mg/kg; may be repeated after 60-90m
	IV	Initial bolus dose 50-100mg. May be repeated in 5m. Do *not* exceed 200-300mg over 1h. Usual maintenance infusion rate 1-4mg/m

PHARMACOKINETICS

Onset		Duration			
IV bolus	IM	IV bolus	IM	Protein binding	Excretion
45-90s	5-15m	10-20m	60-90m	60%-80%	Via urine, 90% as metabolites

SIDE/ADVERSE EFFECTS: CNS: ***twitching convulsions, respiratory depression/arrest***, drowsiness, dizziness, sensation of heat/cold, numbness, disorientation ▪ CV: ***hypotension, bradycardia*** (can induce cardiac arrest/CV collapse) ▪ EENT: blurred vision, tinnitus ▪ GI: vomiting.

INTERACTIONS: Drug: Use c̄ succinylcholine, other surgical muscle relaxants may ↑ neuromuscular blockage ▪ Use c̄ other antiarrhythmics ↑ effects ▪ Use c̄ β blockers, cimetidine ↑ lidocaine serum levels.

NURSING MANAGEMENT PRIORITIES

ADMINISTRATION: Assess for hx of amide-type local anesthetic/tocainide hypersensitivity ▪ IM: inject into deltoid muscle ▪ IV: dilute according to manufacturer's directions; administer bolus dose (over 60s), followed by infusion drip; use infusion-control device; cardiac monitoring; do *not* give c̄ epinephrine, preservatives ▪ Do *not* administer discolored/precipitated solutions ▪ Do *not* use solutions c̄ preservatives for spinal anesthesia ▪ Do *not* add to blood product infusions ▪ Discard solutions w/out preservatives after use ▪ Have emergency support equipment available ▪ Topical (PO): have pt swish in mouth, abstain from food for 60m ▪ Elderly may require ↓ dosage.

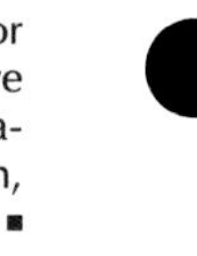

EVALUATION: Monitor VS, esp BP ▪ Monitor respiratory status; auscultate lungs ▪ Observe for neurotoxic effects (confusion, hallucinations, behavioral changes); notify physician, D/C drug ▪ Monitor serum levels of toxicity ▪ Therapeutic blood levels: 1.5-5μg/ml.

EDUCATION: Notify physician/nurse of abnormal rxs (difficult breathing, rash, tremors, lightheadedness, GI distress, blurred vision) ▪ Procedure for topical application.

NOTES:

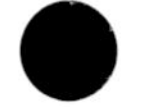

liothyronine sodium (T_3) • (lye-oh-thye-roe-neen)

CATEGORY: *Thyroid hormone* Rx; Preg Cat A

BRAND NAME
Cytomel (SKB)

DOSAGE FORMS
Tablet: 5, 25, 50µg

USE: Treatment of hypothyroidism ▪ Suppression of pituitary TSH in prevention/treatment of various types of goiters ▪ Diagnostic T_3 suppression test for hyperthyroidism.
ACTION: Thyroid hormones regulate general body metabolism by controlling cellular oxidative process; influence growth, tissue differentiation, maturation.

PHARMACOKINETICS

PO absorption	Half-life	Protein binding	Excretion
95%	2½d	99%	Via urine, feces

CONTRAINDICATIONS: Thyrotoxicosis, uncorrected adrenocortical deficiency, acute MI. **CC:** Not indicated for obesity; use as sole agent/in combination c̄ an anorexiant adrenergic can produce serious toxicity, which can be life threatening ▪ Extended use can result in adrenocortical insufficiency ▪ Use in myxedematous pts requires low starting doses.

DOSAGE: Must be individualized.

Cretinism *PO*	Start c̄ 5µg/d. ↑ By 5-µg increments q3-4d until desired effect is obtained
Infants	Usually require 20µg/d
1-3y/o	Usually require 50µg/d
>3y/o	May require full adult dose
Adult *PO*	
Mild hypothyroidism	Usual maintenance dose 25-75µg/d
Myxedema	Usual maintenance dose 50-100µg/d
Simple goiter	Usual dose 75µg/d
T_3 suppression test	75-100µg/d for 7d. Repeat
^{131}I uptake test	Hyperthyroidism, no significant change after 24h. Normal function, significant ↓ in ^{131}I uptake

SIDE/ADVERSE EFFECTS: Usually limited to overdosage; same as symptoms of hyperthyroidism ▪ CNS: headache, insomnia, nervousness, tremors ▪ CV: angina, ***cardiac arrhythmias***, palpitations, tachycardia ▪ GI: diarrhea ▪ Other: intolerance to heat; sweating, weight loss.

INTERACTIONS: Drug: Use c̄ epinephrine in pts c̄ coronary disease may induce coronary insufficiency ▪ Use c̄ PO anticoagulants ↑ their activity, requires lower anticoagulant doses ▪ Use c̄ cholestyramine ↓ PO absorption of thyroid preparations ▪ Use in diabetic pts may require ↑ dosage of hypoglycemic agents.

NURSING MANAGEMENT PRIORITIES

ADMINISTRATION: Assess for hx of hypersensitivity ▪ Administer daily dose before breakfast ▪ Avoid exposure to moisture/light in storage ▪ Elderly may require ↓ dosage.

EVALUATION: Monitor VS, esp heart rate ▪ Observe for signs of OD (chest pain, fever, nervousness, rapid/irregular heartbeat) ▪ Monitor thyroid function tests (T_3, T_4, TSH); evaluate pt use of iodine-containing substances before exam ▪ Diabetics: closely monitor blood glucose (hyperglycemia) ▪ May potentiate anticoagulant effect; assess for bleeding/bruising.

EDUCATION: Take as ordered by physician; do *not* change dose ▪ Avoid high-iodine foods (soybeans, cabbage, shellfish) ▪ Procedure for checking radial pulse ▪ Take pulse on arising qd; notify physician if ↑/irregular; D/C drug ▪ Keep scheduled appointments for lab work/c̄ physician ▪ Do *not* change brand-name preparations ▪ Notify physician *immediately* of difficult breathing, chest pain, rapid/irregular heartbeat; D/C drug ▪ Check c̄ physician/pharmacist before taking OTC preparations ▪ Notify physician/dentist of use before treatment ▪ Store in dry, tightly closed, light-resistant container.

NOTES:

lisinopril • (lye-sin-oh-pril)

CATEGORY: *Antihypertensive:* angiotensin inhibitor — Rx; Preg Cat C/D†

BRAND NAMES
Prinivil (MSD)
Zestril (Zeneca)

DOSAGE FORMS
Tablet: 5, 10, 20, 40mg
Tablet: 5, 10, 20mg

COMBINATION PRODUCTS
Prinzide (MSD) 12.5, 25
Zestoretic (Zeneca) 20/12.5, 20/25

lisinopril/hydrochlorothiazide per tablet: 20mg/12.5mg, 20mg/25mg

USE: Treatment of hypertension as sole agent/in combination c̄ other antihypertensives ▪ Adjunct for heart failure in pts not fully responding to dig & diuretics ▪ Treatment of acute MI in combination c̄ standard MI therapy. **ACTION:** Antihypertensive activity appears related to suppression of renin-angiotensin-aldosterone system by competitive inhibition of ACE, which produces angiotensin II from angiotensin I; this results in ↓ peripheral arterial resistance, aldosterone secretion.

CONTRAINDICATIONS: Hypersensitivity; hx of angioedema c̄ other ACE inhibitors. D/C during pregnancy as soon as possible. **CC:** Risk of anaphylactoid rxs, agranulocytoses, neutropenia c̄ use.

DOSAGE: Normal renal function

Adult *PO*	Initial dose of 10mg/d. Usual dosage range 20-40mg as a single dose/d
Heart failure	Start c̄ 5mg once/d. Usual range 5-20mg/d as single dose c̄ dig/diuretic
Combination product	Usual dose 1-2 tablets (20/12.5)/d or 1 tablet (20/25)/d

PHARMACOKINETICS

PO absorption	Onset	Peak	Half-life	Duration	Excretion
25%	1h	6-7h	12h	24h	As unchanged drug via urine

Note: Side/adverse effects; common in *italic;* serious in ***boldface italic.***

*Available in Canada only.
†1st trimester, C; 2nd & 3rd trimesters, D.

MI Start c̄ 5mg, then 5mg after 24h, 10mg after 48h, & thereafter 10mg/d

SIDE/ADVERSE EFFECTS: CNS: *headache, dizziness,* somnolence, paresthesias ▪ CV: hypotension, tachycardia, palpitations, chest pain, edema ▪ GI: N/V/D, pain, dyspepsia, flatulence, anorexia ▪ MET: gout ▪ INT: rash, pruritus ▪ REN: azotemia, acute renal failure ▪ RESP: bronchitis, sinusitis, pharyngeal pain, angioedema, nasal congestion, dyspnea ▪ Other: blurred vision, joint pain, muscle cramps, impotence, *fatigue.*

INTERACTIONS: Drug: Use c̄ diuretics may produce transient hypotension ▪ Indomethacin, other NSAIA may antagonize therapeutic effects ▪ Use K^+-sparing diuretics c̄ caution (hyperkalemia). **Lab:** ⬆ In liver enzymes & serum bilirubin.

NURSING MANAGEMENT PRIORITIES

ADMINISTRATION: Assess for hx of hypersensitivity ▪ Assess BP; notify physician of extremes ▪ Assess renal function; may require ⬇ dosage if impaired ▪ May crush, administer c̄ liquid; may be administered w/out regard to food ▪ Assess serum Na^+ (normal: 135-145mEq/L); notify physician of abnormalities ▪ Assess for rapid ⬇ in BP w/in 3h after administration of 1st dose (occurs c̄ hyponatremia) ▪ SLE, elderly may require ⬇ dosage ▪ Avoid abrupt withdrawal; D/C gradually.

EVALUATION: Monitor VS, esp BP ▪ Monitor CBC (esp WBC, differential) periodically during therapy ▪ Monitor electrolyte status (⬆ K^+; ⬇ Na^+) ▪ Monitor I&O, daily weight ▪ Assess for edema in extremities.

EDUCATION: Dizziness may occur; use caution in potentially hazardous activities ▪ Avoid changing positions (lying/sitting/standing) rapidly ▪ Notify physician of fever, sore throat, bruising/bleeding, swelling of feet/legs ▪ Take as ordered by physician, even if symptom free; do *not* skip doses ▪ May take w/out regard to food ▪ Do *not* D/C w/out notifying physician ▪ Check c̄ physician/pharmacist before taking OTC/Rx preparations ▪ Avoid high-Na^+ foods (canned soups, lunch meats, cheese) ▪ Avoid high-K^+ foods (bananas, citrus fruits, raisins) ▪ Check c̄ physician before using salt substitutes ▪ Avoid ⬆ exercise, temperature extremes, smoking ▪ Used to control, *not* cure, hypertension ▪ Maintain optimum weight ▪ Keep scheduled appointments c̄ physician; have BP checked at regular intervals ▪ Women: avoid breastfeeding ▪ Full drug effects may require several wks of therapy.

NOTES:

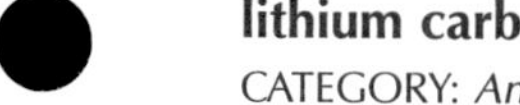

lithium carbonate/lithium citrate▲ • (li-thee-um)

CATEGORY: *Antimanic*

Rx; Preg Cat D

BRAND NAMES	DOSAGE FORMS
Cibalith-S (Ciba)▲	Syrup: 8mEq/5ml
Eskalith (SKB)	Capsule: 300mg
	CR tablet: 450mg
	Tablet: 300mg
Lithobid (Solvay)	Slow-release tablet: 300mg
Lithonate (Solvay)	Capsule: 300mg
Lithotabs (Solvay)	Tablet: 300mg

USE: Treatment of manic depressive illnesses. **ACTION:** Antimanic effect not determined; studies indicate that lithium ions alter Na^{+} transport in nerve cells, which effects shift in catecholamine metabolism; toxic levels of lithium close to therapeutic levels, tolerance greater during acute manic phase, ⬇ when symptoms subside; acute mania usually requires serum level 1.0-1.5mEq/L, desirable long-term maintenance levels 0.6-1.2mEq/L; accurate pt evaluation requires clinical & lab analysis.

PHARMACOKINETICS

PO absorption	Peak	Half-life	Excretion
95%-100%	0.5-3h	Initial 0.8-1.2h	Via urine

CONTRAINDICATIONS: No current absolute contraindications. **CC:** Therapeutic serum levels are close to toxic levels ▪ Use in pts c̄ severe cardiovascular or renal disease, dehydration, sodium depletion ⬆ risk of toxicity & is not generally recommended.

DOSAGE: Must be individualized.

Adult *PO* 600mg tid. Maintenance 900-1200mg/d

SIDE/ADVERSE EFFECTS: Dependent on serum levels; relatively few c̄ <1.5mEq/L; mild-moderate c̄ 1.5-2.5mEq/L; moderate-severe c̄ 2.0-2.5mEq/L ▪ CNS: drowsiness, blackout spells, slurred speech, epileptic-type seizures, psychomotor retardation, choreoathetotic movements ▪ CV: ***cardiac arrhythmias,*** hypotension, peripheral circulatory collapse, inversion of T-waves ▪ END: hypothyroidism ▪ GI: anorexia, N/V/D ▪ INT: alopecia, dry hair, chronic folliculitis, psoriasis ▪ Other: hyperactive deep tendon reflex.

INTERACTIONS: Drug: Use c̄ haloperidol can produce encephalopathic syndrome c̄ irreversible brain damage ▪ Use c̄ ACE-I, calcium blockers, thiazides ⬆ lithium toxicity ▪ Use c̄ NSAIAs ⬆ lithium serum levels ▪ Use c̄ iodine-containing substances ⬆ hypothyroid effect.

Note: Side/adverse effects: common in *italic;* serious in ***boldface italic.***

*Available in Canada only.

NURSING MANAGEMENT PRIORITIES

ADMINISTRATION: Assess for hx of hypersensitivity ▪ Administer c̄ meals; do *not* crush extended-release tablets ▪ Monitor optimum fluid intake (2-3L/d), Na^+ intake (6-10g/d) ▪ Do *not* mix/concurrently administer syrup c̄ other drugs ▪ Avoid exposure to heat/direct light in storage ▪ Elderly may require ↓ dosage.

EVALUATION: Monitor VS, esp BP ▪ Monitor WBC, ECG ▪ Monitor renal function (I&O, daily weight, urine specific gravity [normal: 1.005-1.025]) ▪ Assess for edema in extremities ▪ Diabetics: closely monitor blood glucose ▪ Monitor lithium blood levels 2 times/wk during treatment, q2-3mos when stabilized ▪ Therapeutic blood levels: 1.0-1.5mEq/L; maintenance, 0.6-1.2mEq/L.

EDUCATION: Dizziness/drowsiness may occur; use caution in potentially hazardous activities ▪ Take as ordered by physician; do *not* ↑ dose ▪ ↑ Fluid intake (10-12 glasses/d) ▪ Maintain normal Na^+ intake (6-10g/d) ▪ Diabetics: closely monitor blood/urine glucose ▪ Take c̄ meals; swallow extended-release tablets whole ▪ Avoid caffeinated beverages, ↑ exercise, hot climates, saunas ▪ Keep scheduled appointments c̄ physician/for blood work ▪ Notify physician of symptoms of toxicity (dizziness, blurred vision, trembling, poor coordination) ▪ Women: avoid breastfeeding ▪ Full drug effects may require several wks of therapy.

NOTES:

loperamide hcl • (loe-per-a-mide)

CATEGORY: *Antidiarrheal agent* Rx/OTC▲

BRAND NAMES	DOSAGE FORMS
Imodium (Janssen)	Capsule: 2mg
Imodium A-D▲ (McNeil)	Caplet▲: 2mg
	Liquid▲: 1mg/5ml
Kaopectate II▲ (Upjohn)	Caplet: 2mg
Maalox Antidiarrheal▲ (RPR)	Tablet: 2mg
Pepto Diarrhea Control (P G)	Liquid: 1mg/5ml

USE: Rx: Adjunct in treatment of acute nonspecific diarrhea, chronic diarrhea associated c̄ inflammatory bowel disease ▪ ↓ Ileostomy discharge volume ▪ OTC: Control of diarrhea, incl diarrhea in travelers. **ACTION:** Antidiarrheal effect due to slowing of intestinal motility by direct effect on muscular peristalsis.

PHARMACOKINETICS

PO absorption	Peak	Half-life	Excretion
Adequate	2.5-5h	9.1-14.4h	Primarily via feces as metabolites

CONTRAINDICATIONS: Hypersensitivity, when constipation is contraindicated. **CC:** Use c̄ acute dysentery not indicated.

DOSAGE

Pediatric	*PO*	2.5y/o: 1mg tid d1, followed by 1mg/10kg only after loose stool
		5-8y/o: 2mg bid d1, followed by 1mg/10kg only after loose stool
		8-12y/o: 2mg tid d1, followed by 1mg/10kg only after loose stool
Adult	*PO*	Initial dose 4mg, followed by 2mg after each unformed stool. Do *not* exceed 16mg/d. Usual maintenance dose in chronic diarrhea 4-8mg/d

SIDE/ADVERSE EFFECTS: CNS: drowsiness, dizziness ▪ GI: *N/V, abdominal pain*/distention, constipation, dry mouth ▪ INT: skin rash ▪ Other: tiredness.

INTERACTIONS: Drug: Use c̄ other drugs ↑ their PO absorption.

NOTES:

NURSING MANAGEMENT PRIORITIES

ADMINISTRATION: Assess for hx of hypersensitivity ▪ Assess F/E balance; do *not* administer if severely impaired ▪ Assess hepatic function; ↓ dosage if impaired.

EVALUATION: Monitor bowel function; ↓ dose as diarrhea is controlled ▪ Assess hydration status (I&O, daily weight) ▪ Check for signs of abdominal distention; D/C drug ▪ Monitor children, elderly closely (↑ susceptibility to adverse effects).

EDUCATION: Follow clear liquid/bland diet until diarrhea subsides ▪ Take as directed by physician; do *not* ↑ dose ▪ Dizziness/drowsiness may occur; use caution in potentially hazardous activities ▪ Avoid use c̄ alcohol, CNS depressants ▪ Notify physician if diarrhea persists >48h, fever occurs ▪ Maintain fluid intake (6-8 glasses/d) ▪ Use sugarless gum/hard candy to diminish dry mouth.

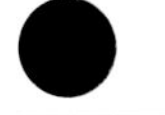

loracarbef • (loe-rah-kar-behf)

CATEGORY: *Antibiotic:* carbacephem, β-lactam Rx; Preg Cat B

BRAND NAME
Lorabid (Lilly)

DOSAGE FORMS
Capsules 200mg, powder for PO suspension 100mg/5ml

USE: Treatment of respiratory infections including bronchitis (acute secondary bacterial or exacerbation of chronic), pneumonia, pharyngitis, sinusitis & tonsillitis, otitis media, uncomplicated skin/skin structure, uncomplicated pyelonephritis caused by susceptible strains of *Escherichia coli, Haemophilus influenzae, Moraxella catarrhalis, Staphylococcus aureus, S. saprophyticus, Streptococcus pyogenes.* **ACTION:** Bactericidal activity due to inhibition of mucopeptide cell wall synthesis in susceptible organisms. Exhibits good resistance to β lactamase produced by various bacterial strains.

PHARMACOKINETICS

PO absorption	Peak	Half-life	Protein binding	Excretion
90%	0.8-1h	1h	25%	Over 90% unchanged via urine

CONTRAINDICATIONS: Hypersensitivity to drug or cephalosporin-type antibiotics. **CC:** Cross-allergenicity can exist c̄ cephalosporins, penicillins, other β-lactam antibiotics ▪ Use can produce pseudomembranous colitis.

DOSAGE

Adult (≥13y/o)	*PO*	Usual dose 200-400mg q12h for 7-10d. Uncomplicated cystitis 200mg q24h for 7d. Pneumonia & uncomplicated pyelonephritis 400mg q12h for 14d
Pediatric (6mo-12y/o)	*PO*	Pharyngitis/tonsillitis, impetigo 15mg/kg/d q12h in divided doses for 7-10d. Acute otitis media 30mg/kg/d q12h in divided doses for 10d

SIDE/ADVERSE EFFECTS: CNS: headache (2.9%), dizziness, nervousness ▪ GI: diarrhea (4.1%), nausea (1.9%), pain (1.4%), anorexia ▪ GU: vaginitis (1.3%) ▪ INT: ***erythema multiforme,*** pruritus, urticaria ▪ MET: ↑ in SGPT,

Note: Side/adverse effects: common in *italic;* serious in ***boldface italic.***

*Available in Canada only.

SGOT, alkaline phosphate, BUN ▪ Other: vasodilation, transient thrombocytopenia, leuokopenia.

INTERACTIONS: Drug: Bacteriostatic antibiotics can antagonize bactericidal activity ▪ Use c̄ PO anticoagulants may ↑ their activity ▪ Use c̄ probenecid will ↓ renal excretion.

NURSING MANAGEMENT PRIORITIES

ADMINISTRATION: Assess for hx of cephalosporin/penicillin hypersensitivity ▪ Obtain C&S before therapy ▪ Assess renal status; ↓ dosage if impaired ▪ Administer 1h ac/2h pc c̄ full glass H_2O at evenly spaced intervals ▪ PO suspension: shake well before using ▪ Use caution c̄ aspirin/anticoagulants ▪ Do *not* administer c̄ alcohol-containing substances.

EVALUATION: Monitor VS, esp temperature ▪ Observe for signs of superinfection (diarrhea, perineal itching, oral ulcers) ▪ Assess for bleeding, monitor bleeding time; administer vitamin K as ordered ▪ Monitor CBC, renal function ▪ Urine glucose: false + c̄ Clinitest; use Clinistix/Diastix.

EDUCATION: Complete full course of therapy ▪ Take on empty stomach at equal intervals around clock to maintain blood levels ▪ Diarrhea may occur; if prolonged, notify physician ▪ Avoid use c̄ alcohol ▪ Report signs of bleeding *immediately* ▪ PO suspension: refrigerate; shake well before use ▪ Store in dry, tightly closed container ▪ Discard outdated preparations ▪ Maintain good personal hygiene, esp perineal, oral ▪ ↑ Fluid intake (8-10 glasses/d) ▪ Use Clinistix/Diastix for urine testing ▪ Notify physician of symptoms of allergic rx (fever, difficult breathing, rash) ▪ Women: avoid breastfeeding ▪ Carry identification (MedicAlert) if cephalosporin allergic.

NOTES:

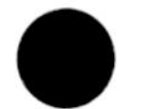

lorazepam/oxazepam • (lor-az-e-pam/ox-az-e-pam)

CATEGORY: *Benzodiazepine:* antianxiety agent, anxiolytic — Rx C-IV; Preg Cat D

BRAND NAMES	DOSAGE FORMS
lorazepam	
Ativan (W-A)	Injection (IM/IV): 1, 2, 4mg/ml Tablet: 0.5, 1, 2mg
**Novolorazem (Novopharm)*	Tablet: 1, 2mg
oxazepam	
**Ox-Pam (ICN)*	Tablet: 10, 15, 30mg
Serax (Wyeth)	Capsule: 10, 15, 30mg Tablet: 15mg
**Zapex (Riva)*	Tablet: 10, 15, 30mg

USE: Treatment of anxiety ▪ Treatment of insomnia, preop sedation (lorazepam) ▪ Treatment of alcohol withdrawal (oxazepam). **ACTION:** Benzodiazepines appear to potentiate the inhibitory effects of gamma aminobutyric acid in central-mediated neurotransmission ▪ Anxiolytic activity due to depression of CNS at brainstem formation, limbic, thalamic areas.

PHARMACOKINETICS

PO absorption	Peak	Half-life	Protein binding	Excretion
lorazepam				
Rapid	2h	12h	85%	Via urine as metabolites
oxazepam				
Good	3h	8.2h	NA	Via urine as metabolites

CONTRAINDICATIONS: Hypersensitivity, narrow-angle glaucoma (lorazepam). **CC:** Risk of physical, psychologic dependence ▪ Lorazepam IV injection must be diluted c̄ an equal amount of diluent ▪ Benzodiazepines are not indicated for psychiatric disorders, esp when anxiety is not a significant symptom.

DOSAGE

lorazepam

Adult

Anxiety	*PO*	2-3mg 2-3 times/d
Insomnia	*PO*	2-4mg at hs

Note: Side/adverse effects: common in *italic;* serious in ***boldface italic.***

*Available in Canada only.

Preop	*IM*	0.05mg/kg to a maximum 4mg
	IV	2-4mg
oxazepam	*PO*	
Adult		
Alcoholism		15-30mg 3-4 times/d
Anxiety		10-15mg 3-4 times/d. Severe cases 15-30mg 3-4 times/d
Geriatric		10mg tid. May ↑ to 15mg 3-4 times/d

SIDE/ADVERSE EFFECTS: CNS: *drowsiness, fatigue, ataxia* ▪ CV: hypotension ▪ HEM: neutropenia (rare) ▪ PSYCH: paradoxic anxiety, hallucinations, hyperexcited states.

INTERACTIONS: Drug: Use c̄ other CNS depressants produces additive effects ▪ Use c̄ MAO-I can produce serious toxic effects.

NURSING MANAGEMENT PRIORITIES

ADMINISTRATION: Assess for hx of benzodiazepine hypersensitivity ▪ Do *not* mix/dilute parenteral preparations (incompatibility); discard discolored/precipitated solution ▪ IM: inject *deep, slowly* into large muscle mass ▪ IV: assess respirations before each dose; administer *slowly* (5mg/ml); keep pt recumbent for 8h ▪ Avoid exposure to heat/moisture/light in storage; avoid plastic for storage of parenteral preparations ▪ Avoid abrupt withdrawal ▪ Have emergency support measures available ▪ Elderly may require ↓ dosage ▪ Problem discussion, sympathetic listening contributes to relief of anxiety.

EVALUATION: Monitor renal, hepatic status ▪ Assess for symptoms of abrupt withdrawal (tremors, abdominal/muscle cramps, convulsions) c̄ prolonged use ▪ Check for signs of dependence (↑ drug request) ▪ Monitor activity status (safety precautions) ▪ Assess for tolerance to therapeutic dose ▪ Assess for paradoxic rxs (CNS stimulation), esp in elderly ▪ Check for depression; suicide precautions prn.

EDUCATION: Drowsiness may occur; use caution in potentially hazardous activities ▪ Avoid use c̄ alcohol, CNS depressants ▪ Indiscriminate use may lead to dependence ▪ Do *not* keep at bedside ▪ Take as ordered by physician, even if symptom free; do *not* ↑ dose ▪ Women: avoid breastfeeding ▪ Check c̄ physician/pharmacist before taking OTC preparations ▪ Practice relaxation exercises, ventilation of feelings.

NOTES:

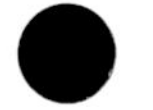

losartan potassium/valsartan • (low-sar-tan/val-sar-tan)

CATEGORY: *Antihypertensive:* angiotensin II antagonist Rx; Preg Cat C/D[†]

BRAND NAMES	**DOSAGE FORMS**
losartan	
Cozaar (Merck)	Tablet: 25, 50mg
valsartan	
Diovan (Novartis)	Capsule: 80, 160mg

COMBINATION PRODUCT

Hyzaar (Merck)	losartan 50mg/hydrochlorothiazide: 12.5mg/tablet

USE: Treatment of hypertension as sole agent/in combination c̄ other antihypertensives. **ACTION:** Antihypertensive effect due to suppression of angiotensin II, a potent vasoactive hormone in renin-angiotensin-aldosterone system, by selectively blocking effects of angiotensin II on angiotensin II receptors (AT_1), resulting in ↓ peripheral arterial resistance, ↓ aldosterone secretion. Drug does not block conversion of angiotensin I by ACE into angiotensin II, has little affinity for angiotensin II (AT_2), receptors. Maximum antihypertensive effects occur in 3-6wks.

PHARMACOKINETICS

PO absorption	Peak	Half-life	Protein binding	Excretion
losartan				
Good	1-4h	2-9h	98%	Via urine, feces
valsartan				
Good	2-4h	6h	95%	Via urine, feces

CONTRAINDICATIONS: Hypersensitivity. **CC:** African Americans do not respond to treatment as well as non-African Americans (losartan) ▪ D/C during pregnancy as soon as possible ▪ Correct volume-depleted conditions before use of losartan or initiate c̄ ↓ dosage ▪ Use c̄ caution c̄ impaired hepatic function. ▪ Safety & efficacy in pts <18y/o not established.

DOSAGE: Adult *PO*

losartan	Initial dose of 50mg once/d, 25mg c̄ diuretic or intravascular volume depletion. Usual range: 25-100mg/d
Hyzaar	Usual dose 1 tablet/d

Note: Side/adverse effects: common in *italic;* serious in ***boldface italic.***

*Available in Canada only.
†1st trimester, C; 2nd & 3rd trimesters, D.

valsartan Initial dose of 80mg once/d in absence of volume depletion. Adjust according to response c̄ a range of 80-320mg/d

SIDE/ADVERSE EFFECTS: CNS: *dizziness*, insomnia ▪ GI: abdominal pain, diarrhea, dyspepsia, dry mouth ▪ RESP: sinus disorders, *URI*, nasal congestion ▪ Other: facial edema, muscle cramps, back pain.

INTERACTIONS: Drug: Use c̄ cimetidine can ↑ losartan levels ▪ Use c̄ phenobarbital can ↓ losartan levels. **Lab:** ↑ Liver enzyme, bilirubin. **Food:** Meals slow down PO absorption.

NURSING MANAGEMENT PRIORITIES

ADMINISTRATION: Assess for hx hypersensitivity ▪ Assess BP; notify physician of extremes ▪ Assess renal function; may require ↓ dosage if impaired & volume depleted ▪ Diuretics may be D/C for 2-3d before beginning drug to avoid hypotension ▪ Administer consistently c̄ or w/out food ▪ Assess serum Na^+ (normal: 135-145mEq/L) ▪ Assess for rapid ↓ in BP w/in 3h after administration of first dose (c̄ hyponatremia) ▪ Avoid abrupt withdrawal; D/C gradually.

EVALUATION: Monitor VS, esp BP ▪ Monitor CBC (esp WBC, differential) throughout therapy ▪ Monitor electrolyte status (↑K^+, ↓Na^+) ▪ Monitor I&O, daily weight ▪ Monitor renal function (proteinuria); notify physician ▪ Assess for edema in extremities.

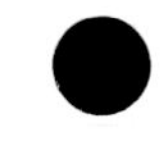

EDUCATION: Dizziness may occur; use caution in potentially hazardous activities ▪ Avoid changing positions (lying/sitting/standing) rapidly ▪ Notify physician of fever, sore throat, bruising/bleeding, swelling of feet/legs ▪ Take as ordered by physician even if symptom free; do *not* skip doses ▪ Take consistently c̄ or w/out food ▪ Do not D/C w/out notifying physician ▪ Check c̄ physician/pharmacist before taking OTC/Rx preparations ▪ Avoid high-Na^+ foods (canned soups, lunch meats, cheese) ▪ Avoid high-K^+ foods (bananas, citrus juices, raisins) ▪ Check c̄ physician/pharmacist before using salt substitutes ▪ Avoid ↑ exercise, temperature extremes, smoking ▪ Used to control, *not* cure, hypertension ▪ Maintain optimum weight ▪ Keep scheduled appointments c̄ physician; have BP checked regularly ▪ Women: notify physician of pregnancy possibility; avoid breastfeeding ▪ Full drug effects may require several wks of therapy.

NOTES:

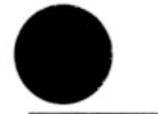

loxapine hcl▲/succinate • (lox-a-peen)

CATEGORY: *Antipsychotic:* tricyclic antipsychotic, neuroleptic Rx; Preg Cat NA

BRAND NAMES
**Loxapac (W-A)*
Loxitane (Lederle)
Loxitane C (Lederle)
Loxitane IM (Lederle)

DOSAGE FORMS
Tablet: 5, 10, 25, 50mg
Capsule: 5, 10, 25, 50mg
PO concentrate▲: 25mg/ml
Injection: 50mg/ml▲

USE: Treatment of psychotic disorders. **ACTION:** Antipsychotic mechanism not established.

SIDE/ADVERSE EFFECTS: CNS: drowsiness, extrapyramidal rxs, tardive dyskinesia ▪ CV: hypotension, tachycardia, hypertension, syncope ▪ EENT: nasal congestion ▪ GI: dry mouth, constipation ▪ GU: urinary retention ▪ INT: dermatitis, seborrhea, photosensitivity, phototoxicity.

INTERACTIONS: Drug: Use c̄ other CNS depressants produces additive depression.

PHARMACOKINETICS

PO absorption	Onset	Peak	Duration	Half-life	Excretion
Complete	20-30m	1.5-3h	12h	5-19h	50% via urine, feces w/in 24h

CONTRAINDICATIONS: Hypersensitivity, coma, presence of large amounts of CNS depressants. **CC:** Use can result in extrapyramidal symptoms, tardive dyskinesia, neuroleptic malignant syndrome.

DOSAGE

Adult	*PO*	Initial dose 10mg bid. Usual maintenance dose 20-100mg/d. Do *not* exceed 250mg/d
	IM	12.5-50mg q4-6h or longer for control

NURSING MANAGEMENT PRIORITIES

ADMINISTRATION: Assess for hx of amoxapine hypersensitivity ▪ Assess for VS, esp BP ▪ Assess IOP, renal function ▪ PO concentrate: dilute before administration c̄ >60ml orange/grapefruit juice; use manufacturer's dropper to measure dose ▪ IM: inject *slowly, deep* into UOQ of buttock; keep pt lying down for ½h after injection ▪ Avoid SC/IV injection ▪ Discard markedly discolored/precipitated solutions ▪ Avoid exposure to moisture/light

Note: Side/adverse effects: common in *italic;* serious in ***boldface italic.***

*Available in Canada only.

in storage; do *not* freeze liquid forms ▪ Avoid abrupt withdrawal; D/C gradually ▪ Maintain hydration ▪ Elderly/debilitated pts may require ↓ dosage.

EVALUATION: Monitor hepatic, ophthalmic, renal status ▪ Monitor BP, CBC ▪ Monitor fluid retention (I&O, daily weight) ▪ Assess for extrapyramidal symptoms (tics/spasms, trembling, shuffling gait) ▪ Seizure precautions in pts c̄ hx of convulsive disorders ▪ Long-term therapy: assess for jaundice, agranulocytosis ▪ Assess for symptoms of abrupt withdrawal (nausea, dyskinesia, trembling, dizziness) ▪ Assess IOP.

EDUCATION: Dizziness/drowsiness may occur; use caution in potentially hazardous activities ▪ Avoid changing positions (lying/sitting/standing) rapidly ▪ Avoid use c̄ alcohol, CNS depressants ▪ Take PO forms c̄ meals ▪ Store in tightly closed, light-resistant container ▪ Use sugarless gum/hard candy to diminish dry mouth ▪ Maintain fluid intake (6-8 glasses/d) ▪ Avoid exposure to direct sunlight, UV light (sunlamps) ▪ Notify physician of fever, sore throat, bruising/bleeding ▪ Notify physician of extrapyramidal symptoms (tics/spasm, trembling, shuffling gait) ▪ Avoid ↑ exercise, temperature extremes ▪ Take as directed by physician ▪ Avoid smoking ▪ Take antacid/antidiarrheal preparations at least 1h before/after drug ▪ Check c̄ physician/pharmacist before taking OTC preparations ▪ Scheduled periodic eye exams ▪ Procedure for PO concentrate administration.

NOTES:

magnesium sulfate (injection) • (mag-nee-zhum sul-fate)

CATEGORY: *Anticonvulsant* Rx; Preg Cat A

AVAILABLE PREPARATIONS
Magnesium sulfate (various)

DOSAGE FORMS
Injection (IM/IV): 10, 12.5, 50%

USE: Anticonvulsant for seizures associated c̄ epilepsy, pregnancy induced hypertension ▪ Treatment of Mg deficiency. **ACTION:** Anticonvulsant activity due to inhibition of peripheral neuromuscular transmission.

PHARMACOKINETICS

	Onset	Duration	Excretion
IV	Immediate	30m	Via urine
IM	1h	3-4h	Via urine

CONTRAINDICATIONS: Heart block/myocardial damage (parenteral), severe renal impairment. **CC:** Use c̄ caution in presence of renal insufficiency ▪ Do not administer w/in 2h before delivery in toxemic pregnant women.

DOSAGE

Anticonvulsant		
Pediatric	*IM*	20-40mg/kg
Adult	*IM*	1-5g prn
	IV	1-4g
	Infusion	4g in 250ml 5% dextrose at <3ml/m
Cerebral edema		To 2.5g IV
Mg deficiency		
Pediatric		2-10mEq/d
Adult		4-24mEq/d

SIDE/ADVERSE EFFECTS: CNS: depression of deep tendon reflexes ▪ CV: hypotension, depressed cardiac function, circulatory collapse ▪ GI: diarrhea ▪ INT: sweating, flushing ▪ RESP: respiratory depression.

INTERACTIONS: Drug: Use c̄ CNS depressants may ↑ effects ▪ Use c̄ great caution in dig pts.

NURSING MANAGEMENT PRIORITIES

ADMINISTRATION: IM: do *not* exceed 50% solution in adults; 1% procaine may be added to ⬇ injection pain; *deep* gluteal injection ▪ IV: do *not* exceed 20% solution, 150mg/m ▪ Assess patellar reflex (knee jerk); hold dose until positive response obtained ▪ Assess respirations; do *not* administer if <16/m ▪ Institute seizure precautions ▪ Do *not* administer discolored/precipitated solutions ▪ Do *not* leave pt unattended ▪ Place pt in left lateral position if pregnant ▪ Assess urinary output (>25ml/h) ▪ Have emergency support equipment available ▪ Avoid abrupt withdrawal ▪ Provide emotional support.

EVALUATION: Monitor CV, renal status ▪ Monitor BP continuously ▪ Monitor serum Mg^{++} levels ▪ Observe for seizure activity; record details (duration, characteristics, pt response) ▪ Monitor respirations (toxicity: <16/m) ▪ Assess patellar reflex; notify physician if hyporeflexic ▪ Monitor urinary output ▪ Assess neonate for Mg^{++} toxicity ▪ Therapeutic serum Mg^{++} concentration: 4-6mEq/L.

EDUCATION: Explain procedure, rationale to pt, family ▪ Safety precautions ▪ Comfort measures.

OVERDOSE MANAGEMENT: Symptoms: hypotension, ⬇ respirations/respiratory paralysis, absence of deep tendon reflexes, ⬇ fetal heart rate ▪ Treatment: administer IV 10ml 10% aqueous solution calcium gluconate over 3m; *Warning*—do *not* give to dig pts (arrhythmias may occur) ▪ Emergency artificial ventilation may be necessary.

NOTES:

mannitol • (man-i-tole)

CATEGORY: *Osmotic diuretic:* urogenital irrigant   Rx; Preg Cat C

BRAND NAMES
Osmitrol (Baxter)
Resectisol Irrigation (Kendall McGaw)

DOSAGE FORMS
Injection (IV): 5, 10, 15, 20%
Solution: 5%

USE: Promotion of diuresis in oliguric phase of acute renal failure ▪ ↓ IOP, vitreous volume before surgery ▪ ↓ ICP, treatment of cerebral edema ▪ Forced excretion of toxic substances ▪ GU irrigant for transurethral surgical procedures. **ACTION:** Diuresis due to ↑ in osmotic pressure of glomerular filtrate, which inhibits tubular reabsorption of H_2O solutes, producing rapid urinary excretion.

PHARMACOKINETICS

Onset	Duration	Half-life	Excretion
30-60m	3-8h	100m	Via urine primarily as unchanged drug

CONTRAINDICATIONS: Hypersensitivity, anuria, severe dehydration/pulmonary congestion, cerebral hemorrhage, severe cardiac/renal dysfunction after institution of therapy. **CC:** Use can result in F/E imbalance ▪ Possible exacerbation of existing hypovolemia ▪ Transurethral irrigating solution must be clear c̄ an unbroken seal.

DOSAGE: Should be administered at rate to produce satisfactory urine flow.

Adult *IV infusion rates*

Renal failure	50-200g/d
ICP	1.5-2g/kg over 30-60m
IOP	1.5-2g/kg over 30-60m
Toxic substances	Suggested loading dose 25g followed by infusion rate to produce at least 100ml/h urine flow
Transurethral irrigation	2.5%-5% solution as required

SIDE/ADVERSE EFFECTS: CNS: headache, ***convulsions*** ▪ CV: anginalike chest pains, edema, ***thrombocytopenia, F/E imbalance***, tachycardia, hypotension, hypertension ▪ EENT: blurred vision ▪ GI: N/V ▪ RESP: ***pulmonary congestion*** ▪ Other: chills, fever.

INTERACTIONS: Drug: Use c̄ lithium salts may ↑ their urinary excretion.

NURSING MANAGEMENT PRIORITIES

ADMINISTRATION: Assess renal function; administer test dose if severely impaired ▪ Use in-line filter for concentrations >15% ▪ Do *not* use crystallized solutions; dissolve according to manufacturer's directions ▪ Do *not* mix c̄ blood components in same IV line ▪ Insert indwelling urinary catheter per physician's order ▪ Follow established guidelines for minimum/maximum rate of infusion, desired urinary output.

EVALUATION: Monitor VS, esp BP, respirations ▪ Monitor I&O, urine specific gravity, CVP qh; daily weight ▪ Monitor serum electrolytes (Na^+, K^+, Cl^-) ▪ Check IV site carefully; avoid extravasation ▪ Monitor for signs of ↑ extracellular fluid volume, esp 8-12h postinfusion for rebound fluid overload.

EDUCATION: Avoid changing positions (lying/sitting/standing) rapidly ▪ Urinary catheter inserted for hourly output determinations.

NOTES:

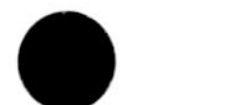

maprotiline hcl • (ma-proe-ti-leen)

CATEGORY: *Tetracyclic antidepressant:* mood elevator — Rx; Preg Cat B

BRAND NAME
Ludiomil (C-G)

DOSAGE FORMS
Tablet: 25, 50, 75mg

USE: Treatment of depressive neurosis (dysthymic disorder), manic depressive states ▪ Treatment of anxiety associated c̄ depression. **ACTION:** Antidepressant activity appears related to inhibition of norepinephrine reuptake in central adrenergic neurons; drug is tetracyclic, extremely close to tricyclic drugs.

PHARMACOKINETICS

PO absorption	Peak	Half-life	Protein binding	Excretion
Slow but complete	8-24h	51h	88%	60%-70% via urine, 30% via feces as metabolites

CONTRAINDICATIONS: Hypersensitivity, MAO-I therapy, MI (acute recovery period), glaucoma. **CC:** Use can cause seizures ▪ Use c̄ extreme caution c̄ a hx or presence of cardiovascular disorders.

DOSAGE

Adult	*PO*	75-225mg/d
Geriatric	*PO*	50-75mg/d

SIDE/ADVERSE EFFECTS: CNS: *drowsiness,* dizziness, headache, incoordination, tremors, extrapyramidal symptoms, paresthesia (extremities), insomnia, seizures ▪ CV: ***arrhythmias,*** MI, stroke, ***heart block,*** postural hypotension ▪ GI: anorexia, N/V/D, stomatitis, cramps, black tongue, dry mouth, constipation ▪ GU: gynecomastia, testicular swelling, galactorrhea, breast enlargement, urinary hesitancy ▪ HEM: ***agranulocytosis,*** eosinophilia, ***thrombocytopenia*** ▪ HEP: cholestatic jaundice ▪ INT: skin rash, photosensitivity, alopecia ▪ PSYCH: disorientation, delusions, hallucinations, exacerbation of psychosis, confusion ▪ Other: parotid swelling.

INTERACTIONS: Drug: Significant depressant effects c̄ alcohol ▪ Use c̄ anticholinergics, chlorpromazine may produce ↑ atropinelike effects; paralytic ileus could occur ▪ Significant ↑ in activity c̄ epinephrine, levarterenol, other adrenergic agents ▪ Significant antagonism to effects of reserpine, clonidine, guanethidine-type antihypertensives ▪ Use c̄ MAO-I best avoided.

NURSING MANAGEMENT PRIORITIES

ADMINISTRATION: Assess for hx of TCA hypersensitivity ▪ Assess for hx of glaucoma, prostatic hypertrophy, renal/hepatic disease; may require ↓ dosage ▪ PO: administer as single dose/d at hs c̄ food ▪ Institute safety precautions ▪ Institute suicide precautions ▪ Dosage is ↑ *slowly*; maintenance dose is lowest dose that will maintain remission of depression ▪ Avoid abrupt withdrawal; D/C gradually ▪ Heavy smokers may require ↑ dosage ▪ Elderly may require ↓ dosage.

EVALUATION: Monitor CV, hepatic, renal status ▪ Monitor VS, esp BP ▪ Monitor CBC, esp long-term ▪ Monitor fluid retention (I&O, daily weight), constipation ▪ Assess for symptoms of abrupt withdrawal (nausea, headache, malaise) ▪ Assess for actual swallowing of PO forms.

EDUCATION: Dizziness/drowsiness may occur; use caution in potentially hazardous activities ▪ Avoid changing positions (lying/sitting/standing) rapidly ▪ Avoid use c̄ alcohol, other CNS depressants for up to 1 wk after end of therapy ▪ Take c̄ food to ↓ GI irritation ▪ Take as directed by physician ▪ Use sugarless gum/hard candy to diminish dry mouth ▪ Constipation may occur; ↑ fluids, bulk-containing foods ▪ Check c̄ physician before taking OTC/Rx preparations ▪ May produce peculiar taste ▪ Notify physician/dentist of use before treatment ▪ Store in tightly closed container ▪ Avoid exposure to direct sunlight, UV light (sunlamps); use sunscreen, protective clothing ▪ Encourage recreational/diversional interests ▪ Notify physician of fever, sore throat, malaise ▪ Keep scheduled appointments c̄ physician ▪ Full drug effects may require several wks of therapy.

NOTES:

medroxyprogesterone acetate • (me-drox-ee-proe-jess-te-rone)

CATEGORY: *Progestational hormone* Rx; Preg Cat X

BRAND NAMES
Amen (Carnick)
Cycrin (Lederle)
Provera (Upjohn)

DOSAGE FORMS
Tablet: 10mg
Tablet: 2.5, 5, 10mg
Tablet: 2.5, 5, 10mg

USE: Amenorrhea ▪ Abnormal uterine bleeding due to hormonal imbalance in absence of organic disease. **ACTION:** Progestational agents affect pituitary gland, uterus, vaginal mucosa, mammary glands; inhibit pituitary gonadotropin, resulting in ovarian suppression; uterine effect incl relaxation of uterine smooth muscle, ↑ secretory phase of endometrial development; vaginal mucosa exhibits ↑ mucification; other effects incl stimulation of mammary tissue growth, progesterone withdrawal resulting in menstruation.

PHARMACOKINETICS: Good PO absorption; excreted as conjugated metabolites via urine.

CONTRAINDICATIONS: Hypersensitivity, hx of thrombophlebitis, thromboembolic disorders, cerebral apoplexy, suspected breast malignancy, liver disease, undiagnosed vaginal bleeding. **CC:** Observe for signs of thrombolytic disorders.

DOSAGE
Adult *PO*

Amenorrhea	5-10mg/d for 5-10d. Withdrawal bleeding usually w/in 3-7d after ending therapy
Uterine bleeding	5-10mg/d for 5-10d beginning on calculated day 16 or 21 of menstrual cycle. Withdrawal bleeding usually w/in 3-7d after ending therapy

SIDE/ADVERSE EFFECTS: CV: edema, ***thrombophlebitis, pulmonary embolism*** ▪ END: galactorrhea ▪ GU: breakthrough bleeding, spotting, menstrual flow change, amenorrhea, cervical erosion/secretions ▪ HEP: cholestatic jaundice ▪ INT: acne, alopecia, hirsutism, urticaria, pruritus, rash ▪ PSYCH: depression.

INTERACTIONS: Drug: Possible ↓ in glucose tolerance; accordingly, antidiabetic agents may require dose adjustments.

NURSING MANAGEMENT PRIORITIES

ADMINISTRATION: Assess for hx of progestin hypersensitivity ▪ PO: administer c̄ meals ▪ Avoid exposure to light in storage.

EVALUATION: Monitor VS, esp BP, pulse ▪ Monitor hydration status (I&O, daily weight) ▪ Assess emotional status (mental depression) ▪ Monitor hepatic status.

EDUCATION: Review package insert c̄ pt ▪ Take as directed by physician ▪ Avoid exposure to direct sunlight, UV light (sunlamps); use sunscreen ▪ Keep scheduled appointments c̄ physician/for Pap/pelvic exams ▪ Notify physician/dentist of use before therapy ▪ Women: avoid breastfeeding, pregnancy; menstrual changes may occur ▪ Procedure for breast self-exam ▪ Symptoms of thrombotic episodes (sudden shortness of breath, migraine headache, chest pain, diplopia).

NOTES:

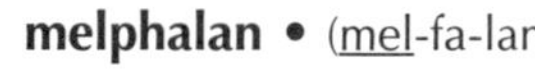

melphalan • (mel-fa-lan)

CATEGORY: *Alkylating agent:* antineoplastic

Rx; Preg Cat D

BRAND NAME	DOSAGE FORM
Alkeran (G-W)	Tablet: 2mg

USE: Treatment of multiple myeloma, epithelial/ovarian cancer. **ACTION:** Antineoplastic activity due to alkylating effect on DNA replication.

PHARMACOKINETICS

PO absorption	Peak	Half-life	Excretion
Incomplete	2h	1.5h	10% unchanged in urine w/in 24h

CONTRAINDICATIONS: Depressed neutrophil/platelet count, recent radiation/similar antineoplastic therapy, hypersensitivity, prior resistance to drug. **CC:** Use requires qualified physician ▪ Use can produce severe bone marrow depression resulting in bleeding or infection ▪ Use ↑ risks of mutagenic effects ▪ Drug is leukemogenic, can cause 2° acute nonlymphocytic leukemia.

DOSAGE

Pediatric/ Adult	*PO*	Usual dose 6mg/d for 2-3wks. D/C drug for up to 4wks. Usual maintenance dose 2mg/d Ovarian cancer: 0.2mg/kg/d for 5d. Can be repeated q4-5wks

SIDE/ADVERSE EFFECTS: GI: *N/V/D,* oral ulcers ▪ HEM: *dose-related depression of bone marrow resulting in anemia, neutropenia,* ***thrombocytopenia*** ▪ INT: *alopecia,* rash ▪ RESP: ***pulmonary fibrosis,*** interstitial pneumonitis.

INTERACTIONS: Drug: Live vaccines contraindicated during therapy ▪ Radiation/other myelosuppressive drugs produce additive bone marrow depression.

NURSING MANAGEMENT PRIORITIES

ADMINISTRATION: Assess for hx of hypersensitivity (incl chlorambucil) ▪ Check pt hx for recent course of radiation/antineoplastic therapy; report to physician ▪ Avoid exposure to moisture/light in storage ▪ Administer antiemetic before therapy ▪ Force liquids (3000ml/d) ▪ Provide emotional support.

EVALUATION: Monitor CBC throughout therapy ▪ Assess for infection, bleeding, anemia ▪ Assess for ↑ serum uric acid levels ▪ Monitor hepatic function during therapy ▪ Assess hydration status (I&O, daily weight).

EDUCATION: Store in tightly closed, light-resistant container ▪ ↑ Fluid intake (10-12 glasses/d) ▪ Avoid exposure to infection ▪ Check c̄ physician before immunization (pt, family) ▪ Diet as tolerated; avoid spicy foods ▪ Maintain good oral hygiene; use soft-bristled toothbrush ▪ Notify physician of symptoms of bone marrow depression (fever, sore throat, bruising, bleeding, lethargy) ▪ Loss of hair may occur (reversible) ▪ Compliance c̄ prescribed dosage regimen ▪ Women: avoid breastfeeding ▪ Encourage ventilation of feelings ▪ Use contraception if sexually active.

NOTES:

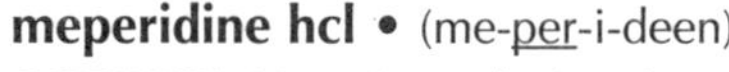

meperidine hcl • (me-per-i-deen)

CATEGORY: *Narcotic:* synthetic opiate — Rx C-II; Preg Cat C

BRAND NAME	DOSAGE FORMS
Demerol HCl (Winthrop)	Injection (IM/IV/SC): 25, 50, 75, 100mg/ml; syrup: 50mg/ml; tablet: 50, 100mg

USE: Relief of moderate/severe pain ▪ Preop sedation, postop analgesia, OB analgesia, support of anesthesia. **ACTION:** Narcotics produce analgesia, euphoria, sedation; equianalgesic doses of meperidine, morphine produce same amount of euphoria, respiratory depression, sedation, addiction liability; PO administration significantly less effective; 70mg equivalent to 10mg morphine.

CONTRAINDICATIONS: Hypersensitivity, c̄ MAO-I therapy, nursing mothers. **CC:** Use can produce dependence; abrupt D/C can result in withdrawal symptoms ▪ Use c̄ caution in presence of head injuries, ⬆ ICP, impaired respiration, supraventricular tachycardias.

DOSAGE

Analgesic		
Pediatric	*PO/IM/SC*	0.5-0.8mg/lb q3-4h prn
Adult	*PO/IM/SC*	50-150mg q3-4h prn
OB	*IM/SC*	50-100mg when pain is regular. May be repeated q1-3h
Anesthesia		Titrated against pt needs by IV injection/continuous infusion
Preop		
Pediatric	*IM/SC*	0.5-1mg/kg 30-90m before anesthesia
Adult	*IM/SC*	50-100mg 30-90m before anesthesia

PHARMACOKINETICS

	Onset	Peak	Duration	Protein binding	Half-life	Excretion
PO	15-20m	60m	2-4h	60%-70%	4-8h	Renal as metabolites, 5% unchanged
IM	10m	40-60m	2-4h	60%-70%	4-8h	
SC	10m	30-50m	2-4h	60%-70%	4-8h	

Note: Side/adverse effects: common in *italic;* serious in ***boldface italic.*** — *Available in Canada only.

SIDE/ADVERSE EFFECTS: CNS: *sedation, lightheadedness*, euphoria, dysphoria, weakness, tremor, disorientation, transient hallucinations ▪ CV: hypotension, palpitation, flushing of face, phlebitis after IV administration ▪ GI: *N/V*, dry mouth, biliary tract spasm, constipation ▪ GU: urinary retention ▪ INT: *sweating*, pruritus, urticaria ▪ RESP: respiratory depression ▪ Other: addiction.

INTERACTIONS: Drug: Use c̄ alcohol, antihistamines, barbiturates, benzodiazepines, methotrimeprazine, phenothiazines, depressants can produce additive CNS depression; ↓ dosage may be required.

NURSING MANAGEMENT PRIORITIES

ADMINISTRATION: Assess for hx of hypersensitivity ▪ Store under double lock/key; document use accurately ▪ Assess quality, intensity, location of pain ▪ Check compatibility chart for mixing preop IM preparations ▪ Do *not* administer if respirations <12/m ▪ IM: inject *deep* into muscle; rotate sites ▪ IV: dilute; administer *slowly* ▪ Have narcotic antagonist, support measures available ▪ Avoid administration in pts c̄ suspected head injury ▪ Administer *before* pt has intense pain ▪ Utilize + power of suggestion ▪ Avoid abrupt withdrawal c̄ long-term use ▪ Elderly may require ↓ dosage.

EVALUATION: Monitor respirations, circulatory function ▪ Assess bowel function, abdominal distention ▪ Assess renal function, urinary retention ▪ Check for signs of dependence (↑ drug request) ▪ Assess for potentiation of CNS depressant effect ▪ Assess for N/V; administer antiemetic ▪ Assess for signs of OD (coma, pinpoint pupils, respiratory depression).

EDUCATION: Avoid changing positions (lying/sitting/standing) rapidly ▪ Avoid excessive sensory stimulation ▪ Keep bedrails up when nonambulatory ▪ Obtain assistance prn when ambulatory ▪ Turn, cough, deep-breathe after surgery ▪ Constipation may occur; ↑ fluids, bulk-containing foods ▪ Avoid potentially hazardous activities ▪ Avoid smoking ▪ Indiscriminate use may lead to severe dependence ▪ Avoid use c̄ alcohol, CNS depressants.

OVERDOSE MANAGEMENT: *See* Narcotics.

NOTES:

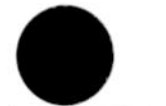

mephobarbital (methylphenobarbital) • (me-foe-<u>bar</u>-bi-tal)

CATEGORY: *Barbiturate:* anticonvulsant, sedative

Rx C-IV; Preg Cat D

BRAND NAME
Mebaral (Sanofi)

DOSAGE FORMS
Tablet: 32, 50, 100mg

USE: Control of grand mal/petit mal seizures ▪ Sedative.
ACTION: Anticonvulsant activity due to depression of motor cortex; after administration, up to 75% converted to phenobarbital by liver.

PHARMACOKINETICS

PO absorption	Onset	Duration	Excretion
50%	30-60m	10-16h	Via urine as metabolites

CONTRAINDICATIONS: Hypersensitivity, severe liver/respiratory impairment, porphyria, addiction. **CC:** Use can produce dependency; abrupt D/C can result in withdrawal symptoms ▪ Use in pts c̄ premonitory signs of hepatic coma not recommended.

DOSAGE

Anticonvulsant

Pediatric	*PO*	<5y/o: 16-32mg 3-4 times/d >5y/o: 32-64mg 3-4 times/d
Adult	*PO*	400-600mg/d

Sedative

Pediatric	*PO*	16-32mg 3-4 times/d
Adult	*PO*	32-100mg 3-4 times/d

SIDE/ADVERSE EFFECTS: CNS: *drowsiness, lethargy,* headache, dizziness, paradoxic restlessness/excitement, *hangover* ▪ GI: N/V ▪ INT: morbilliform rash, ***Stevens-Johnson syndrome***, urticaria ▪ Other: drug tolerance/addiction, asthma, angioneurotic edema.

INTERACTIONS: Drug: Use c̄ alcohol, antihistamines, benzodiazepines, methotrimeprazine, narcotics, tranquilizers ⬆ depressant effects ▪ Barbiturates are enzyme inducers, can ⬇ effect of PO anticoagulants, other drugs ▪ MAO-I ⬆ activity of barbiturates ▪ Barbiturates ⬇ PO absorption of griseofulvin.

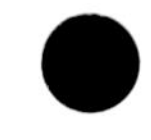

NURSING MANAGEMENT PRIORITIES

ADMINISTRATION: Assess for hx of barbiturate hypersensitivity ▪ Do *not* administer if respirations <12/m ▪ Avoid exposure to moisture in storage ▪ Avoid abrupt withdrawal; institute strict seizure precautions if drug abruptly withdrawn ▪ Elderly may require ⬇ dosage.

EVALUATION: Monitor hepatic, renal, cardiac, respiratory status ▪ Monitor occurrence/characteristics of seizures ▪ Assess for symptoms of abrupt withdrawal (tremors, abdominal/muscle cramps, convulsions) c̄ prolonged use ▪ Assess for actual swallowing of PO forms ▪ Check for signs of dependence (⬆ drug request) ▪ Monitor activity status (safety precautions) ▪ Assess for tolerance/barbiturate cross-tolerance to therapeutic dose ▪ Assess for paradoxic rxs (CNS stimulation), esp in elderly ▪ Observe pt sleep patterns ▪ Check for depression; suicide precautions prn.

EDUCATION: Drowsiness may occur; use caution in potentially hazardous activities ▪ Avoid use c̄ alcohol, other CNS depressants ▪ Indiscriminate use may lead to dependence ▪ Do *not* keep at bedside ▪ Take as ordered by physician; do *not* ⬆ dose ▪ Store in tightly closed container ▪ Safety precautions may be instituted (bedrails) ▪ Do *not* smoke after taking drugs ▪ Practice relaxation exercises, ventilation of feelings ▪ Utilize sleep producers (reading, warm milk, soft music) ▪ Women: avoid breastfeeding ▪ Carry medical identification (MedicAlert) ▪ Do *not* omit daily dose.

OVERDOSE MANAGEMENT: Principal symptoms: exaggerated CNS depression ▪ Respiration depressed, pupils may be constricted, shock, coma ▪ Emergency medical treatment: remove drug by lavage/emesis, maintain respiration; administer IV fluids, vasopressor to maintain BP; force renal excretion c̄ osmotic diuretics; hemodialysis if indicated.

NOTES:

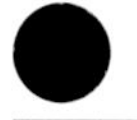

mercaptopurine (6-mp) • (mer-cap-toe-pyoor-een)

CATEGORY: *Antineoplastic: antimetabolite, purine antagonist* Rx; Preg Cat D

BRAND NAME	DOSAGE FORM
Purinethol (G-W)	Tablet: 50mg

USE: Treatment of acute lymphatic & myelogenous leukemia. **ACTION:** Antimetabolitic activity due to competitive inhibition c̄ hypoxanthine & guanine for the enzyme hypoxanthine guanine phosphoribosyltransferase, resulting in the intracellular conversion of 6-MP into a purine antagonist nucleotide with a subsequent ⬇ in both RNA & DNA synthesis. Drug exhibits strong immunosuppressive activity.

PHARMACOKINETICS

PO absorption	Half-life	Protein binding	Excretion
Variable	Adult 47m, children 21m	19%	Via urine as unchanged drug, metabolites

CONTRAINDICATIONS: Known to resistance to drug. **CC:** 6-MP is not effective for CNS leukemia ▪ Complete cross-resistance between 6-MP & thioguanine is usually present ▪ Use requires confirmed leukemia diagnosis ▪ Use will result in dose-related bone marrow suppression (myelosuppression) ▪ 6-MP is hepatotoxic.

DOSAGE

Children/Adult	*PO*	Starting dose of 2.5mg/kg/d; ⬆ to 5mg/kg/d after 4wks if required. Usual maintenance range is 1.5-2.5mg/kg/d

SIDE/ADVERSE EFFECTS: CNS: ***hepatic encephalopathy*** ▪ GI: anorexia, N/V/D, intestinal ulceration ▪ HEP: intrahepatic cholestasis, jaundice, ***parenchymal cell necrosis*** ▪ HEM: anemia, leukopenia, ***thrombocytopenia*** ▪ INT: hyperpigmentation, rash ▪ Other: hyperuricemia, rare drug fever.

INTERACTIONS: Drug: Use c̄ allopurinol will ⬆ 6-MP toxicity ▪ Use c̄ hepatotoxic drug will produce additive toxicity.

NURSING MANAGEMENT PRIORITIES

ADMINISTRATION: Check pt hx for recent course of radiation/antineoplastic agents ▪ Assess PO cavity for ulceration; notify physician ▪ Assess renal function; may

Note: Side/adverse effects: common in *italic;* serious in ***boldface italic.*** *Available in Canada only.

require ↓ dosage if impaired ▪ Administer antiemetic before therapy ▪ Provide emotional support ▪ Avoid exposure to moisture/light in storage.

EVALUATION: Monitor hepatic, renal function; CBC, esp WBC, platelets throughout therapy; notify physician if ↓ ▪ Assess for infection, bleeding, anemia ▪ May produce ↑ serum uric acid level ▪ Assess hydration status (I&O, daily weight) ▪ Monitor for hepatic toxicity (jaundice, clay-colored stools).

EDUCATION: Store in dry, tightly closed, light-resistant container ▪ ↑ Fluid intake (8-10 glasses/d) ▪ Avoid exposure to infection ▪ Check c̄ physician before immunization (pt, family) ▪ Diet as tolerated; avoid spicy food ▪ Maintain good oral hygiene; use soft-bristled toothbrush ▪ Notify physician of symptoms of bone marrow depression (fever, sore throat, bruising, bleeding, lethargy) ▪ Compliance c̄ prescribed dosage regimen ▪ Women: avoid breastfeeding ▪ Check c̄ physician/pharmacist before taking OTC preparations ▪ Avoid use c̄ alcohol ▪ Use contraception if sexually active.

NOTES:

meropenem • (meh-row-pen-em)

CATEGORY: *Carbapenum antibiotic:* β-lactam antibiotic Rx; Preg Cat B

BRAND NAME	**DOSAGE FORMS**
Merrem (Zeneca)	IV powder for injection: 500-mg, 1-g vial

USE: Treatment of intraabdominal infections (eg, complicated appendicitis, peritonitis) caused by susceptible strains of *Bacteroides fragilis/thetaiotaomicron, Escherichia coli, Klebsiella pneumoniae, Peptostreptococcus* spp, *Pseudomonas aeruginosa, Streptococcus viridans* group ▪ Treatment of pediatric (≥3mo of age) bacterial meningitis caused by susceptible strains of *Haemophilus influenzae, Neisseria meningitis, S. pneumoniae.* **ACTION:** Bactericidal activity due to inhibition of mucopeptide cell wall synthesis in susceptible organisms. Drug has good resistance to action of β-lactamases c̄ exception of metallo-β-lactamases.

PHARMACOKINETICS: meropenem has a half-life of 1-1.5h, protein binding is 2%, 70% is excreted unchanged in urine over 12h.

CONTRAINDICATIONS: Hypersensitivity to drug, β-lactams or in pts c̄ anaphylactic rx to β-lactams. **CC:** Use of β-lactams has caused serious/fatal hypersensitivity rxs, esp in pts c̄ a hx or sensitivity to multiple antigens ▪ Use can result in seizures, pseudomembranous colitis ▪ Continue anticonvulsant therapy in pts c̄ seizure disorders during meropenem treatment ▪ Not indicated for methicillin-resistant Staphylococci infection.

DOSAGE: For normal renal function c̄ a maximum dose of 2g q8h.

Adult	*IV*	1g q8h by infusion over 15-30m or as a bolus injection (5-20ml) over 3-5m
Pediatric (≥3mo of age or <50kg)	*IV*	20mg/kg q8h for intraabdominal infections, 40mg/kg q8h for meningitis by infusion or bolus injection. Do *not* exceed maximum dose of 2g q8h
>50 kg		1g q8h for intraabdominal infections, 2g q8h for meningitis by infusion or bolus injection

SIDE/ADVERSE EFFECTS: CNS: ***seizures,*** headache, depression, insomnia, confusion, dizziness ▪ CV: BP changes, bradycardia, tachycardia, cardiac irregularities

■ GI: N/V/D, anorexia, flatulence, abdominal pain, thrush, constipation ■ Other: anemia, dysuria ■ Local: inflammation, pain, edema, phlebitis/thrombophlebitis at injection site.

INTERACTIONS: Drug: Bacteriostatic antibiotics can antagonize bactericidal activity ■ Use c̄ probenecid will ↓ renal excretion & use is not recommended ■ Use c̄ PO anticoagulants may ↑ their activity. **Lab:** ↑ In ALT, AST, alkaline phosphatase, LDH, bilirubin ■ Possible false results c̄ Coombs' test.

NURSING MANAGEMENT PRIORITIES

ADMINISTRATION: Assess for hx of β-lactam hypersensitivity ■ Obtain C&S before therapy ■ Assess renal function; ↓ dosage if impaired ■ Reconstitute, dilute according to manufacturer's directions ■ Administer via IV infusion over 20-30m period or IV bolus over 3-5m ■ Do *not* mix c̄ any solutions containing other drugs ■ Do *not* administer cloudy solutions; yellow-amber color does *not* indicate ↓ potency ■ Have support equipment available for anaphylaxis.

EVALUATION: Monitor VS, esp temperature ■ Monitor renal, hepatic status ■ Observe for signs of superinfection (diarrhea, itching, oral ulcers) ■ Assess for tremors, seizures; notify physician (may ↓ dose or D/C).

EDUCATION: ↑ Fluid intake (8-10 glasses/d) ■ Maintain good personal hygiene (esp perineal, oral) ■ Diarrhea may occur; check c̄ physician before taking any antidiarrheal agents ■ Notify nurse/physician of symptoms of allergic rx (difficult breathing, rash) ■ Carry identification (MedicAlert) if β-lactam allergic.

NOTES:

metaproterenol sulfate • (met-a-proe-ter-e-nole)

CATEGORY: *Sympathomimetic:* β2 adrenergic, bronchodilator — Rx; Preg Cat C

BRAND NAME
Alupent (B-I)

DOSAGE FORMS
Inhaler: 0.65mg/dose
Solution: 0.4, 0.6, 5%
Syrup: 10mg/5ml
Tablet: 10, 20mg

USE: Treatment of bronchial asthma; reversible bronchospasm associated c̄ bronchitis, emphysema. **ACTION:** Sympathomimetic activity at β_2-adrenergic receptors produces bronchodilation.

PHARMACOKINETICS

PO absorption	Onset	Peak	Excretion
Good	15m	1h	Via urine primarily as metabolites

CONTRAINDICATIONS: Hypersensitivity, cardiac arrhythmia associated c̄ tachycardia. **CC:** Inhalation administration can produce life-threatening, paradoxic bronchospasm.

DOSAGE

Pediatric	*PO*	6-9y/o: 10mg 3-4 times/d >9y/o: 20mg 3-4 times/d
Adult	*PO*	20mg 3-4 times/d
Pediatric/ Adult	*Inhalation*	Inhaler: single dose (2-3 inhalations) q3-4h Bulb nebulizer: 10 inhalations 5% solution: 0.3ml c̄ IPPB

SIDE/ADVERSE EFFECTS: CNS: nervousness, tremors, headache, drowsiness ▪ CV: ⬆ heart rate, palpitations ▪ GI: N/V ▪ MS: muscle cramps.

INTERACTIONS: Drug: Use c̄ nonselective β blockers (eg, propranolol) antagonizes bronchodilation ▪ Use c̄ MAO-I requires supervision ▪ Use c̄ other sympathomimetics best avoided.

NURSING MANAGEMENT PRIORITIES
ADMINISTRATION: Assess for hx of catecholamine hypersensitivity (incl sulfites) ▪ Avoid concurrent administration of epinephrine, other sympathomimetic agents ▪ PO: administer c̄ food to ⬇ GI upset ▪ Inhalation: consult manufacturer's directions; excessive use may ⬇ effective-

ness; rinse mouth c̄ H_2O after administration ▪ Avoid exposure to heat/light in storage ▪ Elderly may require ↓ dosage ▪ Administer adrenocorticoid inhalations 15m before this aerosol for ↑ effectiveness (if ordered).

EVALUATION: Monitor VS, esp BP, heart rate; D/C drug if >120 beats/m ▪ Monitor respiratory rate, sputum ▪ Monitor I&O.

EDUCATION: Tolerance to drug effect may develop; report to physician ▪ Take as ordered by physician; do *not* ↑ dose ▪ Notify physician *immediately* of rapid/"skipped" heartbeats, chest pain, tremors; D/C drug ▪ Report to physician failure to respond to usual dose (tolerance) ▪ Store in tightly closed, light-resistant container ▪ Procedure for inhalation administration (shake well; exhale via nose; administer while inhaling deeply through mouth; exhale slowly after 10s; wait 2m before next dose) ▪ Inhalation: may produce unpleasant taste; excessive use of aerosol may cause paradoxic (rebound) bronchospasm ▪ Check c̄ physician/pharmacist before taking OTC preparations.

NOTES:

metaraminol bitartrate • (met-a-ram-i-nole)

CATEGORY: *Sympathomimetic:* vasopressor — Rx; Preg Cat C

BRAND NAME	DOSAGE FORMS
Aramine (Merck)	Injection (IM/IV/SC): 10mg/ml

USE: Prevention/treatment of acute hypotension due to spinal anesthesia ▪ Adjunct in hypotension due to drugs, hemorrhage, surgical complications, shock associated c̄ brain damage. **ACTION:** Adrenergic effect due to α-, β_1-adrenergic agonist activity, resulting in vasoconstriction, positive inotropic cardiac effect.

PHARMACOKINETICS: Onset of pressor activity about 10m IM, 5-20m SC, 1-2m IV; excretion via urine.

CONTRAINDICATIONS: Hypersensitivity. **CC:** Injection contains sodium bisulfite, which can cause allergic rxs.

DOSAGE

Adult *IM/SC*	2-10mg. Wait 10m before giving additional dosage
IV infusion	15-100mg in 500ml solution, administered at rate to maintain satisfactory BP. Severe shock may require direct IV injection 0.5-5mg followed by infusion

SIDE/ADVERSE EFFECTS: CV: ***ventricular tachycardia, other arrhythmias*** ▪ Other: tissue necrosis.

INTERACTIONS: Drug: Avoid use c̄ cyclopropane, halothane, MAO-I, TCAs, reserpine, guanethidine.

NURSING MANAGEMENT PRIORITIES

ADMINISTRATION: Assess for hx of catecholamine hypersensitivity (incl sulfites) ▪ Assess circulatory status; do *not* administer SC if impaired ▪ Assess F/E balance; correct deficiencies ▪ IV: infuse into large vein; use microdrip/infusion pump; do *not* mix c̄ other drugs in solution; keep vein open after D/C in case therapy must be reinstituted (⬇ BP) ▪ Have atropine (for bradycardia), phentolamine (⬇ pressor effect), emergency support equipment available ▪ Do *not* leave pt unattended ▪ Avoid exposure to heat/light in storage ▪ Withdraw drug *gradually*.

EVALUATION: Monitor VS, esp BP (q5m until stable, then q15m) ▪ Monitor I&O q1h ▪ Monitor serum electrolytes (Na^+, K^+) ▪ Cardiac monitoring ▪ Check IV site carefully; avoid extravasation ▪ Continue monitoring BP after D/C; resume if ⬇ BP ▪ Diabetics: monitor blood glucose carefully.

EDUCATION: Notify physician/nurse of abnormal rxs (difficult breathing, chest pain, irregular heartbeat).

NOTES:

metaraminol bitartrate

metformin hcl • (met-form-in)

CATEGORY: *Oral hypoglycemic:* biguanide derivative — Rx C-II; Preg Cat B

BRAND NAME
Glucophage (B-MS)

DOSAGE FORMS
Tablet: 500, 850mg

USE: Management of type II (noninsulin-dependent) diabetes that cannot be controlled by diet alone. **ACTION:** Antidiabetic activity not fully determined. Drug lowers basal, postprandial plasma glucose levels. Antihyperglycemic effect may be due to ⬇ gluconeogenesis (hepatic glucose production), delayed or ⬇ PO absorption of glucose, ⬆ insulin sensitivity.

PHARMACOKINETICS

PO absorption	Half-life	Protein binding	Excretion
Good	6.2h	Negligible	Via urine as unchanged drug

CONTRAINDICATIONS: Hypersensitivity, acute or metabolic acidosis, renal impairment, radiologic studies using iodinated contrast diagnostics. **CC:** Metformin accumulation can result in lactic acidosis.

DOSAGE

Adult	*PO*	Start c̄ 500mg bid or 850mg/d. Adjust to pt needs. Do *not* exceed 2550mg/d

SIDE/ADVERSE EFFECTS: GI: anorexia, N/V/D, flatulence, transient metallic taste ▪ HEM: ⬇ vitamin B_{12} serum level, possible (rare) ***megaloblastic anemia*** ▪ MET: ***lactic acidosis.***

INTERACTIONS: Drug: Use c̄ iodinated contrast diagnostics contraindicated ▪ Use c̄ alcohol c̄ ⬆ lactate metabolism ▪ Use c̄ cimetidine will ⬆ metformin plasma levels ▪ Nifedipine will ⬆ metformin PO absorption. **Food:** Meals will prolong peak plasma levels by approximately 35m.

NURSING MANAGEMENT PRIORITIES

ADMINISTRATION: Assess for hx of hypersensitivity ▪ Assess for metabolic acidosis; do *not* use if present ▪ Assess for renal, hepatic function; may require ⬇ dosage if impaired, use caution ▪ Administer in single AM dose/divided doses c̄ meals ▪ Avoid exposure to moisture/light in storage

■ Withhold 2d before/following radiologic studies involving contrast material (↓ renal function) ■ Elderly may require ↓ dosage.

EVALUATION: Monitor hepatic, renal, hematologic status ■ Monitor FBS ■ Evaluate pt closely during first wk to assess effectiveness ■ Monitor for signs of hypoglycemia/hyperglycemia ■ Monitor electrolyte status, blood pH, serum lactate levels (lactic acidosis).

EDUCATION: Compliance c̄ special diet therapy ■ Take c̄ meals as directed by physician ■ Blood/urine glucose/ketone testing procedure ■ Symptoms of hypoglycemia (anxiety, headache, fatigue, nausea, sweating); notify physician *immediately* ■ Always carry lump of sugar/candy for quick use (hypoglycemia) ■ Avoid use c̄ alcohol ■ Check c̄ physician before taking OTC preparations ■ Notify physician *immediately* of symptoms of hyperglycemia (excessive hunger, thirst, urination, rapid pulse, sweet-smelling breath, weight loss) ■ Notify physician *immediately* of excessive weakness/tiredness, muscle pain, difficulty breathing, stomach discomfort, dizziness, irregular heartbeats ■ Maintain good personal hygiene ■ Carry medical identification (MedicAlert) ■ Store in tightly closed container ■ Keep scheduled appointments c̄ physician/for blood glucose determinations ■ Schedule periodic eye exams ■ Maintain optimum body weight ■ Avoid exposure to direct sunlight, UV light (sun lamps); use sunscreen, protective clothing ■ Women: notify physician of possible pregnancy (insulin use recommended); avoid breastfeeding ■ PO hypoglycemic needs may change c̄ ↑ stress, ↑ exercise, ↓ appetite; notify physician ■ Report skin rash, itching to physician.

NOTES:

methadone hcl • (meth-a-doan)

CATEGORY: *Narcotic:* synthetic opiate

Rx C-II; Preg Cat NA

BRAND NAMES	DOSAGE FORMS
Dolophine HCl (Lilly)	Injection (IM/SC): 10mg/ml Tablet: 5, 10mg
generic (Roxane)	PO concentrate: 10mg/ml PO solution: 5, 10mg/5ml

USE: Relief of severe pain ▪ Detoxification of narcotic addiction ▪ Methadone maintenance of narcotic addiction.

ACTION: Narcotics produce analgesia, euphoria, sedation; methadone has high misuse potential/addiction liability; very long half-life, which makes it suitable for addiction maintenance programs.

CONTRAINDICATIONS: Hypersensitivity; use c̄ extreme caution in head injuries. **CC:** Use can produce dependence; abrupt D/C can result in withdrawal ▪ D/C of maintenance treatment will result in withdrawal symptoms ▪ Use c̄ caution in presence of head injuries, ↑ ICP, impaired respiration.

DOSAGE

Adult *PO/IM/SC*

Analgesic	2.5-10mg q3-4h
Detoxification	≥40mg once/d. Gradually ↓ dose every few days
Maintenance	≥40-120mg once/d

PHARMACOKINETICS

PO absorption	Onset	Duration	Methadone maintenance duration	Protein binding	Excretion
Complete	10-15m	4-6h	22-48h	High	Via urine, feces

SIDE/ADVERSE EFFECTS: CNS: *sedation, lightheadedness*, euphoria, dysphoria, tremors, disorientation, ⬇ convulsive threshold ▪ CV: hypotension, palpitations, flushing of face ▪ EENT: miosis ▪ GI: *N/V*, dry mouth, constipation, biliary tract spasm ▪ GU: urine retention ▪ INT: pruritus, urticaria ▪ RESP: ***respiratory depression***.

INTERACTIONS: Drug: Use c̄ alcohol, antihistamines, barbiturates, benzodiazepines, methotrimeprazine, phenothiazines, other CNS depressants produces additive CNS depression; dosage ⬇ may be required ▪ Use c̄ TCAs may produce additive respiratory depression.

NURSING MANAGEMENT PRIORITIES

ADMINISTRATION: Assess for hx of opioid hypersensitivity ▪ Assess quality, intensity, location of pain ▪ Store under double lock/key; document use accurately ▪ Check compatibility for mixing c̄ other drugs in solution ▪ Do *not* administer if respirations are <12/m ▪ IM: inject *deep* into muscle; rotate sites ▪ Have narcotic antagonist (naloxone), support measures available ▪ Avoid administration in pts c̄ suspected head injuries ▪ Administer *before* pt has intense pain ▪ Administer around clock to pt c̄ severe, chronic pain ▪ Utilize + power of suggestion ▪ Avoid abrupt withdrawal c̄ long-term use ▪ Elderly may require ⬇ dosage.

EVALUATION: Monitor respirations, circulatory function, esp BP ▪ Assess bowel function, abdominal distention ▪ Assess renal function, urinary retention ▪ Check for signs of dependence (⬆ drug request) ▪ Assess for potentiation of CNS depressant effect ▪ Assess for N/V; administer antiemetic ▪ Assess for signs of OD (coma, pinpoint pupils, respiratory depression) ▪ SC: check for tissue irritation ▪ May produce ⬆ CSF pressure.

EDUCATION: Avoid changing positions (lying/sitting/standing) rapidly ▪ Avoid excessive sensory stimulation ▪ Keep bedrails up when nonambulatory ▪ Turn, cough, deep-breathe after surgery ▪ Constipation may occur; ⬆ fluids, bulk-containing foods ▪ Avoid potentially hazardous activities ▪ Avoid smoking ▪ Indiscriminate use may lead to severe dependence ▪ Avoid use c̄ alcohol, other CNS depressants ▪ Women: avoid breastfeeding ▪ Take as ordered by physician; do *not* ⬆ dose ▪ Notify physician/dentist of use before treatment.

OVERDOSE MANAGEMENT: *See* Narcotics.

NOTES:

methimazole/propylthiouracil • (meth-im-a-zole/proe-pill-thye-oh-yoor-a-sill)

CATEGORY: *Antithyroid* — Rx; Preg Cat D

BRAND NAMES	DOSAGE FORMS
methimazole	
Tapazole (Jones)	Tablet: 5, 10mg
propylthiouracil (generic)	Tablet: 50mg

USE: Treatment of hyperthyroidism ▪ Amelioration of hyperthyroidism in preparation for subtotal thyroidectomy, radioactive iodine therapy. **ACTION:** Antithyroid activity due to interference c̄ oxidation of iodide to active iodine & by inhibition of coupling of iodotyrosines, resulting in ↓ thyroid hormone synthesis; drug does not inactivate existing thyroid hormones.

PHARMACOKINETICS

	PO absorption	Peak	Excretion
methimazole	Rapid	1h	12% of dose via urine in 24h
propylthiouracil	Rapid	1-1.5h	35% of dose excreted via urine in 24h as metabolites, unchanged drug

CONTRAINDICATIONS: Hypersensitivity, nursing mothers. **CC:** D/C c̄ significant signs of hepatic toxicity ▪ ↓ Dosage c̄ ↑ TSH levels.

DOSAGE: *PO*

methimazole		
	Pediatric	0.4mg/kg/d in 3 divided doses at 8-h intervals. Maintenance dose is ½ initial dose
	Adult	15-60mg in 3 divided doses at 8-h intervals. Maintenance dose is 5-15mg/d
propylthiouracil		
	Pediatric	6-10y/o: Starting dose 50-150mg/d at 8-h intervals. Maintenance dose dependent on response >12y/o: Starting dose 150-300mg/d. Maintenance dose dependent on response
	Adult	Starting dose 300mg/d. Severe cases may require 600-900mg/d. Usual maintenance dose 100-150mg/d

SIDE/ADVERSE EFFECTS: CNS: headache, neuritis, paresthesias ▪ GI: N/V, epigastric distress ▪ GU: nephritis ▪ HEM: ***agranulocytosis*** ▪ HEP: hepatitis ▪ INT: urticaria, pruritus, skin pigmentation ▪ MS: arthralgia ▪ Other: fever.

INTERACTIONS: Drug: Use c̄ bone marrow depressants can ↑ development of agranulocytosis ▪ Use c̄ PO anticoagulants may ↑ their activity.

NURSING MANAGEMENT PRIORITIES

ADMINISTRATION: Assess for hx of hypersensitivity ▪ Administer c̄ meals at equal intervals around clock ▪ Physician may order concurrent administration of Lugol's (iodine) solution 1-1½wks before thyroid surgery to ↓ vascularity of gland ▪ Avoid exposure to light in storage.

EVALUATION: Monitor CBC throughout therapy ▪ Monitor thyroid function tests ▪ Assess for signs of hypothyroidism (N/V/D, muscle spasms, weight gain, cold sensation); D/C drug, notify physician ▪ Monitor pt receiving anticoagulant therapy; may potentiate bleeding.

EDUCATION: Take c̄ meals ▪ Take as ordered by physician ▪ Notify physician of fever, sore throat, bruising/bleeding ▪ Procedure for checking radial pulse ▪ Check radial pulse, weight 2-3 times/wk ▪ Check c̄ physician/pharmacist before taking OTC preparations ▪ Women: avoid breastfeeding ▪ Store in light-resistant container ▪ Notify physician *immediately* of skin rash, swollen neck glands; ▪ D/C drug ▪ Check c̄ physician before using iodized salt, eating shellfish ▪ Keep scheduled appointments c̄ physician/for blood work ▪ Notify physician/dentist of use before treatment ▪ Full drug effect may require several days of therapy.

NOTES:

methotrexate/methotrexate sodium▲ (amethopterin, mtx) • (meth-oh-trex-ate)

CATEGORY: *Antineoplastic:* antimetabolic, folic acid antagonist — Rx; Preg Cat X

BRAND NAMES	DOSAGE FORMS
Folex, PFS (Adria)	Injection: 25mg/ml
Methotrexate (Immunex)	Injection: 25mg/ml Powder for injection: 20, 50, 100mg, 1g/vial Tablet: 25mg
Rheumatrex dose pack (Immunex)	Tablet: 2.5mg

USE: Treatment of gestational choriocarcinoma, chorioadenoma destruens, hydatidiform mole, lymphoblastic/meningeal leukemias ▪ Treatment of breast cancer, epidermoid cancer of head/neck, lung cancer ▪ Treatment of Burkitt lymphoma, advanced states (III, IV) of lymphosarcoma, advanced mycosis fungoides, disabling psoriasis ▪ Selected adult rheumatoid arthritis. **ACTION:** Antimetabolic activity due to competitive inhibition of dehydrofolate reductase, which inhibits folic acid synthesis.

PHARMACOKINETICS: PO peak 1-2h; excreted unchanged.

CONTRAINDICATIONS: Psoriasis in pregnant pts or pts c̄ preexisting blood dyscrasias, liver, kidney impairment.

CC: Use requires qualified physicians, has been associated c̄ fatalities.

DOSAGE: Must be individualized.

Arthritis	7.5mg once/wk *PO* or 2.5mg at 12-h intervals for 3 doses once/wk. Then adjust. Do *not* exceed 20mg/wk
Trophoblastic tumor	15-30mg/d *PO/IM* for 5d, repeated 3-5 times c̄ ≥1wk of rest between courses
Lymphoblastic leukemia	3.3mg/m² c̄ prednisone 60mg/m²/d. After remission, 30mg/m² *PO/ IM* twice/wk or 2.5mg/kg *IV* q14d
Meningeal leukemia	12mg/m² intrathecal q2-5d
Lymphoma	10-25mg/d *PO* for 4-8d for several courses c̄ 7-10d rest period
Mycosis fungoides	2.5-10mg/d *PO* for wks or mos
Psoriasis	10-25mg/wk as single *PO/IM/IV* dose. Do *not* exceed dose of 50mg/wk. Single dose of 10-25 mg/wk or 2.5-5mg *PO* at 12-h intervals doses once/ wk. Do *not* exceed 30mg/wk

SIDE/ADVERSE EFFECTS: CNS: headache, drowsiness, aphasia, paresis, ***convulsions***, blurred vision ■ GI: *N/V/D*, *abdominal distress*, ***ulcerative stomatitis***, anorexia, gingivitis, ***bleeding, hematemesis*** ■ GU: ***renal failure***, azotemia, cystitis, ***hematuria***, menstrual dysfunction, abortion, fetal teratogenesis, severe nephropathy ■ HEM: ***bone marrow depression***, *leukopenia*, ***thrombocytopenia***, anemia, ***hypogammaglobulinemia***, hemorrhage, septicemia ■ HEP: hepatic toxicity ■ INT: erythematous rash, pruritus, urticaria, photosensitivity, depigmentation, alopecia ■ RESP: ***interstitial pneumonitis, chronic interstitial obstructive pulmonary disease.***

INTERACTIONS: Drug: Use c̄ PO hypoglycemics, phenylbutazone, salicylates, sulfonamide, thiazides can ↑ methotrexate (MTX) toxicity due to protein storage site displacement ■ Use c̄ alcohol, other hepatotoxic drugs ↑ toxic effect ■ Salicylates, probenecid ↓ MTX renal excretion ■ Folic acid preparations (vitamins) can antagonize antineoplastic effect ■ Use c̄ PO anticoagulants may enhance their effects.

NURSING MANAGEMENT PRIORITIES

ADMINISTRATION: Check pt hx for recent course of radiation/antineoplastic agents ■ Assess PO cavity for ulceration ■ Assess renal function; may require ↓ dosage if impaired ■ Administer antiemetic before therapy ■ PO: administer 1h ac/2h pc ■ Parenteral: dilute according to manufacturer's directions; administer by *slow* IV push ■ Avoid exposure to moisture/light in storage.

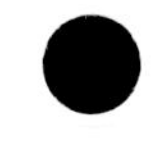

EVALUATION: Monitor CBC & neurologic, hepatic function ■ Assess for infection, bleeding, anemia ■ May produce hyperglycemia; monitor diabetics closely ■ Assess hydration status.

EDUCATION: Store in dry, tightly closed, light-resistant container ■ ↑ Fluid intake (8-10 glasses/d) ■ Avoid exposure to infection ■ Check c̄ physician before immunization ■ Diet as tolerated; avoid spicy foods ■ Maintain good oral hygiene; use soft-bristled toothbrush ■ Notify physician of symptoms of bone marrow depression (fever, sore throat, bruising, bleeding, lethargy) ■ Avoid exposure to direct sunlight, UV light ■ Loss of hair may occur (reversible) ■ Compliance c̄ prescribed dosage regimen ■ Women: avoid breastfeeding ■ Check c̄ physician/pharmacist before taking OTC preparations ■ Avoid use c̄ alcohol ■ Use contraception (during & for up to 8wks after therapy).

NOTES:

methoxamine hcl • (meth-<u>ox</u>-a-meen)

CATEGORY: *Sympathomimetic:* vasopressor — Rx; Preg Cat C

BRAND NAME
Vasoxyl (G-W)

DOSAGE FORMS
Injection (IM/IV): 20mg/ml

USE: Maintaining BP during anesthesia ▪ Termination of some episodes of paroxysmal supraventricular tachycardia. **ACTION**: Adrenergic effect due to α-agonist activity, resulting in peripheral vasoconstriction w/out ⬆ cardiac irritability.

PHARMACOKINETICS: Onset of pressor effects 15-20m IM; duration 1-1.5h.

CONTRAINDICATIONS: Hypersensitivity, hypertension. **CC:** Injection contains sodium bisulfite, which can cause allergic rxs ▪ Use c̄ caution in presence of arteriosclerosis, bradycardia, hyperthyroidism, myocardial disease, partial heart block.

DOSAGE

Adult		
Spinal anesthesia	*IM*	Usual dose 10-15mg shortly before/at time of spinal anesthesia administration. Subsequent doses may be required
Hypotension	*IV*	3-5mg for emergencies
	IM	Usual dose 10-15mg. Usual postop dose for moderate hypotension 5-10mg
Paroxysmal supraventricular tachycardia	*IV*	10mg

SIDE/ADVERSE EFFECTS: ***Sustained hypertension c̄ headache,*** projectile vomiting, urinary frequency/desire to void, pilomotor response.

INTERACTIONS: Drug: Use c̄ MAO-I, TCAs, vasopressin, ergot alkaloids ↑ pressor effects ▪ Use c̄ halothane, other halogenated general anesthetics can induce cardiac arrhythmias ▪ Use c̄ β blockers, guanethidine, reserpine may result in significant hypertension.

NURSING MANAGEMENT PRIORITIES

ADMINISTRATION: Assess for hx of catecholamine hypersensitivity (incl sulfites) ▪ Assess F/E balance; correct deficiencies ▪ IV: administer via *slow* (2-3m) injection if systolic BP <60mmHg ▪ IM: may administer after IV dose for prolonged effect; doses 15m apart ▪ Do *not* leave pt unattended ▪ Have atropine available for bradycardia ▪ Avoid exposure to light in storage ▪ Elderly may require ↓ dosage.

EVALUATION: Monitor VS, esp BP, heart rate (bradycardia) ▪ Monitor I&O (urinary retention) ▪ Check IV site carefully; avoid extravasation.

EDUCATION: Notify physician/nurse of abnormal rxs (difficult breathing, severe headache, severe faintness/dizziness).

NOTES:

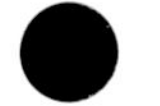

methyldopa/methyldopate hcl▲ • (meth-ill-doe-pa)

CATEGORY: *Antihypertensive*

Rx; Preg Cat B

BRAND NAME
Aldomet (Merck)

DOSAGE FORMS
Injection (IV)▲: 250mg/vial
PO suspension: 250mg/5ml
Tablet: 125, 250, 500mg

COMBINATION PRODUCTS

Aldoril 15, 25, 30, 50 (Merck)	methyldopa/hydrochlorothiazide per tablet: 250mg/15mg, 250mg/25mg, 500mg/30mg, 500mg/50mg

USE: Treatment of hypertension as sole agent/in combination c̄ thiazide diuretic. **ACTION:** Antihypertensive effect probably due to conversion to α-methylnorepinephrine, which stimulates central inhibitory α-adrenergic receptors, resulting in ⬇ BP.

PHARMACOKINETICS

PO absorption	Peak	Half-life	Excretion
Up to 50%	3-6h	1.7h	Via urine primarily as metabolites

CONTRAINDICATIONS: Hypersensitivity, active hepatic disease associated c̄ previous therapy. **CC:** Use associated c̄ rare fatal hepatic necrosis ▪ Use c̄ caution in pts c̄ previous liver impairment ▪ PO suspension contains sodium bisulfite, which can cause allergic rxs.

DOSAGE

Pediatric	*PO*	Initial dose 10mg/kg/d in 2-4 doses. Maximum dose 65mg/kg or 3g/d, whichever less
	IV	20-40mg/kg/d divided q6h. Maximum dose 65mg/kg or 3g/d, whichever less
Adult	*PO*	Initial dose 250mg 2-3 times/d for 2d. ⬆ At intervals of at least 2d. Usual maintenance range 500mg-2g in 2-4 doses/d
	IV	250-500mg q6h prn. Do *not* exceed 1g q6h
Aldoril	*PO*	1-2 tablets (any combination) 2-3 times/d for 2d. ⬆ At intervals of at least 2d until satisfactory response obtained

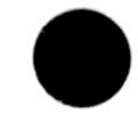

SIDE/ADVERSE EFFECTS: CNS: *sedation, headache, dizziness,* symptoms of cerebrovascular insufficiency, Parkinson's disease, Bell's palsy, psychic disturbances ▪ CV: bradycardia, edema, orthostatic hypotension, exacerbation of angina, prolonged carotid sinus hypersensitivity ▪ GI: N/V/D, colitis, *dry mouth,* ***pancreatitis,*** sore/black tongue ▪ HEM: ***hemolytic anemia,*** leukopenia, ***thrombocytopenia*** ▪ HEP: jaundice, ↑ serum AST, ALT, alkaline phosphatase, *hepatitis* ▪ INT: eczema rashes, ***toxic epidermal necrolysis*** ▪ Other: breast enlargement, lactation, gynecomastia, nasal congestion, impotence.

INTERACTIONS: Drug: Use c̄ MAO-I can antagonize antihypertensive effect ▪ Use c̄ levodopa, phenothiazines, TCAs can produce additive hypotensive effects ▪ Use c̄ lithium can produce ↑ lithium toxicity. **Lab:** False + Coombs' test.

NURSING MANAGEMENT PRIORITIES

ADMINISTRATION: Assess for hx of hypersensitivity ▪ PO suspension: shake well before pouring ▪ IV: dilute c̄ 5% dextrose solution; administer *slowly* (30-60m) ▪ Do *not* administer SC/IM ▪ Elderly may require ↓ dosage.

EVALUATION: Monitor VS, esp BP ▪ Monitor F/E balance, esp Na^+, K^+, Cl^- ▪ Monitor hepatic, CV, renal, hemopoietic status c̄ long-term use ▪ Monitor I&O, daily weight ▪ Assess for edema in extremities.

EDUCATION: Dizziness/drowsiness may occur; use caution in potentially hazardous activities ▪ Avoid changing positions (lying/sitting/standing) rapidly ▪ Take as ordered by physician, even if symptom free; do *not* change dose ▪ Used to control, *not* cure, hypertension ▪ Avoid use c̄ alcohol, CNS depressants ▪ Avoid ↑ exercise, temperature extremes, smoking ▪ Notify physician of muscle cramps, difficult breathing, cold extremities, fever, prolonged tiredness ▪ Keep scheduled appointments c̄ physician; have BP checked regularly ▪ Maintain optimum weight ▪ Avoid high-Na^+ foods (canned soups, lunch meats, cheese) ▪ Check c̄ physician/pharmacist before taking OTC preparations ▪ Notify physician/dentist of use before treatment ▪ Do *not* D/C drug w/out checking c̄ physician ▪ Carry identification (MedicAlert) if hypertensive ▪ May produce ↓ libido, impotence ▪ May darken urine if left standing.

NOTES:

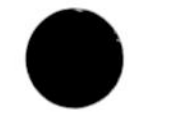

methylprednisolone/methylprednisolone acetate▲ •

(meth-ill-pred-niss-oh-lone)

CATEGORY: *Glucosteroid:* corticosteroid — Rx; Preg Cat NA

BRAND NAMES	**DOSAGE FORMS**
Depo-Medrol▲ *(Upjohn)*	Injection suspension: 20, 40, 80mg/ml
Medrol (Upjohn)	ADT Pak, Dosepak, tablet: 2, 4, 8, 24, 32mg; retention enema▲

USE: Treatment of adrenocortical deficiency, adrenogenital syndrome, other endocrine disorders; allergic states, collagen diseases, dermatologic diseases, GI diseases, hematologic disorders, ophthalmologic diseases; respiratory diseases, rheumatic disorders ▪ Treatment of tuberculous meningitis, neurologic/myocardial involvement associated c̄ trichinosis ▪ Remission of proteinuria in nephrotic syndrome; acute exacerbation of multiple sclerosis ▪ Palliative management of leukemia, lymphomas. **ACTION:** Glucosteroids cause a variety of pharmacologic activities; two major effects are potent antiinflammatory effect, inhibition of immune response.

PHARMACOKINETICS: PO administration usually produces peak effect in 1-2h, duration of about 1.5d.

CONTRAINDICATIONS: Systemic fungal infections. **CC:** *See* cortisone.

DOSAGE

Adult	*PO*	2-60mg/d
	Injection/suspension	10-80mg IM qd. Intraarticular, intralesional; 4-80mg/dose
	Enema	1 enema 3-7 times/wk for ≥2wks. Can be administered by continuous drip

SIDE/ADVERSE EFFECTS: CNS: ***convulsions***, headache, psychic impairment, vertigo, mood swings; pseudotumor cerebri may develop after treatment ▪ CV: edema due to Na^+ retention, CHF, hypertension ▪ EENT: ↑ IOP, glaucoma, posterior subcapsular cataracts, exophthalmos ▪ END: Cushingoid states, growth suppression in children, menstrual irregularities, 2° adrenocortical/pituitary unresponsiveness, hyperglycemia, carbohydrate intolerance ▪ GI: peptic ulcer/***possible perforation, pancreatitis***, abdominal distention, ulcerative esophagitis ▪ INT: poor wound healing, fragile skin, petechiae; ecchymoses, fa-

Note: Side/adverse effects: common in *italic;* serious in ***boldface italic.*** — *Available in Canada only.

cial erythema, ↑ sweating, urticaria, hirsutism ▪ MET: negative nitrogen balance, hypokalemic alkalosis ▪ MS: muscle weakness/loss of mass, fracture of long bones, osteoporosis.

INTERACTIONS: Drug: Severe hypokalemia can occur c̄ diuretics (nonpotassium sparing) ▪ Use c̄ ulcerogenic drugs (aspirin, indomethacin) can produce additive effects ▪ Use c̄ antidiabetic agents may require ↑ doses of antidiabetic drugs.

NURSING MANAGEMENT PRIORITIES

ADMINISTRATION: Assess for hx of hypersensitivity ▪ Administer single daily/alternate-day dose *before* 9AM; multiple doses at equal intervals ▪ PO: administer c̄ food, milk, antacids ▪ IM: shake well; do *not* freeze; inject into gluteal UOQ (avoid deltoid); rotate sites ▪ IV (succinate salt only): (direct) reconstitute according to manufacturer's directions c̄ compatible diluent, administer *slowly* (1m); (infusion) further dilute c̄ 5% dextrose/normal saline, administer at prescribed rate; stable w/in 48h of reconstitution; do *not* use discolored/precipitated solutions ▪ Rectal: administer via continuous drip or retention enema; shake bottle q30m ▪ Avoid abrupt withdrawal ▪ Avoid exposure to heat in storage ▪ Elderly may require ↓ dosage; monitor BP.

EVALUATION: Monitor VS, esp BP ▪ Diabetics: closely monitor blood/urine glucose (hyperglycemia) ▪ Assess mental/emotional status; avoid TCAs if depression induced ▪ Monitor serum electrolytes (esp CA^{++}, K^{+}, Na^{+}), vision/IOP, stools for occult blood c̄ prolonged use ▪ Monitor hydration status (I&O, daily weight).

EDUCATION: Take c̄ food/milk (single daily dose *before* 9AM; multiple doses at equal intervals) ▪ Take as ordered by physician; do *not* ↑ dose/stop taking ▪ Eat foods high in K^{+}, high in protein; avoid black licorice ▪ Follow diet low in Na^{+} ▪ Check c̄ physician before immunization (pt, family) ▪ Avoid exposure to infection ▪ Report following symptoms *immediately* to physician: anorexia, difficult breathing, weakness, dizziness; may appear during periods of ↑ stress/trauma ▪ Notify physician if experiencing black/tarry stools, slow wound healing, blurred vision, bruising/bleeding, weight gain, emotional changes ▪ Diabetics: closely monitor blood/urine glucose ▪ Notify physician/dentist of use before treatment ▪ Keep appointments c̄ physician/for blood work/for eye exams ▪ Women: avoid breastfeeding ▪ Body image changes may occur c̄ prolonged use (reversible).

NOTES:

methyltestosterone • (meth-ill-tess-toss-te-rone)

CATEGORY: *Androgenic hormone* Rx; Preg Cat X

BRAND NAME	DOSAGE FORMS
Oreton Methyl (Schering)	Buccal tablet, tablet

USE: Treatment of conditions due to androgen deficiency, incl eunuchoidism, eunuchism, male climacteric 2° to androgen deficiency, postpubertal cryptorchidism ▪ Prevention of postpartum breast engorgement ▪ Palliation of androgen-responsive, advancing, inoperable postmenopausal mammary cancer ▪ Treatment of delayed male puberty, impotence. **ACTION:** Androgens required for development, maintenance of male reproductive system, 2° sex characteristics; initiate specific RNA, protein synthesis in responsive tissue.

PHARMACOKINETICS

Peak	Half-life	Excretion
1-2h	1h initially 3.5h after 3-4h	Urine, feces, 10% unchanged

CONTRAINDICATIONS: Known/suspected carcinoma of prostate gland/male breast; prepubertal boys; pregnant/breastfeeding women; cardiac, renal, hepatic decompensation. **CC:** Androgen therapy for breast cancer or immobilized pts may cause hypercalcemia ▪ Extensive use can result in hepatic neoplasms, oligospermia, peliosis hepatis ▪ Use c̄ caution in pts c̄ preexisting cardiac, hepatic, or renal dysfunction, epilepsy.

DOSAGE: Buccal administration produces effects at half PO dose; PO dose about twice buccal dose.

Buccal

Androgen deficiencies	5-20mg or more qd
Postpartum breast engorgement	40mg/d for 3-5d
Breast cancer	25-100mg/d

SIDE/ADVERSE EFFECTS: END: virilization in women, oligospermia, gynecomastia, priapism, amenorrhea ▪ HEP: hepatocellular neoplasms (rare), peliosis hepatis ▪ INT: acne, edema, hirsutism, stomatitis c̄ buccal preparations ▪ MET: hypercalcemia.

INTERACTIONS: Drug: Use c̄ PO anticoagulants can significantly ⬆ anticoagulant activity.

NOTES:

NURSING MANAGEMENT PRIORITIES

ADMINISTRATION: Assess for pregnancy; do *not* administer ▪ Assess for hx of CV, hepatic, renal dysfunction; notify physician ▪ Place buccal tablets in upper/lower buccal pouch between gum, cheek; allow 30m to dissolve ▪ PO: administer c̄ food ▪ Avoid exposure to moisture/light in storage.

EVALUATION: Assess CV, hepatic, renal status ▪ Observe for signs of jaundice; D/C drug, notify physician ▪ Observe for edema, weight gain ▪ Assess for hypercalcemia ▪ Diabetics: monitor for hypoglycemia ▪ Assess for stomatitis (buccal).

EDUCATION: Store in tightly closed, light-resistant container ▪ Proper use of buccal tablets; do *not* swallow; avoid eating, drinking, smoking; maintain good oral hygiene ▪ Notify physician immediately of jaundice, edema ▪ Women: masculinizing effects may occur; notify physician ▪ Men: overstimulation of sexual function may occur; notify physician ▪ Exercise regimen (esp for immobilized pts) to ⬇ hypercalcemia ▪ Take PO forms c̄ meals ▪ Diabetics: monitor blood/urine glucose carefully.

metoclopramide hcl • (met-oh-kloe-pra-mide)

CATEGORY: *GI stimulant:* peristaltic stimulant

Rx; Preg Cat B

BRAND NAMES	DOSAGE FORMS
**Emex (Beecham)*	Tablet: 10mg
**Maxeran (Nordic)*	Injection (IV): 5mg/ml PO solution: 1mg/ml Tablet: 5mg
Maxolon (SKB)	Tablet: 10mg
Octamide PFS (Adria)	Injection (IV): 5mg/ml
Reglan (Robins)	Injection (IV): 5, 10mg/ml Syrup: 5mg/5ml Tablet: 5, 10mg

USE: Treatment of symptomatic gastroesophageal reflux not responsive to conventional therapy ▪ Treatment of symptoms associated c̄ acute/recurrent diabetic gastroparesis ▪ Antiemetic for cancer chemotherapy ▪ Facilitation of small bowel intubation ▪ Facilitation of barium removal after radiologic exam. **ACTION:** Peristaltic stimulation appears related to upper gut sensitizing to acetylcholine, ↑ gastric tone, amplitude contraction, relaxation of pyloric sphincter, resulting in accelerated emptying; drug causes release of prolactin.

PHARMACOKINETICS

PO absorption	Peak	Half-life	Protein binding	Excretion
Complete	1-2h	2.5-5h	13%-22%	Via urine, feces primarily as metabolites

CONTRAINDICATIONS: GI hemorrhage, obstruction, perforation; hypersensitivity, pheochromocytoma, epilepsy c̄ drugs that induce extrapyramidal symptoms. **CC:** Use can result in rare cases of depression, extrapyramidal symptoms, tardive dyskinesia.

DOSAGE

Pediatric		
Intubation	*IV*	<6y/o: 0.1mg/kg 6-14y/o: 2.5-5mg
Adult		
Reflux	*PO*	10-15mg 30m ac, at hs. Single 20-mg dose before provoking condition
Diabetic gastroparesis	*PO*	10mg 30m ac, at hs for 2-8wks
	IV	Severe symptoms: 10mg

Note: Side/adverse effects: common in *italic;* serious in ***boldface italic.***

*Available in Canada only.

Antiemetic

Chemotherapy	*IV*	1-2mg/kg
Postop	*IM*	10-20mg
Intubation	*IV*	10mg
Barium removal	*IV*	10mg

SIDE/ADVERSE EFFECTS: CNS: *drowsiness, restlessness, lassitude,* dizziness, headache, insomnia, extrapyramidal rxs, akathisia, extrapyramidal rxs (rare) ▪ EENT: visual disturbances ▪ END: galactorrhea, amenorrhea, gynecomastia, impotence ▪ GI: nausea, bowel disturbances (diarrhea) ▪ INT: rash ▪ RESP: ***bronchospasm*** ▪ Other: porphyria.

INTERACTIONS: Drug: Use c̄ anticholinergics/narcotics can antagonize stimulant effect ▪ Use c̄ CNS depressants produces additive depression ▪ Insulin adjustment may be required for diabetics ▪ Use c̄ other drugs ↑ their PO absorption from intestine.

NURSING MANAGEMENT PRIORITIES

ADMINISTRATION: Assess for hx of hypersensitivity ▪ Assess renal function; may require ↓ dosage if impaired ▪ PO: administer 30m ac, at hs ▪ IV: dilute according to manufacturer's directions; administer *slowly* (direct injection 1-2m, infusion >15m); discard unused portions ▪ Avoid exposure to heat/light in storage; cover IV bags c̄ aluminum foil ▪ Na^+ content: 0.14mEq/ml (IV); calculate in Na^+-restricted diets ▪ Elderly may require ↓ dosage.

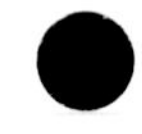

EVALUATION: Monitor VS, daily weight, I&O ▪ Observe for extrapyramidal symptoms (muscle spasms, tremors, shuffling gait); notify physician ▪ Monitor serum electrolytes (↓ K^+, ↑ Na^+), blood glucose ▪ Observe for potentiation of CNS depressant effect.

EDUCATION: Drowsiness may occur; use caution in potentially hazardous activities ▪ Take on empty stomach (30m ac, at hs) ▪ Take as ordered by physician; do *not* ↑ dose ▪ Avoid use c̄ alcohol, other CNS depressants.

NOTES:

metolazone • (me-tole-a-zone)

CATEGORY: *Diuretic:* antihypertensive

Rx; Preg Cat B

BRAND NAMES
Mykrox† *(Fisons)*
Zaroxolyn (Fisons)

DOSAGE FORMS
Tablet: 0.5mg
Tablet: 2.5, 5, 10mg

USE: Treatment of hypertension as sole agent/in combination c̄ other antihypertensives ▪ Treatment of edema due to renal dysfunction ▪ Adjunct in treatment of edema due to CHF. **ACTION:** Diuretic activity due to excretion of H_2O, Na, Cl, other electrolytes by inhibiting tubular reabsorption at cortical diluting site, proximal convoluted tubules.

CONTRAINDICATIONS: Hypersensitivity, hepatic precoma/coma. **CC:** Use can result in rare episodes of potassium, sodium depletion ▪ Do not interchange various dosage formulations during treatment.

DOSAGE

Adult *PO*	2.5-20mg/d

SIDE/ADVERSE EFFECTS: CNS: dizziness, drowsiness, fainting, headache, paresthesia ▪ CV: orthostatic hypotension, ***venous thrombosis***, palpitations ▪ EENT: blurred vision; dry nose/throat ▪ GI: constipation, N/V, anorexia, epigastric distress ▪ HEM: ***aplastic anemia,*** leukopenia, ***agranulocytosis, thrombocytopenia*** ▪ HEP: cholestatic jaundice, hepatitis ▪ INT: urticaria, purpura, necrotizing angiitis ▪ Other: gout attack.

PHARMACOKINETICS

PO absorption	Onset	Peak	Duration	Protein binding	Excretion
Incomplete	1h	2h	12-24h	Approximately 35% >50% bound to RBC	Via urine, primarily as unchanged drug

*Available in Canada only.
†More completely absorbed and not therapeutically equivalent to other formulations. Usual dose 0.5-1mg/d.

Note: Side/adverse effects: common in *italic;* serious in ***boldface italic.***

INTERACTIONS: Drug: ↑ Dig toxicity due to hypokalemia ▪ Use c̄ corticosteroids produces ↑ hypokalemia ▪ Antidiabetic agents may require dose adjustments ▪ Use c̄ diazoxide can produce significant diabetogenic effects ▪ Use c̄ lithium salts is best avoided.

NURSING MANAGEMENT PRIORITIES

ADMINISTRATION: Assess for hx of hypersensitivity (incl sulfonamides) ▪ Assess renal function; do *not* administer if severely impaired ▪ Administer c̄ food/milk on arising ▪ Assess serum K^+ (normal level: 3.5-5mEq/L) ▪ Elderly may require ↓ dosage.

EVALUATION: Monitor F/E, hepatic, renal status ▪ Monitor VS, esp BP, pulse ▪ Monitor serum for ↑ BUN, creatinine, uric acid; ↓ K^+ ▪ Diabetics: closely monitor blood sugar (hyperglycemia) ▪ Monitor fluid retention (I&O, daily weight) ▪ Monitor digitalized pts closely (↓ K^+: ↑ dig toxicity).

EDUCATION: Expect ↑ urine output; have bathroom facilities easily accessible ▪ May cause weakness, lethargy ▪ Take c̄ food ▪ Take on waking, at same time qd ▪ Take even if symptom free ▪ Used to control, *not* cure, hypertension ▪ Notify physician of signs of hypokalemia (muscle cramps, lethargy, nausea) ▪ Avoid changing positions (lying/sitting/standing) rapidly ▪ Take as directed by physician; do *not* skip doses ▪ Eat foods high in K^+ (bananas, fruit juices, raisins); avoid black licorice ▪ Avoid high-Na^+ foods (canned soups, lunch meats, cheese) ▪ Maintain optimum weight ▪ Diabetics: check blood/urine glucose carefully ▪ Avoid smoking ▪ Use sugarless gum/hard candy to diminish dry mouth.

NOTES:

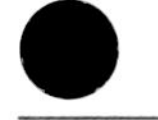

metoprolol tartrate • (me-toe-proe-lole)

CATEGORY: *β-adrenergic blocker:* antihypertensive — Rx; Preg Cat B

BRAND NAMES	**DOSAGE FORMS**
**Betaloc (ASTRA)*	
Lopressor (Novartis)	Injection (IV): 5mg/vial, syringe Tablet: 50, 100mg
Toprol XL (Astra)	Extended release tablet: 50, 100, 200mg

COMBINATION PRODUCTS

Lopressor HCT (Novartis)	metoprolol/hydrochlorothiazide per tablet: 50mg/25mg, 100mg/25mg, 100mg/50mg

USE: Treatment of hypertension as sole agent/in combination c̄ other antihypertensives (esp thiazide diuretics) ▪ To ↓ mortality rate in MI ▪ Long-term treatment of angina. **ACTION:** Blocks access of catecholamine neurotransmitter to β_1 receptors located in heart; antihypertensive effect not determined.

PHARMACOKINETICS

PO absorption	Peak	Half-life	Protein binding	Excretion
95%	1h	3-7h	12%	95% as metabolites via urine

CONTRAINDICATIONS: Hypersensitivity, cardiogenic shock, heart block >1°, overt cardiac failure, sinus bradycardia. **CC:** Abrupt D/C can exacerbate ischemic heart disease ▪ Use can result in possible cardiac failure c̄ ↓ myocardial contractility ▪ Use c̄ caution in presence of bronchospastic disease, diabetes, peripheral vascular disease ▪ Tachycardia of hyperthyroidism can be masked, abrupt D/C may induce thyrotoxicosis.

DOSAGE

Adult

Angina	*PO*	100-400mg/d
Hypertension	*PO*	100-450mg/d
MI early	*IV/PO*	3 bolus injections of 5mg at 2-m intervals followed in 15m by 50mg PO q6h for 48h. Thereafter 100mg bid
MI late	*PO*	100mg bid
Lopressor HCT		
50/25		2 tablets/d
100/25		1-2 tablets/d
100/50		1 tablet/d

Note: Side/adverse effects: common in *italic;* serious in ***boldface italic.***

*Available in Canada only.

SIDE/ADVERSE EFFECTS: CNS: *tiredness, dizziness,* depression, mental confusion ▪ CV: bradycardia, palpitations, shortness of breath, cold extremities, CHF ▪ GI: N/D, gastric pain, constipation, flatulence ▪ INT: pruritus, rash ▪ Other: wheezing, Peyronie's disease (1/100,000).

INTERACTIONS: Drug: Use c̄ reserpine, other catecholamine-depleting drugs can result in serious adrenergic blockage ▪ Nonselective β adrenergics antagonize therapeutic response.

NURSING MANAGEMENT PRIORITIES

ADMINISTRATION: Assess for hx of β-blocker hypersensitivity ▪ Assess BP, apical pulse; if <60/m, hold drug, notify physician ▪ Assess hepatic function, I&O ▪ Do *not* administer in presence of respiratory distress (asthma, CHF, COPD) ▪ PO: administer c̄ food ▪ IV: cardiac monitor ▪ Avoid exposure to heat/moisture/light in storage ▪ Avoid abrupt withdrawal ▪ Elderly may require ↓ dosage.

EVALUATION: Monitor hepatic, renal, respiratory status ▪ Monitor BP, pulse ▪ Monitor CBC, FBS (diabetics) ▪ Assess for depression ▪ May produce alteration in blood glucose levels (hypoglycemia); may mask signs of hypoglycemia.

EDUCATION: Check pulse before taking; if <60/m, do *not* take drug, notify physician ▪ Take as directed by physician; do *not* skip doses ▪ Take c̄ food ▪ Do *not* D/C drug w/out notifying physician ▪ Check c̄ physician/pharmacist before taking OTC/Rx preparations ▪ Dizziness/drowsiness may occur; use caution in potentially hazardous activities ▪ Diabetics: carefully monitor blood/urine glucose levels ▪ May experience ↑ sensitivity to cold ▪ Notify physician of respiratory distress, leg edema ▪ Notify physician/dentist of β blocker use before treatment ▪ Maintain optimum weight ▪ Keep scheduled appointments c̄ physician ▪ Follow low-Na^+ diet ▪ Store in tightly closed, light-resistant container ▪ Avoid ↑ exercise, cold, smoking ▪ Women: avoid breastfeeding.

NOTES:

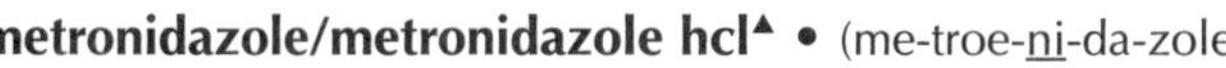

metronidazole/metronidazole hcl▲ • (me-troe-ni-da-zole)

CATEGORY: *Antiprotozoan:* antibacterial — Rx; Preg Cat B

BRAND NAMES / **DOSAGE FORMS**

Brand names	Dosage forms
Flagyl (Searle) (Rhone-Poulenc [Canada])	Powder for injection (IV): 500mg/vial▲ IV; IVRTU: 500mg/100ml▲ Tablet: 250, 500mg
MetroGel (Galderma)	Gel: 0.75%
MetroGel-Vaginal (3M)	Gel: 0.75%
Protostat (Ortho)	Tablet: 250, 500mg Vaginal insert: 500mg
**Novonidazol (Novopharm)*	Tablet: 250mg Vaginal insert: 500mg

USE: Treatment of symptomatic/asymptomatic trichomoniasis ▪ Treatment of amebic dysentery, amebic liver abscesses ▪ Treatment of anaerobic bacterial infections caused by susceptible strains of *Bacteroides* spp, *Clostridium* spp, *Eubacterium* spp, *Fusobacterium* spp, *Peptococcus* spp, *Peptostreptococcus* spp ▪ Treatment of rosacea (gel), bacterial vaginitis (vaginal gel). **ACTION:** Antimicrobial activity appears related to inhibition of hydrogen release in metabolic pathways in susceptible organisms.

PHARMACOKINETICS

PO absorption	Peak	Half-life	Protein binding	Excretion
80%	1-3h	8h	20%	60%-80% via urine as metabolites

CONTRAINDICATIONS: Hypersensitivity, 1st trimester of pregnancy (trichomoniasis). **CC:** Avoid unnecessary use due to carcinogenic potential ▪ Use can result in seizures, peripheral neuropathy.

DOSAGE

Pediatric

Amebiasis	*PO*	30-50mg/kg/d in 3 doses for 10d

Adult

Amebiasis	*PO*	750mg tid for 5-10d. Amebic liver abscess: 500 or 750mg tid for 5-10d
Bacterial	*PO*	7.5mg/kg q6h for 7-10d. Do *not* exceed 4g/d
	IV	Loading dose 15mg/kg infused over 1h, $\bar{c}$ maintenance dose after 6h of 7.5mg/kg infused over 1h q6h. Do *not* exceed 4g/d. Switch to PO when clinically indicated

Note: Side/adverse effects: common in *italic;* serious in ***boldface italic.***

*Available in Canada only.

	For surgical prophylaxis, 15mg/kg infused over 30-60m, completed 1h before surgery. 7.5mg/kg infused over 30-60m at 6 & 12h after initial dose
Rosacea	Cover affected areas in AM & PM after washing
Trichomoniasis	
PO	2g for 1d or 250mg tid for 7d
Vaginitis	1 applicatorful bid for 5d

SIDE/ADVERSE EFFECTS: CNS: ***convulsive seizures***, peripheral neuropathy, dizziness, incoordination, headache ▪ CV: ECG T-wave flattening ▪ EENT: nasal congestion ▪ GI: anorexia, N/V/D, cramps, metallic taste ▪ GU: dysuria, cystitis, polyuria, dark urine ▪ INT: urticaria, erythematous rash, overgrowth of monilia.

INTERACTIONS: Drug: Use c̄ PO anticoagulants may ↑ PT ▪ Use c̄ alcohol produces abdominal distress, N/V, flushing, headache ▪ Use c̄ phenobarbital/phenytoin ↑ metronidazole metabolism ▪ Use c̄ disulfiram may cause acute psychotic rx ▪ Use c̄ lithium may ↑ its toxicity ▪ Use c̄ astemizole not recommended.

NURSING MANAGEMENT PRIORITIES

ADMINISTRATION: Assess for hx of hypersensitivity ▪ Obtain C&S before therapy ▪ PO: administer c̄ food/milk; may crush tablets ▪ Administer at equal intervals around clock to maintain blood levels ▪ Do *not* administer direct IV bolus ▪ IV: avoid contact c̄ aluminum-containing products; do *not* mix c̄ other drugs; do *not* refrigerate neutralized solution.

EVALUATION: Monitor VS, esp temperature; CBC, esp WBCs; stools for amebae (3mo) ▪ Assess for neurotoxic effects (paresthesias, tremors, incoordination); D/C drug.

EDUCATION: Take c̄ food/milk to ↓ GI distress; may crush tablets ▪ Take as ordered by physician even if symptom free ▪ Notify physician *immediately* of tremors, alteration in sensation, incoordination; D/C drug ▪ Avoid alcohol ▪ Trichomoniasis: have partner use condom c̄ sexual intercourse during therapy; identify all sexual contacts for treatment; maintain good perineal hygiene ▪ May turn urine red/brown ▪ Women: avoid breastfeeding ▪ May cause metallic taste.

NOTES:

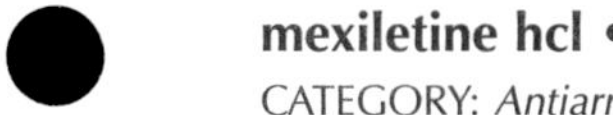

mexiletine hcl • (mex-ill-e-teen)

CATEGORY: *Antiarrhythmic* Rx; Preg Cat C

BRAND NAME
Mexitil (B-I)

DOSAGE FORMS
Capsules: 150, 200, 250mg

USE: Treatment of symptomatic ventricular arrhythmias including frequent PVC, tachycardia, & unifocal & multifocal couplets. **ACTION:** Antiarrhythmic effect due to inhibition of inward Na current, which ⬇ phase 0 action potential. The drug is a class IB antiarrhythmic & ⬇ the effective refractory period in Purkinje fibers.

PHARMACOKINETICS

PO absorption	Peak	Half-life	Protein binding	Excretion
90%	2-3h	10-12h	50%-60%	10% as unchanged drug via urine

CONTRAINDICATIONS: Hypersensitivity, cardiogenic shock, preexisting 2°/3° AV block (in the absence of a pacemaker). **CC:** Use can produce acute liver dysfunction esp in pts c̄ CHF or ischemia ▪ Use c̄ caution in presence of severe CHF, hypotension ▪ Use can exacerbate arrhythmias.

DOSAGE: Initial dose of 200mg q8h. A minimum of 2-3d is required between dosage adjustments, which are in 50- or 100-mg increments up or down. For rapid control the loading dose is 400mg, followed by 200mg in 8h. Stabilized pts may be put on a q12h schedule, with a maximum dose of 450mg q12h.

SIDE/ADVERSE EFFECTS: CNS: *dizziness, tremor, nervousness, difficult coordination*, sleep irregularities, headache, paresthesias, depression, confusion ▪ CV: palpitations, anginal pain, PVC, hypotension, edema ▪ EENT: tinnitus, blurred vision ▪ GI: *N/V, heartburn*, diarrhea, constipation, dry mouth, changes in appetite ▪ Other: rash, arthralgia, dyspnea, fever, fatigue, ***rare blood dyscrasias.***

INTERACTIONS: Drug: Use c̄ enzyme inducers incl phenytoin, rifampin, barbiturates can ⬇ mexiletine blood levels ▪ Use c̄ cimetidine requires monitoring because of erratic mexiletine blood levels ▪ Renal excretion rates will ⬆ c̄ acidifiers & ⬇ c̄ alkalizing agents. **Lab:** ⬆ In SGOT.

NURSING MANAGEMENT PRIORITIES

ADMINISTRATION: Assess for hx of hypersensitivity, incl amide-type anesthetics ▪ Administer c̄ food, milk, antacid to ⬇ GI distress ▪ Assess for CHF, hepatic dysfunction; may require ⬇ dosage ▪ Administer first dose; 6-12h after quinidine, disopyramide; 3-6h after procainamide; 8-12h after tocainide ▪ ⬇ Dose/withdraw lidocaine after starting drug ▪ Assess for hx of seizures; institute precautions ▪ Dosage may be ⬆/⬇ q2-3d by 50-100mg/dose ▪ Heavy smokers may require ⬆ dosage ▪ Avoid exposure to heat/moisture/light in storage.

EVALUATION: Monitor VS, esp BP, heart rate (hypotension, heart block) ▪ Assess neurologic status; notify physician if impaired ▪ Monitor CBC (leukopenia), platelets (thrombocytopenia); notify physician ▪ Monitor I&O, daily weight ▪ May ⬆ serum AST; + antinuclear antibody titer.

EDUCATION: Dizziness may occur; use caution in potentially hazardous activities ▪ Take c̄ food, milk, antacids to ⬇ GI irritation ▪ Take as ordered by physician, even if symptom free ▪ Notify physician/dentist of use before treatment ▪ Keep scheduled appointments c̄ physician ▪ Notify physician *immediately* of chest pain, difficult breathing, seizures, bleeding/bruising, swelling of legs/feet ▪ Store in dry, tightly closed, light-resistant container ▪ Women: avoid breastfeeding.

NOTES:

mezlocillin sodium • (mez-loe-sill-in)

CATEGORY: *Extended-spectrum penicillin:* antibiotic — Rx; Preg Cat B

BRAND NAME
Mezlin (Bayer)

DOSAGE FORMS
Powder for injection (IM/IV): 1-, 2-, 3-, 4-g vials

USE: Treatment of infections due to susceptible strains of *Bacteroides* spp, *Escherichia coli,* group A hemolytic streptococci, *Haemophilus influenzae, Klebsiella* spp, *Morganella morganii, Neisseria gonorrhoeae, Peptococcus* spp, *Peptostreptococcus* spp, *Proteus mirabilis, Pseudomonas* spp, *Serratia* spp, *Streptococcus faecalis, S. pneumoniae* ▪ In combination c̄ aminoglycoside in treating serious *Pseudomonas aeruginosa* infections. **ACTION:** Bactericidal activity due to inhibition of mucopeptide cell wall synthesis in susceptible organisms.

PHARMACOKINETICS

PO absorption	Peak	Half-life	Protein binding	Excretion
65%	45m	1-1.5h	16%-42%	55% via urine in 6h

CONTRAINDICATIONS: Hypersensitivity to any penicillin/cephalosporin. **CC:** Penicillins can produce serious/fatal (anaphylaxis) hypersensitivity rxs ▪ Possible cross allergenicity c̄ cephalosporins, other β-lactam antibiotics ▪ Use c̄ caution perioperatively c̄ vecuronium.

DOSAGE

Pediatric	*IV/IM*	≥1mo: 50mg/kg q4h
Adult	*IV/IM*	Usual range 6-18g/d divided given q4-6h. Do *not* exceed 2g/IM injection site. Usual maximum IV dose 24g/d

SIDE/ADVERSE EFFECTS: CNS: ***possible convulsions***, neuromuscular irritability ▪ GI: N/V/D, abnormal taste ▪ HEM: anemia, eosinophilia, leukopenia, neutropenia, ***thrombocytopenia*** ▪ HEP: ↑ serum AST, ALT, bilirubin ▪ INT: rash, pruritus, urticaria ▪ Other: localpain/***thrombophlebitis*** at injection site, ***anaphylactic rxs***, ↓ K^+ level.

INTERACTIONS: Drug: Use c̄ bacteriostatic antibiotics can lead to antibiotic antagonism ▪ PO anticoagulant therapy may require dose adjustments ▪ Use c̄ vecuronium can ↑, prolong its neuromuscular activity.

NURSING MANAGEMENT PRIORITIES

ADMINISTRATION: Assess for hx of penicillin/cephalosporin hypersensitivity ▪ Obtain C&S before therapy ▪ Have support equipment available for anaphylaxis ▪ Do *not* mix c̄ aminoglycosides, other antibacterial solutions ▪ Reconstitute according to manufacturer's directions ▪ Maintain blood levels; administer at equal intervals around clock ▪ IM: inject *deep, slowly* into gluteal UOQ ▪ IV: administer by *slow* direct injection, IVPB (30m infusion) ▪ Na^+ content: 1.9mEq (43mg)/g; calculate in Na^+-restricted diets.

EVALUATION: Monitor VS, esp temperature ▪ Monitor hepatic, renal status (I&O) ▪ Assess for hypokalemia; may require supplemental K^+ ▪ Observe for signs of superinfection (diarrhea, perineal itching, oral ulcers) ▪ Assess for hypersensitivity rxs (fever, difficult breathing, rash) ▪ Monitor blood cultures, WBC, differential for drug effectiveness.

EDUCATION: Diarrhea may occur ▪ Maintain good personal hygiene (esp perineal, oral) ▪ Maintain fluid intake (6-8 glasses/d) ▪ Avoid concurrent ingestion of highly acidic substances (fruit juices) ▪ Carry identification (MedicAlert) if penicillin allergic.

NOTES:

miconazole/miconazole nitrate▲ • (mi-kon-a-zole)

CATEGORY: *Antifungal* Rx-OTC; Preg Cat C

BRAND NAMES	DOSAGE FORMS
Micatin▲ (Ortho)	OTC topical preparations
Monistat 3▲ (Ortho)	Vaginal suppository: 200mg
Monistat 7▲ (Ortho)	Vaginal cream: 2%
	Vaginal suppository: 100mg
Monistat-Derm▲ (Ortho)	Rx topical preparations
Monistat IV (Janssen)	Injection (IV): 10mg/ml

USE: Treatment of systemic infections caused by susceptible strains of *Candida albicans, Coccidioides immitis, Cryptococcus neoformans, Paracoccidioides brasiliensis, Petriellidium boydii* ▪ Topical treatment of cutaneous/vaginal moniliasis, dermatophytes (tinea infections). **ACTION:** Antifungal activity due to alteration in cell membrane permeability, resulting in leakage of vital intracellular components.

PHARMACOKINETICS: After IV administration, drug metabolized in liver, excreted as metabolites via urine, feces.

CONTRAINDICATIONS: Hypersensitivity. **CC:** Possible anaphylaxis or cardiopulmonary arrest c̄ IV administration.

DOSAGE

Pediatric	*IV infusion*	20-40mg/kg/d. Do *not* exceed 15mg/kg/infusion
Adult	*IV infusion*	
Coccidioidomycosis		1800-3600mg/d
Cryptococcosis		1200-2400mg/d
Candidiasis		600-1800mg/d
Paracoccidioidomycosis		200-1200mg/d
Petriellidiosis		600-3000mg/d
	Topical	
Vaginal moniliasis		One applicatorful/suppository into vagina once/d for 3d (Monistat 3) or 7d (Monistat 7)
Dermatophytes/ cutaneous moniliasis		Apply preparation at least twice/d

SIDE/ADVERSE EFFECTS: Phlebitis, pruritus, nausea, fever, chills, rash, ***thrombophlebitis;*** local topical application can produce irritation, burning.

INTERACTIONS: Drug: Use c̄ PO anticoagulants ↑ their activity, dosage adjustment may be required ▪ Use c̄ amphotericin B may result in antimicrobial antagonism ▪ Use c̄ astemizole not recommended ▪ IV use c̄ cisapride can produce fatal cardiac arrhythmias.

NURSING MANAGEMENT PRIORITIES

ADMINISTRATION: Assess for hx of hypersensitivity ▪ Obtain C&S before therapy ▪ IV: dilute in 5% dextrose/normal saline solution; stable for 48h at room temperature; administer *slowly* (30-60m); do *not* mix c̄ other IV drugs ▪ Do *not* administer discolored/precipitated solutions ▪ Administer antiemetic/antihistamine as ordered before IV dose (↓ nausea) ▪ Cleanse areas for application well before administration ▪ Shake topical preparations well before administering ▪ Use lotion on skinfold areas (toes, fingers) ▪ Avoid occlusive dressings.

EVALUATION: Monitor VS, esp temperature ▪ Monitor CBC (H&H), serum electrolytes, lipids ▪ Monitor skin, mucous membranes for redness, swelling, irritation ▪ May potentiate anticoagulant effect; assess for bleeding.

EDUCATION: Take as ordered by physician; complete full course of therapy ▪ Keep affected areas dry, exposed to air; avoid occlusive dressings ▪ Maintain good hygiene, esp in affected area; keep towels, personal items separate from those of others to avoid spread of infection ▪ Vaginal: use sanitary napkin to prevent staining of clothing; avoid sexual intercourse during therapy (prevent reinfection) ▪ Avoid contact c̄ eyes ▪ Procedure for topical/vaginal application ▪ Full drug effects may require 1-2wks.

NOTES:

minoxidil • (mi-nox-i-dill)

CATEGORY: *Antihypertensive*

Rx/OTC▲; Preg Cat C

BRAND NAMES
Loniten (Upjohn)
Rogaine▲ (Upjohn)

DOSAGE FORMS
Tablet: 2.5, 10mg
Topical solution for men: 2%, 5%
Topical solution for women: 2%

CONTRAINDICATIONS: Hypersensitivity, pheochromocytoma. **CC:** Use should be restricted to pts who do not respond adequately to maximum therapeutic doses of other antihypertensives ▪ Use requires concurrent use of a suitable diuretic ▪ Use can result in pericardial effusion c̄ rare episodes of tamponade, exacerbation of angina.

USE: Limited to treatment of severe hypertension that is symptomatic or associated c̄ target organ damage & cannot be controlled c̄ diuretic plus two other antihypertensive drugs c̄ maximum dosage. Topical solution treats male/female baldness of the scalp (vertex).
ACTION: Antihypertensive effect due to direct peripheral vasodilation, resulting in ⬇ of peripheral vascular resistance; drug has recently received much publicity for restoring hair growth when applied topically (usually as pharmacy-prepared suspension made from crushed tablets).

PHARMACOKINETICS

PO absorption	Peak	Half-life	Protein binding	Excretion
90%	2-8h	4.2h	None	90% metabolized excreted primarily via urine

DOSAGE: *PO*

Pediatric	
<12/yo	Initial dose 0.2mg/kg as single daily dose. Usual effective maintenance dose 0.25-1mg/kg/d. Do *not* exceed 50mg/d
Adult/Children	
>12y/o	Initial dose 5mg as single daily dose. Usual dose 5mg as single daily dose. Usual effective maintenance dose 10-40mg/d. Do *not* exceed 100mg/d
Topical solution	Apply 1ml to scalp & rub in. Do *not* exceed 2ml/d

Note: Side/adverse effects: common in *italic;* serious in ***boldface italic.***

*Available in Canada only.

SIDE/ADVERSE EFFECTS: CV: temporary edema, ***ECG, T-wave changes in direction/magnitude, pericardial effusion/tamponade,*** possible exacerbation of angina pectoris ▪ END: breast tenderness ▪ GI: N/V ▪ HEM: leukopenia, ***thrombocytopenia*** ▪ INT: skin rash, *hypertrichosis.*

INTERACTIONS: **Drug:** Use c̄ guanethidine can result in significant orthostatic effects.

NURSING MANAGEMENT PRIORITIES

ADMINISTRATION: Assess for hx of hypersensitivity ▪ Avoid abrupt withdrawal; D/C gradually ▪ Elderly may require ↓ dosage ▪ Topical: Apply to dry hair/scalp, wash hands afterward; do *not* use if scalp is irritated or sunburned.

EVALUATION: Monitor VS, esp BP (lying/sitting/standing), apical pulse ▪ Monitor I&O, daily weight ▪ Monitor CV, hepatic, renal status ▪ Assess for edema; auscultate lungs (rales).

EDUCATION: Review package insert c̄ pt ▪ Take as ordered by physician even if symptom free; do *not* skip/change dose ▪ Do *not* D/C drug w/out notifying physician ▪ Maintain optimum weight ▪ Keep scheduled appointments c̄ physician; have BP checked regularly ▪ Follow low-Na^+ diet ▪ Avoid ↑ exercise, temperature extremes, smoking, alcohol ▪ Notify physician *immediately* of shortness of breath, chest pain, fluid retention, dizziness, bruising/bleeding ▪ Used to control, *not* cure, hypertension ▪ Check c̄ physician/pharmacist before taking OTC/Rx preparations ▪ Procedure for checking radial pulse ▪ Take pulse daily; report any ↑ of >20 beats/m to physician *immediately* ▪ Notify physician/dentist of use before treatment ▪ ↑ Body hair growth/darkening may occur several wks after therapy started (reversible); depilatory may be used ▪ Procedure for topical application ▪ Full drug effects may require several mos of therapy.

NOTES

mirtazapine • (mer-taz-e-peen)

CATEGORY: *Antidepressant*

Rx; Preg Cat C

BRAND NAME
Remeron (Organon)

DOSAGE FORMS
Tablet: 15, 30mg

USE: Treatment of depression. **ACTION:** Antidepressant activity not fully determined & appears related to an ↑ in central noradrenergic & serotonergic activity. Mirtazapine antagonizes central presynaptic alpha 2 adrenergic inhibitory autoreceptors & heteroreceptors resulting in an ↑ in noradrenergic & serotonergic central activity. Drug also exhibits strong H-l antihistaminic, moderate peripheral anti-alpha-1 & antimuscarinic activity.

CONTRAINDICATIONS: Hypersensitivity. **CC:** Do not use c̄ MAO-I or w/in 14d of initiating or D/C c̄ an MAO-I ▪ Use has resulted in extremely rare cases of agranulycytosis, activation of mania/hypomania & seizures ▪ Use for >6wks not evaluated ▪ Use c̄ caution c̄ conditions/diseases that affect metabolism or hemodynamic response.

DOSAGE

Adult	*PO*	Starting dose of 15mg/d as a single dose at hs c̄ a range of 15-45mg/d

SIDE/ADVERSE EFFECTS: CNS: somnolence (most frequent), dizziness, abnormal dreams/thinking, tremor, confusion ▪ CV: hypertension, vasodilation, bradycardia, rare abnormal ECG changes ▪ GI: dry mouth, ↑ appetite, constipation, nausea, anorexia ▪ RESP: dyspnea, ↑ cough Other: back pain, urinary frequency/infection, rare hypothyroidism.

INTERACTIONS: Drug: Use c̄ alcohol & other CNS depressants will produce additional depression. **Lab:** ↑ In cholesterol, triglycerides, ALT serum levels.

PHARMACOKINETICS

PO absorption	Peak	Half-life	Protein binding	Excretion
Complete	2h	20-40h	85%	Via urine (75%), feces (25%) primarily as metabolites

Note: Side/adverse effects: common in *italic;* serious in ***boldface italic.***

*Available in Canada only.

NURSING MANAGEMENT PRIORITIES

ADMINISTRATION: Assess for hx of hypersensitivity, glaucoma, prostatic hypertrophy, renal/hepatic disease ▪ Administer c̄ food ▪ Institute suicide/safety precautions ▪ Administer at hs before sleep ▪ Avoid abrupt withdrawal.

EVALUATION: Monitor hepatic, renal status; BP, CBC, I&O, daily weight, constipation ▪ Assess for symptoms of abrupt withdrawal (nausea, headache, malaise) ▪ Assess for actual swallowing of PO forms.

EDUCATION: Dizziness/drowsiness may occur; use caution in potentially hazardous activities ▪ Avoid changing positions (lying/sitting/standing) rapidly ▪ Avoid use c̄ alcohol, CNS depressants for up to 1wk after end of therapy ▪ Take c̄ food to ↓ GI irritation ▪ Use sugarless gum/hard candy to diminish dry mouth ▪ Constipation may occur; ↑ fluids, bulk-containing foods Check c̄ physician/pharmacist before taking OTC/Rx preparations ▪ Notify physician/dentist of use before treatment ▪ Notify physician of fever, sore throat, malaise ▪ Full drug effects may require several wks of therapy.

NOTES:

misoprostol • (mis-oh-prost-ole)

CATEGORY: *Gastric antisecretory:* synthetic prostaglandin E analog — Rx; Preg Cat X

BRAND NAME
Cytotec (Searle)

DOSAGE FORMS
Tablet: 100, 200μg

USE: Prevention of gastric ulcers during NSAIA therapy in pts at high risk of developing gastric ulcers. **ACTION:** Drug is converted in body into prostaglandin F analogs, which inhibit gastric acid secretion & ↑ mucus & bicarbonate production in stomach. Stimulation of uterus resulting in contraction is also produced.

CONTRAINDICATIONS: Hypersensitivity to drug/prostaglandins, pregnancy. **CC:** Females must avoid pregnancy during treatment, must be given PO/written warnings concerning miscarriage.

DOSAGE

Adult *PO*	200μg qid c̄ meals, at hs for duration of NSAIA therapy. A ↓ dose of 100μg qid c̄ meals, at hs can be used if higher dose cannot be tolerated

SIDE/ADVERSE EFFECTS: CNS: headache (2.4%), drowsiness, dizziness, anxiety ▪ CV: chest pain, edema, BP changes ▪ EENT: abnormal vision, conjunctivitis, earache, tinnitus ▪ GI: diarrhea (13%), pain (7%), nausea (3.2%), flatulence (2.9%), dyspepsia (2%), vomiting (1.3%), abnormal taste ▪ GU: cramps, menstrual disorders, spotting, polyuria, dysuria ▪ INT: alopecia, rash, dermatitis ▪ Other: fatigue, fever, URI, bronchospasm, anemia, thrombocytopenia.

PHARMACOKINETICS

PO absorption	Onset	Duration	Half-life	Protein binding	Excretion
Extensive	30m	3h	20-40m	90%	Via urine

INTERACTIONS: Drug: Use c̄ antacids ↓ misoprostol availability.

NURSING MANAGEMENT PRIORITIES

ADMINISTRATION: Assess for hx of prostaglandin hypersensitivity ▪ Assess for pregnancy; do *not* administer ▪ Administer c̄ meals & at hs ▪ Use c̄ caution in pts c̄ seizure disorders ▪ Avoid concurrent administration c̄ antacids.

EVALUATION: Monitor VS, esp BP ▪ Monitor GI status; notify physician of abdominal pain.

EDUCATION: Take c̄ meals & at hs ▪ Do *not* take antacids w/in 2h of drug; avoid Mg^{++}-containing antacids (diarrhea) ▪ Take as directed by physician, usually not for >4wks ▪ Diarrhea may occur ▪ Women: notify physician of pregnancy possibility; avoid breastfeeding; D/C if pregnant.

NOTES:

montelukast sodium • (mon-tea-lew-cast)

CATEGORY: *Antiasthmatic:* leukotriene modifier

Rx; Preg Cat B

BRAND NAME
Singulair (Merck)

DOSAGE FORMS
Chewable tablet: 5mg
Tablet: 10mg

USE: Prophylaxis & treatment for adults/children >6y/o c̄ chronic asthma. **ACTION:** Antiasthmatic activity due to modification of physiologic activities of leukotriene agonists in pathogenesis of asthma. Leukotrienes produce broncho-constriction, edema, inflammation, mucus secretions. Montelukast is a selective antagonist of leukotrienic activity at leukotrienic receptor sites on respiratory smooth muscle, resulting in antagonized muscular constriction.

CONTRAINDICATIONS: Hypersensitivity. **CC:** Not indicated for acute asthma attacks ▪ Chewable tablets contain phenylalanine ▪ Safety & efficacy in pediatric pts <6y/o not established.

DOSAGE

Adult/children >15y/o	*PO*	10mg once/d in PM
Children 6-14y/o	*PO*	5mg once/d in PM

SIDE/ADVERSE EFFECTS: CNS: dizziness, headache ▪ GI: abdominal pain, dyspepsia, gastroenteritis ▪ RESP: nasal congestion, cough, influenza ▪ Other: rash, fever, asthenia.

PHARMACOKINETICS

PO absorption	Peak	Half-life	Protein binding	Excretion
Rapid	3-4h (2-2.5h for chewable tabs)	2.7-5.5h	99%	Via feces as metabolites

INTERACTIONS: Drug: Use c̄ caution c̄ barbiturates, rifampin due to enzyme induction. **Lab:** ↑ In ALT, AST, pyuria.

NURSING MANAGEMENT PRIORITIES

ADMINISTRATION: Assess for hx of hypersensitivity, incl aspirin, NSAIAs ▪ Assess respiratory function, patency of nasal passages ▪ Avoid abrupt withdrawal ▪ Avoid exposure to heat/light in storage.

EVALUATION: Assess respiratory status, adequate inhalation ▪ Monitor frequency of asthmatic attacks.

EDUCATION: Take as directed by physician; do *not* abruptly D/C drug ▪ Notify physician/dentist of use before treatment ▪ Notify physician *immediately* of wheezing, respiratory distress ▪ Do *not* use for acute asthma attacks (prophylaxis only) ▪ Full drug effects may require several wks of therapy.

NOTES:

morphine sulfate • (mor-feen)

CATEGORY: *Narcotic:* opium alkaloid

Rx C-II; Preg Cat C

AVAILABLE PREPARATIONS
Injection (IM/IV/SC): 2, 4, 8, 10, 15mg/ml
PO solution: 10mg/5ml, 20mg/ml, 20mg/5ml, 20mg/10ml
Suppository: 5, 10, 20mg
Tablet: 10, 15, 30mg

USE: Relief of pain ▪ Sedation, hypnosis when pain is present ▪ Preop/postop sedation/analgesia. **ACTION:** Narcotics produce analgesia, euphoria, sedation; morphine sulfate has high misuse potential, addiction liability.

CONTRAINDICATIONS: Hypersensitivity; use c̄ extreme caution in head injuries. **CC:** Use can produce dependence, abrupt D/C can result in withdrawal symtoms ▪ Use c̄ caution in pts c̄ head injuries, ↑ ICP, impaired respiration.

DOSAGE

Pediatric	*SC*	0.1-0.2mg/kg/dose. Do *not* exceed single dose 15mg
Adult	*PO*	10-30mg q4h
	IM	5-20mg q4h
	IV	2.5-15mg/dose
	SC	5-20mg q4h
	Rectal	10-20mg q4h

PHARMACOKINETICS

	Onset	Peak Analgesia	Duration	Half-life	Protein binding	Excretion
PO	15-20m	60m	4-7h	2.25h	35%	Approximately 90% excreted in urine primarily as metabolites
IM	10m	30-60m	6-7h	2.25h	35%	
IV	1-3m	20m	6-7h	2.25h	35%	
SC	10m	50-90m	6-7h	2.25h	35%	
Rectal	15-20m	60m	6-7h	2.25h	35%	

SIDE/ADVERSE EFFECTS: CNS: *sedation, lightheadedness,* euphoria, dysphoria, tremors, disorientation, ↓ convulsive threshold ▪ CV: hypotension, palpitations, flushing of face, phlebitis of IV site ▪ EENT: miosis ▪ GI: *N/V*, dry mouth, constipation, biliary tract spasm ▪ GU: urine retention ▪ INT: pruritus, urticaria ▪ RESP: ***respiratory depression***.

INTERACTIONS: Drug: Use c̄ alcohol, antihistamines, barbiturates, benzodiazepines, methotrimeprazine, phenothiazines, other CNS depressants produces additive CNS depression; ↓ dosage may be required ▪ Use c̄ TCAs may produce additive respiratory depression.

NURSING MANAGEMENT PRIORITIES

ADMINISTRATION: Assess for hx of opioid hypersensitivity ▪ Assess quality, intensity, location of pain ▪ Store under double lock/key; document use accurately ▪ Check compatibility for mixing c̄ other drugs in solution ▪ PO liquid: dilute c̄ juice to mask disagreeable taste ▪ Do *not* administer if respirations are <12/m ▪ IM: inject *deep* into muscle; rotate sites ▪ IV: dilute; administer *slowly* (3-5m); keep pt supine for 2h ▪ Have narcotic antagonist (naloxone), support measures available ▪ Avoid administration in pts c̄ suspected head injury ▪ Administer *before* pt experiences intense pain ▪ Avoid abrupt withdrawal c̄ long-term use ▪ Administer around clock to pts c̄ severe chronic pain ▪ Elderly may require ↓ dosage.

EVALUATION: Monitor respirations, circulatory function, esp BP ▪ Assess bowel function, abdominal distention, renal function, urinary retention ▪ Check for signs of dependence ▪ Assess for potentiation of CNS depressant effect ▪ Assess for N/V; administer antiemetic ▪ Assess for signs of OD (coma, pinpoint pupils, respiratory depression) ▪ SC: check for tissue irritation.

EDUCATION: Avoid changing positions (lying/sitting/standing) rapidly ▪ Avoid excessive sensory stimulation ▪ Keep bedrails up when nonambulatory ▪ Turn, cough, deep breathe after surgery ▪ Constipation may occur; ↑ fluids, bulk-containing foods ▪ Avoid potentially hazardous activities ▪ Avoid smoking ▪ Avoid use c̄ alcohol, other CNS depressants ▪ Women: avoid breastfeeding ▪ Take as ordered ▪ PO liquid: may mix c̄ juice; do *not* freeze ▪ Notify physician/dentist of use before treatment.

OVERDOSE MANAGEMENT: *See* Narcotics.

NOTES:

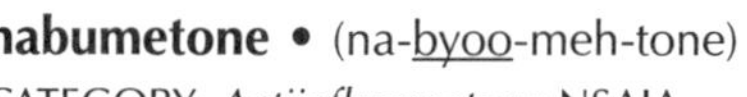

nabumetone • (na-byoo-meh-tone)

CATEGORY: *Antiinflammatory:* NSAIA — Rx; Preg Cat C

BRAND NAME
Relafen (SKB)

DOSAGE FORMS
Tablet: 500, 750mg

USE: Treatment of acute & chronic osteoarthritis/ rheumatoid arthritis. **ACTION:** Drug is converted by hepatic biotransformation into 6-methyoxy-2 naphthylacetic acid (6 MNA), a potent inhibitor of prostaglandin synthesis resulting in an antiinflammatory effect.

PHARMACOKINETICS

PO absorption	Peak	Half-life	Protein binding	Excretion
Good	2.5-4h	22.5-30h	99%	Via urine, feces as metabolites

CONTRAINDICATIONS: Hypersensitivity, pts c̄ aspirin- or other NSAIA-induced allergies (asthma, urticaria). **CC:** Use can ↑ risk of GI bleeding, ulcers, perforation, photosensitivity.

DOSAGE

Adult *PO* — Initial dose of 1000mg as a single dose w/out regard to meals c̄ a maximum dose of 2000mg/d.

SIDE/ADVERSE EFFECTS: CNS: Dizziness, headache, fatigue, somnolence, insomnia, asthenia, nightmares ▪ CV: edema, vasculitis ▪ EENT: tinnitus ▪ GI: diarrhea (14%), dyspepsia (13%), abdominal pain (12%), N/V, dry mouth, anorexia, ulcers, bleeding, ↑ appetite, melena ▪ GU: azotemia, dysuria, hematuria, renal stones ▪ HEM: anemia, leukopenia, granulocytopenia, ***thrombocytopenia*** ▪ INT: acne, alopecia, photosensitivity, pruritus, rash, sweating, ***erythema multiforme, Stevens-Johnson syndrome*** ▪ Other: fever, chills, hypokalemia.

INTERACTIONS: Drug: Use c̄ ulcerogenic drugs produces additive effects ▪ Use c̄ warfarin, other high-protein–binding drugs can ↑ their activity due to protein displacement.

NURSING MANAGEMENT PRIORITIES

ADMINISTRATION: Assess for hx of NSAIA hypersensitivity ▪ Avoid administration to individuals c̄ hx of asthma, bleeding disorders, salicylate hypersensitivity ▪ Assess for hepatic, renal status; ↓ dosage if impaired ▪ May be administered c̄ food/milk; encourage upright position for 15-30m ▪ Avoid exposure to moisture/light in storage ▪ Elderly may require ↓ dosage.

Note: Side/adverse effects: common in *italic;* serious in ***boldface italic.*** — *Available in Canada only.

EVALUATION: Monitor hematologic, hepatic, renal status c̄ prolonged use ▪ Monitor pt receiving anticoagulant therapy; may potentiate bleeding ▪ Monitor I&O, daily weight c̄ prolonged use ▪ Assess for edema in extremities, GI bleeding ▪ Assess for visual disturbances, skin rash; D/C drug, notify physician.

EDUCATION: Dizziness/drowsiness may occur; use caution in potentially hazardous activities ▪ Take c̄ food/milk; maintain upright position for 15-30m ▪ Take as ordered by physician; do *not* ↑ dose ▪ Notify physician *immediately* of bleeding, ↑ urine output, swelling of feet/legs, lethargy, GI distress, jaundice, visual disturbance ▪ Avoid taking c̄ aspirin, other NSAIAs ▪ Avoid use c̄ alcohol ▪ Check c̄ physician/pharmacist before taking OTC preparations ▪ Notify physician/dentist of use before treatment ▪ Store in tightly closed container ▪ Full drug effects may require several wks of therapy.

NOTES:

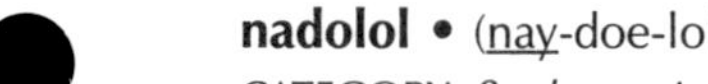

nadolol • (nay-doe-lole)

CATEGORY: *β-adrenergic blocker:* antianginal, antihypertensive Rx; Preg Cat C

BRAND NAME	**DOSAGE FORMS**
Corgard (B-MS)	Tablet: 20, 40, 80, 120, 160mg

COMBINATION PRODUCTS

Corzide 40/5, 80/5 (B-MS)	Nadolol/bendroflumethiazide per tablet: 40mg/5mg, 80mg/5mg

USE: Treatment of angina pectoris ▪ Treatment of hypertension as sole agent/in combination c̄ other antihypertensives (esp thiazide diuretics). **ACTION:** Blocks access of catecholamines to β_1, β_2 receptors, resulting in bronchial constriction, ⬇ heart rate, ⬇ myocardial contractility; antihypertensive effect not determined.

PHARMACOKINETICS

PO absorption	Peak	Half-life	Protein binding	Excretion
30%	3-4h	20-24h	30%	Via urine as unchanged drug

CONTRAINDICATIONS: Hypersensitivity, bronchial asthma, cardiogenic shock, overt cardiac failure, sinus bradycardia, heart block >1°. **CC:** Abrupt D/C can exacerbate ischemic heart disease ▪ Possible cardiac failure c̄ ⬇ myocardial contractility ▪ Tachycardia of hyperthyroidism may be masked, abrupt D/C may induce thyrotoxicosis ▪ Use c̄ caution in presence of bronchospastic, peripheral vascular disease.

DOSAGE

Adult *PO*

Angina	20-240mg/d as single dose
Hypertension	40-320mg/d as single dose. Up to 640mg/d may be required
Corzide 40/5, 80/5	Usual dose 1 tablet/d

SIDE/ADVERSE EFFECTS: CNS: dizziness, fatigue, paresthesias, sedation, behavioral changes ▪ CV: bradycardia (≤60), hypotension, ***cardiac failure,*** peripheral vascular insufficiency ▪ EENT: dry eyes, nasal congestion, tinnitus, blurred vision ▪ GI: N/D, anorexia, abdominal discomfort, flatulence, dry mouth ▪ GU: impotence ▪ RESP: bronchospasm ▪ Other: weight gain.

INTERACTIONS: Drug: Use c̄ reserpine, other catecholamine-depleting drugs can result in serious adrenergic blockage ▪ Nonselective β adrenergics antagonize therapeutic response.

NURSING MANAGEMENT PRIORITIES

ADMINISTRATION: Assess for hx of β-blocker hypersensitivity ▪ Assess BP, apical pulse; if <60/m, hold drug, notify physician ▪ Assess hepatic function, I&O ▪ Do *not* administer in presence of respiratory distress (asthma, CHF, COPD) ▪ Administer c̄ food ▪ Avoid exposure to heat/ moisture/light in storage ▪ Avoid abrupt withdrawal ▪ Elderly may require ⬇ dosage.

EVALUATION: Monitor hepatic, renal, respiratory status ▪ Monitor BP, pulse ▪ Monitor CBC, FBS (diabetics) ▪ Assess for depression ▪ May produce alteration in blood glucose levels (hypoglycemia); may mask signs of hypoglycemia.

EDUCATION: Check pulse before taking; if <60/m, do *not* take drug, notify physician ▪ Take as directed by physician; do *not* skip doses ▪ Take c̄ food ▪ Do *not* D/C drug w/out notifying physician ▪ Check c̄ physician/pharmacist before taking OTC/Rx preparations ▪ May cause drowsiness; use caution in potentially hazardous activities ▪ Diabetics: carefully monitor blood/urine glucose levels ▪ May experience ⬆ sensitivity to cold ▪ Notify physician of respiratory distress, leg edema ▪ Notify physician/ dentist of β-blocker use before treatment ▪ Maintain optimum weight ▪ Keep scheduled appointments c̄ physician ▪ Follow low-Na^+ diet ▪ Store in tightly closed, light-resistant container ▪ Avoid ⬆ exercise, cold, smoking ▪ Women: avoid breastfeeding.

NOTES:

nafcillin sodium • (naf-sill-in)

CATEGORY: *Penicillinase-resistant penicillin:* antibiotic — Rx; Preg Cat NA

BRAND NAMES	**DOSAGE FORMS**
Nallpen (SKB)	Powder for injection (IM/IV): 0.5-, 1-, 2-, 10-g vial
Unipen (W-A)	Capsule: 250mg

USE: Treatment of infections due to susceptible strains of penicillinase-producing staphylococci. **ACTION:** Bactericidal activity due to inhibition of mucopeptide cell wall synthesis in susceptible organisms.

PHARMACOKINETICS

PO absorption	Peak	Half-life	Protein binding	Excretion
Adequate	0.5-2h	0.5-1.5h	70%-90%	Via urine as unchanged drug, metabolites

CONTRAINDICATIONS: Hypersensitivity to any penicillin. **CC:** Serious/fatal (anaphylaxis) allergic rxs have occurred c̄ penicillin use ▪ Possible cross-allergenicity c̄ cephalosporins ▪ Resistance to any penicillin-resistant penicillin should be interpreted as resistance to all. Cross-resistance c̄ cephalosporins occurs frequently.

DOSAGE

Neonate	*PO*	10mg/kg 3-4 times/d
	IM	10mg/kg bid
Pediatric	*PO*	50mg/kg/d in 4 doses
	IM	25mg/kg bid
Adult	*PO*	250-500mg q4-6h. Severe infections may require 1g q4-6h
	IM	500mg q6h. Severe infections may require 500mg q4h
	IV	500mg q4h. Severe infections may require 1g q4h

SIDE/ADVERSE EFFECTS: CNS: neuropathy usually associated c̄ high parenteral doses ▪ GI: *N/V/D, epigastric distress, black hairy tongue,* flatulence, smell/taste disturbances ▪ GU: ***interstitial nephritis*** (rare) ▪ HEM: anemia, eosinophilia, leukopenia, neutropenia, ***thrombocytopenia*** ▪ HEP: ↑ serum levels of AST, ALT, LDH ▪ INT: rash, pruritus, urticaria ▪ MS: arthralgia ▪ Other: *local irritation at injection site*, fever, ***anaphylaxis.***

INTERACTIONS: Drug: Bacteriostatic antibiotics c̄ any penicillin can lead to antibiotic antagonism ▪ PO anticoagulant therapy may require dose adjustments.

NURSING MANAGEMENT PRIORITIES

ADMINISTRATION: Assess for hx of penicillin/cephalosporin hypersensitivity ▪ Obtain C&S ▪ Maintain blood levels; administer at equal intervals around clock ▪ PO: administer 1h ac/2h pc ▪ Reconstitute powder according to manufacturer's directions c̄ sterile or bacteriostatic H_2O for injection/0.9% NaCl injection; stable for 3d at room temperature, 7d refrigerated ▪ IM: administer by *deep* intragluteal injection (vastus lateralis <3y/o) ▪ IV: (direct) dilute in 15-30ml sterile H_2O for injection/NaCl injection, administer over 5-10m; (infusion) mix c̄ diluent recommended by manufacturer; use only 24-48h because of possibility of thrombophlebitis (esp elderly) ▪ Do *not* administer bacteriostatic agents w/in 1h ▪ Do *not* administer discolored/precipitated solutions ▪ Have support equipment available for anaphylaxis ▪ Na^+ content: 2.9mEq (67mg)/g; calculate in Na^+-restricted diets.

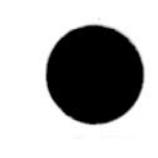

EVALUATION: Monitor pt c̄ allergies/asthma (high risk for hypersensitivity) ▪ Monitor VS, renal, hepatic, hemopoietic status ▪ Observe for signs of superinfection ▪ Check IV insertion site; rotate q48h.

EDUCATION: Complete full course of therapy (usually 10d) even if symptom free ▪ Take on empty stomach at equal intervals ▪ Take c̄ H_2O, *not* c̄ acidic beverage (orange juice, carbonated beverages) ▪ Diarrhea may occur ▪ Store in dry, tightly closed container ▪ Discard outdated preparations ▪ Maintain good personal hygiene (esp perineal, oral) ▪ Maintain fluid intake (6-8 glasses/d) ▪ Notify physician of symptoms of allergic rxs (fever, difficult breathing, rash) ▪ Carry identification (MedicAlert) if penicillin allergic.

NOTES:

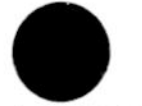

nalbuphine hcl • (<u>nal</u>-byoo-feen)

CATEGORY: *Analgesic:* opioid agonist-antagonist — Rx; Preg Cat C

BRAND NAME	DOSAGE FORMS
Nubain (Du Pont)	Injection (IM/IV/SC): 10, 20mg/ml

USE: Relief of moderate/severe pain ▪ Preop sedation, obstetric analgesia, adjunct to surgical anesthesia. **ACTION:** Analgesic mechanism not determined; possible site of activity may be in subcortical areas of brain; narcotic agonist activity equivalent to morphine (mg/mg); narcotic antagonist activity 1/4 that of nalorphine, 10 times pentazocine.

PHARMACOKINETICS

Onset IV	Onset IM/SC	Duration	Half-life	Excretion
2-3m	15m	3-6h	5h	Via urine, feces as unchanged drug, metabolites

CONTRAINDICATIONS: Hypersensitivity. **CC:** Use in narcotic-dependent pts can produce withdrawal symptoms.

DOSAGE

Adult *IM/IV/SC*	10mg/70kg weight, repeat q3-6h. Do *not* exceed single dose 20mg, daily total 160mg in nontolerant pts

SIDE/ADVERSE EFFECTS: CNS: *sedation*, dizziness, vertigo, headache, dreams, depression ▪ CV: hypertension, hypotension, bradycardia, tachycardia ▪ EENT: blurred vision ▪ GI: bitter taste, cramps, dyspepsia, dry mouth ▪ GU: urinary retention ▪ INT: urticaria, rash ▪ Other: autonomic responses (sweating/clammy sensation, flushing, warmth).

INTERACTIONS: Drug: Use c̄ CNS depressants produces additive effects ▪ Use in narcotic-dependent pts can produce withdrawal symptoms.

NURSING MANAGEMENT PRIORITIES

ADMINISTRATION: Assess for hx of opioid hypersensitivity ▪ Check compatibility chart for mixing preop IM preparations ▪ Do *not* administer if respirations are <12/m ▪ IM: inject *deep* into muscle; rotate sites ▪ IV: dilute; administer *slowly* ▪ Have narcotic antagonist, support measures available ▪ Avoid administration in pts c̄ suspected head injury ▪ Administer *before* pt has intense pain ▪ Avoid light/freezing in storage ▪ Utilize + power of suggestion ▪ Avoid abrupt withdrawal ▪ Elderly may require ↓ dosage.

EVALUATION: Monitor respirations, circulatory function ▪ Assess bowel function, abdominal distention ▪ Assess renal function, urinary retention ▪ Check for signs of dependence c̄ prolonged use (↑ drug request) ▪ Assess for potentiation of CNS depressant effect ▪ Assess for signs of OD (coma, pinpoint pupils, respiratory depression).

EDUCATION: Avoid changing positions (lying/sitting/standing) rapidly ▪ Avoid excessive sensory stimulation ▪ Keep bedrails up when nonambulatory ▪ Obtain assistance prn when ambulatory ▪ Turn, cough, deep-breathe after surgery ▪ Constipation may occur; ↑ fluid, bulk-containing foods ▪ Avoid potentially hazardous activities ▪ Avoid smoking while taking drug ▪ Indiscriminate use may lead to dependence ▪ Avoid use c̄ alcohol, other CNS depressants.

OVERDOSE MANAGEMENT: naloxone hcl is specific antidote in conjunction c̄ support therapy using oxygen, IV fluids, vasopressors.

NOTES:

naloxone hcl • (nal-ox-own)

CATEGORY: *Narcotic antagonist* Rx; Preg Cat B

BRAND NAME
Narcan (Du Pont)

DOSAGE FORMS
Injection (IM/IV/SC): 0.4, 1mg/ml
Neonatal injection (IM/IV/SC): 0.02mg/ml

USE: Induce complete/partial reversal of narcotic depression (incl respiratory) induced by natural/synthetic narcotics, propoxyphene, narcotic agonist/antagonist, nalbuphine, pentazocine, butorphanol ▪ Diagnosis of suspected acute opioid OD. **ACTION:** Narcotic antagonism primarily due to competition c̄ narcotics for CNS receptor sites.

PHARMACOKINETICS: IM/SC onset 2-5m, IV 1-2m; half-life 60-90m in adults, longer in infants; excreted via urine primarily as metabolites.

CONTRAINDICATIONS: Hypersensitivity. **CC:** Not intended for nonopioid respiratory depression ▪ Use c̄ caution, esp c̄ newborns of known or suspected opioid-dependent mothers.

DOSAGE

Pediatric *IM/IV/SC*	
Overdose	0.01mg/kg IV. Subsequent dose 0.1mg/kg may be given IV prn
Postop	0.005-0.01mg/kg IV. Repeat at 2-3m intervals to desired degree of reversal
	Neonate: 0.01mg/kg. Repeat at 2-3m intervals to desired degree of reversal
Adult *IM/IV/SC*	
Overdose	0.4-2mg IV. Repeat at 2-3m intervals to desired degree of reversal
Postop	0.1-0.2mg/kg IV. Repeat at 2-3m intervals to desired degree of reversal

SIDE/ADVERSE EFFECTS: GI: N/V (rare) c̄ high doses postop ▪ Other: withdrawal symptoms in narcotic-dependent pts.

NURSING MANAGEMENT PRIORITIES

ADMINISTRATION: Mix c̄ sterile H_2O for injection prn ▪ Do *not* leave pt unattended ▪ Have emergency support equipment available ▪ Store in original container; avoid exposure to light.

EVALUATION: Monitor VS, esp respirations ▪ Observe for ⬇ respirations after treatment because duration of action of narcotic may be longer than that of naloxone ▪ Observe for signs of narcotic withdrawal (restlessness, muscle spasms, ⬆ VS, lacrimation) ▪ Assess for ⬆ PTT ▪ Assess ABGs.

EDUCATION: Explain procedure, rationale to pt, family ▪ Safety precautions ▪ Comfort measures.

NOTES:

naproxen/naproxen sodium▲ • (na-prox-en)

CATEGORY: *Antiinflammatory:* analgesic

Rx/OTC†; Preg Cat B

BRAND NAMES	DOSAGE FORMS
Aleve (P-G)†	Tablet: 200mg
Anaprox▲ *(Syntex)*	Tablet: 275mg
Anaprox DS▲ *(Syntex)*	Tablet: 550mg
Naprelan (W-A)	Tablet: 375, 500mg
Naprosyn (Syntex)	PO suspension: 125mg/5ml Tablet: 250, 375, 500mg (also 125mg in Canada)
Naproxen EC (Syntex)	Delayed release tablet: 375, 500mg
**Naxen (SynCare)*	Tablet: 125, 250, 375, 500mg

USE: Treatment of rheumatoid/osteoarthritis, ankylosing spondylitis, acute gout, tendinitis, bursitis ▪ Relief of mild/moderate pain, primary dysmenorrhea. **ACTION:** Antiinflammatory, analgesic activity appears related to inhibition of prostaglandin synthesis.

PHARMACOKINETICS

PO absorption	Peak	Half-life	Protein binding	Excretion
Complete	2-4h	13h	99%	95% via urine primarily as unchanged drug

CONTRAINDICATIONS: Hypersensitivity, aspirin/other antiinflammatory agent hypersensitivity. **CC:** Use ↑ risk of GI bleeding, ulcers, perforation.

DOSAGE

Adult *PO*

Pain, dysmenorrhea, tendinitis, bursitis	Naproxen 500mg followed by 250mg q6-8h, c̄ maximum dose 1.25g/d. Naproxen sod-ium 550mg followed by 275mg q6-8h, c̄ maximum dose 1.375g/d
Acute gout	Naproxen 750mg followed by 250mg q8h until remission. Naproxen sodium 825mg followed by 275mg q8h until remission

Note: Side/adverse effects: common in *italic;* serious in ***boldface italic.***

*Available in Canada only.

Juvenile arthritis	10mg/kg/d in 2 divided doses
Arthritis, spondylitis	Naproxen 250-375mg bid, adjust, c̄ maximum dose 1g/d. Naproxen sodium 275mg bid, adjust, c̄ maximum dose 1.1g/d
OTC dose	200mg q8-12h. Do *not* exceed 600mg/d

SIDE/ADVERSE EFFECTS: CNS: headache, dizziness, drowsiness ▪ CV: edema, palpitations, CHF ▪ EENT: tinnitus, ⬇ hearing, blurred vision ▪ GI: *constipation, abdominal pain, nausea,* vomiting, stomatitis ▪ GU: ***glomerular nephritis,*** hematuria, ***interstitial nephritis,*** nephrotic syndrome ▪ HEM: ***agranulocytosis, aplastic anemia, hemolytic anemia*** ▪ INT: rash, alopecia, pruritus, purpura, urticaria ▪ Other: thirst, eosinophilic pneumonia.

INTERACTIONS: Drug: Use c̄ ulcerogenic drugs produces additive effects ▪ Use c̄ PO anticoagulants may ⬆ their activity ▪ Aspirin will ⬇ naproxen plasma levels.

NURSING MANAGEMENT PRIORITIES

ADMINISTRATION: Assess for hx of NSAIA hypersensitivity ▪ Avoid administration to pts c̄ hx of asthma, bleeding disorders, salicylate hypersensitivity ▪ Assess for hx of peptic ulcer; use c̄ caution ▪ Assess hematologic, renal, hepatic function; use caution if impaired ▪ Administer c̄ food/milk to ⬇ GI irritation; encourage upright position for 15-30m ▪ Avoid exposure to moisture in storage ▪ Elderly may require ⬇ dosage.

EVALUATION: Monitor hepatic, renal status c̄ prolonged use ▪ Monitor pt receiving anticoagulant therapy; may potentiate bleeding ▪ Monitor I&O, daily weight ▪ Assess for edema in extremities ▪ Assess for visual/hearing disturbances; D/C drug, notify physician.

EDUCATION: Dizziness/drowsiness may occur; use caution in potentially hazardous activities ▪ Take c̄ food/milk to ⬇ GI distress; maintain upright position for 15-30m ▪ Take as ordered by physician, do *not* ⬆ dose ▪ Notify physician *immediately* of bleeding, ⬇ urine output, swelling of feet/legs, lethargy, GI distress, jaundice, visual disturbance ▪ Avoid taking c̄ aspirin/other NSAIAs ▪ Avoid use c̄ alcohol ▪ Check c̄ physician/pharmacist before taking OTC preparations ▪ Notify physician/dentist of use before treatment ▪ Store in tightly closed container ▪ Schedule eye exams c̄ prolonged use ▪ Full drug effects may require several wks of therapy.

NOTES:

naratriptan • (nare-ah-trip-tan)

CATEGORY: *Antimigraine agent:* serotonin receptor agonist — Rx; Preg Cat C

BRAND NAME
Amerge (G-W)

DOSAGE FORMS
Tablet: 1, 2.5mg

USE: Treatment of acute migraine c̄ or w/out aura
ACTION: Migraine is associated c̄ selective cerebral vasodilation & release of sensory neuropeptides from the trigemovascular system that includes substance P, neurokinin A, & other vasoactive peptides.

Antimigraine activity of naratriptan, a serotonin 5HT-1 receptor agonist, appears related to specific agonist activity on selected cerebral blood vessels containing 5HT-1 receptors, resulting in vasoconstriction & inhibition of sensory neuropeptide release from the trigemovascular system.

CONTRAINDICATIONS: Hypersensitivity, w/in 24h after administration of an ergot-type medication, incl dihydroergotamine, ergotamine, methysergide, current use &/or w/in 2wks of D/C MAO-I therapy, severe cardiovascular/peripheral syndrome, & hepatic/renal impairment. **CC:** Use of 5HT-1 agonists requires a + diagnosis of migraine ▪ Use can produce significant cardiovascular events, incl MI, ventricular tachycardia/fibrillation, cardiac arrest, death ▪ Use in geriatric pts c̄ ↓ renal function requires caution ▪ Use c̄ caution in pts c̄ hepatic impairment ▪ Safety & efficacy in children not established.

DOSAGE

Adult	*PO*	1 or 2.5mg as a single dose & repeated if needed once q4h to a maximum of 5mg in 24h

PHARMACOKINETICS

PO absorption	Peak serum	Half-life	Protein binding	Excretion
High	3-4h	2.8-3.7h	28%-31%	Via feces, urine primarily as metabolites

Note: Side/adverse effects: common in *italic;* serious in ***boldface italic.*** — *Available in Canada only.

SIDE/ADVERSE EFFECTS: CNS: dizziness, sleep disorders, tremors, aggression ▪ CV: ***abnormal EKG, atrial/ventricular arrhythmias,*** hypotension ▪ GI: N/V/D, dyspepsia, gastroenteritis, constipation, hyposalivation ▪ GU: bladder inflammation, ***urinary hemorrhage***, vaginal inflammation ▪ HEM: ↑ WBC, ***thrombocytopenia*** ▪ INT: rash, pruritus, urticaria, photosensitivity ▪ RESP: bronchitis, cough, pneumonia ▪ Other: muscle pain, chills, fever.

INTERACTIONS: Drug: Use c̄ PO contraceptives can ↓ naratriptan metabolism & clearance.

NURSING MANAGEMENT PRIORITIES

ADMINISTRATION: Assess for hx of hypersensitivity to serotonin 5HT-1 receptor agonists ▪ Assess CV, hepatic, renal function; use caution if impaired ▪ Assess severity of headache, associated symptoms ▪ Administer c̄ fluids at onset of attack ▪ Maintain quiet environment.

EVALUATION: Monitor neurologic, CV, hepatic, renal status; notify physician if abnormal ▪ Monitor severity of headache when relief is obtained ▪ Observe pt for signs of ↑ bleeding.

EDUCATION: Dizziness may occur, use caution in potentially hazardous activities ▪ Avoid foods containing tyramine (aged & fermented foods) ▪ Notify physician *immediately* of abnormal rxs (burning, numbness, tingling, bleeding) ▪ Check c̄ physician/pharmacist before taking any OTC preparations ▪ Women: avoid breastfeeding.

NOTES:

nefazodone hcl • (neh-faz-oh-doan)

CATEGORY: *Antidepressant* Rx; Preg Cat C

BRAND NAME
Serzone (B-MS)

DOSAGE FORMS
Tablet: 100, 150, 200, 250mg

USE: Treatment of depression. **ACTION:** Antidepressant activity not determined.

PHARMACOKINETICS

PO absorption	Peak	Half-life	Protein binding	Excretion
Complete	1h	2-4h	99%	Via urine as metabolites

CONTRAINDICATIONS: Hypersensitivity, use c̄ astemizole, terfenadine. **CC:** Long-term use (>6wk) requires periodic reevaluation, use c̄ MAO-I can result in fatal rxs.

DOSAGE

Adult	*PO*	Start c̄ 100mg bid. Thereafter dosage may be ↑ by 100-200mg at least q1wk at 1-wk intervals to a maximum of 600mg/d
Geriatrics	*PO*	Start c̄ 50mg bid & adjust

SIDE/ADVERSE EFFECTS: CNS: headache, somnolence, dizziness, lightheadedness, confusion, agitation ▪ CV: ***sinus bradycardia,*** peripheral edema ▪ EENT: blurred vision, tinnitus ▪ GI: dry mouth, N/V/D, constipation, dyspepsia, taste changes ▪ GU: urinary frequency & infection, vaginitis ▪ INT: pruritus, rash ▪ Other: pharyngitis, fever.

INTERACTIONS: Drug: Use c̄ astemizole, MAO-I, contraindicated ▪ Use c̄ other high-protein–bound drugs can result in displacement from inactive protein binding sites ▪ Use c̄ alprazolam, astemizole, terfenadine, triazolam can ↑ their plasma levels ▪ Use c̄ propranolol ↓ its plasma levels. **Food:** Meals can ↓ PO absorption.

NURSING MANAGEMENT PRIORITIES

ADMINISTRATION: Assess for hx of hypersensitivity ▪ Assess for hx of seizures; use caution ▪ Assess hepatic, renal status; ↓ dosage if impaired ▪ Administer pc ▪ Institute safety, seizure precautions ▪ Institute suicide precautions ▪ Avoid abrupt withdrawal; D/C gradually ▪ Avoid moisture/heat/direct light in storage ▪ Elderly may require ↓ dosage.

EVALUATION: Monitor BP (hypotension c̄ antihypertensive therapy) ▪ Monitor CV, hepatic, renal status ▪ Monitor fluid retention (I&O, daily weight), constipation ▪ Assess for weight loss (anorectic effect) ▪ Assess for symptoms of abrupt withdrawal (nausea, headache, malaise) ▪ Assess for actual swallowing of PO forms ▪ Assess for skin rash, hives; notify physician, D/C drug.

EDUCATION: Dizziness/drowsiness may occur; use caution in potentially hazardous activities ▪ Avoid changing positions (lying/sitting/standing) rapidly ▪ Avoid use c̄ alcohol, other CNS depressants for up to 1wk after end of therapy ▪ Take shortly pc ▪ Take as directed by physician ▪ Use sugarless gum/hard candy to diminish dry mouth ▪ Constipation may occur; ↑ fluids, bulk-containing foods ▪ Notify physician of skin rash, hives; D/C drug ▪ Check c̄ physician/pharmacist before taking OTC/Rx preparations ▪ Notify physician/dentist of use before treatment ▪ Store in a tightly closed, light-resistant container ▪ Encourage recreational/diversional interests ▪ Notify physician of weight loss, fever, sore throat, malaise ▪ Keep scheduled appointments c̄ physician ▪ Women: notify physician of pregnancy possibility; avoid breastfeeding ▪ Full drug effects may require several wks of therapy.

NOTES:

neostigmine bromide/neostigmine methylsulfate • (nee-oh-stig-meen)

CATEGORY: *Anticholinesterase:* cholinergic, parasympathomimetic   Rx; Preg Cat C

BRAND NAMES	DOSAGE FORMS
Prostigmin Bromide (ICN)	Tablet: 15mg
Prostigmin Methylsulfate (ICN)	Injection (IM/IV/SC): 0.25, 0.5, 1mg/ml (2.5mg/ml in Canada)

USE: Symptomatic control of myasthenia gravis ▪ Prevention/treatment of postoperative distention, urinary retention ▪ Antidote for tubocurarine-like drugs (nondepolarizing agents). **ACTION:** Anticholinesterase drugs inhibit acetylcholinesterase enzyme, resulting in higher levels of acetylcholine, producing nicotinic effect at autonomic ganglia, skeletal muscle myoneural junctions, muscarinic effect at postganglionic fibers in parasympathetic nervous system.

PHARMACOKINETICS

PO absorption	Peak	Half-life	Protein binding	Excretion
Poor	1-2	42-60m	15%-25%	80% via urine in 24h

CONTRAINDICATIONS: Hypersensitivity, mechanical bowel/urinary tract obstruction, peritonitis. **CC:** Use c̄ caution in pts c̄ bradycardia, bronchial asthma, cardiac arrhythmias, coronary occlusion, epilepsy, hyperthyroidism, peptic ulcer, vagotonia.

DOSAGE

Pediatric/Adult	*PO*	Dosage must be individualized for myasthenia gravis, varies from 15-375mg/d
Adult		
Myasthenia gravis	*SC/IM*	0.5mg. Subsequent doses dependent on response
Postop	*SC/IM*	0.25mg as soon as possible after surgery. May be repeated q4-6h for 2-3d for prevention of urinary retention
Urinary retention	*SC/IM*	0.5mg. If urination does not occur w/in 1h, catheterize. After urine voiding, continue doses of 0.5mg q3h for at least 5 injections
Antidote	*IV*	0.5-2mg by slow injection. Recommended that atropine sulfate 0.6-1.2mg also be given IV by separate syringe

SIDE/ADVERSE EFFECTS: CNS: dizziness, drowsiness, headache, ***convulsions*** ▪ CV: bradycardia, tachycardia, ***AV block,*** hypotension ▪ EENT: miosis, vision change ▪ GI: N/V, flatulence, cramps ▪ GU: urinary frequency ▪ INT: rash, urticaria ▪ RESP: ↑ secretion, dyspnea, ***bronchospasm,*** depression ▪ Other: diaphoresis.

INTERACTIONS: Drug: Use c̄ anticholinergics antagonizes cholinergic effects.

NURSING MANAGEMENT PRIORITIES

ADMINISTRATION: Assess for hx of hypersensitivity ▪ Do *not* administer c̄ other cholinergic drugs ▪ Largest dose scheduled before periods of ↑ fatigue ▪ PO: administer c̄ food/milk to ↓ GI irritation ▪ Document response after each dose ▪ Have atropine, support equipment available.

EVALUATION: Monitor VS, esp pulse, respirations ▪ Monitor muscle strength ▪ Assess for excessive cholinergic manifestations (↑ sweating, ↑ salivation, muscle tremors) ▪ Monitor GI status (flatus, abdominal distention) ▪ Assess for urinary retention; catheterize if no voiding w/in 1h of first dose.

EDUCATION: Take c̄ food/milk to ↓ GI distress ▪ Take as ordered by physician; do *not* change dose ▪ Space daily activities to ↓ fatigue, conserve energy ▪ Adhere to scheduled coughing & deep-breathing, ROM activities ▪ Record high, low points of muscle strength ▪ Rectal tube may be inserted after administration to help expel gas related to postop abdominal distention ▪ Carry medical identification (MedicAlert) for myasthenia gravis.

NOTES:

netilmicin sulfate • (ne-til-mye-sin)

CATEGORY: *Aminoglycoside:* antibiotic

Rx; Preg Cat D

BRAND NAME	**DOSAGE FORMS**
Netromycin (Schering)	Injection (IM/IV): 100mg/ml

USE: Indicated for infections caused by susceptible strains of *Citrobacter* spp, *Enterobacter* spp, *Escherichia coli, Klebsiella pneumoniae, Proteus* spp, *Pseudomonas aeruginosa, Serratia* spp ▪ Alternate for penicillin-resistant staphylococcal infections.

ACTION: Bactericidal activity due to inhibition of ribosomal protein synthesis in susceptible organisms.

PHARMACOKINETICS

IM peak	Half-life	Excretion
0.5-1h	2-2.5h	80% unchanged in urine in 24h

CONTRAINDICATIONS: Hypersensitivity, previous aminoglycoside toxicity (possible). **CC:** Use of aminoglycosides during pregnancy can result in bilateral congenital deafness ▪ Use can produce serious ototoxicity, nephrotoxicity ▪ Use aminoglycosides c̄ caution in pts c̄ neuromuscular disorders ▪ Injection contains sodium metabisulfite, which can cause allergic rxs.

DOSAGE: *IM/IV*. For pts c̄ impaired renal function, adjust dose according to manufacturer's recommendations.

Neonate <6wks	4-6.5mg/kg/d given as 2-3.25mg/kg q12h
Pediatric 6wk-12y/o	5.5-8mg/kg/d given as 1.8-2.7mg/kg q8h or 2.74mg/kg q12h
Adult	3-4mg/kg/d given as 1.5-2mg/kg q8-12h. More serious infection may require 4-6.5mg/kg/d

SIDE/ADVERSE EFFECTS: CNS: paresthesias ▪ CV: palpitations, hypotension ▪ EENT: ***ototoxicity*** (auditory vestibular damage: dizziness, vertigo, tinnitus, roaring in ears, hearing loss), blurred vision ▪ GI: V/D ▪ GU: ***nephrotoxicity*** (casts, proteinuria, ↑ BUN, ↑ serum creatinine) ▪ HEM: anemia, leukopenia, ***thrombocytopenia*** ▪ HEP: ↑ alkaline phosphatase, bilirubin, AST, ALT ▪ MET: hypokalemia.

INTERACTIONS: Drug: Avoid use c̄ neurotoxic/nephrotoxic drugs (eg, other aminoglycosides, colistin, ethacrynic acid, furosemide, polymyxin B, vancomycin) ▪ Dimenhydrinate can mask aminoglycoside ototoxicity ▪ ↑ Succinylcholine/tubocurarine activity; Ca salts can reverse blockade ▪ PO anticoagulant activity may ↑ due to ↓ intestinal vitamin K synthesis.

NURSING MANAGEMENT PRIORITIES

ADMINISTRATION: Assess for hx of aminoglycoside hypersensitivity ▪ Obtain C&S before therapy ▪ Obtain pt weight for dosage calculation ▪ Determine creatinine clearance before administration ▪ IV: single dose may be diluted in 50-200ml parenteral solution; infuse over ½-1h; use less diluent for pediatric IV ▪ Store solution in glass containers for up to 72h ▪ IM: administer by *deep, slow* injection; rotate sites; avoid inflamed areas ▪ Maintain hydration.

EVALUATION: Assess for hearing dysfunction ▪ Monitor hepatic, renal, VIII CN function during therapy ▪ Assess for edema in extremities ▪ Assess for neuromuscular blockade, respiratory paralysis, nephrotoxicity ▪ Observe for signs of superinfection (diarrhea, URI, coated tongue) ▪ Assess for hypersensitivity rx (fever, difficult breathing, rash) ▪ Assess peak (<16µg/ml), trough (<4µg/ml) serum concentrations.

EDUCATION: Report hearing, balance difficulties to physician at once ▪ ↑ Fluid intake (10-12 glasses/d) ▪ Women: avoid breastfeeding.

NOTES:

nicardipine hcl • (nye-card-i-peen)

CATEGORY: *Calcium blocker:* antianginal, antihypertensive, slow channel blocker Rx; Preg Cat C

BRAND NAMES
Cardene (Roche)

Cardene IV (W-A)

DOSAGE FORMS
Capsule: 20, 30mg
SR capsule: 30, 45, 60mg
IV injection 2.5mg/ml

USE: Treatment as a sole agent/in combination c̄ a β blocker for chronic stable angina pectoris; treatment for hypertension as a sole agent/in combination c̄ other antihypertensives. **ACTION:** Antianginal & antihypertensive effect due to inhibition of extracellular calcium-ion transmembrane migration in cardiac, vascular smooth muscle via slow channel passageway, resulting in coronary dilation; ↑ myocardial oxygen supply, ↓ oxygen consumption. Slow channel effect is greater in vascular smooth muscle.

CONTRAINDICATIONS: Hypersensitivity, advanced aortic stenosis. **CC:** Possible exacerbation of angina c̄ use ▪ Use c̄ caution in pts c̄ CHF, in combination c̄ a β blocker.

DOSAGE: Normal hepatic & renal function

Adult *PO*	
Angina/hypertension	20-40mg tid. Dosage ↑ requires 3-d intervals. SR capsule usual dose is 30-60mg bid
Adult *IV*	
Hypertension	Usual infusion dose 5mg/h & then adjusted

PHARMACOKINETICS

PO absorption	Onset	Peak	Half-life	Protein binding	Excretion
Complete	20m	0.5-2h	2-4h	95%	As metabolites via urine (60%), feces (35%)

SIDE/ADVERSE EFFECTS: CNS: *headache, dizziness,* tremor, paresthesia, flushing, somnolence ▪ CV: *pedal edema,* palpitations, tachycardia, angina, abnormal ECG ▪ GI: *nausea, dyspepsia, dry mouth,* constipation, vomiting ▪ Other: rash, dyspnea, myalgia, malaise, *asthenia.*

INTERACTIONS: Drug: Calcium blockers may ↑ dig serum level ▪ Use c̄ β blockers is well tolerated ▪ Cimetidine ↑ nicardipine serum levels ▪ Nicardipine may ↑ cyclosporine serum levels.

NURSING MANAGEMENT PRIORITIES

ADMINISTRATION: Assess for hx of hypersensitivity ▪ Assess for hx of heart failure; use c̄ caution ▪ Assess BP, heart rate; if apical pulse <60/m, hold dose, notify physician ▪ Assess hepatic, renal function; ↓ dosage if impaired ▪ Assess dietary intake (avoid high-fat meals) ▪ Avoid exposure to light/moisture in storage ▪ Elderly may require ↓ dosage.

EVALUATION: Monitor VS, esp BP (2h & 8h after administration), heart rate ▪ Monitor I&O ▪ Assess for CHF (dyspnea, peripheral edema, ↑ weight); notify physician ▪ Monitor hepatic, renal status.

EDUCATION: Dizziness may occur; use caution in potentially hazardous activities ▪ Avoid changing positions (lying/sitting/standing) rapidly ▪ Avoid high-fat meals during therapy ▪ Procedure for checking radial pulse ▪ If pulse slow (<60/m) or irregular, notify physician ▪ Avoid caffeine ▪ Check c̄ physician/pharmacist before taking OTC preparations ▪ Take as ordered by physician; do *not* change dose ▪ Notify physician of difficult breathing, chest pain, swelling of hands/legs ▪ Keep scheduled appointments c̄ physician; have BP checked regularly ▪ Continue to use sublingual nitroglycerin (if ordered) to relieve sudden chest pain or for prophylaxis before exertion ▪ Avoid use c̄ alcohol ▪ Avoid smoking ▪ Carry identification (MedicAlert) if hypertensive ▪ Women: avoid breastfeeding.

NOTES:

DESCRIPTION: Small group of drugs used in treatment of angina, arrhythmias; also called calcium antagonists, slow channel blockers, calcium channel blocking agents.

DRUGS: amlodipine *(Norvasc),* bepridil *(Vascor),* diltiazem hcl *(Cardizem),* felodipine *(Plendil),* isradipine *(DynaCirc),* mibefradil dihydrochloride *(Posicar),* nicardipine hcl *(Cardene),* nifedipine *(Procardia),* nimodipine *(Nimotop),* nisoldipine *(Sular),* verapamil hcl *(Calan, Isoptin, Verelan).*

THERAPEUTIC USE: Treatment of vasospastic angina: amlodipine, diltiazem, nifedipine, verapamil ▪ **Chronic stable angina:** amlodipine, bepridil, diltiazem, mibefradil, nicardipine, nifedipine, verapamil ▪ **Hypertension:** amlodipine, diltiazem (only SR dosage forms), felodipine, isradipine, mibefradil, nicardipine, nifedipine (only SR dosage forms), nisoldipine, verapamil (only SR dosage forms) ▪ **Arrhythmias:** verapamil (control of rapid ventricular rate in atrial flutter/fibrillation & prophylaxis of repetitive paroxysmal supraventricular tachycardia) ▪ **Spasm of subarachnoid hemorrhage:** nimodipine.

PHARMACOKINETICS

	Absorption		Onset	Peak	Half-life	Protein binding	Excretion
amlodipine	PO	NA	NA	6-12h	30-50h	93%	Via urine
bepridil	PO	100%	1h	2-3h	24h	99%	Via urine
diltiazem	PO	80%	30m	2-3h	3.5-9h	70%-85%	Via urine
felodipine	PO	100%	2-5h	2-5h	11-16h	99%	Via urine
isradipine	PO	90%-95%	20m	1.5h	1.5-8h	95%	Via urine
nicardipine	PO	100%	20m	0.5-2h	2-4h	>95%	Via urine, feces
nifedipine	PO	90%	20m	30m	2h	92%-98%	Via urine
nimodipine	PO	NA	NA	1h	1-2h	95%	Via urine
nisoldipine	PO	NA	NA	6-12h	7-12h	99%	Via urine
verapamil	PO	90%	30m	1-2h	2-8h	90%	Via urine
	IV	—	3-5m	5m	2-8h	90%	Via urine

MECHANISM OF ACTION: Antianginal effect due to inhibition of extracellular calcium-ion transmembrane migration in cardiac, vascular smooth muscle via slow channel pathway, resulting in coronary dilation; in addition, ↑ myocardial O_2 supply, ↓ O_2 consumption. Antiarrhythmic effect of verapamil due to effect on SA node, prolongation of atrioventricular refractory period.

DOSAGE: Usual adult dosage range

amlodipine	*PO*	5-10mg once/d
bepridil	*PO*	200-400mg/d
diltiazem	*PO*	180-240mg divided, 3-4 times/d
felodipine	*PO*	5-10mg/d
isradipine	*PO*	5-20mg/d divided
mibefradil	*PO*	50-100mg once/d
nicardipine	*PO*	20-40mg tid
nifedipine	*PO*	10-20mg tid
nimodipine	*PO*	60mg q4h for 21d
nisoldipine	*PO*	20-60mg once/d
verapamil	*PO*	320-480mg divided
	IV	5-10mg bolus over 2m

NURSING MANAGEMENT PRIORITIES

ASSESS: Hx of hypersensitivity ▪ Apical pulse, BP, ECG ▪ Lung sounds ▪ CAUTION: hepatic disease, heart failure ▪ **ndx: Therapeutic effects**: ↓ Cardiac output ▪ Pain ▪ Altered tissue perfusion ▪ **Adverse effects:** Risk for activity intolerance ▪ Anxiety ▪ Ineffective breathing patterns ▪ ↓ Cardiac output ▪ Constipation ▪ Fluid volume excess ▪ Pain. **PLAN:** Prevent postural hypotension ▪ Institute cardiac monitoring (IV, initial PO) ▪ Administer at equal intervals around clock to maintain blood levels ▪ **Special considerations:** G: caution, ↓ dosage (renal impairment, prolonged half-life) ▪ P: caution, ↓ dosage (↑ hemodynamic effect) ▪ OB: caution if pregnant, breastfeeding not recommended ▪ **Dietary management**: Avoid caffeine, use c̄ alcohol, high-Na^+ foods ▪ **Lab test evaluation**: Serum digoxin levels (digitalized pts). **IMPLEMENT:** Assess apical pulse for 1m ▪ Monitor F/E status (I&O, daily weight, peripheral edema) ▪ **Patient education:** Procedure for checking radial pulse ▪ Comply c̄ prescribed drug regimen ▪ Take safety precautions c̄ ambulation, hazardous activity ▪ Report abnormal rxs to physician (chest pain; difficult breathing; rapid, irregular heart rate) ▪ Avoid sudden position changes (postural hypotension) ▪ Check c̄ physician/pharmacist before taking OTC preparations ▪ Keep appointments c̄ physician. **EVALUATE: Observe for therapeutic effects:** ↓ Cardiac arrhythmias ▪ Normal heart rate, rhythm ▪ ↓ BP.

nifedipine • (nye-fed-i-peen)

CATEGORY: *Calcium blocker:* antianginal, slow channel blocker — Rx; Preg Cat C

BRAND NAMES | **DOSAGE FORMS**

BRAND NAMES	DOSAGE FORMS
Adalat (Bayer)	Capsule 10, 20mg
Adalat CC (Bayer)	Extended release tablets: 30, 60, 90mg
Procardia (Pratt)	*Capsule, 10, 20mg* XL tablet: 30, 60, 90mg

USE: Treatment of chronic, stable, vasospastic angina pectoris ▪ Nonlabeled OB uses include prophylaxis of preterm labor ▪ Treatment of hypertension as a sole agent/in combination (XL only). **ACTION:** Antianginal effect due to inhibition of extracellular calcium-ion transmembrane migration in cardiac, vascular smooth muscle via slow channel passageway, resulting in coronary dilation; in addition, ↑ myocardial oxygen supply, ↓ oxygen consumption.

CONTRAINDICATIONS: Hypersensitivity. **CC:** Use can result in exacerbation of angina or acute MI ▪ Observe for excessive hypotensive effects, possible ↑ bleeding time due to ↓ in platelet aggregation.

DOSAGE

Adult *PO*	Initial dose 10mg tid. Usual daily range 10-20mg tid. Do *not* exceed 30mg/dose or 180mg/d OB (labor) dose is usually 10mg tid as required XL tablets: start c̄ 30 or 60mg once/d & adjust over 7-14d. Do *not* exceed 120mg/d CC tablets: start c̄ 30mg once/d & adjust over 7-14d. Do *not* exceed 90mg/d

PHARMACOKINETICS

PO absorption	Onset	Peak	Half-life	Protein binding	Excretion
90%	20m	30m	2h	92%-98%	80% via urine as unchanged drug, metabolites

SIDE/ADVERSE EFFECTS: CNS: *dizziness*, headache, nervousness ▪ CV: *peripheral edema*, transient hypotension, palpitations ▪ EENT: nasal congestion, sore throat, blurred vision, gingival hyperplasia (rare) ▪ GI: *nausea*, diarrhea, cramps, flatulence, constipation ▪ HEM: anemia, leukopenia, purpura ▪ INT: urticaria, dermatitis, pruritus ▪ MS: muscle cramps, tremor, joint stiffness ▪ Other: flushing, weakness.

INTERACTIONS: Drug: Use c̄ dig may ↑ dig body levels ▪ Use c̄ antihypertensives may ↑ hypotensive effects ▪ Use c̄ β blockers may occasionally ↑ possibility of CHF, severe hypotension, angina attacks. **Lab:** ↑ In creatine phosphokinase, serum glutamate oxaloacetate transaminase, serum glutamate pyruvate transaminase, + Coombs' test.

NURSING MANAGEMENT PRIORITIES

ADMINISTRATION: Assess for hx of hypersensitivity ▪ Assess for hx of heart failure; use c̄ caution ▪ Assess BP, heart rate; if apical pulse <60, hold dose, notify physician ▪ May puncture capsule c̄ needle, deposit solution sublingually or in buccal pouch for rapid action ▪ Avoid exposure to light/moisture in storage ▪ Elderly may require ↓ dosage.

EVALUATION: Monitor VS, esp BP, heart rate ▪ Monitor I&O ▪ Assess for CHF (dyspnea, peripheral edema, ↑ weight); notify physician ▪ Monitor hepatic, renal status ▪ Diabetics: closely monitor blood glucose ▪ Digitalized pts: assess for dig toxicity (bradycardia, anorexia, palpitations).

EDUCATION: Dizziness may occur; use caution in potentially hazardous activities ▪ Avoid changing positions (lying/sitting/standing) rapidly ▪ Procedure for checking radial pulse ▪ If pulse slow (<60) or irregular, do *not* take drug; notify physician ▪ Avoid caffeine ▪ Check c̄ physician/pharmacist before taking OTC preparations ▪ Take as ordered by physician; do *not* change dose ▪ Notify physician of difficult breathing, chest pain, swelling of hands/ legs; D/C drug ▪ Keep scheduled appointments c̄ physician ▪ Continue to use sublingual nitroglycerin (if ordered) to relieve sudden chest pain or for prophylaxis before exertion ▪ Avoid use c̄ alcohol ▪ Avoid smoking ▪ Diabetics: monitor blood or urine glucose carefully; keep scheduled lab appointments.

NOTES:

nitrofurantoin • (nye-troe-fyoor-an-toyn)

CATEGORY: *Antiinfective:* urinary antimicrobial — Rx; Preg Cat B

BRAND NAMES	DOSAGE FORMS
Furadantin (P-G)	Suspension: 25mg/5ml Tablet: 50, 100mg
Macrobid (P-G)	Capsule: 100mg
Macrodantin (P-G)	Capsule: 25, 50, 100mg
**Nephronex (Cortunon)*	Tablet: 50, 100mg
**Novoturan (Novopharm)*	Suspension: 25mg/5ml Tablet: 50, 100mg

USE: Treatment of UTIs caused by susceptible strains of *Enterobacter* spp, enterococci, *Escherichia coli, Klebsiella* spp, *Proteus* spp, *Staphylococcus aureus* (not indicated for treatment of associated renal cortical/perinephric abscesses). **ACTION:** Bacteriostatic activity due to possible interference c̄ several enzyme systems incl coenzyme A in susceptible organisms.

PHARMACOKINETICS

PO absorption	Half-life	Protein binding	Excretion
Good	20m	25%-60%	Via urine as unchanged drug, metabolites

CONTRAINDICATIONS: Hypersensitivity, anuria, oliguria, significant renal dysfunction, pregnancy at term, infants <1mo. **CC:** Use associated c̄ acute/subacute/chronic pneumonitis/pulmonary fibrosis or both & chronic active hepatitis/necrosis ▪ Possible severe/irreversible neuropathy ▪ Use can result in pseudomembranous colitis.

DOSAGE

Pediatric	*PO*	5-7mg/kg/d in 4 equal doses c̄ food
Adult	*PO*	50-100mg qid c̄ food

SIDE/ADVERSE EFFECTS: CNS: peripheral neuropathy, headache, dizziness, drowsiness ▪ EENT: nystagmus ▪ GI: diarrhea, *anorexia, N/V,* pain, ***pancreatitis*** ▪ HEM: ***hemolytic anemia***, granulocytopenia, ***agranulocytosis***, leukopenia, ***thrombocytopenia, megaloblastic anemia,*** eosinophilia ▪ HEP: cholestatic jaundice, hepatitis ▪ INT: pruritus, urticaria, maculopapular rash, ***exfoliative dermatitis, erythema multiforme,*** alopecia ▪ MS: arthralgia ▪ RESP: acute, subacute, chronic diffuse ***interstitial pneumonitis/pulmonary fibrosis;*** asthma attack ▪ Other: ***anaphylaxis,*** drug fever.

INTERACTIONS: Drug: Probenecid/sulfinpyrazone ↓ renal excretion, ↑ toxicity ▪ Use c̄ nalidixic acid best avoided ▪ Use c̄ magnesium trisilicate antacid ↓ PO absorption of nitrofurantoin.

NURSING MANAGEMENT PRIORITIES

ADMINISTRATION: Assess for hx of hypersensitivity ▪ Assess creatinine clearance; if <40ml/m, do *not* administer ▪ Obtain C&S before therapy ▪ Administer c̄ food/milk to ↓ GI irritation; do *not* crush (may stain teeth); have pt rinse mouth after administration ▪ PO suspension: shake well before pouring ▪ Avoid exposure to light/metals (except stainless steel, aluminum) in storage.

EVALUATION: Monitor VS, esp temperature ▪ Monitor respiratory status ▪ Monitor I&O, CBC, urine pH (acidity ↑ drug effect) ▪ Assess for UTI (cloudy, foul-smelling urine; painful urination) ▪ Urine glucose: false + c̄ Clinitest; use Clinistix/Diastix.

EDUCATION: Take c̄ food/milk to ↓ GI distress ▪ Take as ordered by physician; Rx will be continued for 3d after sterile urine specimens obtained ▪ Notify physician *immediately* of numbness, tingling, ↓ muscle strength; D/C drug ▪ Use Clinistix/Diastix for urine testing ▪ May turn urine brown ▪ Store in amber glass container ▪ Women: avoid breastfeeding ▪ Check c̄ physician/pharmacist before taking antacids.

NOTES:

nitroglycerin (glyceryl trinitrate) formulations • (nye-troe-gli-ser-in)

CATEGORY: *Antianginal:* coronary vasodilator Rx; Preg Cat C

FORMULATIONS/BRAND NAMES

Capsule:	*Nitro-Bid Plateau (Marion), Nitrocine (Schwartz), Nitrostat (P-D)*
IV injection:	*Nitrol (Rorer), Nitro-Bid IV (Marion), Nitrostat (IV) (P-D), Tridil (Du Pont)*
Lingual aerosol:	*Nitrolingual (RPR)*
Tablet:	*Nitrong (RPR)*
Sublingual tablet:	*Nitrostat (P-D), generic (various manufacturers)*
Ointment:	*Nitro-Bid (Marion), Nitrol (Adria)*
Transdermal:	*Deponit (Schwartz), Minitran (3M), Nitrodisc (Searle), Nitro-Dur (Key), Transderm-Nitro (Summit)*
Translingual spray:	*Nitrolingual (RPR)*
Transmucosal:	*Nitrogard (Forest)*

USE: Prevention/treatment of angina pectoris ▪ Control of BP during surgery (IV) ▪ CHF associated c̄ acute MI (IV).
ACTION: Nitrates relax smooth muscle in small blood vessels, dilate arteries/capillaries, esp in coronary circulation, relieving myocardial ischemia & thereby ⬇ anginal pain.

PHARMACOKINETICS

	Onset	Duration
Sublingual tablet	2-3m	25-30m
Extended action:	20-60m	Several hours to maximum
Capsule, ointment, transdermal		24h depending on dosage, release system

CONTRAINDICATIONS: Hypersensitivity, severe anemia, glaucoma, recent MI, ⬆ cranial pressure, uncorrected hypovolemia (IV). **CC:** Use lowest effective dose due to possibility of tolerance.

DOSAGE: Must be individualized

Adult	*IV*	Non-PVC sets: 5μg/m c̄ 5μg/m increments q3-5m until response obtained. PVC sets require larger doses because drug penetrates plastic
	Ointment	A ribbon of 1-5in q8h
	PO	2.5-6.5mg q8-12h
	Sublingual	0.15-0.6mg

Transdermal	2.5mg, 5mg, 7.5mg, 10mg, 15mg/24h) should produce greatest clinical response c̄ minimum adverse effects
Translingual	Spray 1-2 doses (0.4-0.8mg) on or under tongue
Transmucosal	1mg q3-5h while awake

SIDE/ADVERSE EFFECTS: CNS: *transient headache*, dizziness, apprehension ▪ CV: hypotension, tachycardia, flushing ▪ GI: N/V ▪ INT: rash, local contact dermatitis c̄ topical systems.

INTERACTIONS: Drug: Additive hypotensive effects c̄ calcium blockers, alcohol, phenothiazines, β blockers, other antihypertensives.

NURSING MANAGEMENT PRIORITIES

ADMINISTRATION: Assess for hx of nitrate/nitrite hypersensitivity ▪ Sublingual: assess BP; administer c̄ pt sitting/lying; pt should let tablet dissolve under tongue, should *not* swallow saliva ▪ Administer extended-release preparations whole ▪ Spray: hold canister vertically, spray on tongue; have pt close mouth *immediately*, not inhale spray ▪ IV: dilute in 5% dextrose/normal saline solution; use special non-PVC tubing; do *not* use in-line filters; administer via infusion pump ▪ Ointment: measure proper dose on special applicator paper; do *not* touch medication; spread on skin via paper in thin, uniform layer ▪ Transdermal: apply to clean, hairless area; rotate sites ▪ Avoid exposure to heat/air/ moisture/light in storage.

EVALUATION: Monitor VS, esp BP, heart rate; hemodynamic status (IV) ▪ Assess for transient headache, burning under tongue (sublingual); indicates potency ▪ Assess angina pain characteristics, duration; effectiveness.

EDUCATION: Dizziness, lightheadedness may occur; use caution in potentially hazardous activities ▪ Avoid changing positions (lying/sitting/standing) rapidly ▪ Notify physician *immediately* of dry mouth, blurred vision; D/C drug ▪ Sublingual: use *before* activities known to trigger angina attacks, to relieve acute attacks; burning sensation should occur when sublingual tablet placed under tongue (indicates potency); if pain *not* relieved c̄ 3 tablets/15m, notify physician/go to emergency room ▪ Transient headache expected ▪ Procedure for administration of various preparations; warn pt (esp c̄ impaired vision, taste)/family of potential for mistaking nitrate ointment for toothpaste ▪ Store in original amber glass container, avoid metal/plastic, remove cotton; replace c̄ fresh supply w/in 3-6mos after opening ▪ Carry medical identification (MedicAlert).

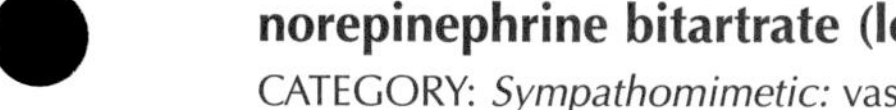

norepinephrine bitartrate (levarterenol bitartrate) • (nor-ep-i-nef-rin)

CATEGORY: *Sympathomimetic:* vasopressor

Rx; Preg Cat NA

BRAND NAME
Levophed (S-W)

DOSAGE FORM
Injection (IV): 1mg/ml

USE: Treatment of acute hypotensive states ▪ Adjunct in cardiac arrest. **ACTION:** Adrenergic activity produces powerful vasoconstriction (α activity), cardiac stimulation (β activity), dilation of coronary arteries (β activity), resulting in ↑ systemic BP, coronary artery circulation. **USE:** Treatment of acute hypotensive states ▪ Adjunct in cardiac arrest.

PHARMACOKINETICS: Duration of activity extremely short; excretion via urine primarily as metabolites.

CONTRAINDICATIONS: Hypotensive states due to deficient blood volume except as emergency measure, mesenteric/peripheral vascular thrombosis unless life threatening, cyclopropane/halothane anesthesia. **CC:** Possible hypertension, extravasation at site of administration ▪ Injection contains sodium metabisulfite, which can cause allergic rxs.

DOSAGE

Pediatric	*IV*	Usual infusion rate 2μg/m
Adult	*IV*	Usual infusion rate 8-12μg/m

SIDE/ADVERSE EFFECTS: Occasional bradycardia, headache.

INTERACTIONS: Drug: Use c̄ α, β blockers will antagonize pressor, cardiac effects of norepinephrine ▪ Use c̄ MAO-I, TCAs produces significant hypertension.

NURSING MANAGEMENT PRIORITIES

ADMINISTRATION: Assess for hx of catecholamine hypersensitivity (incl sulfites) ▪ Assess F/E balance; correct deficiencies ▪ Administer via infusion pump ▪ Dilute c̄ dextrose/saline solution (do *not* administer in NaCl solution alone); infuse into large vein; avoid use of leg veins, esp in elderly, pts c̄ vascular disease ▪ Do *not* administer SC/IM ▪ Do *not* mix c̄ blood components in same IV line ▪ Do *not* use discolored/precipitated solutions ▪ Avoid exposure to light in storage ▪ Have emergency support equipment available ▪ Do *not* leave pt unattended ▪

Withdraw drug *gradually* ▪ Elderly may require ↓ dosage.

EVALUATION: Monitor VS, esp BP (q2-3m until stable, then q5m) ▪ Monitor I&O q1h ▪ Assess respiratory status, ABGs, circulatory overload ▪ Assess CV status (ECG, heart rate, skin color/temperature) ▪ Check IV site carefully; avoid extravasation.

EDUCATION: Notify physician/nurse of abnormal rxs (difficult breathing, chest pain, irregular heartbeat).

NOTES:

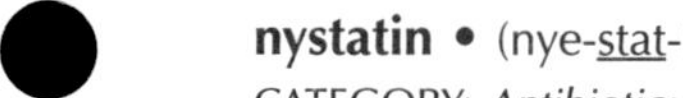

nystatin • (nye-stat-in)

CATEGORY: *Antibiotic:* antimonilial antibiotic — Rx; Preg Cat C

BRAND NAMES	DOSAGE FORMS
Mycostatin (B-MS)	Cream, ointment, powder: 100,000U/g PO suspension: 100,000U/ml PO tablets: 500,000U PO troches: 200,000U/pastille Vaginal tablet: 100,000U
**Nadostine (Nadeau)*	PO suspension: 100,000U/ml PO tablet: 500,000U
Nilstat (Lederle)	Cream, ointment: 100,000U/g PO suspension: 100,000U/ml PO tablet: 500,000U Vaginal tablet: 100,000U

USE: Treatment of cutaneous, mucocutaneous, vulvovaginal, intestinal, PO infections caused by susceptible strains of *Candida* (moniliasis, candidiasis); antibiotic exhibits no appreciable PO absorption. **ACTION:** Antimonilial activity due to drug binding to cell membrane sterols, altering cell membrane permeability & allowing leakage of vital intracellular components; drug exhibits no PO absorption.

PHARMACOKINETICS: Not applicable.

CONTRAINDICATIONS: Hypersensitivity. **CC:** Not effective for systemic *Candida* infections ▪ D/C topical application c̄ appearance of irritation or sensitization rxs.

DOSAGE

Oral candidiasis (thrush) *PO*		
	Infants	200,000U (PO suspension) in PO cavity qid
	Children/Adult	400,000U (PO suspension) in PO cavity qid
Intestinal candidiasis *PO*		
	Adult	0.5-1 million U (tablet) tid
Topical candidiasis		Various dosage forms (cream, etc) applied 2-3 times/d to infected area. Vaginal tablet inserted once/d for 2wks

SIDE/ADVERSE EFFECTS: GI: large PO doses occasionally cause N/V/D, distress ▪ INT: local irritation c̄ topical use.

INTERACTIONS: Drug: None currently reported.

NURSING MANAGEMENT PRIORITIES

ADMINISTRATION: Assess for hx of hypersensitivity ▪ Obtain C&S before therapy ▪ PO suspension: instruct pt to retain on each side of mouth for as long as possible ▪ Troche: instruct pt to dissolve in mouth; do *not* chew or swallow ▪ Cleanse areas for application well before administration ▪ Avoid occlusive dressings ▪ Store vaginal tablets in refrigerator ▪ Avoid exposure to heat/moisture/light in storage.

EVALUATION: Monitor VS, esp temperature ▪ Monitor skin, mucous membranes for redness, swelling, irritation ▪ Monitor GI status.

EDUCATION: Contact dermatitis may occur ▪ Keep affected areas dry, exposed to air; avoid occlusive dressings ▪ May require several wks/mos of treatment; take until lab tests normal ▪ Maintain good hygiene; esp in affected area ▪ Avoid use of mouthwash if taking nystatin for PO candidiasis ▪ Avoid reinfection (use condoms, separate laundering, avoid tight clothing).

NOTES:

olanzapine • (oh-lanz-e-peen) 238

CATEGORY: *Antipsychotic:* neuroleptic Rx; Preg Cat C

BRAND NAME
Zyprexa (Lilly)

DOSAGE FORMS
Tablet: 5, 7.5, 10mg

USE: Management of psychotic disorders. **ACTION:** Antipsychotic activity appears associated c̄ dopamine & serotonin antagonism, resulting in tranquilizing effect in psychotic pts. Drug is relatively free of extrapyramidal symptoms & exhibits antiadrenergic & antihistaminic activity.

PHARMACOKINETICS

PO absorption	Peak	Half-life	Protein binding	Excretion
Good	6h	30h	93%	Via urine, feces primarily as metabolites

CONTRAINDICATIONS: Hypersensitivity. **CC:** Use can induce seizures (0.9%), tardive dyskinesia (1%), neuroleptic malignant syndrome (NMS), hyperprolactinemia, orthostatic hypotension ■ Use c̄ caution c̄ liver impairment ■ Safety & effectiveness in pts <18y/o not established ■ Safety of doses >20mg/d not established.

DOSAGE

Adults *PO* Initial dose of 5-10mg once/d c̄ target dose of 10mg/d w/in several days. Further ↑ should occur at intervals of not <1wk in 5-mg increments. Usual maintenance range is 10-15mg once/d

SIDE/ADVERSE EFFECTS: CNS: drowsiness, agitation, nervousness, dizziness, headache, anxiety ■ CV: orthostatic hypotension, palpitations, tachycardia ■ GI: N/V, dry mouth, constipation, ↑ appetite, taste changes ■ INT: vesiculobullous rash, eczema, urticaria ■ Other: amblyopia, premenstrual syndrome, hematuria.

INTERACTIONS: Drug: Use c̄ alcohol is best avoided ■ Use antihypertensives can produce ↑ hypotension ■ Use c̄ CNS depressants will cause additive sedative effects ■ Use c̄ carbamazepine can ↓ olanzapine effects. **Lab:** ↑ In AST, ALT, GGT values.

NURSING MANAGEMENT PRIORITIES

ADMINISTRATION: Assess for hx of hypersensitivity ▪ Assess VS, esp BP ▪ Assess hepatic, renal function; may require ↓ dosage if impaired ▪ Assess for hx of seizures; use caution ▪ Institute safety, seizure, suicide precautions ▪ Avoid abrupt withdrawal; D/C gradually ▪ Elderly/debilitated pts may require ↓ dosage.

EVALUATION: Monitor CV, hepatic, renal status ▪ Monitor BP, constipation ▪ Assess for extrapyramidal rx ▪ Seizure precautions in pts c̄ hx of convulsive disorders.

EDUCATION: Dizziness/drowsiness may occur; use caution in potentially hazardous activities ▪ Avoid changing positions (lying/sitting/standing) rapidly ▪ Avoid use c̄ alcohol, other CNS depressants ▪ Store in tightly closed, light-resistant container ▪ Use sugarless gum/hard candy to diminish dry mouth ▪ Constipation may occur; ↑ fluids, bulk-containing foods ▪ Women: avoid breastfeeding ▪ Notify physician of fever, sore throat, tics/spasms, trembling, shuffling gait ▪ Avoid ↑ exercise, temperature extremes ▪ Check c̄ physician/pharmacist before taking OTC preparations ▪ Full drug effects may require several wks of therapy.

NOTES:

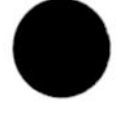

olsalazine sodium • (ole-sal-a-zeen)

CATEGORY: *Salicylate:* colon antiinflammatory Rx; Preg Cat C

BRAND NAME	**DOSAGE FORM**
Dipentum (Pharmacia)	Capsules: 250mg

ACTION: Drug is converted by colon bacteria into active metabolite mesalamine (5-aminosalicylic acid; 5-ASA) where it exerts a topical antiinflammatory effect in ulcerative colitis. **USE:** Maintenance of ulcerative colitis remission in pts unable to take sulfasalazine.

PHARMACOKINETICS

PO absorption	Peak	Half-life	Protein binding	Excretion
Poor	1h	0.9h	99%	1% in urine

CONTRAINDICATIONS: Salicylate hypersensitivity. **CC:** Use can result in possible exacerbation of colitis ▪ Use may produce renal tubular damage, esp in pts c̄ preexisting renal disease.

DOSAGE

Adult *PO* Usual maintenance dose is 1g/d in 2 divided doses

SIDE/ADVERSE EFFECTS: CNS: headache (5%), drowsiness, lethargy, fatigue, depression, dizziness, insomnia ▪ GI: diarrhea (17%), pain/cramps (10%), N/V, dyspepsia, anorexia, stomatitis ▪ INT: rash, itching ▪ Other: arthralgia, URI.

INTERACTIONS: Drug: Use c̄ PO anticoagulants can ↑ PT.

NURSING MANAGEMENT PRIORITIES

ADMINISTRATION: Assess for hx of salicylate hypersensitivity ▪ Assess renal status; ↓ dosage if impaired ▪ Administer c̄ food at evenly spaced intervals ▪ Assess abdominal pain, characteristics of stools.

EVALUATION: Monitor renal status ▪ Assess for rash, fever; D/C drug, notify physician ▪ May ↑ serum ALT, AST.

EDUCATION: Take c̄ food ▪ Take at evenly spaced intervals around the clock ▪ Take as directed by physician ▪ Diarrhea may occur; notify physician ▪ Keep scheduled appointments c̄ physician for proctoscopy/sigmoidoscopy.

NOTES:

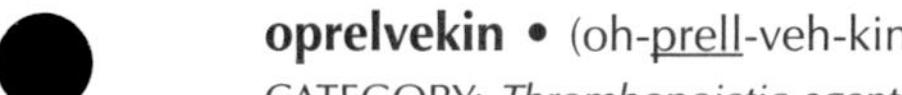

oprelvekin • (oh-prell-veh-kin) 240

CATEGORY: *Thrombopoietic agent:* recombinant interleukin Rx; Preg Cat C

BRAND NAME	DOSAGE FORM
Neumega (Genetics Institute)	Powder for SC injections: 5mg/vial

USE: Stimulation of thrombocyte production to prevent thrombocytopenia/thrombocyte transfusion in pts following myelosuppressive chemotherapy c̄ nonmyeloid neoplasms. **ACTION:** Oprelvekin is a human interleukin II hemopoietic growth factor obtained from *Escherichia coli* bacteria c̄ recombinant DNA. Interleukin II induces a strong thrombopoietic effect, resulting in ⬆ platelet production c̄ thrombocytes that have normal structure, activity, life span.

PHARMACOKINETICS

Peak serum	Half-life	Excretion
3.2h	6.9h	Via urine primarily as metabolites

CONTRAINDICATIONS: Hypersensitivity. **CC:** Administer 6-24h following completion of chemotherapy ▪ Use c̄ caution in pts c̄ CHF/possible CHF development/hx of cardiac insufficiency due to drug-induced fluid retention ▪ Monitoring of fluid balance is required during treatment ▪ Use c̄ caution in pts c̄ hx of atrial arrhythmias after careful clinical consideration due to arrhythmia-inducing properties of the drug ▪ Not indicated for myeloablative chemotherapy ▪ Use c̄ caution in pts c̄ preexisting CNS-associated tumors/papilledema due to possible exacerbation during treatment.

DOSAGE

Adult/Children	*SC*	50µg/kg for adults & 75-100µg/kg for children once/d

SIDE/ADVERSE EFFECTS: CNS: dizziness, insomnia, headache ▪ CV: atrial arrhythmias, edema, palpitations, tachycardia, vasodilation ▪ vasodilation ▪ GI: N/V/D, mucositis, thrush ▪ HEM: transient ⬇ in hematocrit/RBC, neutropenic fever ▪ RESP: ⬆ cough, dyspnea, pleural effusion, pharyngitis, rhinitis ▪ Other: transient, blurred vision, rash.

INTERACTIONS: None currently reported.

NOTES:

NURSING MANAGEMENT PRIORITIES

ADMINISTRATION: Assess for hx of hypersensitivity ▪ Obtain CBC, differential & platelet counts, electrolytes, chest x-ray before administration ▪ Assess CV, pulmonary function; notify physician if impaired ▪ Reconstitute according to manufacturer's directions; use w/in 3h of administration; do *not* shake vigorously or freeze ▪ Administer SC (abdomen, thigh, hip, upper arm).

EVALUATION: Monitor VS ▪ Monitor hematologic, renal function ▪ Monitor fluid retention (I&O, daily weight).

EDUCATION: Dizziness may occur; use caution c̄ ambulation ▪ Notify physician *immediately* of abnormal rxs (peripheral edema, shortness of breath, fever, palpitations) ▪ May produce visual alterations ▪ Women: avoid breastfeeding ▪ Use contraception if sexually active.

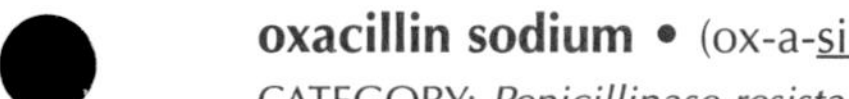

oxacillin sodium • (ox-a-sill-in)

CATEGORY: *Penicillinase-resistant penicillin:* antibiotic — Rx; Preg Cat B

BRAND NAMES

Bactocill (SKB)

DOSAGE FORMS

Powder for injection (IM/IV): 0.5-, 1-, 2-, 4-, 10-g vial

USE: Treatment of infections due to susceptible strains of penicillinase-producing staphylococci. **ACTION:** Bactericidal activity due to inhibition of mucopeptide cell wall synthesis in susceptible organisms.

PHARMACOKINETICS

PO absorption	Peak	Half-life	Protein binding	Excretion
30%-35%	30-60m	20-48m	92%-96%	Via urine as unchanged drug, metabolites

CONTRAINDICATIONS: Hypersensitivity to any penicillin. **CC:** Serious/fatal (anaphylaxis) allergic rxs have occurred c̄ penicillin use ▪ Possible cross-allergenicity c̄ cephalosporins ▪ Resistance to any penicillinase-resistant penicillin should be interpreted as resistance to all: cross-resistance c̄ cephalosporins occurs frequently.

DOSAGE

Premature/Neonate	*IM/IV*	25mg/kg/d divided
Pediatric (<40g)	*PO/IM/IV*	50mg/kg/d divided q4h. Severe infections 100mg/kg/d divided q4-6h
Adult	*PO*	500mg q4-6h. Severe infections 1g q4 6h
	IM/IV	250-500mg q4-6h. Severe infections 1g q4-6h

SIDE/ADVERSE EFFECTS: CNS: neuropathy usually associated c̄ high parenteral doses ▪ GI: PO incl *N/V/D, epigastric distress,* black hairy tongue, flatulence, smell/taste disturbances ▪ GU: ***interstitial nephritis*** (rare) ▪ HEM: anemia, eosinophilia, leukopenia, neutropenia, ***thrombocytopenia*** ▪ HEP: ↑ serum levels of AST, ALT, LDH ▪ INT: rash, pruritus, urticaria ▪ MS: arthralgia ▪ Other: *local irritation at injection site,* fever, ***anaphylaxis***.

INTERACTIONS: Drug: Bacteriostatic antibiotics c̄ any penicillin can lead to antibiotic antagonism ▪ PO anticoagulant therapy may require dose adjustments ▪ Probenecid inhibits tubular secretion of penicillin.

NURSING MANAGEMENT PRIORITIES

ADMINISTRATION: Assess for hx of penicillin/cephalosporin hypersensitivity ▪ Obtain C&S before therapy ▪ Maintain blood levels; administer at equal intervals around clock ▪ PO: administer 1h ac/2h pc ▪ Avoid exposure to moisture in storage ▪ Reconstitute powder according to manufacturer's directions c̄ sterile H_2O for injection; shake well; do *not* administer discolored/precipitated solutions; check product information for stability (parenteral/PO solution) ▪ IM: administer by *deep* intragluteal injection ▪ IV: (direct) dilute according to manufacturer's directions; administer *slowly* (10m); (infusion) mix c̄ diluent recommended by manufacturer ▪ Do *not* administer bacteriostatic agents w/in 1h or mix c̄ aminoglycosides ▪ Have support equipment available for anaphylaxis ▪ Na^+ content: 2.8-3.1mEq (64-71mg)/g; calculate in Na^+-restricted diets.

EVALUATION: Monitor pts c̄ allergies/asthma (high risk for hypersensitivity) ▪ Observe for signs of superinfection (diarrhea, perineal itching, oral ulcers) ▪ Monitor VS, esp temperature; renal, hepatic, hematologic status ▪ Check IV insertion site; rotate q48h.

EDUCATION: Complete full course of therapy (usually 10d) even if symptom free ▪ Take on empty stomach ▪ Take c̄ H_2O, *not* c̄ acidic beverage (orange juice, carbonated beverage) ▪ Take at equal intervals ▪ Diarrhea may occur ▪ Store in dry, tightly closed container ▪ Discard outdated preparations ▪ Maintain good personal hygiene (esp perineal, oral) ▪ Maintain fluid intake (6-8 glasses/d) ▪ Notify physician of symptoms of allergic rx (fever, difficult breathing, rash) ▪ Women: avoid breastfeeding ▪ Carry identification (MedicAlert) if penicillin allergic.

NOTES:

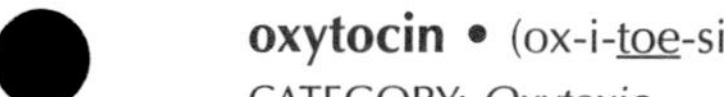

oxytocin • (ox-i-toe-sin)

CATEGORY: *Oxytoxic*

Rx; Preg Cat C

BRAND NAMES

Pitocin (P-D)

Syntocinon (Sandoz) (Sandoz Pharma [Canada])

DOSAGE FORMS

Injection (IM/IV): 5U/0.5ml, 10U/ml

Injection (IM/IV): 10U/ml

Nasal spray: 40U/ml (2, 5ml bottle)

USE: Antepartum: initiation/augmentation of uterine contractions ▪ Stimulate uterine contractions during stage 3 of labor, control postpartum hemorrhage ▪ Initiate milk let-down reflex (spray). **ACTION:** Oxytoxic effect due to ↑ sodium ion permeability in uterine smooth muscle cells, which ↑ number of contracting myofibrils, enables uterus to contract; uterine sensitivity to oxytocin gradually ↑ during pregnancy, reaching peak before parturition.

PHARMACOKINETICS

IM absorption	Onset	Duration	Excretion
Excellent	3-5m	2-3h	Via urine primarily as metabolites

CONTRAINDICATIONS: Hypersensitivity, cephalopelvic disproportion, unfavorable fetal position, obstetric emergencies that favor surgical intervention, fetal distress when delivery not imminent, prolonged use in uterine inertia/severe toxemia, hypertonic uterine patterns when vaginal delivery is contraindicated; nasal spray during pregnancy. **CC:** Induction &/or stimulation of labor must be given by IV route.

DOSAGE

Adult *IM/IV*

Antepartum	Start c̄ infusion rate 1-2mU/m. Slowly ↑ until contractions reach desired rate, intensity
Postpartum	10-40U in 100ml, infused at sufficient rate to control uterine atony. 3-10U after delivery of placenta
Nasal spray	1 spray in one/both nostrils 2-3m before nursing/pumping breasts

SIDE/ADVERSE EFFECTS: CV: ***cardiac arrhythmia,*** postpartum hemorrhage, fetal bradycardia ▪ GI: N/V ▪ GU: pelvic hematoma; uterine hypertonicity, spasms, tetanic contractions, rupture.

Note: Side/adverse effects: common in *italic;* serious in ***boldface italic.***

*Available in Canada only.

INTERACTIONS: Drug: Use c̄ vasopressors can produce severe hypertension.

NOTES:

NURSING MANAGEMENT PRIORITIES

ADMINISTRATION: Fetal monitoring: assess fetal maturity, position ▪ Administer by only *one* route, *not* simultaneous routes ▪ IV: use infusion pump; do *not* give IV push ▪ Place pt in left lateral position ▪ Do *not* leave pt unattended ▪ Have emergency support equipment available ▪ Avoid overstimulation of uterus ▪ Do *not* administer discolored/precipitated solutions ▪ Parenteral: store in original container, avoid freezing.

EVALUATION: Monitor BP, pulse q15m ▪ Monitor fetal heart rate, intrauterine pressure ▪ Assess uterine rupture, fetal distress ▪ Monitor uterine contractions; stop if very frequent (<q2m)/prolonged ▪ Monitor I&O; assess hydration status (continuous infusion, PO fluids can lead to H_2O intoxication) ▪ Postpartum: monitor fundal height/ tone.

EDUCATION: Explain procedure, rationale to pt, family ▪ Occurrence of contractions ▪ Relaxation techniques ▪ Comfort measures ▪ Procedure for use of nasal spray.

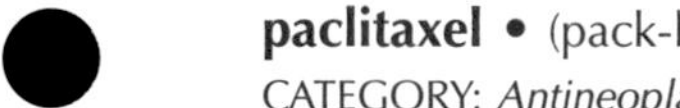

paclitaxel • (pack-lih-tax-el)

CATEGORY: *Antineoplastic:* antimicrotubule agent Rx; Preg Cat D

BRAND NAME	**DOSAGE FORM**
Taxol (BM-ONC)	IV concentrate injection: 6mg/ml

USE: Treatment of metastatic breast & ovarian cancer not responsive to other chemotherapeutic agents ▪ Treatment (2nd line) of AIDS-related Kaposi's sarcoma. **ACTION:** Natural antineoplastic obtained from the Western yew shrub. Antineoplastic activity is related to antimicrotubule activity resulting in cell replication inhibition. Paclitaxel promotes synthesis of stable & nonfunctional microtubules that cannot be reorganized into a functional microbtubule network, which is an essential part of the mitotic spindle in the late G_2 and M-phase of the cell cycle.

PHARMACOKINETICS: Pharmacokinetics have not been fully determined. Following IV administration there is an initial rapid decline in plasma concentrations & extensive clearance of the drug from the body, which is followed by a second & slow influx of the drug from peripheral body compartments into plasma. Drug exhibits 88%-98% protein binding & is metabolized in the liver.

CONTRAINDICATIONS: Hypersensitivity, <1500 baseline neutrophil counts. **CC:** Use requires qualified physicians ▪ Use requires baseline neutrophil counts >1500/mm^3 ▪ Use of PVC equipment to prepare infusion from undiluted concentrate not recommended ▪ Administration requires an in-line filter c̄ a microporous membrane not >0.22 microns ▪ Use can produce severe conduction abnormalities (<19%) c̄ subsequent pacemaker requirements.

DOSAGE: All pts should be premedicated c̄ a steroid, antihistamine, H_2 blocker to prevent severe hypersensitivity rxs. Suggested drugs: dexamethasone 20mg PO 12h & 6h before surgery, diphenhydramine 50mg IV 30-60m before surgery, cimetidine 300mg IV, or ranitidine 50mg IV 30-60m before surgery

Adult *IV*

Breast cancer	175mg/m^2 over 3h q3wks
Ovarian cancer	135 or 175mg/m^2 over 3h q3wks
Kaposi's sarcoma	135mg/m^2 over 3h q3wks or 100mg/m^2 over 3h q2wks

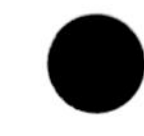

SIDE/ADVERSE EFFECTS: CNS: peripheral neuropathy (mild paresthesia most frequent) ▪ CV: bradycardia & hypotension during administration, ***abnormal ECG including nonspecific*** repolarization abnormalities, sinus tachycardia, premature beats ▪ GI: N/V/D, mucositis ▪ HEP: ↑ levels of bilirubin, alkaline phosphatase, AST ▪ HEM: Bone marrow suppression including anemia, *neutropenia*, ***leukopenia***, ***thrombocytopenia*** ▪ Other: alopecia, myalgia, arthralgia.

INTERACTIONS: Drug: Use c̄ other bone marrow depressants will produce additive effects ▪ Use c̄ ketoconazole is best avoided.

NURSING MANAGEMENT PRIORITIES

ADMINISTRATION: Assess for hx of hypersensitivity ▪ Assess hematologic status; do *not* administer if neutropenic ▪ Do *not* administer c̄ PVC equipment ▪ Premedicate c̄ glucocorticoids before infusion to prevent severe hypersensitivity ▪ Dilute according to manufacturer's directions; infuse via in-line filter ▪ Avoid contact c̄ skin; wash thoroughly c̄ soap & water ▪ Provide emotional support.

EVALUATION: Monitor VS, esp heart rate, BP ▪ Check IV site closely; avoid extravasation ▪ Monitor neurologic, hepatic, renal function ▪ Monitor CBC throughout therapy, esp WBCs ▪ Assess for infection, bleeding, anemia ▪ Assess for development of neuropathy (numbness, tingling, pain in distal extremities) ▪ Assess hydration status (I&O, daily weight).

EDUCATION: ↑ Fluid intake (10-12 glasses/d) ▪ Avoid exposure to infection ▪ Check c̄ physician before immunization (pt, family) ▪ Diet as tolerated; avoid spicy foods ▪ Maintain good oral hygiene; use soft-bristled toothbrush ▪ Notify physician of symptoms of bone marrow depression (fever, sore throat, bruising, bleeding, lethargy) ▪ Women: avoid breastfeeding ▪ Encourage ventilation of feelings ▪ Use contraception if sexually active.

NOTES:

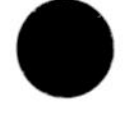

paroxetine hcl • (pair-ox-eh-teen)

CATEGORY: *Antidepressant:* selective serotonin reuptake inhibitor (SSRI) Rx; Preg Cat B

BRAND NAME
Paxil (SKB)

DOSAGE FORMS
Tablet: 20, 30mg

USE: Treatment of depression. Long-term use requires reevaluation of clinical effectiveness. **ACTION:** Antidepressant activity appears related to inhibition of serotonin reuptake in CNS.

PHARMACOKINETICS

PO absorption	Peak	Half-life	Protein binding	Excretion
Complete	5.2h	21d	95%	Via urine, feces as metabolites

CONTRAINDICATIONS: Hypersensitivity, pts taking MAO-I. **CC:** Use can activate rare cases of mania/hypomania ▪ Do not administer w/in 14d of D/C MAO-I treatment; allow at least 14d after D/C of paroxetine treatment before initiating MAO-I therapy.

DOSAGE

Adult *PO* — Initial dose 20mg once/d. Usual daily range 20-50mg. Dose changes require interval of at least 1wk. Do *not* exceed 40mg/d for hepatic, renal impairment & elderly

SIDE/ADVERSE EFFECTS: CNS: headache, drowsiness, dizziness, insomnia, nervousness, anxiety, tremor, paresthesia, agitation ▪ CV: palpitation, vasodilation, postural hypotension ▪ EENT: blurred vision ▪ GI: N/V/D, dry mouth, ⬇ appetite, flatulence, dyspepsia, taste changes, abdominal pain ▪ GU: ejaculation delay, urinary frequency, female anorgasmia ▪ INT: rash, sweating ▪ Other: fever, chest, back pain, myopathy, asthenia, cough.

INTERACTIONS: Drug: Use c̄ MAO-I contraindicated ▪ Use c̄ tryptophan not recommended ▪ Use c̄ PO anticoagulants may ⬆ their activity ▪ Use c̄ enzyme inducers &/or inhibitors can alter therapeutic results ▪ Use c̄ procyclidine can ⬆ anticholinergic effects ▪ Use c̄ other high-protein–bound drugs can result in displacement from inactive protein binding sites.

NURSING MANAGEMENT PRIORITIES

ADMINISTRATION: Assess for hx of hypersensitivity ▪ Assess for hx of seizures; use caution ▪ Assess hepatic, renal status; ⬇ dosage if impaired ▪ Administer consistently c̄ or w/out food in AM or PM ▪ Institute safety, seizure precautions ▪ Institute suicide precautions ▪ Avoid abrupt withdrawal; ⬇ gradually ▪ Avoid exposure to moisture/ heat/direct light in storage ▪ Elderly may require ⬇ dosage.

EVALUATION: Monitor CV, hepatic, renal status ▪ Monitor fluid retention (I&O, daily weight), constipation ▪ Assess for weight loss (anorectic effect) ▪ Monitor F/E status (hyponatremia) ▪ Assess for symptoms of abrupt withdrawal (nausea, headache, malaise) ▪ Assess for actual swallowing of PO forms ▪ Assess for skin rash, hives; notify physician, D/C drug.

EDUCATION: Dizziness/drowsiness may occur; use caution in potentially hazardous activities ▪ Avoid changing positions (lying/sitting/standing) rapidly ▪ Avoid use c̄ alcohol, other CNS depressants for up to 1wk after end of therapy ▪ Take consistently c̄ or w/out food ▪ Take as directed by physician ▪ Use sugarless gum/hard candy to diminish dry mouth ▪ Constipation may occur; ⬆ fluids, bulk-containing foods ▪ Notify physician/dentist of use before treatment ▪ Store in tightly closed, light-resistant container ▪ Encourage recreational/diversional interests ▪ Notify physician of weight loss, fever, sore throat, malaise ▪ Keep scheduled appointments c̄ physician ▪ Women: notify physician of possibility of pregnancy; avoid breastfeeding ▪ Full drug effects may require several wks of therapy.

NOTES:

penicillin g benzathine/penicillin g procaine • (pen-i-sill-in)

CATEGORY: *Natural repository penicillin:* antibiotic Rx; Preg Cat NA

BRAND NAMES	DOSAGE FORMS
penicillin g benzathine	Suspension (IM)
Bicillin L-A, C-R, C-R 900/300 (Wyeth), Permapen (Roerig)	
penicillin g procaine	Suspension (IM)
Crysticillin 300 AS (Apothecon)	
Pfizerpen-AS (Roerig)	
Wycillin (W-A)	

USE: penicillin g/v drug of choice for most strains of *Actinomyces,* α-hemolytic streptococci, *Bacillus anthracis, Bacteroides* (except *B. fragilis*), *Clostridium perfringens, C. tetani* (c̄ antitoxins), *Erysipelothrix rhusiopathiae, Fusobacterium* (Vincent angina), group A β-hemolytic streptococci, *Neisseria gonorrhoeae, N. meningitidis, Pasteurella multocida,* staphylococci (non-penicillinase producing), *Streptobacillus moniliformis,* streptococci (groups C, G, H, L, M), *Streptococcus pneumoniae, Treponema pallidum* (syphilis), *T. pertenue* (yaws) ▪ Prophylaxis of group A strep infections in pts c̄ rheumatic fever, prevention of recurrence ▪ Prevention of bacterial endocarditis in pts c̄ congenital/rheumatic heart lesions who require dental procedure, upper respiratory tract surgery, instrumentation ▪ Prevention of bacteremia after tooth extraction. **ACTION:** Bactericidal activity due to inhibition of mucopeptide cell wall synthesis in susceptible organisms; sterile aqueous suspension after deep IM injection produces tissue repository from which drug is slowly absorbed.

PHARMACOKINETICS

PO absorption	Peak	Protein binding	Excretion
Very slow	Varies up to 24h	45%-68%	Via urine by tubular excretion

CONTRAINDICATIONS: Hypersensitivity to any penicillin. **CC:** Serious/fatal (anaphylaxis) allergic rxs have occurred even c̄ PO dosage forms of penicillin ▪ Possible cross-allergenicity c̄ cephalosporins, other β-lactam antibiotics.

DOSAGE: Variable due to severity of infection

penicillin g benzathine *IM*

Pediatric	600,000-1.2 million U usually as single dose

Note: Side/adverse effects: common in *italic;* serious in ***boldface italic.*** *Available in Canada only.

Adult		1.2-2.4 million U usually as single dose
penicillin g procaine	*IM*	
Pediatric		500,000-1 million U/d
Adult		600,000-1.2 million U/d

SIDE/ADVERSE EFFECTS: GI: N/V/D, epigastric distress, black hairy tongue ▪ HEM: ***hemolytic anemia,*** leukopenia, ***thrombocytopenia*** ▪ HEP: ↑ serum AST, bilirubin ▪ INT: maculopapular rash, urticaria, ***exfoliative dermatitis*** ▪ Other: Jarisch-Herxheimer rx (arthralgia, chills, fever, headache, sore throat, sweating, altered BP), local pain at injection site, ***anaphylaxis,*** overgrowth of nonsusceptible organisms.

INTERACTIONS: Drug: Use c̄ bacteriostatic antibiotics can produce antibiotic antagonism ▪ Antacid, antidiarrheal suspension ↓ PO absorption ▪ Probenecid delays penicillin excretion ▪ Avoid administration c̄ strong acidic/alkaline substances (can inactivate penicillin).

NURSING MANAGEMENT PRIORITIES

ADMINISTRATION: Assess for hx of penicillin/cephalosporin hypersensitivity (incl procaine) ▪ Obtain C&S before therapy ▪ IM: dilute according to manufacturer's directions; shake well; inject *slowly* into gluteal UOQ ▪ Refrigerate parenteral preparations ▪ Do *not* administer w/in 1h of bacteriostatic agents ▪ Avoid exposure to moisture in storage ▪ Have support equipment available for anaphylaxis.

EVALUATION: Monitor pts c̄ allergies/asthma (high risk for hypersensitivity) ▪ Monitor renal, hepatic, hematologic status ▪ Observe for signs of superinfection (diarrhea, perineal itching, oral ulcers) ▪ Monitor VS, esp temperature.

EDUCATION: Diarrhea may occur ▪ Maintain good personal hygiene (esp perineal, oral) ▪ Maintain fluid intake (6-8 glasses/d) ▪ Women: avoid breastfeeding ▪ Notify physician of symptoms of allergic rx (fever, difficult breathing, rash) ▪ Carry identification (MedicAlert) if penicillin allergic ▪ IM injection may be painful.

NOTES:

penicillin g potassium/penicillin v potassium • (pen-i-sill-in)

CATEGORY: *Natural penicillin:* antibiotic

Rx; Preg Cat B

BRAND NAMES
penicillin g potassium
Pfizerpen (Roerig)
penicillin v potassium
Beepen-VK (SKB)
Betapen-VK (Apothecon)
Pen Vee K (W-A)
V-Cillin K (Lilly)
Veetids (Apothecon)

DOSAGE FORMS: Many PO/parenteral dosage forms.

USE: penicillin g/v drug of choice for most strains of *Actinomyces,* α-hemolytic streptococci, *Bacillus anthracis, Bacteroides* (except *B. fragilis*), *Clostridium perfringens, C. tetani* (c̄ antitoxin), *Corynebacterium diphtheriae* (c̄ antitoxins), *Erysipelothrix rhusiopathiae, Fusobacterium* (Vincent angina), group A β-hemolytic streptococci, *Neisseria gonorrhoeae, N. meningitidis, Pasteurella multocida,* staphylococci (non-penicillinase producing), *Streptobacillus moniliformis,* streptococci (groups C, G, H, L, M), *Streptococcus pneumoniae, Treponema pallidum* (syphilis), *T. pertenue* (yaws) ▪ Prophylaxis of group A strep infections in pts c̄ rheumatic fever, prevention of recurrence ▪ Prevention of bacterial endocarditis in pts c̄ congenital/rheumatic heart lesions who require dental procedure, upper respiratory tract surgery, instrumentation ▪ Prevention of bacteremia after tooth extraction. **ACTION:** Bactericidal activity due to inhibition of mucopeptide cell wall synthesis in susceptible organisms; PO preparations limited to microorganisms c̄ sensitivity to penicillin v potassium w/in range of serum levels attainable by PO administration. The severity of infection dictates PO administration (V) or parenteral IM (G procaine) or IV (G potassium).

CONTRAINDICATIONS: Hypersensitivity to any penicillin. **CC:** Serious/fatal (anaphylaxis) allergic rxs have occurred even c̄ PO dosage forms of penicillin ▪ Possible cross-allergenicity c̄ cephalosporins, other β-lactam antibiotics.

PHARMACOKINETICS: Penicillin g poorly absorbed PO & acid labile. Use penicillin v for PO use.

DOSAGE: Highly variable due to severity of infection
penicillin g
Pediatric *PO* 25,000-90,000 U/kg in 3-6 doses

	IM/IV	300,000-1.2 million U/d. Up to 10 million U/d may be required. Usual dose for premature/full-term infants 30,000U/kg bid
Adult	*IM/IV*	300,000-8 million U/d. Up to 60 million U/d may be required
penicillin v		
Pediatric	*PO*	<12y/o: 15-50mg/kg/d in 3-6 doses
Adult	*PO*	250-500mg 3-4 times/d

SIDE/ADVERSE EFFECTS: GI: N/V/D, epigastric distress, black hairy tongue ▪ HEM: ***hemolytic anemia***, leukopenia, ***thrombocytopenia*** ▪ HEP: ↑ serum AST, bilirubin ▪ INT: maculopapular rash, urticaria, ***exfoliative dermatitis*** ▪ Other: Jarisch-Herxheimer rx (arthralgia, chills, fever, headache, sore throat, sweating, alterations in BP); local pain at injection site; anaphylaxis, overgrowth of nonsusceptible organisms.

INTERACTIONS: Drug: Use c̄ bacteriostatic antibiotics can produce antibiotic antagonism ▪ Antacid/antidiarrheal suspension ↓ PO absorption ▪ Probenecid delays penicillin excretion ▪ Avoid PO administration c̄ strong acidic/alkaline substances (can inactivate penicillin).

NURSING MANAGEMENT PRIORITIES

ADMINISTRATION: Assess for hx of penicillin/cephalosporin hypersensitivity ▪ Obtain C&S before therapy ▪ PO: administer on empty stomach (1h ac/2h pc); avoid citrus juices, carbonated beverages ▪ IV: dilute according to manufacturer's directions; administer by *slow* direct infusion/IVPB ▪ IM: dilute according to manufacturer's directions; shake well; inject *slowly* into gluteal UOQ ▪ Refrigerate parenteral preparations ▪ Do *not* administer w/in 1h of bacteriostatic agents ▪ Avoid exposure to moisture in storage ▪ Have support equipment available for anaphylaxis ▪ Na^+ content: 0.3mEq (6.9mg)/1 million U; calculate in Na^+-restricted diet.

EVALUATION: Monitor pts c̄ allergies/asthma (risk for hypersensitivity) ▪ Monitor renal, hepatic, hemopoietic status ▪ Observe for signs of superinfection (diarrhea, itching, coated tongue) ▪ Monitor VS, esp temperature.

EDUCATION: Take at equal intervals around clock to maintain blood levels ▪ Diarrhea may occur ▪ Maintain good personal hygiene (esp perineal, oral) ▪ Maintain fluid intake (6-8 glasses/d) ▪ Women: avoid breastfeeding ▪ Notify physician of symptoms of allergic rx (fever, difficult breathing, rash) ▪ Carry identification (MedicAlert) if penicillin allergic ▪ IM injection may be painful.

NOTES:

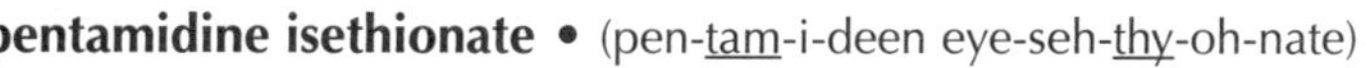

pentamidine isethionate • (pen-tam-i-deen eye-seh-thy-oh-nate)

CATEGORY: *Antiprotozoan agent* — Rx; Preg Cat C

BRAND NAMES
NebuPent (Fujisawa)
Pentam 300 (Fujisawa)

DOSAGE FORMS
Powder for aerosol: 300mg/vial
Powder for injection (IM/IV): 300-mg vials

USE: Treatment of *Pneumocystis carinii* pneumonia (PCP). Has been used to treat African sleeping sickness (trypanosomiasis) & visceral leishmaniasis (not approved by the Food and Drug Administration). **ACTION:** Antiprotozoan activity not established. The drug may inhibit protein & nucleic acid synthesis in susceptible organisms.

PHARMACOKINETICS: Few studies have been done. A daily dose of 4mg/kg over 12d produced a plasma concentration of 0.3-0.5µg/ml. Complete excretion via urine required 6-8wks after drug was withdrawn.

CONTRAINDICATIONS: Hypersensitivity, esp to inhalation therapy. **CC:** Powder for aerosal administration must be reconstituted only c̄ sterile H_2O for injection, must not be mixed c̄ other drugs ▪ Inhalation administration can produce bronchospasm, cough & does not preclude PCP development ▪ Parenteral administration has been associated c̄ cardiac arrhythmias, hypoglycemia, hypotension, acute pancreatitis.

DOSAGE

Pediatric/Adult

IM/IV	4mg/kg once/d for 14d. Infuse IV dose over 60m
Inhalation	300mg administered until nebulizer is empty (30-45m) q4wks

SIDE/ADVERSE EFFECTS: CNS: confusion/hallucinations, dizziness ▪ CV: ***fatal episodes of cardiac arrhythmias** & hypotension* ▪ GI: *N/V*, bad taste, diarrhea, *anorexia* ▪ HEM: severe leukopenia & ***thrombocytopenia,*** anemia ▪ INT: *rash,* ***Stevens-Johnson syndrome*** ▪ Renal: nephrotoxicity (25%) is most common, ***acute renal failure*** ▪ Other: local phlebitis, hypoglycemia, ↑ AST (serum glutamate oxaloacetate transaminase), ALT (serum glutamate pyruvate transaminase) levels, hypocalcemia, bronchospasm (inhalation administration), fever.

INTERACTIONS: Drug: Use c̄ nephrotoxic drugs, including aminoglycosides, amphotericin B, colistin, & vancomycin, can result in significant toxicity.

NURSING MANAGEMENT PRIORITIES

ADMINISTRATION: Assess for hx of hypersensitivity ▪ Obtain C&S before therapy ▪ Assess renal function; may require ⬇ dosage if impaired ▪ Administer by deep IM injection c̄ pt lying down (hypotension); monitor BP afterward q5-15m until stable ▪ IM: add 3ml sterile H_2O for injection to each 300-mg vial; rotate injection sites ▪ IV: add 3-5ml sterile H_2O for injection or D_5W injection to each 300-mg vial; dilute in 50-250ml D_5W injection, administer over 60-m period; stable for 24h (room temperature); discard unused portion.

EVALUATION: Monitor VS, CBC ▪ Avoid extravasation; assess for pain, redness at site ▪ Diabetics: monitor blood glucose (hypoglycemia/hyperglycemia) ▪ Monitor renal function (nephrotoxicity); notify physician ▪ Monitor ECG throughout therapy (arrhythmias) ▪ May ⬆ serum ALT, AST, creatinine, K^+; ⬇ Ca^{++}.

EDUCATION: Dizziness/drowsiness may occur; use caution in potentially hazardous activities ▪ Complete full course of therapy as directed by physician ▪ Notify nurse/physician of pain, redness at IV injection site ▪ Notify physician *immediately* of bleeding/bruising, difficult breathing, rash, severe GI distress ▪ Maintain good personal hygiene ▪ May produce unpleasant, metallic taste.

NOTES:

pentazocine lactate[▲]/pentazocine hcl • (pen-taz-oh-seen)

CATEGORY: *Analgesic:* opioid agonist-antagonist Rx C-IV; Preg Cat C

BRAND NAME	DOSAGE FORMS
Talwin (S-W)	Injection (IM/IV/SC)▲ 30mg/ml

COMBINATION PRODUCTS

Talwin Compound (S-W)	pentazocine hcl/aspirin per tablet: 12.5mg/325mg
Talwin NX (S-W)	pentazocine hcl/naloxone per tablet: 50mg/0.5mg

USE: Relief of moderate/severe pain ▪ Preop sedation, obstetric analgesia, adjunct to surgical anesthesia.
ACTION: Analgesic mechanism not determined; possible site of activity may be in subcortical areas of brain; narcotic agonist activity in 30-mg dose equivalent to 10mg morphine, 75mg meperidine; narcotic antagonist activity equivalent to 1/50 that of nalorphine; drug has low misuse potential, weak addiction liability.

CONTRAINDICATIONS: Hypersensitivity. **CC:** Use in narcotic-dependent pts can result in withdrawal symptoms ▪ Use c̄ caution in pts c̄ head injuries, ↑ ICP, impaired respiration ▪ Use can result in rare cases of dependence, esp in pts c̄ a hx of drug abuse.

DOSAGE

Adult *IM/IV/SC*

Analgesic	30mg q3-4h. Do *not* exceed 60mg IM/SC, 30mg IV. Do *not* exceed 360mg/d
Obstetric	30mg IM, 20mg IV
Talwin Compound	2 tablets PO 3-4 times/d
Talwin NX	1-2 tablets PO q3-4h. Do *not* exceed 12 tablets/d

PHARMACOKINETICS

Onset					
IV	IM/SC	Duration	Half-life	Protein binding	Excretion
2-3m	15m	1-2h	2-3h	60%	Via urine, feces as unchanged drug, metabolites

Note: Side/adverse effects: common in *italic;* serious in ***boldface italic.***

▲Available in Canada only.

SIDE/ADVERSE EFFECTS: CNS: *dizziness, lightheadedness, euphoria*, mood change, sedation, depression ▪ CV: tachycardia, edema of face ▪ EENT: blurred vision, nystagmus, miosis ▪ GI: *vomiting*, dry mouth, constipation ▪ GU: urinary retention ▪ INT: soft tissue induration, nodules, cutaneous depression at injection site, multiple-dose sclerosis of tissue, ***toxic epidermal necrolysis.***

INTERACTIONS: Drug: Use c̄ CNS depressants produces additive effects ▪ Use in narcotic-dependent pts can produce withdrawal symptoms ▪ Use c̄ MAO-I can result in severe excitation, rigidity, hypertension.

NURSING MANAGEMENT PRIORITIES

ADMINISTRATION: Assess for hx of opioid hypersensitivity ▪ Check compatibility chart for mixing preop preparations ▪ Do *not* administer if respirations are <12/m ▪ IM: inject *deeply* into muscle; rotate sites ▪ IV: dilute; administer *slowly* ▪ Have narcotic antagonist, support measures available ▪ Avoid administration in pts c̄ suspected head injury ▪ Administer *before* pt has intense pain ▪ Avoid light/freezing in storage ▪ Utilize + power of suggestion ▪ Avoid abrupt withdrawal ▪ Elderly may require ↓ dosage.

EVALUATION: Monitor respirations, circulatory function ▪ Assess bowel function, abdominal distention ▪ Assess renal function, urinary retention ▪ Check for signs of dependence (↑ drug request) ▪ Assess for potentiation of CNS depressant effect ▪ Check for signs of OD (coma, pinpoint pupils, respiratory depression).

EDUCATION: Avoid changing positions (lying/sitting/standing) rapidly ▪ Avoid excessive sensory stimulation ▪ Keep bedrails up when nonambulatory ▪ Obtain assistance prn when ambulatory ▪ Turn, cough, deep-breathe after surgery ▪ Constipation may occur; ↑ fluid, bulk-containing foods ▪ Avoid potentially hazardous activities ▪ Avoid smoking while taking drug ▪ Indiscriminate use may lead to dependence ▪ Avoid use c̄ alcohol, other CNS depressants.

NOTES:

pentobarbital/pentobarbital sodium▲ • (pen-toe-bar-bi-tal)

CATEGORY: *Barbiturate*

Rx C-II; Preg Cat D

BRAND NAMES

Nembutal (Abbott)
Nembutal Sodium▲ (Abbott)
**Novopentobarb*
**Pentogen*

DOSAGE FORMS

Elixir
Capsule, injection (IM/IV), suppository

USE: Sedative, hypnotic ▪ Treatment of acute convulsive conditions. **ACTION:** Sedative, hypnotic activity due to depression of midbrain reticular formation; anticonvulsant properties due to depression of motor cortex.

DOSAGE

Pediatric	*IM*	2-6mg/kg. Do *not* exceed 100mg
	PO	2-6mg/kg/24h divided
	Rectal	2mo-1y/o: 30mg at hs 1-4y/o: 30-60mg at hs 5-12y/o: 60mg at hs 12-14y/o: 60-120mg at hs
Adult	*IM*	150-200mg
	IV	150mg/70kg weight suggested
	PO	100-200mg at hs
	Rectal	120-200mg at hs

PHARMACOKINETICS

PO absorption	Onset	Duration	Half-life	Protein binding	Excretion
90%-95%	10-15m	3-4h	4h	35%-45%	98%-99% in urine as metabolites

CONTRAINDICATIONS: Hypersensitivity, severe liver/respiratory impairment, porphyria, addiction. **CC:** Barbiturates are habit forming. Dependence, tolerance can occur c̄ sustained use ▪ Abrupt D/C in barbiturate-dependent pts will induce withdrawal symptoms.

SIDE/ADVERSE EFFECTS: CNS: *drowsiness, lethargy, hangover,* headache, dizziness, paradoxic restlessness/excitement ▪ GI: N/V ▪ INT: morbilliform rash, ***Stevens-Johnson syndrome***, urticaria ▪ Other: drug tolerance/addiction, asthma, angioneurotic edema.

INTERACTIONS: Drug: Use c̄ alcohol, antihistamines, benzodiazepines, methotrimeprazine, narcotics, tranquilizers produces ↑ depressant effects ▪ Barbiturates are enzyme inducers, can ↓ effect of PO anticoagulants, other drugs ▪ MAO-I ↑ activity of barbiturates ▪ Barbiturates ↓ PO absorption of griseofulvin.

NURSING MANAGEMENT PRIORITIES

ADMINISTRATION: Assess for hx of barbiturate hypersensitivity ▪ Administer PO hypnotic dose 15-30m before hs ▪ IM: inject *deeply, slowly* into large muscle mass ▪ IV: inject *slowly*, wait 1m for full effect; additional small increments may be given to total 200-500mg in normal adults ▪ Avoid abrupt withdrawal ▪ Elderly may require ↓ dosage.

EVALUATION: IV: observe for coughing, chest wall spasm, hiccoughs, laryngospasm, pain at injection site, excessive CNS depression, thrombophlebitis ▪ Monitor hepatic, renal, cardiac, respiratory status ▪ Assess for symptoms of abrupt withdrawal (tremors, abdominal/muscle cramps, convulsions) c̄ prolonged use ▪ Assess for actual swallowing of PO forms ▪ Check for signs of dependence (↑ drug request) ▪ Monitor activity status (safety precautions) ▪ Assess for tolerance/barbiturate-cross-tolerance to therapeutic dose ▪ Assess for paradoxic rxs (CNS stimulation), esp in elderly ▪ Observe pt sleep patterns ▪ Check for depression; suicide precautions prn.

EDUCATION: Drowsiness may occur; use caution in potentially hazardous activities ▪ Avoid use c̄ alcohol, other CNS depressants ▪ Indiscriminate use may lead to dependence ▪ Do *not* keep at bedside ▪ Take as ordered by physician ▪ Do *not* smoke after taking drug ▪ Women: avoid breastfeeding.

OVERDOSE MANAGEMENT: *See* Barbiturates.

NOTES:

pentosan polysulfate sodium • (pen-toe-san)

CATEGORY: *Urinary analgesics* Rx; Preg Cat B

BRAND NAME	DOSAGE FORM
Elmiron-100 (Baker Norton)	Capsule: 100mg

DOSAGE

Adult	*PO*	100mg tid c̄ H_2O 1h ac or 2h pc

USE: Symptomatic treatment of bladder pain associated c̄ interstitial cystitis. **ACTION:** Urinary analgesic mechanism not determined. Drug appears to adhere to bladder mucosal membrane, resulting in a barrier that prevents irritating urinary solutes from reaching mucosal cells.

PHARMACOKINETICS

PO absorption	Half-life	Excretion
3%	4.8h	Via urine

CONTRAINDICATIONS: Hypersensitivity. **CC:** Drug exhibits heparinlike anticoagulant activity (about 6.5% of heparin) & can produce bleeding complications incl ecchymosis, epistaxis, bleeding gums ▪ Use c̄ caution in pts c̄ hx of heparin-induced thrombocytopenia, existing coagulation irregularities, hepatic impairment.

SIDE/ADVERSE EFFECTS: CNS: dizziness, headache ▪ GI: N/V/D, dyspepsia, abdominal pain ▪ HEM: ↑ PT, leukopenia, ***thrombocytopenia*** ▪ INT: alopecia, photosensitivity, pruritus, rash ▪ MET: liver function abnormalities ▪ Other: conjunctivitis, visual disorders.

INTERACTIONS: Drug: Use c̄ anticoagulants can produce additive effects.

NURSING MANAGEMENT PRIORITIES

ADMINISTRATION: Assess for hx of hypersensitivity ▪ Assess renal function; do *not* administer if impaired ▪ Administer 1h ac/2h pc c̄ full glass of H_2O.

EVALUATION: Monitor renal status ▪ Assess for jaundice, bleeding; D/C drug, notify physician.

EDUCATION: Take on empty stomach c̄ full glass of H_2O ▪ Notify physician *immediately* of yellow skin/eyeballs, bleeding; D/C drug ▪ D/C when pain, other symptoms disappear ▪ Hair loss may occur ▪ Do *not* use tablets for future symptoms w/out checking c̄ physician.

NOTES:

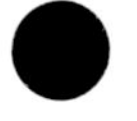

pentoxifylline • (pen-tox-if-i-lin)

CATEGORY: *Hemorrheologic agent* Rx; Preg Cat C

BRAND NAME	**DOSAGE FORM**
Trental (H-M-R)	CR tablet: 400mg

USE: Symptomatic treatment of intermittent claudication associated c̄ peripheral arterial disease ▪ Investigational agent for symptomatic treatment of acute/chronic cerebrovascular insufficiency. **ACTION:** Hemorrheologic effect due to ⬇ blood viscosity, enhancement of erythrocyte flexibility, resulting in significant ⬆ in tissue oxygen levels in pts c̄ peripheral arterial disease.

PHARMACOKINETICS

PO absorption	Peak	Half-life	Excretion
Almost complete	1h	0.4-0.8h	Primarily via urine as metabolites

CONTRAINDICATIONS: Intolerance to drug/methylxathines (caffeine, theophylline, theobromine), recent cerebral/retinal bleeding. **CC:** Use can result in rare cases of arrhythmias, hypotension ▪ Drug/metabolites are excreted in breast milk ▪ Possible toxicity due to ⬇ renal clearance in pts c̄ renal impairment ▪ Use c̄ caution in pts c̄ hemorrhage risk possibilities.

DOSAGE

Adult *PO* 400mg tid c̄ meals

SIDE/ADVERSE EFFECTS: CNS: *dizziness, drowsiness,* headache, tremor ▪ CV: anginal chest pain ▪ EENT: blurred vision ▪ GI: dyspepsia, N/V, bloating, flatulence ▪ HEM: leukopenia ▪ INT: pruritus, rash, urticaria ▪ Other: flulike symptoms.

INTERACTIONS: Drug: Use c̄ PO anticoagulants may ⬆ PT.

NURSING MANAGEMENT PRIORITIES

ADMINISTRATION: Assess for hx of xanthine hypersensitivity ▪ Administer c̄ food to ⬇ GI irritation; swallow tablet whole ▪ Assess renal function; ⬆ dose if impaired ▪ Avoid exposure to heat/moisture in storage.

EVALUATION: Monitor VS, esp BP ▪ Monitor renal status ▪ Observe for CNS effects (drowsiness, flushing, fainting), notify physician *immediately.*

EDUCATION: Drowsiness/dizziness may occur, use caution in potentially hazardous activities ▪ Take c̄ meals; do *not* crush/chew tablets; swallow whole ▪ Notify physician of drowsiness, flushing, fainting ▪ Avoid smoking ▪ May require several wks for therapeutic effect; do *not* D/C.

NOTES:

perphenazine • (per-fen-a-zeen)

CATEGORY: *Phenothiazine:* antipsychotic, neuroleptic Rx; Preg Cat C

BRAND NAMES
**Phenazine (ICN)*
Trilafon (Schering)

DOSAGE FORMS
Tablet: 2, 4, 8, 16mg
Injection (IM/IV): 5mg/ml
PO concentrate: 16mg/5ml
Tablet: 2, 4, 8, 16mg

COMBINATION PRODUCTS
Etrafon (Schering), **PMS Levazine (Pharmascience),* *Triavil (Merck)* — *See* perphenazine/amitriptyline hcl

USE: Treatment of psychotic states ▪ Treatment of N/V, intractable hiccoughs. **ACTION:** Antipsychotic activity associated c̄ a ⬇ in central dopamine-dependent pathways, which results in a tranquilizing effect: drug exhibits anti-α-adrenergic, anticholinergic, antiemetic, antiserotonin, ganglionic blocking activity.

PHARMACOKINETICS: Drug has good PO absorption, exhibits high protein binding, & is excreted via urine as metabolites.

CONTRAINDICATIONS: Hypersensitivity, comatose states, bone marrow depression, presence of large amounts of CNS depressants, subcortical brain damage. **CC:** Extended use can result in extrapyramidal symptoms, tardive dyskinesia, neuroleptic malignant syndrome.

DOSAGE

Psychiatric		
Adult	*PO*	6-64mg/d divided
	IM	5-10mg. Do *not* exceed 30mg/d
Nausea/vomiting		
Adult	*PO*	8-16mg/d divided
	IM	5-10mg for rapid control
	IV	Do *not* exceed 5mg/dose for severe symptoms

SIDE/ADVERSE EFFECTS: CNS: drowsiness, extrapyramidal rxs, tardive dyskinesia, ***seizures*** ▪ CV: postural hypotension, tachycardia, ECG changes ▪ EENT: blurred vision, corneal/lenticular changes, pigmentary retinopathy ▪ END: lactation, moderate breast enlargement in women ▪ HEM: ***agranulocytosis,*** leukopenia ▪ HEP: cholestatic jaundice ▪ INT: urticaria, photosensitivity, exfoliative dermatitis ▪ PSYCH: adverse behavioral changes incl catatonic-like states ▪ Other: fever, hemolytic anemia, hypothermia.

INTERACTIONS: Drug: Al/Mg antacid preparations ↓ absorption ▪ Use c̄ narcotics, barbiturates, other CNS depressants ↑ CNS depression ▪ Guanethidine, other related antihypertensives antagonized.

NURSING MANAGEMENT PRIORITIES

ADMINISTRATION: Assess for hx of phenothiazine hypersensitivity ▪ PO: administer c̄ food; do *not* crush/break SR tablets ▪ PO concentrate: dilute before administration c̄ >60ml fluid ▪ IM: inject *slowly*, deeply into UOQ of buttock; keep pt lying down for 30m after injection ▪ IV: dilute according to manufacturer's directions; administer 1mg/injection at 1-2m intervals; monitor BP; maintain pt supine for 30m ▪ Avoid skin contact c̄ liquid forms (contact dermatitis) ▪ Position vomiting pt to prevent aspiration ▪ Avoid abrupt withdrawal ▪ Heavy smokers may require ↑ dosage ▪ Elderly/debilitated pts may require ↓ dosage.

EVALUATION: Monitor hepatic, ophthalmic, renal status; BP, CBC, I&O, weight, constipation ▪ Assess for extrapyramidal symptoms (tics/spasms, trembling, shuffling gait) ▪ Seizure precautions in pts c̄ hx of convulsive disorders ▪ Long-term therapy: assess for jaundice, agranulocytosis ▪ Assess for symptoms of abrupt withdrawal (nausea, dyskinesia, trembling, dizziness).

EDUCATION: Use caution in potentially hazardous activities ▪ Avoid changing positions (lying/sitting/standing) rapidly ▪ Avoid use of alcohol, other CNS depressants ▪ Store in tightly closed, light-resistant container ▪ Use sugarless gum/hard candy to diminish dry mouth ▪ Constipation may occur; ↑ fluids, bulk-containing foods ▪ May turn urine pink/red/brown ▪ Avoid contact c̄ liquid forms ▪ Take PO forms c̄ meals; swallow SR tablets whole ▪ Use sunscreen, protective clothing ▪ Notify physician of fever, sore throat, bruising/bleeding, extrapyramidal symptoms ▪ Take as directed by physician ▪ Avoid smoking ▪ Check c̄ physician before taking OTC preparations ▪ Do *not* take antacids/antidiarrheals w/in 2h of drug ▪ Full drug effects may require several wks of therapy.

OVERDOSE MANAGEMENT: *See* Phenothiazines.

NOTES:

phenazopyridine hcl • (fen-az-oh-peer-i-deen)

CATEGORY: *Urinary analgesic* Rx; Preg Cat B

BRAND NAMES
**Phenazo (ICN)*
Phenazodine (Lannett)
Pyridium (P-D)
**Pyronium (ProDoc)*

DOSAGE FORMS
Tablet: 100mg
Tablet: 100mg
Tablet: 100, 200mg

USE: Symptomatic treatment of pain, burning, urgency, frequency, other discomfort arising from irritation of lower urinary tract associated c̄ endoscopic procedures, infection, passage of sounds/catheters, surgery, trauma. **ACTION:** Urinary analgesic mechanism not determined.

PHARMACOKINETICS: Not applicable.

CONTRAINDICATIONS: Hypersensitivity, renal insufficiency. **CC:** Use c̄ caution in pts c̄ impaired renal function. Consider D/C c̄ appearance of drug accumulation (yellow tinge of skin/sclera).

DOSAGE: *PO*

Pediatric	4mg/kg tid pc
Adult	200mg tid pc

SIDE/ADVERSE EFFECTS: GI: GI disturbances ▪ GU: renal toxicity ▪ HEM: ***hemolytic anemia,*** methemoglobinemia ▪ HEP: hepatic toxicity.

INTERACTIONS: Drug: None currently reported.

NURSING MANAGEMENT PRIORITIES
ADMINISTRATION: Assess for hx of hypersensitivity ▪ Assess renal function; do *not* administer if impaired ▪ Administer pc.

EVALUATION: Monitor renal status ▪ Assess for jaundice; D/C drug, notify physician ▪ Urine glucose: may produce false + c̄ Clinistix/Diastix; use Clinitest ▪ May interfere c̄ excretion, urine tests ▪ Diabetics: closely monitor blood/urine glucose, ketones.

EDUCATION: Take pc ▪ Discolors urine orange/red; may stain clothing ▪ Notify physician *immediately* of yellow skin/eyeballs; D/C drug ▪ D/C when pain, other symptoms disappear ▪ Diabetics: use Clinitest for urine testing ▪ Do *not* use tablets for future symptoms w/out checking c̄ physician.

Note: Side/adverse effects: common in *italic;* serious in ***boldface italic.*** *Available in Canada only.

NOTES:

phenazopyridine hcl

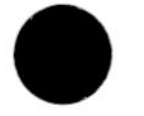

phenobarbital/phenobarbital sodium▲ • (fee-noe-bar-bi-tal)

CATEGORY: *Barbiturate*

Rx C-IV; Preg Cat D

BRAND NAMES

**Gardenal*
Luminal, Luminal Sodium▲ *(S-W)*
Solfoton (Poythress)

DOSAGE FORMS

Capsule, elixir, injection (IM/IV), tablet

DOSAGE

Pediatric		
Anticonvulsant	*PO*	15-50mg 2-3 times/d
	IM/IV	3-5mg/kg
Sedative	*PO*	2mg/kg tid
	IM/IV	2mg/kg
Adult		
Anticonvulsant	*PO*	50-100mg 2-3 times/d
	IM/IV	200-300mg
Sedative	*IM/IV*	30-120mg/d divided
Hypnotic	*PO*	100-320mg at hs
	IM/IV	130-200mg at hs

USE: Sedative, hypnotic ▪ Anticonvulsant for grand mal, status epilepticus, fever-, drug-, tetanus-induced convulsions ▪ Treatment of hyperbilirubinemia in neonates, Gilbert syndrome. **ACTION:** Sedative, hypnotic activity due to depression of midbrain reticular formation; anticonvulsant properties due to depression of motor cortex.

PHARMACOKINETICS

PO absorption	Onset	Duration	Half-life	Protein binding	Excretion
75%-90%	24-40m	6-8h	2-6d	20%-45%	75% in urine as metabolites

CONTRAINDICATIONS: Hypersensitivity, severe liver/respiratory impairment, porphyria, addiction. **CC:** Barbiturates are habit forming. Dependence, tolerance can develop c̄ sustained use ▪ Abrupt D/C in dependent pts will induce withdrawal symptoms.

SIDE/ADVERSE EFFECTS: CNS: *drowsiness, lethargy, hangover,* dizziness, paradoxic restlessness/excitement ▪ GI: N/V ▪ INT: morbilliform rash, ***Stevens-Johnson syndrome,*** urticaria ▪ Other: drug tolerance/addiction, asthma, angioneurotic edema.

Note: Side/adverse effects: common in *italic;* serious in ***boldface italic.***

*Available in Canada only.

INTERACTIONS: Drug: Use c̄ alcohol, antihistamines, benzodiazepines, methotrimeprazine, narcotics, tranquilizers ↑ depressant effects ■ Barbiturates are enzyme inducers, can ↓ effect of PO anticoagulants, other drugs ■ MAO-I ↑ activity of barbiturates ■ Barbiturates ↓ PO absorption of griseofulvin.

NURSING MANAGEMENT PRIORITIES

ADMINISTRATION: Assess for hx of barbiturate hypersensitivity ■ Do *not* administer if respirations <12/m ■ Administer hypnotic dose 1h before hs ■ Avoid exposure to moisture/light (elixir) in storage ■ Avoid abrupt withdrawal ■ Elderly may require ↓ dosage ■ ↓ Environmental stimuli.

EVALUATION: Monitor hepatic, renal, cardiac, respiratory status ■ Assess for symptoms of abrupt withdrawal (tremors, abdominal/muscle cramps, convulsions) c̄ prolonged use ■ Assess for actual swallowing of PO forms ■ Check for signs of dependence (↑ drug request) ■ Monitor serum concentrations; therapeutic blood levels: 10-40μg/ml ■ Monitor activity status (safety precautions) ■ Assess for tolerance/barbiturate cross-tolerance to therapeutic dose ■ Assess for paradoxic rxs (CNS stimulation), esp in elderly ■ Observe pt sleep patterns ■ Check for depression; suicide precautions prn.

EDUCATION: Drowsiness may occur; use caution in potentially hazardous activities ■ Avoid use c̄ alcohol, other CNS depressants ■ Indiscriminate use may lead to dependence ■ Do *not* keep at bedside ■ Take as ordered by physician ■ Store in tightly closed, light-resistant container (elixir) ■ Safety precautions may be instituted (raise bedrails) ■ Do *not* smoke after taking drug ■ Women: avoid breastfeeding ■ Practice relaxation exercises, ventilation of feelings ■ Utilize sleep producers (reading, warm milk, soft music).

OVERDOSE MANAGEMENT: Principal symptoms: ↑ CNS depression ■ Respiration depressed, pupils may be constricted, shock, coma ■ Emergency medical treatment: remove drug by lavage/emesis, maintain respiration; administer IV fluids, vasopressor to maintain BP; diuresis beneficial c̄ normal renal function; hemodialysis if indicated (anuria, shock).

NOTES:

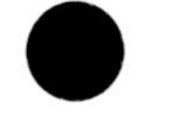

phenoxybenzamine hcl/phentolamine mesylate •

(fen-ox-se-ben-za-meen/fen-tule-a-meen)

CATEGORY: α-*adrenergic blocker:* antihypertensive, sympatholytic Rx; Preg Cat C

BRAND NAMES	**DOSAGE FORMS**
phenoxybenzamine	
Dibenzyline (SKB)	Capsule: 10mg
phentolamine	
Regitine (Novartis)	Powder for injection (IM/IV) 5mg/vial

USE: Treatment of hypertensive episodes due to pheochromocytoma ▪ Possibly effective for vasospastic peripheral vascular disorders, incl Raynaud's syndrome, acrocyanosis, frostbite sequelae (phenoxybenzamine) ▪ Control of hypertension during pheochromocytoma surgery (phentolamine) ▪ Treatment of dermal necrosis after norepinephrine administration, dx of pheochromocytoma (phentolamine).
ACTION: Antihypertensive effect due to noncompetitive blocking of α-adrenergic receptors, resulting in ↓ peripheral vascular resistance, reflex tachycardia.

PHARMACOKINETICS

Half-life	Duration	Excretion
24h	3-4d after single dose	Up to 50% in 12h, 80% in 24h; in urine, bile

CONTRAINDICATIONS: Any condition in which ↓ BP may be undesirable. **CC:** Adrenergic blocking agents can exacerbate symptoms of respiratory infections ▪ Use c̄ caution in pts c̄ cerebral/coronary arteriosclerosis or renal impairment ▪ Use can induce angina, coronary insufficiency, MI.

DOSAGE

phenoxybenzamine		
Adult	*PO*	Start c̄ 10mg bid. May be ↑ by 10mg qod, usually to 20-40mg 2-3 times/d
phentolamine		
Pediatric/Adult		
Surgery	*IM/IV*	Preop: 1mg q1-2h in children, 5mg q1-2h in adults. Repeat prn Surgery: 1mg prn in children, 5mg prn in adults
Necrosis		Prevention: 10mg/L of norepinephrine Treatment: 5-10mg into extravasation area w/in 12h

Note: Side/adverse effects: common in *italic;* serious in ***boldface italic.*** *Available in Canada only.

Hypertensive crisis	15mg
Pheochromocytoma dx	1mg in children, 5mg in adults. Inject, record BP at 30-s intervals for 3m, 60-s intervals for next 7m

SIDE/ADVERSE EFFECTS: CV: postural hypotension, tachycardia ▪ EENT: nasal congestion, miosis ▪ GI: GI irritation ▪ GU: inhibition of ejaculation.

INTERACTIONS: Drug: Use c̄ nonselective adrenergic agents may produce significant hypotension, tachycardia.

NURSING MANAGEMENT PRIORITIES

ADMINISTRATION: Assess BP ▪ Avoid exposure to moisture in storage ▪ Prevent postural hypotension ▪ Elderly may require ⬇ dosage.

EVALUATION: Monitor BP; observe for hypotension ▪ Observe pt for at least 4d before each dose ⬆ ▪ Assess peripheral circulation (skin color, temperature, pulse) ▪ Assess renal, respiratory status.

EDUCATION: Avoid changing positions (lying/sitting/standing) rapidly ▪ Dizziness, lightheadedness may occur; use caution in potentially hazardous activities ▪ Avoid smoking ▪ Compliance c̄ prescribed drug regimen ▪ Store in tightly closed container ▪ Men: disturbance of sexual function may occur ▪ Avoid use c̄ alcohol, constrictive clothing, extremely hot objects ▪ Check c̄ physician before taking OTC cold/cough/allergy preparations ▪ Nasal stuffiness may occur ▪ Avoid positions that may impair peripheral circulation ▪ Use sugarless gum/hard candy to diminish dry mouth ▪ Full therapeutic effect requires several wks.

NOTES:

phenylephrine hcl • (fen-ill-ef-rin)

CATEGORY: *Sympathomimetic:* decongestant, vasopressor Rx/OTC; Preg Cat C

BRAND NAMES	DOSAGE FORMS
**Mydfrin (Alcon)*	Ophthalmic solution
Neo-Synephrine (S-W) (Sterling [Canada])	Injection (IM/IV/SC), ophthalmic solution, viscous ophthalmic solution
	OTC: jelly, nasal drops, spray

USE: Maintain BP during spinal/inhalation anesthesia; prolong spinal anesthesia ▪ Treatment of hypotension due to drugs, hypersensitivity, shock ▪ Ophthalmic, nasal decongestant. **ACTION:** Sympathomimetic effect primarily α response, producing peripheral vasoconstriction, ⬇ heart rate, ⬆ BP, no β-adrenergic effect on heart at normal doses.

PHARMACOKINETICS

IM/SC absorption	IM/SC onset	Duration	Excretion
Good	10-15m	1-2h	Probably via urine

CONTRAINDICATIONS: Hypersensitivity, ophthalmic solutions in narrow-angle glaucoma, 10% solution c̄ aneurysms or in infants, parenteral use c̄ hypertension or ventricular tachycardia may be contraindicated. **CC:** Use c̄ caution in pts c̄ bradycardia, severe arteriosclerosis, hyperthyroidism, myocardial disease, partial heart block, the elderly ▪ Excessive use of nasal products can result in a "rebound effect" & ⬆ congestion.

DOSAGE

Injection

Hypotension	Usual dose 2-5mg IM/SC. Usual range 1-10mg. Do *not* exceed initial dose 5mg
Severe hypotension	Add 10mg to 100-ml infusion solution. For rapid response start infusion at 100-180gtt/m. Maintenance rate 40-60gtt/m
Spinal anesthesia	3mg, or 2mg for lower anesthesia levels, SC/IM 3-4m before administration of anesthetic. For hypotensive emergencies, 0.2mg IV recommended. Subsequent doses should *not* exceed previous dose by >0.1-0.2mg, c̄ single maximum dose 0.5mg

Paroxysmal supraventricular tachycardia	Initial dose up to 0.5mg by rapid IV injection (15-20s). Subsequent doses should *not* exceed previous dose by >0.1-0.2mg c̄ single maximum dose 1mg
Topical ophthalmic	
Vasoconstriction, pupil dilation	1gtt suitable topical anesthetic followed by 1gtt 10% ophthalmic solution on upper limbus. May be repeated in 1h
Surgery	Apply 2.5%/10% solution 30-60m before surgery
Ophthalmic exam	1gtt 2.5% solution in each eye
Topical nasal	Apply 1-2gtt/spray or small amount of jelly in each nostril q2-4h

SIDE/ADVERSE EFFECTS: CNS: headache, excitement, restlessness ▪ CV: ***arrhythmias*** (rare) ▪ INT: local irritation (topical preparations).

INTERACTIONS: Drug: Concurrent/sequential use c̄ MAO-I produces significant hypertension ▪ Use c̄ halothane can cause arrhythmias ▪ Use c̄ oxytoxic drugs can cause persistent hypertension.

NURSING MANAGEMENT PRIORITIES

ADMINISTRATION: Assess for hx of sympathomimetic, sulfite hypersensitivity ▪ Ophthalmic, place pressure on lacrimal sacs for 1m after administration ▪ IV: dilute according to manufacturer's directions; do *not* freeze, expose to light; titrate according to findings following physician's guidelines; use infusion pump; avoid abrupt withdrawal, D/C gradually ▪ Do *not* use discolored/precipitated solutions ▪ Have phentolamine available for OD (parenteral preparations) ▪ Elderly may require ⬇ dosage.

EVALUATION: Monitor VS, esp BP (IV: q2-3m, then q5m when stable) ▪ IV: monitor ECG, heart rate, respirations ▪ Check IV insertion site carefully; avoid extravasation.

EDUCATION: Take as ordered by physician; do *not* ⬆ dose ▪ Ophthalmic: blurred vision may occur; use caution in potentially hazardous activities; wear dark glasses ▪ Notify physician *immediately* of rapid/irregular heart rate, numbness/tingling of arms & legs, headache ▪ Procedure for ophthalmic, intranasal administration.

NOTES:

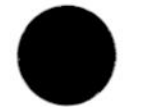

phenytoin/phenytoin sodium* • (fen-i-toyn)

CATEGORY: *Anticonvulsant:* antiepileptic — Rx; Preg Cat NA

BRAND NAME
Dilantin (P-D)

DOSAGE FORMS
Capsules, Infatabs*, injection (IM/IV), PO suspension*

USE: Treatment of grand mal, psychomotor seizures ▪ Prevention/treatment of seizures during neurosurgery ▪ Pain associated c̄ trigeminal neuralgia, migraine. **ACTION:** Anticonvulsant activity due to inhibition of seizure activity in motor cortex; drug tends to stabilize threshold against hyperexcitability caused by excessive stimulation/environmental changes; ⬇ maximum activity of brain for tonic phase of grand mal seizures; phenytoin exhibits antiarrhythmic activity, esp due to dig toxicity.

PHARMACOKINETICS

PO absorption	Peak: Prompt	Peak: Extended	Half-life	Excretion
Complete	1.5-3h	4-12h	22h	Via urine, feces

CONTRAINDICATIONS: Hypersensitivity, IV use in sinus bradycardia, SA block, Adams-Stokes syndrome, 2°/3°AV block. **CC:** Abrupt D/C can induce status epilepticus ▪ IM route not intended for status epilepticus ▪ Use c̄ caution in presence of hypotension, myocardial insufficiency.

DOSAGE

Pediatric *PO*	Initial dose 5mg/kg/d in 2-3 doses. Usual maintenance range 4-mg/kg/d
Adult *PO*	Initial dose 100mg tid, then individualize dose. Usual maintenance range 300-400mg/d, c̄ maximum dose 600 mg
Status epilepticus	
Pediatric	15-20mg/kg by slow IV injection. Do *not* exceed 1-3mg/kg/m
Adult	10-15mg/kg by slow IV injection. Do *not* exceed 50mg/m
Arrhythmias	100mg IV at 5-m intervals until satisfactory response or total 1g given
Neurosurgery	100-200mg IM at 4-h intervals, continued during postop period

SIDE/ADVERSE EFFECTS: CNS: headache, ataxia, nystagmus, ⬇ coordination, mental confusion, slurred speech,

Note: Side/adverse effects: common in *italic;* serious in ***boldface italic.***

*Available in Canada only.

dizziness, insomnia, sensory peripheral polyneuropathy c̄ long-term treatment ▪ CV: ***atrial, ventricular conduction, depression*** ▪ GI: constipation ▪ HEM: ***agranulocytosis,*** leukopenia, ***thrombocytopenia***, pancytopenia, ***megaloblastic anemia*** ▪ INT: morbilliform rash, ***exfoliative dermatitis, lupus erythematosus, Stevens-Johnson syndrome*** ▪ Other: gingival hyperplasia, enlargement of lips, local/injection site irritation.

INTERACTIONS: Drug: Use c̄ dicumarol is best avoided ▪ Disulfiram, isoniazid, valproic acid, many other drugs can inhibit phenytoin metabolism, resulting in ↑ phenytoin toxicity ▪ Use c̄ TCAs can induce seizures.

NURSING MANAGEMENT PRIORITIES

ADMINISTRATION: Assess for hx of hydantoin hypersensitivity ▪ Assess hepatic, hemopoietic, renal function; use caution if impaired ▪ PO: may crush tablet/empty capsule, mix c̄ food/liquid ▪ PO suspension: shake well before pouring ▪ IV: preferred parenteral route; administer *slowly* (<50mg/m); flush c̄ 0.9% NaCl solution; do *not* administer cloudy solutions; do *not* mix c̄ 5% dextrose solutions; do *not* mix c̄ other IV infusions ▪ Maintain seizure precautions ▪ Have emergency support equipment available ▪ Avoid abrupt withdrawal ▪ Elderly may require ↓ dosage ▪ Therapeutic blood levels: 10-20µg/ml.

EVALUATION: Monitor occurrence/characteristics of seizures ▪ Monitor BP; hepatic, renal, hematologic status; activity ▪ Assess oral cavity for gingival hyperplasia ▪ Assess for skin rash; D/C drug, notify physician ▪ Check IV insertion site carefully; avoid extravasation.

EDUCATION: Drowsiness may occur ▪ Maintain good oral hygiene (overgrowth of gum tissue) ▪ Take at equal intervals; do *not* omit doses ▪ Take c̄/immediately after meals ▪ May color urine pink/red/brown ▪ Avoid use c̄ alcohol ▪ Notify physician/dentist of use before treatment ▪ Use sugarless gum/hard candy to diminish dry mouth ▪ Keep appointments for dental exams/c̄ physician ▪ Avoid changing generic-name preparations ▪ Do *not* D/C drug w/out checking c̄ physician ▪ Carry medical identification (MedicAlert).

NOTES:

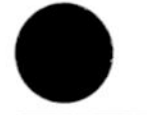

pilocarpine hcl • (pye-loe-kar-peen)

CATEGORY: *Parasympathomimetic: cholinergic,* muscarinic — Rx; Preg Cat C

BRAND NAMES
*Adsorbocarpine (Alcon), Akarpine (Akorn), *Carpine Nitrate (Allergan), Isopto Carpine (Alcon), *Minims (Sandu), *Miocarpine (Cooper Vision), Ocusert Pilo (Alza), Pilocar (Cooper Vision), Pilopine HS (Alcon), Piloptic (Optopics)*

AVAILABLE PREPARATIONS
Sterile ophthalmic solutions 0.25%-10%, ocular therapeutic systems (Ocusert)

USE: Main therapeutic use is to treat glaucoma by producing miosis, ⬇ of IOP by topical application. **ACTION:** Direct-acting parasympathomimetic produces ⬆ GI motility, profuse sweating/secretions, contractions of pupils/ciliary muscle, causing ⬇ IOP.

PHARMACOKINETICS: After instillation of 1% solution, onset is about 10-30m, usual duration 4-10h.

CONTRAINDICATIONS: Hypersensitivity, undesirable papillary constriction (eg, acute inflammatory disease of anterior segment of eye). **CC:** Miotics have been associated c̄ retinal detachment, esp c̄ preexisting retinal disease ▪ Use c̄ caution in presence of bronchial asthma, cardiac insufficiency, GI spasms, hypotension/hypertension, Parkinson's disease, peptic ulcers, recent MI, urinary tract obstruction.

DOSAGE: Must be individualized to clinical needs of pt.

SIDE/ADVERSE EFFECTS: Contact allergy/follicles in conjunctiva after prolonged use, ciliary spasm.

INTERACTIONS: Drug: Anticholinergics, antihistamines, hydroxyzine, TCAs can antagonize therapeutic effects.

NURSING MANAGEMENT PRIORITIES
ADMINISTRATION: Assess for hx of hypersensitivity ▪ Wash hands thoroughly before administration ▪ Carefully check label ("For ophthalmic use"), % of solution ▪ Avoid contamination of solution, dropper tip ▪ Apply pressure to

lacrimal sac 1-2m after instillation; instruct pt to keep eyes closed for 3-5m after insertion of gtt ▪ Store ocular system in refrigerator ▪ Avoid exposure to moisture/light in storage.

EVALUATION: Monitor IOP ▪ Assess for systemic cholinergic manifestations (↑ sweating, ↑ salivation, muscle tremors) ▪ Assess for altered mental status, esp in pts c̄ dementia ▪ Assess for signs of contact allergy.

EDUCATION: Will produce blurred vision, ↓ night/ distance vision; avoid potentially hazardous activities ▪ Take as ordered by physician; do *not* ↑ dose ▪ Notify physician *immediately* of eye irritation; D/C drug ▪ Keep scheduled appointments c̄ ophthalmologist ▪ Procedure for ocular system insertion; store in refrigerator ▪ Tolerance may develop to brow pain.

NOTES:

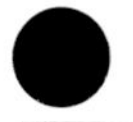

pimozide • (pim-oh-zide)

CATEGORY: *Antipsychotic* Rx; Preg Cat C

BRAND NAME
Orap (Gate)

DOSAGE FORM
Tablet: 2mg

USE: Suppression of motor tics associated c̄ Tourette's disorder that is unresponsive to standard treatment. **ACTION:** Suppression of motor, phonic tics appears related to blockage of CNS dopaminergic receptors.

PHARMACOKINETICS

PO absorption	Peak	Half-life	Excretion
>50%	4-12h	55h	Via urine primarily as metatolites

CONTRAINDICATIONS: Hypersensitivity, pts c̄ cardiac arrhythmias or congenital long QT syndrome or taking drugs that prolong QT interval of ECG, tics not associated c̄ Tourette's disorder, severe toxic CNS depression, or any comatose state. **CC:** Use can result in extrapyramidal symptoms, tardive dyskinesia, neuroleptic malignant syndrome (NMS) ▪ Use c̄ caution in pts c̄ convulsive disorders, liver/kidney impairment.

DOSAGE: *PO*

Adult/Children ≥12y/o: Starting dose of 1-2mg/d in divided doses c̄ subsequent ↓ qod. Usual maintenance dose <0.2mg/kg/d. Do not exceed 0.2mg/kg/d or 10mg/d

SIDE/ADVERSE EFFECTS: CNS: drowsiness, extrapyramidal rxs, *tardive dyskinesia*, ***neuroleptic malignant syndrome,*** akathisia, dizziness ▪ CV: postural hypotension, tachycardia, ECG changes in QT waves ▪ EENT: blurred vision, cataracts ▪ GI: dry mouth, N/V/D ▪ GU: impotence, urinary frequency, nocturia ▪ HEM: *hemolytic anemia* ▪ INT: rash, sweating ▪ PSYCH: adverse behavioral changes ▪ Other: asthenia, chest pain, muscle cramps, weight changes.

INTERACTIONS: Drug: Use c̄ other CNS depressants produces additive depression ▪ Use c̄ drugs (phenothiazines, antiarrhythmics) that prolong the QT interval is best avoided ▪ Use c̄ anticholinergics can produce additive effects ▪ Use c̄ anticonvulsants can ↓ their effect.

NURSING MANAGEMENT PRIORITIES

ADMINISTRATION: Assess for hx of neuroleptic agent hypersensitivity ▪ Assess VS, esp BP ▪ Obtain baseline ECG ▪ Administer c̄ food ▪ Assess hepatic, renal status; ⬇ dosage if impaired ▪ Avoid exposure to moisture/light in storage ▪ Avoid abrupt withdrawal (c̄ long-term therapy); D/C gradually ▪ Maintain hydration ▪ Elderly/debilitated pts may require ⬇ dosage.

EVALUATION: Monitor hepatic, renal status ▪ Monitor BP, CBC, fluid retention (I&O, daily weight), constipation, ECG ▪ Assess for extrapyramidal rxs (difficulty swallowing, muscle spasms) ▪ Seizure precautions in pts c̄ hx of convulsive disorders ▪ Long-term therapy: assess for jaundice, agranulocytosis ▪ Assess for symptoms of abrupt withdrawal (nausea, dyskinesia, trembling, dizziness if on long-term therapy) ▪ Assess for NMS (fever, convulsions, muscle rigidity, sweating); D/C drug, notify physician.

EDUCATION: Dizziness/drowsiness may occur; use caution in potentially hazardous activities ▪ Avoid changing positions (lying/sitting/standing) rapidly ▪ Avoid use c̄ alcohol, other CNS depressants ▪ Take as directed by physician ▪ Take c̄ meals ▪ Store in tightly closed, light-resistant container ▪ Use sugarless gum/hard candy to diminish dry mouth ▪ Maintain fluid intake (6-8 glasses/d) ▪ Avoid exposure to direct sunlight, UV light (sunlamps); use sunscreen, protective clothing ▪ Notify physician of fever, sore throat, bruising/bleeding ▪ Notify physician of extrapyramidal symptoms (tics/spasms, trembling, shuffling gait) ▪ Avoid ⬆ exercise, temperature extremes ▪ Avoid smoking ▪ Check c̄ physician/pharmacist before taking OTC preparations ▪ Do *not* take antacids/antidiarrheals w/in 2h of drug ▪ Full drug effects may require several wks of therapy.

NOTES:

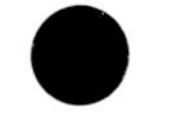

piperacillin sodium/piperacillin sodium-tazobactam sodium •

(pi-per-a-sill-in)

CATEGORY: *Extended-spectrum penicillin:* antibiotic: β-lactamase resistant combination

Rx; Preg Cat B

BRAND NAMES

piperacillin sodium

Pipracil (Lederle)

piperacillin-tazobactam

Zosyn (Lederle)

DOSAGE FORMS

Powder for injection (IM/IV): 2-, 3-, 4-g vial

Powder for injection (IV) 2/0.125, 3/0.357, 4g/0.5g per vial

PHARMACOKINETICS

IM absorption	Peak	Half-life	Protein binding	Excretion
70%-80%	30m	0.5-1.1h	16%-22%	60%-80% via urine in 24h as unchanged drug

USE: piperacillin: treatment of infections due to susceptible strains of *Acinetobacter, Bacteroides, Clostridium* spp, *Enterobacter* spp, *Enterococci, Escherichia coli, Haemophilus influenzae, Klebsiella* spp, *Neisseria gonorrhoeae, Pseudomonas aeruginosa, Proteus* spp, *Serratia* spp, *Streptococcus pneumoniae* ▪ In combination c̄ aminoglycoside, esp in pts c̄ impaired immune response. Piperacillin-tazobactam: extends the effective spectrum to susceptible β-lactamase strains of *E. coli, Bacteroides, H. influenzae, Staphylococcus aureus.* **ACTION:** piperacillin: bactericidal activity due to inhibition of mucopeptide cell wall synthesis in susceptible organisms. Tazobactam is a β-lactamase inhibitor.

CONTRAINDICATIONS: Hypersensitivity to any penicillin/cephalosporin. **CC:** Penicillins can produce serious/fatal (anaphylaxis) allergic rxs ▪ Possible cross-allergenicity c̄ cephalosporins, other β-lactam antibiotics ▪ Use can result in pseudomembranous colitis.

DOSAGE

piperacillin

Adult *IM/IV*
- Usual range 6-18g divided
- Gonorrhea: usual dose 2g IM c̄ 1g probenecid PO
- Do *not* exceed 2g/IM injection site

piperacillin-tazobactam

Adult *IV* 12g/1.5g/d divided q6h (3g/0.375g). Dosage must be ↓ in renal impairment

SIDE/ADVERSE EFFECTS: CNS: dizziness, headache ▪ GI: N/V/D, ***pseudomembranous colitis*** ▪ HEM: eosinophilia, leukopenia, neutropenia, ***thrombocytopenia*** ▪ HEP: cholestatic hepatitis, ↑ serum AST, ALT, LDH ▪ INT: rash, pruritus, vesicular eruptions ▪ Other: local pain/***thrombophlebitis*** at injection site, ***anaphylactic rxs.***

INTERACTIONS: Drug: Use c̄ bacteriostatic antibiotics can lead to antibiotic antagonism ▪ PO anticoagulant therapy may require dose adjustment ▪ Use c̄ probenecid will ↓ renal excretion of piperacillin & tazobactam.

NURSING MANAGEMENT PRIORITIES

ADMINISTRATION: Assess for hx of penicillin/cephalosporin hypersensitivity ▪ Obtain C&S before therapy ▪ Have support equipment available for anaphylaxis ▪ Do *not* mix c̄ aminoglycosides, other antibacterial solutions ▪ Reconstitute according to manufacturer's directions ▪ Maintain blood levels; administer at equal intervals around clock ▪ IM: inject *deep, slowly* into gluteal UOQ ▪ IV: administer by *slow* direct injection, IVPB (30m infusion) ▪ Na^+ content: 1.98mEq (45.5mg)/g; calculate in Na^+-restricted diets.

EVALUATION: Monitor VS, esp temperature ▪ Monitor hepatic, renal status (I&O) ▪ Assess for hypokalemia; may require supplemental K^+ ▪ Observe for signs of superinfection (diarrhea, perineal itching, oral ulcers) ▪ Assess for hypersensitivity rxs (fever, difficult breathing, rash) ▪ Monitor blood cultures, WBC, differential for drug effectiveness.

EDUCATION: Diarrhea may occur ▪ Maintain good personal hygiene (esp perineal, oral) ▪ Maintain fluid intake (6-8 glasses/d) ▪ Carry identification (MedicAlert) if penicillin allergic.

NOTES:

piroxicam • (peer-ox-i-kam)

CATEGORY: *Antiinflammatory:* NSAIA

Rx; Preg Cat NA

BRAND NAME
Feldene (Pfizer)

DOSAGE FORMS
Capsule: 10, 20mg

USE: Treatment of rheumatoid arthritis/osteoarthritis. **ACTION:** Antiinflammatory activity appears related to inhibition of prostaglandin synthesis.

PHARMACOKINETICS

PO absorption	Peak	Half-life	Excretion
Good	3-5h	50h	Via urine, feces as metabolites (95%)

CONTRAINDICATIONS: Hypersensitivity; aspirin, other antiinflammatory agent hypersensitivity. **CC:** Use ↑ risk of GI bleeding, ulcers, perforation ▪ Use has been associated c̄ jaundice, fatal hepatitis ▪ Use c̄ caution in pts c̄ CHF, hypertension, other preexisting fluid-retention conditions.

DOSAGE

Adult *PO* Initial dosage 20mg/d as single daily dose or divided. Adjust according to response

SIDE/ADVERSE EFFECTS: CNS: dizziness, drowsiness, vertigo, confusion, dream abnormalities ▪ CV: edema, ***exacerbation of CHF,*** angina ▪ EENT: tinnitus, blurred vision, eye irritations ▪ GI: N/V/D, anorexia, constipation, flatulence, abdominal pain ▪ GU: hematuria, ***interstitial nephritis, nephrotic syndrome,*** dysuria ▪ HEM: ↓ hemoglobin/hematocrit, anemia, eosinophilia, leukopenia ▪ HEP: jaundice, hepatitis ▪ INT: photosensitivity ▪ MET: hypoglycemia, hyperglycemia ▪ Other: ***anaphylaxis.***

INTERACTIONS: Drug: Use c̄ aspirin ↓ plasma levels ▪ Use c̄ lithium may ↑ its plasma levels ▪ May displace/be displaced by other drugs that are highly protein bound (eg, anticoagulants, sulfonamides); dosage adjustment may be required. **Lab:** Positive antinuclear antibody test (ANA).

NURSING MANAGEMENT PRIORITIES

ADMINISTRATION: Assess for hx of NSAIA hypersensitivity ▪ Avoid administration in pts c̄ hx of asthma, bleeding disorders, salicylate hypersensitivity ▪ Assess renal, hepatic function; use c̄ caution if impaired ▪ Administer c̄ food/milk, at same time qd; encourage upright position for 15-30m ▪ Avoid exposure to moisture/light in storage ▪ Elderly may require ↓ dosage.

EVALUATION: Monitor hematologic, hepatic, renal status c̄ prolonged use ▪ Monitor serum for ↑ BUN, creatinine, K^+; hold drug, notify physician ▪ Monitor pt receiving anticoagulant therapy; may potentiate bleeding ▪ Monitor I&O, daily weight ▪ Assess for edema in extremities ▪ Assess for visual, hearing disturbances; D/C drug, notify physician.

EDUCATION: Dizziness/blurred vision may occur; use caution in potentially hazardous activities ▪ Take c̄ food/milk to ↓ GI distress; maintain upright position for 15-30m ▪ Take as ordered by physician; do *not* skip dose ▪ Store in tightly closed, light-resistant container ▪ Avoid exposure to direct sunlight, UV light (sunlamps); usesunscreen, protective clothing ▪ Notify physician *immediately* of bleeding, rash, flulike symptoms, swelling of feet/legs, GI distress, jaundice, visual/hearing disturbance ▪ Avoid taking c̄ aspirin, other NSAIAs ▪ Avoid use c̄ alcohol ▪ Check c̄ physician/pharmacist before taking OTC preparations ▪ Keep scheduled appointments c̄ physician/for blood work/for eye exams ▪ Women: avoid breastfeeding ▪ Full drug effects may require several wks of therapy.

NOTES:

potassium chloride

CATEGORY: *Electrolyte:* mineral

Rx; Preg Cat C

BRAND NAMES
Kaon (Adria)
K-Lease (Adria)
K-Lor (Abbott)
Klorvess (Sandoz)
Klotrix (Bristol)
K-Lyte (Apothecon)
K-Tab (Abbott)
Micro-K Extencaps (Robins)
Rum-K (Fleming)
Slow-K (Summit)

DOSAGE FORMS
Capsule, injection (IV), pediatric injection (IV), PO solution, powder for PO solution, tablet (enteric-coated, extended-release)

USE: Prevention/treatment of K^+ deficiency ▪ Treatment of dig-induced cardiac arrhythmias. **ACTION:** Potassium is essential electrolyte required for nerve transmission, contraction of muscle tissue, gastric secretion, carbohydrate metabolism, acid-base balance; main intracellular cation; potassium chloride has 13.4mEq K^+/g.

PHARMACOKINETICS: Well absorbed PO; excreted primarily via urine.

CONTRAINDICATIONS: Existing conditions that result in ↑ K^+ levels (eg, renal impairment of potassium excretion, untreated Addison's disease, acute dehydration, heat cramps), conditions that result in extensive tissue necrosis. **CC:** Use of CR formulations should be restricted to pts c̄ compliance problems c̄ regular (non-CR) formulations due to ↑ risk of bleeding, ulceration ▪ Enteric-coated formulations are associated c̄ small bowel lesions ▪ Alkalinizing potassium salt (acetate, bicarbonate) should be employed to correct hypokalemia in presence of metabolic acidosis.

DOSAGE: Must be individualized. Normal daily adult requirement 40-80mEq. Usual daily supplemental dose 20mEq; 40-100mEq for potassium depletion.

SIDE/ADVERSE EFFECTS: GI: N/V/D, abdominal discomfort, ulceration, **hemorrhage** ▪ Other: tissue necrosis, phlebitis, vasospasm at parenteral injection site.

INTERACTIONS: Drug: Use c̄ potassium-sparing diuretics may result in severe hyperkalemia ▪ Use c̄ captopril, enalapril will ↑ potassium retention.

NURSING MANAGEMENT PRIORITIES

ADMINISTRATION: Assess renal function; do *not* adminiter if impaired ▪ Assess ECG, serum electrolytes, esp K^+ (normal levels: 3.5-5mEq/L); notify physician of abnormalities ▪ PO: do *not* crush/chew tablets; do *not* remove foil wrapper until ready to use; administer c̄ pt in upright position, c̄ full glass of liquid or c̄ food ▪ IV: dilute according to manufacturer's directions; infuse *slowly* (10-20mEq/L); do *not* exceed 40mEq/L ▪ Do *not* administer discolored/precipitated solutions ▪ Do *not* administer IM or IV push ▪ Chloride salt is preferred salt.

EVALUATION: Monitor VS, esp heart rate ▪ Monitor I&O, GI status ▪ Monitor serum electrolytes (K^+ levels) ▪ Monitor ECG for U waves (hypokalemia), tented T waves (hyperkalemia) ▪ Assess for symptoms of hypokalemia (muscle cramps, lethargy, nausea), hyperkalemia (difficult breathing, tingling in extremities, nervousness, irregular heartbeat) ▪ Check IV insertion site carefully (phlebitis); avoid extravasation.

EDUCATION: Take as ordered by physician; do *not* skip doses ▪ Swallow tablets whole; do *not* crush; take c̄ food/full glass of liquid ▪ Dilute liquid, powder preparations c̄ H_2O; sip slowly when eating ▪ Notify physician *immediately* of ↓ muscle strength, restlessness, irregular heart rate ▪ Avoid using c̄ salt substitutes, low-Na^+ milk (↑ K^+) ▪ Check c̄ physician/pharmacist before taking OTC preparations ▪ Use caution c̄ OTC laxatives (hypokalemia) ▪ Notify physician/dentist of use before treatment ▪ Avoid changing brand-name preparations ▪ Keep scheduled appointments c̄ physician/for blood work.

NOTES:

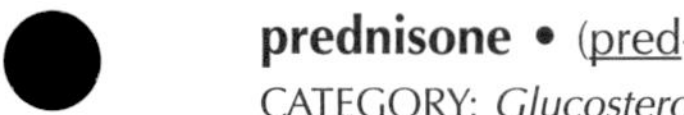

prednisone • (pred-ni-sone)

CATEGORY: *Glucosteroid:* corticosteroid — Rx; Preg Cat NA

BRAND NAMES	DOSAGE FORMS
Deltasone (Upjohn)	Tablet: 2.5, 5, 10, 20, 50mg
Liquid Pred (Muro)	Syrup: 5mg/5ml
Meticorten (Schering)	Tablet: 1mg
Orasone (Solvay)	Tablet: 1, 5, 10, 20, 50mg

USE: Treatment of adrenocortical deficiency, adrenogenital syndrome, other endocrine disorders, allergic states, collagen diseases, dermatologic diseases, GI diseases, hematologic disorders, ophthalmologic diseases, respiratory diseases, rheumatic disorders ▪ Treatment of tuberculous meningitis, neurologic/myocardial involvement associated $\bar{c}$ trichinosis ▪ Remission of proteinuria in nephrotic syndrome, acute exacerbation of multiple sclerosis ▪ Palliative management of leukemias, lymphomas. **ACTION:** Glucosteroids cause a wide variety of pharmacologic activity; two major effects are potent antiinflammatory effect, inhibition of immune response.

PHARMACOKINETICS: PO administration usually produces peak effect in 1-2h, duration about 1.5d.

CONTRAINDICATIONS: Systemic fungal infection. **CC:** 2° adrenocortical deficiency can result from abrupt D/C ▪ Corticosteriods mask symptoms of infection, can activate latent amebiases ▪ Extended use may produce glaucoma, subcapsular cataracts ▪ Use during pregnancy must consider benefits vs. hazards, which include ↑ risk of cleft palate, spontaneous abortion, fetal growth retardation.

DOSAGE

Pediatric	*PO*	0.1-0.15mg/kg/d
Adult	*PO*	5-60mg/d, $\bar{c}$ maximum 250mg if needed

SIDE/ADVERSE EFFECTS: CNS: ***convulsions,*** headache, psychic impairment, vertigo, mood swings; pseudotumor cerebri may develop after treatment ▪ CV: edema due to Na^+ retention, CHF, hypertension ▪ EENT: ↑ IOP, glaucoma, posterior subcapsular cataracts, exophthalmos ▪ END: cushingoid states, growth suppression in children, menstrual irregularities, 2° adrenocortical/pituitary unresponsiveness, hyperglycemia, carbohydrate intolerance ▪ GI: peptic ulcer/***possible perforation, pancreatitis***, abdominal distention, ulcerative esophagitis ▪ INT: poor wound healing, fragile skin, petechiae/ecchymoses, facial erythema,

↑ sweating, urticaria, hirsutism ▪ MET: negative nitrogen balance, hypokalemic alkalosis ▪ MS: muscle weakness/loss of mass, pathologic fracture of long bones, osteoporosis.

INTERACTIONS: Drug: Severe hypokalemia can occur c̄ diuretics (nonpotassium sparing) ▪ Use c̄ ulcerogenic drugs (eg, aspirin, indomethacin) can produce additive effects ▪ Use c̄ antidiabetic agents may require ↑ doses of antidiabetic drugs ▪ Use c̄ live viral vaccines best avoided. **Food:** Excessive consumption of licorice can ↑ hypokalemia.

NURSING MANAGEMENT PRIORITIES

ADMINISTRATION: Assess for hx of hypersensitivity ▪ Administer single daily/alternate-day dose *before* 9AM; multiple doses at equal intervals ▪ Administer c̄ food ▪ Avoid abrupt withdrawal; ↓ gradually ▪ Avoid exposure to heat/light in storage; do *not* freeze ▪ Elderly may require ↓ dosage; monitor BP.

EVALUATION: Monitor VS, esp BP ▪ Diabetics: closely monitor blood/urine glucose (hyperglycemia) ▪ Assess mental/emotional status; avoid TCAs if depression induced ▪ Monitor serum electrolytes (esp K^+, Na^+), ophthalmologic exams, stools for occult blood c̄ prolonged use ▪ Monitor hydration status (I&O, daily weight).

EDUCATION: Take c̄ food/milk (single daily dose *before* 9AM; multiple doses at equal intervals) ▪ Take as ordered by physician; do *not* ↑ dose; D/C drug ▪ Eat foods high in K^+, protein; avoid black licorice ▪ Follow diet low in Na^+ ▪ Check c̄ physician before immunization (pt, family) ▪ Avoid exposure to infection ▪ Report following symptoms *immediately* to physician: anorexia, difficult breathing, weakness, dizziness; may appear during periods of ↑ stress/trauma ▪ Notify physician of black/tarry stools, slow wound healing, blurred vision, bruising/bleeding, emotional changes ▪ Diabetics: carefully monitor blood/urine glucose ▪ Store in tightly closed, light-resistant container ▪ Keep scheduled appointments c̄ physician/for blood work/for eye exams ▪ Women: avoid breastfeeding ▪ Body image changes (full face, ↑ facial hair, ↑ fat deposit) may occur c̄ prolonged use (reversible).

NOTES:

probenecid • (proe-ben-e-sid)

CATEGORY: *Antigout agent:* uricosuric

Rx; Preg Cat C

BRAND NAMES	DOSAGE FORMS
Benemid (Merck)	Tablet: 0.5g
**Benuryl (ICN)*	Tablet: 0.5g

COMBINATION PRODUCT

ColBenemid (MSD)	probenecid/colchicine per tablet: 500mg/0.5mg

USE: Treatment of hyperuricemia associated c̄ gout, gouty arthritis ▪ Adjunct to penicillin therapy. **ACTION:** Uricosuric activity due to inhibition of tubular urate reabsorption in kidney; drug used in combination c̄ penicillins because it inhibits tubular penicillin excretion.

PHARMACOKINETICS

PO absorption	Peak	Half-life	Protein binding	Excretion
Complete	2-4h	4-17h	75%	Via urine primarily as metabolites

CONTRAINDICATIONS: Hypersensitivity, known blood dyscrasias, uric acid kidney stones, children <2y/o; do not start therapy until acute gouty attack subsides. **CC:** Use can exacerbate gout ▪ Urine alkalization c̄ ↑ fluid intake will ↓ possibility of costovertebral pain, hematuria, renal colic, uric acid stones.

DOSAGE: *PO*

Adult	250mg bid for 1wk. Subsequent dose 500mg bid thereafter or suitable dose to maintain normal uric acid level
Adjunct to penicillin/ cephalosporin therapy	
Pediatric 2-14y/o	25mg/kg, maintenance dose of 40mg/kg/d in 4 doses
Adult/Children >50kg	1-2g/d
ColBenemid	
Adult	1-2 tablets for 1wk, then 1 bid. Do not exceed 4 tablets/d

SIDE/ADVERSE EFFECTS: CNS: headache, dizziness ▪ GI: sore gums, anorexia, N/V ▪ GU: nephrotic syndrome, exacerbation of uric acid stones, hematuria, renal colic ▪ HEM: ***hemolytic anemia,*** aplastic anemia ▪ INT: dermatitis, pruritus ▪ Other: exacerbation of gout, fever, flushing, ***anaphylaxis***.

INTERACTIONS: Drug: Salicylates, pyrazinamide antagonize uricosuric activity ▪ Use c̄ methotrexate may ↑ methotrexate toxicity ▪ Probenecid inhibits renal excretion of penicillins, indomethacin, cephalosporins, sulfonamides, sulfonylureas ▪ Use c̄ methotrexate will ↑ its plasma concentration.

NURSING MANAGEMENT PRIORITIES

ADMINISTRATION: Assess for hx of hypersensitivity ▪ Administer c̄ food/milk/antacid ▪ Force liquids (3000ml/d) ▪ Avoid exposure to moisture in storage ▪ Normal serum uric acid: 2.5-6.0mg/dl ▪ Start only after initial gout attack subsides.

EVALUATION: Monitor hepatic, renal status ▪ Monitor CBC, serum uric acid, I&O ▪ Assess joint, mobility status ▪ Diabetics: monitor blood glucose levels closely (hypoglycemia) ▪ Use Clinistix/Diastix for urine testing.

EDUCATION: Take as directed by physician ▪ ↑ Fluid intake (8-10 glasses/d) ▪ Avoid use c̄ alcohol ▪ Avoid use c̄ aspirin-containing products (may take acetaminophen) ▪ Store in tightly closed container ▪ Notify physician of bruising/bleeding, lethargy, jaundice, sore throat ▪ Keep scheduled appointments for serum uric acid determinations ▪ ↓ Intake of high-purine foods (organ meats, legumes) ▪ Check c̄ physician/pharmacist before taking OTC preparations.

NOTES:

procainamide hcl • (proe-kane-a-mide)

CATEGORY: *Antiarrhythmic* Rx; Preg Cat C

BRAND NAMES
Procan SR (P-D)
Pronestyl (Apothecon)

DOSAGE FORMS
SR tablet: 250, 500, 750mg, 1g
Capsule: 250, 375, 500mg
Injection (IM/IV): 100, 500mg/ml
SR tablets: 500mg
Tablet: 250, 375, 500mg

USE: Treatment of arrhythmias incl atrial flutter, fibrillation, paroxysmal atrial tachycardia, PVCs, ventricular tachycardia ▪ Arrhythmias associated c̄ surgery. **ACTION:** Antiarrhythmic activity due to depression of cardiac automaticity, excitability, conductivity, resulting in widening QRS complex; PR, QT intervals prolonged; exhibits anticholinergic activity, produces effects similar to quinidine.

PHARMACOKINETICS

PO absorption	Peak	Half-life	Protein binding	Excretion
75%-95%	90-120m	2.5-7.5h	15%-30%	Via urine

CONTRAINDICATIONS: Hypersensitivity, hypersensitivity to procainelike anesthetics, complete heart block, lupus erythematosus, 2°/3° heart block w/out pacemaker. **CC:** Use c̄ caution in presence of 1° heart block, arrhythmias associated c̄ dig toxicity, cardioverted/digitalized atrial flutter/fibrillation, myasthenia gravis, renal insufficiency.

DOSAGE

Adult *PO*

Atrial arrhythmia	Loading dose 1.25g, followed by 0.75g in 1h. Additional doses 0.5-1g may be given until satisfactory response/tolerance limit reached. Usual maintenance dose 0.5-1g q4-6h
PVCs	50mg/kg/d divided q3h, then adjusted
Ventricular tachycardia	Loading dose 1g, followed by total daily dose 50mg/kg divided q3h, then adjusted. Extended-action tablets should be used for maintenance therapy only
IM	0.5-1g q4-8h for arrhythmias, 100-500mg for arrhythmias during surgery
IV	25-50mg/m

IV infusion	500-600mg over 30m, followed by maintenance infusion rate 2-6 mg/m

SIDE/ADVERSE EFFECTS: CNS: dizziness, mental depression, rare psychosis episodes ▪ CV: hypotension, ***ventricular arrhythmias*** (IV), ***2° heart block*** ▪ GI: N/V/D, anorexia, bitter taste ▪ HEM: neutropenia, ***hemolytic anemia, thrombocytopenia, agranulocytosis*** (rare) ▪ INT: *pruritus, urticaria,* maculopapular rash ▪ Other: ***SLE,*** angioneurotic edema.

INTERACTIONS: Drug: Use c̄ anticholinergics, antihypertensives, antiarrhythmics produces additive effects ▪ Use c̄ surgical neuromuscular blocking agents ⬆ their effects ▪ Use in pts c̄ myasthenia gravis is best avoided; drug antagonizes therapeutic response. **Lab:** Positive antinuclear antibody test.

NURSING MANAGEMENT PRIORITIES

ADMINISTRATION: Assess for hx of hypersensitivity ▪ Assess cardiac, renal function; may require ⬇ dosage ▪ May be administered c̄ food; *best* on empty stomach; tablets may be crushed/capsules opened; administer SR tablets whole ▪ Avoid exposure to moisture in storage ▪ Maintain blood levels; administer at equal intervals ▪ Have emergency support equipment available ▪ Solution may be clear/pale yellow ▪ IV: (direct) dilute 100mg c̄ 10ml 5% dextrose for injection; use cardiac monitoring; administer *slowly* (25-50mg/m); keep pt recumbent; (infusion) mix 1g in 250-500ml 5% dextrose; infuse 2-6mg/m via infusion control device; monitor BP q5-15m.

EVALUATION: Monitor VS, esp BP, heart rate & ECG (IV); notify physician of BP ⬇ >15mmHg ▪ Monitor CBC, blood levels, I&O, daily weight ▪ Assess for SLE c̄ prolonged use; D/C drug, notify physician ▪ Assess for edema in extremities ▪ Therapeutic blood levels: 4-8μg/ml.

EDUCATION: Dizziness may occur; use caution in potentially hazardous activities ▪ May take c̄ food to ⬇ GI irritation; *best* on empty stomach; swallow SR tablets whole ▪ Take as ordered by physician at equal intervals around clock ▪ Avoid caffeine ▪ Procedure for checking radial pulse ▪ Notify physician *immediately* of lethargy, fever, sore throat, swelling of feet/legs, irregular/changed pulse, bruising/bleeding ▪ Notify physician/dentist of use before treatment.

NOTES:

prochlorperazine▲/edisylate△/maleate◆ • (proe-klor-pair-a-zeen)

CATEGORY: *Phenothiazine:* antiemetic, antipsychotic Rx; Preg Cat C

BRAND NAMES

Compazine (SKB)

**Stemetil (Rhone-Poulenc)*

DOSAGE FORMS

Compazine:
Injection (IM)△: 5mg/ml
Spansule◆: 10, 15, 30mg
Suppository▲: 2.5, 5, 25mg
Syrup△: 5mg/5ml
Tablet◆: 5, 10, 25mg

Stemetil:
Injection (IM)△: 5mg/ml
Suppository▲: 10mg
Tablet◆: 5, 10mg

USE: Treatment of psychotic disorders ▪ Treatment of N/V. **ACTION:** Antipsychotic activity associated c̄ a ⬇ in central dopamine-dependent pathways, which results in a tranquilizing effect; exhibits good antiemetic properties.

PHARMACOKINETICS

PO absorption	Onset	Duration	Excretion
Good	30-40m	10-12h	Via urine

CONTRAINDICATIONS: Hypersensitivity; comatose states, bone marrow depression, presence of large amounts of CNS depressants, pediatric surgery. **CC:** Extended use can produce extrapyramidal symptoms, tardive dyskinesia, possible neuroleptic malignant syndrome.

DOSAGE

Psychiatric			
	Pediatric	*PO/Rectal*	2.5mg 2-3 times/d. ⬆ According to response 2-5y/o: Do *not* exceed 20mg/d 6-12y/o: Do *not* exceed 25mg/d
		IM	0.6mg/lb for control
	Adult	*PO*	15-150mg/d divided
		IM	10-20mg repeated q2-4h prn
Nausea/Vomiting			
	Pediatric	*PO/Rectal*	20-29lb: 2.5mg 1-2 times/d. Do *not* exceed 7.5mg/d 30-39lb: 2.5mg 2-3 times/d. Do *not* exceed 10mg/d 40-85lb: 2.5mg tid/5mg bid. Do *not* exceed 15mg/d
		IM	0.6mg/lb
	Adult	*PO*	5-10mg 3-4 times/d
		Rectal	25mg bid
		IM	5-10mg q3-4h. Do *not* exceed 40mg/d

SIDE/ADVERSE EFFECTS: CNS: drowsiness, extrapyramidal rxs, tardive dyskinesia ▪ CV: postural hypotension, tachycardia, ECG changes ▪ EENT: blurred vision, lens opacity, nasal congestion ▪ END: amenorrhea, galactorrhea ▪ GI: dry mouth, constipation ▪ HEM: ***agranulocytosis***, leukopenia ▪ HEP: cholestatic jaundice ▪ INT: urticaria, photosensitivity, skin pigmentation ▪ PSYCH: adverse behavior changes ▪ Other: fever, hyperpyrexia, ***neuroleptic malignant syndrome.***

INTERACTIONS: Drug: Antacids ⬇ absorption ▪ Use c̄ narcotics, barbiturates, other CNS depressants ⬆ CNS depression ▪ Guanethidine, related antihypertensives will be antagonized.

NURSING MANAGEMENT PRIORITIES

ADMINISTRATION: Assess for hx of phenothiazine hypersensitivity ▪ PO: administer c̄ food; do *not* crush/break SR capsules ▪ IM: inject *slowly, deeply* into UOQ of buttock; keep pt lying down for 30m after injection ▪ Do *not* mix c̄ other drugs in same syringe ▪ Avoid subcutaneous injection ▪ IV: add to infusion solution 15-30m before administration ▪ Avoid skin contact c̄ liquid forms (contact dermatitis) ▪ Avoid abrupt withdrawal ▪ Heavy smokers may require ⬆ dosage ▪ Elderly/debilitated pts may require ⬇ dosage.

EVALUATION: Monitor hepatic, renal status; BP, CBC; I&O, weight, constipation ▪ Seizure precautions in pts c̄ hx of convulsive disorders ▪ Long-term therapy: assess for jaundice, agranulocytosis ▪ Assess for symptoms of abrupt withdrawal (nausea, dyskinesia, trembling, dizziness).

EDUCATION: Use caution in potentially hazardous activities ▪ Avoid changing positions (lying/sitting/standing) rapidly ▪ Avoid use c̄ alcohol, other CNS depressants ▪ Use sugarless gum/hard candy to diminish dry mouth ▪ Constipation may occur; ⬆ fluids, bulk-containing foods ▪ May turn urine pink/red/brown ▪ Avoid skin contact c̄ liquid forms ▪ Take PO forms c̄ meals; swallow SR capsules whole ▪ Use sunscreen, protective clothing ▪ Notify physician of fever, sore throat, bruising/bleeding, extrapyramidal symptoms ▪ Check c̄ physician before taking OTC preparations ▪ Do *not* take antacids/antidiarrheals w/in 2h of drug ▪ Full drug effects may require several wks of therapy.

OVERDOSE MANAGEMENT: *See* Phenothiazines.

NOTES:

promethazine hcl • (proe-meth-a-zeen)

CATEGORY: *Antihistamine:* H_1 blocker

Rx; Preg Cat C

BRAND NAMES

**Histanil*
Phenergan (W-A)
**Rhinaris*
**Secaris*

DOSAGE FORMS: Injection, suppository, syrup, tablet.

USE: Symptomatic treatment of allergic disorders mediated by histamine ▪ Treatment of N/V, motion sickness ▪ Sedation for obstetrics, surgery ▪ Adjunct c̄ epinephrine in anaphylactic rxs, c̄ narcotics for postop pain. **ACTION:** H_1 antihistaminic activity due to competitive inhibition of histamine at H_1 histamine receptors on peripheral cells; drug exhibits good anticholinergic, antiemetic, antipruritic, sedative properties.

PHARMACOKINETICS

PO absorption	Onset PO	Onset IV	Duration	Excretion
Almost complete	20m	3-5m	4-6h	Via urine mainly as metabolites

CONTRAINDICATIONS: Hypersensitivity, neonates, nursing mothers, lower respiratory tract symptoms. **CC:** Use c̄ caution in presence of cardiovascular/convulsive disorders, liver dysfunction, narrow-angle glaucoma, pyloroduodenal/urinary bladder obstruction, stenosing peptic ulcer.

DOSAGE

Allergy		
Pediatric	*PO/IM/IV*	6.25-12.5mg tid. 25mg at hs
Adult	*PO*	12.5-25mg tid. 25mg at hs
	IM/IV	25mg, repeat in 2h prn
Motion sickness	*PO*	
Pediatric		12.5-25mg ½h before travel
Adult		25mg ½h before travel
Sedation	*PO/IM/Rectal*	
Pediatric		12.5-25mg at hs
Adult		25-50mg at hs
Nausea/Vomiting	*PO/IM/Rectal*	
Pediatric		12.5-25mg q4-6h prn
Adult		25mg q4-6h prn
Obstetric	*IM*	Early labor, 50mg Labor, 25-75mg

Preop	PO/IM/IV	
Pediatric		0.5mg/kg
Adult		25-50mg

SIDE/ADVERSE EFFECTS: CNS: *drowsiness*, dizziness, fatigue, euphoria, blurred vision ▪ CV: hypotension, palpitations, tachycardia, extrasystole ▪ GI: N/V ▪ HEM: ***agranulocytosis, thrombocytopenia*** ▪ HEP: cholestatic jaundice ▪ INT: drug rash, photosensitivity ▪ Other: anticholinergic effects, thickening of bronchial secretions.

INTERACTIONS: Drug: Use c̄ anticholinergics, CNS depressants, TCAs produces additive effects ▪ MAO-I can ↑ anticholinergic effects of antihistamines **Lab:** Unreliable results c̄ human chorionic gonadotropin/antihuman chorionic gonadotropin pregnancy test ▪ Possible ↑ in blood glucose.

NURSING MANAGEMENT PRIORITIES

ADMINISTRATION: Use caution in pts c̄ peptic ulcer, open-angle glaucoma, bladder obstruction, prostatic hypertrophy ▪ PO: administer c̄ food ▪ IM: preferred parenteral route; inject *deeply* into large muscle mass ▪ IV: avoid concentrations >25mg/ml; administer *slowly* (<25mg/m); avoid perivascular extravasation, intraarterial injection; protect from light c̄ foil covering ▪ Do *not* use discolored/precipitated solutions ▪ Avoid subcutaneous administration ▪ Incompatible c̄ strong alkaline drugs ▪ Have support equipment available for anaphylaxis ▪ Avoid exposure to moisture/light in storage ▪ Maintain hydration.

EVALUATION: Monitor VS, esp BP; serum for ↑ ALT, AST, bilirubin ▪ Assess for excessive drowsiness, dizziness, weakness ▪ False +/− pregnancy test ▪ May ↑ glucose tolerance ▪ Assess for athetoidlike movements of arms in pts c̄ acute pain after parenteral administration; additional analgesics may be required ▪ Monitor children for paradoxic rxs (CNS stimulation) ▪ Assess for tolerance to therapeutic dose.

EDUCATION: Dizziness, drowsiness, lightheadedness may occur ▪ Avoid use c̄ alcohol, other CNS depressants ▪ Take PO forms c̄ meals ▪ Store in tightly closed, light-resistant container ▪ Use sugarless gum/hard candy to diminish dry mouth ▪ ↑ Fluid intake (8-10 glasses/d) ▪ Notify physician of symptoms of allergic rx (fever, difficult breathing, rash) ▪ Carry identification (MedicAlert) if allergic ▪ Women: avoid breastfeeding ▪ Avoid prolonged exposure to direct sunlight, UV light ▪ May discolor urine.

NOTES:

propoxyphene hcl/napsylate▲ • (proe-pox-i-feen)

CATEGORY: *Analgesic*

Rx C-IV; Preg Cat NA

BRAND NAMES / **DOSAGE FORMS**

Brand names	Dosage forms
Darvon (Lilly)	Capsule: 65mg
Darvon-N▲ (Lilly)	PO suspension: 50mg/ml Tablet: 100mg
Dolene (Lederle)	Capsule: 65mg
**Novopropoxyn (Novopharm)*	Capsule: 65mg
**642 (Frosst)*	Tablet: 65mg

COMBINATION PRODUCTS

Darvocet-N 50, 100 (Lilly)	propoxyphene napsylate/acetaminophen per tablet: 50mg/325mg, 100mg/650mg
Darvon Compound-65 (Lilly)	propoxyphene hcl/aspirin/caffeine per capsule: 65mg/389mg/32.4mg

USE: Relief of mild/moderate pain. **ACTION:** Propoxyphene raises pain threshold by undetermined centrally acting mechanism; drug has no antiinflammatory/antipyretic activity; low schedule rating for misuse potential, addiction liability.

PHARMACOKINETICS

PO absorption	Peak	Duration	Half-life	Excretion
Good	2-3h	4-6h	6-12h	Via urine as metabolites, unchanged drug

CONTRAINDICATIONS: Hypersensitivity to drug, aspirin, caffeine. **CC:** Addiction-prone or suicidal pts should not receive the drug ▪ Extensive use c̄ ↑ doses can produce dependence; abrupt D/C may result in withdrawal symptoms ▪ Use c̄ caution in pts c̄ hepatic/renal impairment.

DOSAGE FORMS

Adult *PO*	65mg q4h prn. Do *not* exceed 390mg/d. Dose for napsylate salt 100mg q4h c̄ maximum of 600mg/d
Darvocet-N	One tablet (50 or 100) q4h prn
Darvon Compound-65	One capsule q4h prn

SIDE/ADVERSE EFFECTS: CNS: *dizziness, sedation,* euphoria ▪ EENT: minor visual disturbances ▪ GI: *N/V,* constipation, abdominal pain ▪ INT: skin rashes.

INTERACTIONS: Drug: Use c̄ alcohol, other CNS depressants produces additive sedation.

NURSING MANAGEMENT PRIORITIES

ADMINISTRATION: Assess for hx of hypersensitivity ▪ Assess quality, intensity, location of pain ▪ Assess emotional status; do *not* use in pts c̄ suicidal tendencies ▪ Administer c̄ food if GI irritation occurs; capsules may be opened, mixed c̄ food/liquid ▪ Administer *before* pt has intense pain ▪ Utilize + power of suggestion ▪ Avoid abrupt withdrawal c̄ prolonged use; D/C gradually ▪ Elderly may require ⬇ dosage.

EVALUATION: Monitor respirations, circulatory function ▪ Assess bowel function, abdominal distention ▪ Assess renal function, urinary retention ▪ Check for signs of dependence (⬆ drug request) ▪ Assess for potentiation of CNS depressant effect ▪ Assess for N/V; administer antiemetic ▪ Assess for signs of OD (coma, pinpoint pupils, respiratory depression).

EDUCATION: Dizziness/drowsiness may occur; use caution in potentially hazardous activities ▪ Avoid changing positions (lying/sitting/standing) rapidly ▪ Avoid excessive sensory stimulation ▪ Keep bedrails up when nonambulatory ▪ Turn, cough, deep breathe after surgery ▪ Constipation may occur; ⬆ fluids, bulk-containing foods ▪ Avoid smoking ▪ Indiscriminate use may lead to severe dependence ▪ Avoid use c̄ alcohol, other CNS depressants ▪ Women: avoid breastfeeding ▪ Take as ordered by physician; do *not* ⬆ dose ▪ Notify physician/dentist of use before treatment.

NOTES:

propranolol hcl • (proe-pran-oh-lole)

CATEGORY: *β-adrenergic blocker*

Rx; Preg Cat C

BRAND NAMES

**Detensol (Desbergers)*
Inderal (W-A)

DOSAGE FORMS

LA capsule: 60, 80, 120, 160mg
Injection (IV): 1mg/ml
Tablet: 10, 20, 40, 60, 80mg

COMBINATION PRODUCTS

Inderide (W-A)	propranolol hcl/hydrochlorothiazide combinations: 40/25, 80/25 tablet & 80/50, 120/50, 160/50 LA capsule

USE: Treatment of angina pectoris ▪ Treatment of hypertension ▪ Treatment of cardiac arrhythmias incl paroxysmal atrial tachycardia, atrial flutter/fibrillation, ventricular tachycardia, dig intoxication ▪ To ↓ mortality rate in stable pts after MI ▪ Management of hypertrophic subaortic stenosis & essential tremor ▪ Migraine prophylaxis ▪ Adjunct in pheochromocytoma. **ACTION:** Blocks access of catecholamines to β_1, β_2 receptors, resulting in bronchial constriction, ↓ heart rate, myocardial contractility ▪ Antihypertensive effect not determined.

PHARMACOKINETICS

PO absorption	Peak	Half-life	Protein binding	Excretion
90%	1-1½h	3.5-6h	90%	Via urine, feces

CONTRAINDICATIONS: Hypersensitivity, cardiogenic shock, bronchial asthma, sinus bradycardia, heart block, CHF unless secondary to tachyarrhythmia treatable c̄ propranolol. *See* carteolol.

DOSAGE FORMS

Adult *PO*

Angina	Initial dose 10-20mg 3-4 times/d. Usual effective dose 160mg/d. Do *not* exceed 320mg/d
Hypertension	Initial dose 80mg/d divided, may ↑ until desired effect is obtained. Usual range 120-240mg/d, c̄ doses up to 650mg
Arrhythmia	10-30mg 3-5 times/d
MI prevention	180-240mg/d divided

Hypertrophic subaortic stenosis	20-40mg 3-4 times/d
Essential tremor	120-320mg/d
Migraine	160-240mg/d divided
Pheochromocytoma	60mg/d divided, for 3d before surgery, c̄ α-adrenergic blocking agent
IV	1-3mg for serious arrhythmia
Inderide	Dosage usually 1 LA formulation/d or 1-2 tablet formulations/d

SIDE/ADVERSE EFFECTS: CNS: dizziness, mental depression, fatigue, hallucinations ▪ CV: bradycardia, CHF, hypotension, peripheral vascular insufficiency, heart block ▪ EENT: dry mouth/eyes, visual disturbances ▪ GI: N/V/D, constipation, ischemic colitis ▪ GU: impotence ▪ HEM: ***agranulocytosis,*** thrombocytopenic purpura ▪ INT: alopecia ▪ RESP: bronchospasm.

INTERACTIONS: Drug: Use c̄ reserpine, other catecholamine-depleting drugs can result in serious adrenergic blockage ▪ Nonselective β adrenergics antagonize therapeutic effects ▪ Usually contraindicated c̄ furazolidone, general anesthetics, MAO-I.

NURSING MANAGEMENT PRIORITIES

ADMINISTRATION: Assess for hx of hypersensitivity ▪ Assess apical pulse: if <60/m hold drug, notify physician ▪ PO: administration ac, at hs; may crush tablet; do *not* crush SR capsule, administer whole ▪ IV: inject *slowly* (direct, 1mg/m; infusion, 1mg/10-15m); use cardiac monitoring ▪ Avoid abrupt withdrawal ▪ Elderly may require ↓ dosage.

EVALUATION: Monitor VS, esp BP, heart rate; I&O, weight, blood glucose in diabetics (hypoglycemia).

EDUCATION: Use caution in potentially hazardous activities ▪ Avoid changing positions rapidly ▪ Take ac, at hs; swallow SR capsules whole ▪ Take as ordered by physician even if symptom free; do *not* change dose/D/C ▪ Check pulse before taking: if <60/m do *not* take drug, notify physician ▪ Do *not* abstain from food for >12h (low blood sugar) ▪ Avoid use c̄ alcohol ▪ Notify physician of muscle cramps, difficult breathing, cold extremities, leg edema ▪ Avoid high-Na^+ foods ▪ Check c̄ physician/pharmacist before taking OTC preparations ▪ Diabetics: monitor blood/urine glucose levels; observe for symptoms of hypoglycemia (headache, ↑ sweating, hunger, weakness) ▪ Notify physician/dentist of use before treatment ▪ Carry identification (MedicAlert) if taking propranolol.

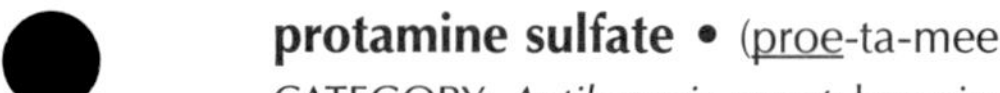

protamine sulfate • (proe-ta-meen)

CATEGORY: *Antiheparin agent:* heparin antagonist Rx; Preg Cat C

BRAND NAME
Protamine Sulfate (Lilly)

DOSAGE FORMS
Injection (IV): 50mg of activity/5-ml vial, 250mg of activity/25-ml vial

USE: Treatment of heparin OD. **ACTION:** Interacts c̄ heparin to form inactive complex w/in 5m of IV administration.

PHARMACOKINETICS: Neutralization of heparin occurs w/in 5m after IV administration. Metabolic rate not determined.

CONTRAINDICATIONS: Hx of previous intolerance. **CC:** Doses >100mg administered over a short period require caution due to anticoagulant effect ▪ Rapid administration can result in hypotensive rx ▪ Use in pts c̄ a cardiopulmonary bypass undergoing cardiovascular surgery has been associated c̄ noncardiogenic pulmonary edema ▪ Use can result in severe myocardial dysfunction, circulatory collapse ▪ Hemorrhage has been observed after complete inactivation of heparin by protamine in a small number of pts following cardiac surgery.

DOSAGE: *IV:* dosage must be individualized; 1mg protamine sulfate neutralizes 90 USP units heparin derived from lung tissue, 110 USP units of heparin derived from intestinal tissue; specific dose depends on heparin origin & severity of heparin OD.

SIDE/ADVERSE EFFECTS: CV: bradycardia, hypotension (sudden) ▪ RESP: dyspnea ▪ Other: possible cross-allergenicity in pts allergic to fish.

INTERACTIONS: Drug: Possible heparin rebound.

NURSING MANAGEMENT PRIORITIES

ADMINISTRATION: Assess for hypersensitivity to fish ▪ Administer by *slow* IV injection; do *not* exceed 50mg in any 10m ▪ Store in refrigerator; avoid freezing.

EVALUATION: Monitor VS, esp BP ▪ Monitor APTT, coagulation studies.

EDUCATION: Report bleeding/bruising *immediately*.

NOTES:

protamine sulfate

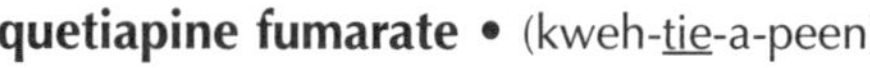

quetiapine fumarate • (kweh-tie-a-peen)

CATEGORY: *Antipsychotic:* neuroleptic

Rx; Preg Cat C

BRAND NAME
Seroquel (Zeneca)

DOSAGE FORMS
Tablet: 25, 100, 200mg

USE: Treatment of psychotic disorders. **ACTION:** Antipsychotic activity appears associated c̄ ↓ in dopamine & serotonin pathways, esp in limbic area, resulting in tranquilizing effect in psychotic pts. Drug Is moderately free of extrapyramidal symptoms & exhibits α-1 antiadrenergic & antihistaminic activity.

PHARMACOKINETICS

PO absorption	Peak	Half-life	Protein binding	Excretion
Rapid	1.5h	6h	83%	Via urine (77%), feces (20%) as metabolites

CONTRAINDICATIONS: Hypersensitivity. **CC:** Use can induce hypothyroidism, neuroleptic malignant syndrome, seizure (0.8%), orthostatic hypotension, tardive dyskinesia ▪ Use >6wks not evaluated ▪ Safety & efficacy in pediatric pts not established ▪ Breastfeeding is not recommended ▪ Use in pts c̄ hepatic impairment may require ↓ dosage.

DOSAGE

Adult	*PO*	Initial dose of 25mg bid c̄ increments of 25-50mg bid on days 2 & 3 c̄ further increments q2d or more. Maintenance dose is 150-750mg/d

SIDE/ADVERSE EFFECTS: CNS: dizziness, postural hypotension, headache, somnolence, extrapyramidal symptoms ▪ CV: tachycardia, palpitations, peripheral edema, vasodilation, ECG changes ▪ GI: dry mouth, dyspepsia, constipation, anorexia, taste disorders ▪ HEM: leukopenia, ***rare thrombocytopenia*** ▪ Other: sweating, pharyngitis, visual disturbances, tinnitus, dysmenorrhea, hypothyroidism, weight gain.

INTERACTIONS: Drug: Use c̄ alcohol is best avoided ▪ Use c̄ antihypertensives can produce additive hypotension ▪ Use c̄ enzyme inducers, barbiturates, carbamazepine, glucosteroids, phenytoin, rifampin can reduce serum levels of quetiapine & ↑ doses may be required ▪ Use c̄ thioridazine ↑ clearance of quetiapine ▪ Use c̄ erythromycin, fluconazole, itraconazole, ketoconazole requires caution due to possible enzyme inhibition of quetiapine metabolism. **Lab:** ↑ Levels of ALT, prolactin.

Note: Side/adverse effects: common in *italic;* serious in ***boldface italic.***

*Available in Canada only.

NURSING MANAGEMENT PRIORITIES

ADMINISTRATION: Assess for hx of hypersensitivity ▪ Assess VS, esp BP ▪ Assess hepatic, renal function; may require ↓ dosage if impaired ▪ Assess for hx of seizures; use caution ▪ Institute safety, seizure, suicide precautions ▪ Avoid abrupt withdrawal; D/C gradually ▪ Elderly/debilitated pts may require ↓ dosage.

EVALUATION: Monitor CV, hepatic, renal status ▪ Monitor BP, CBC, fluid retention (I&O, daily weight), constipation ▪ Assess for extrapyramidal rx ▪ Seizure precautions in pts c̄ hx of convulsive disorders.

EDUCATION: Dizziness/drowsiness may occur; use caution in potentially hazardous activities ▪ Avoid changing positions (lying/sitting/standing) rapidly ▪ Avoid use c̄ alcohol, other CNS depressants ▪ Store in tightly closed, light-resistant container ▪ Use sugarless gum/hard candy to diminish dry mouth ▪ Constipation may occur; ↑ fluids, bulk-containing foods ▪ Women: avoid breastfeeding ▪ May produce alteration in taste ▪ Notify physician of fever, sore throat, bruising/bleeding, tics/spasms, trembling, shuffling gait ▪ Avoid ↑ exercise, temperature extremes ▪ Check c̄ physician/pharmacist before taking OTC preparations ▪ Full drug effects may require several wks of therapy.

NOTES:

quinidine salts • (kwin-i-deen)

CATEGORY: *Antiarrhythmic* Rx; Preg Cat C

BRAND NAMES
quinidine gluconate
Quinaglute Dura Tabs (Berlex), Quinalan (Lannett)
quinidine polygalacturonate
Cardioquin (P-F)
quinidine sulfate
Quinidex Extentabs (Robins)

DOSAGE FORMS: Capsule, injection (IM/IV), tablets.

USE: Treatment of atrial flutter, established atrial fibrillation, after electric conversion of atrial flutter/fibrillation; paroxysmal atrial fibrillation, atrial tachycardia, atrioventricular junction rhythm, ventricular tachycardia not associated c̄ complete heart block; premature atrial/ventricular contraction. **ACTION:** Main antiarrhythmic effect appears related to prolongation of effective refractory period, ⬆ action potential duration in cardiac muscle, His-Purkinje system; drug anticholinergic activity also contributes to cardiac effects.

PHARMACOKINETICS

PO absorption	Peak	Half-life	Protein binding	Excretion
Almost complete	1-2h	3-16h	80%	Via urine, feces

CONTRAINDICATIONS: Hypersensitivity, thrombocytopenic purpura associated c̄ previous therapy, intraventricular conduction defects, AV block/aberrant impulses, abnormal rhythms due to escape mechanisms. **CC:** Use for atrial flutter can result in ⬆ ventricular rates ▪ D/C use c̄ toxicity development ▪ Use c̄ caution in pts c̄ cardiac, hepatic, renal dysfunction.

DOSAGE: Adult

Gluconate	*PO*	324-648mg q8-12h
Gluconate	*IM*	Initial dose 600mg. Subsequent doses 400mg can be repeated as often as q2h
	IV	≤330mg for most cases, c̄ maximum 500-700mg
Polygalacturonate	*PO*	Initial dose 275-825mg. Usual maintenance dose 275mg 3-4 times/d

Sulfate	*PO*
Atrial flutter	Dosage individualized after pt digitalization
Conversion of atrial fibrillation	0.2g q2-3h for 5-8 doses, c̄ subsequent daily dose ↑ until sinus rhythm restored or toxic effects occur
Premature atrial/ ventricular contractions	0.2-0.3g 3-4 times/d
Paroxysmal supraventricular tachycardia	0.4-0.6g q2-3h until paroxysm stops

SIDE/ADVERSE EFFECTS: CNS: headache, dizziness ▪ CV: ***widening of QRS complex, cardiac asystole, ventricular ectopic beats, paradoxic tachycardia, atrial embolism*** ▪ EENT: blurred vision, tinnitus, optic neuritis ▪ GI: *N/V/D*, abdominal pain ▪ HEM: ***acute hemolytic anemia, hypothrombinemia, thrombocytopenic purpura, agranulocytosis*** ▪ INT: pruritus.

INTERACTIONS: Drug: Use c̄ PO anticoagulants may require anticoagulant dosage adjustment ▪ Use c̄ urinary alkalizer may inhibit quinidine excretion, which can ↑ toxicity ▪ Use c̄ verapamil can produce significant hypotensive effects ▪ Use c̄ anticholinergics can produce additive vagolytic effect ▪ Use c̄ dig glycosides can result in cardiac toxicity.

NURSING MANAGEMENT PRIORITIES

ADMINISTRATION: Assess for hx of hypersensitivity ▪ Assess BP, apical pulse; notify physician, D/C drug if abnormal ▪ Test dose may be administered; check c̄ physician ▪ PO: administer c̄ full glass H_2O 1h ac/2h pc; may administer c̄ food to ↓ GI irritation ▪ Administer SR tablets whole ▪ Do *not* use discolored/precipitated solution.

EVALUATION: Monitor VS, esp BP; apical pulse; F/E, renal, hepatic, hematologic status ▪ Cardiac monitoring; report ventricular abnormalities to physician (widened QRS, PVCs) ▪ Observe for diarrhea ▪ Monitor blood levels for toxicity ▪ Therapeutic blood levels: 3-6µg/ml.

EDUCATION: Dizziness may occur; use caution in potentially hazardous activities ▪ Avoid changing positions rapidly ▪ Take as ordered by physician ▪ May take c̄ food to ↓ GI distress ▪ Do *not* crush/chew SR tablets ▪ Notify physician of shortness of breath, chest pain, "skipped" heart beats, sensory disturbances; D/C drug ▪ Check c̄ physician/pharmacist before taking OTC preparations ▪ Avoid use c̄ alcohol, caffeine ▪ Keep appointments c̄ physician/for lab work ▪ Carry medical identification (MedicAlert).

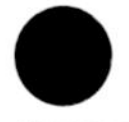

raloxifene • (ray-<u>lox</u>-ih-feen)

CATEGORY: *Antiosteoporosis agent:* selective estrogen receptor modulator Rx; Preg Cat X

BRAND NAME	**DOSAGE FORM**
Evista (Lilly)	Tablet: 60mg

USE: Prevention of osteoporosis in postmenopausal females. **ACTION:** Antiosteoporosis effect due to selective estrogen receptor modulation (SERM), resulting in estrogenlike ↑ in bone density ▪ Drug ↓ resorption & turnover of bone tissue & is devoid of estrogenlike effects in breasts & uterus.

PHARMACOKINETICS

PO absorption	Half-life	Protein binding	Excretion
Rapid	27-32h	≥95%	Via feces as metabolites

CONTRAINDICATIONS: Hypersensitivity, pregnancy, hx of venous thromboembolic conditions. **CC:** Use can result in thromboembolic events incl deep vein thrombosis, pulmonary embolism, retinal vein thrombosis, esp during first 4mo of treatment ▪ Use in premenopausal females not recommended ▪ Supplemental calcium intake required if daily consumption is inadequate ▪ Safety & efficacy not evaluated for use in pts c̄ severe hepatic impairment.

DOSAGE

PO 60mg once/d

SIDE/ADVERSE EFFECTS: CNS: depression, insomnia ▪ GI: N/V, dyspepsia, flatulence ▪ GU: vaginitis, leukorrhea, UTI ▪ HEM: ***thromboembolic events*** ▪ MS: arthralgia, myalgia, arthritis, leg cramps ▪ RESP: chest pain, sinusitis, pharyngitis, cough exacerbation, ***pneumonia*** ▪ Other: infection, rash, flu symptoms, weight gain.

INTERACTIONS: Drug: Use can effect drugs c̄ ↑ protein-binding capabilities & incl clofibrate, diazoxide, diazepam, ibuprofen, naproxen. **Lab:** Use can ↓ cholesterol, LDL, fibrinogen serum levels ▪ Modest ↑ in corticosteroid, estrogen, thyroxine globulin binding.

NURSING MANAGEMENT PRIORITIES

ADMINISTRATION: Assess for hx of hypersensitivity ▪ Assess hepatic function; use caution if impaired ▪ Should *not* be used in premenopausal women or in women on systemic estrogen/hormone replacement therapy ▪ D/C 72h before/during prolonged immobilization.

EVALUATION: Monitor CV status (DVTs) ▪ Monitor hepatic status ▪ Observe pt for signs of bleeding; notify physician.

EDUCATION: Hot flashes may occur when beginning therapy ▪ Supplement calcium & vitamin D if diet is inadequate ▪ Avoid use c̄ alcohol & cigarette smoking ▪ Avoid prolonged restriction of movement (↑ risk of clot formation) ▪ Notify physician *immediately* of abnormal rxs (chest pain, bleeding, difficulty breathing) ▪ Women: avoid pregnancy, breastfeeding ▪ Use contraception if sexually active.

NOTES:

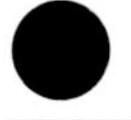

repaglinide • (reh-pag-leh-nide)

CATEGORY: *Oral hypoglycemic*

Rx; Preg Cat C

BRAND NAME
Prandin (Novo Nordisk)

DOSAGE FORMS
Tablet: 0.5, 1, 2mg

USE: Management of type II (noninsulin-dependent) diabetes that cannot be controlled by diet alone ▪ In combination c̄ metformin. **ACTION:** Antidiabetic activity due to stimulation of insulin release from functioning β-cells of pancreas.

PHARMACOKINETICS

PO absorption	Peak	Half-life	Protein binding	Excretion
Complete	1h	1-1.4h	98%	Primarily via feces as metabolites

CONTRAINDICATIONS: Hypersensitivity, diabetic ketoacidosis c̄ /w/out coma. **CC:** Use may be associated c̄ ↑ rate of cardiovascular mortality ▪ Possible loss of glucose control can occur c̄ excessive body stress (infection, trauma) ▪ Prolonged use can lead to ↓ hyperglycemic control (secondary failure) ▪ Safety & efficacy in pediatric pts not established.

DOSAGE

Adult	*PO*	Must be individualized. Usual maintenance range is 0.5-4mg 2-4 times/d. Do *not* exceed 16mg/d

SIDE/ADVERSE EFFECTS: CNS: headache ▪ CV: rare ischemia ▪ GI: N/V/D, dyspepsia ▪ MET: hypoglycemia ▪ RESP: infection (URI), sinusitis, rhinitis, bronchitis ▪ Other: arthralgia, back pain, UTI.

INTERACTIONS: Drug: Use c̄ β-adrenergic blockers, chloramphenicol, MAO-I, NSAIAs, PO anticoagulants, probenecid, salicylates, sulfonamides can ↑ hypoglycemic effects ▪ Use c̄ antifungals (ie, ketoconazole), erythromycin ↓ repaglinide metabolism ▪ Use c̄ enzyme inducers, barbiturates, carbamazepine, rifampin, troglitazone ↑ rapaglinide metabolism ▪ Use c̄ adrenergics, calcium blockers, corticosteroids, estrogens, isoniazid, nicotinic acid, PO contraceptives, phenothiazines, phenytoin, thiazides, thyroid preparations ↓ hypoglycemic effects.

NURSING MANAGEMENT PRIORITIES

ADMINISTRATION: Assess for hx of hypersensitivity ▪ Assess for metabolic acidosis; to *not* use if present ▪ Assess for renal, hepatic function; may require ↓ dosage if impaired, use caution ▪ Avoid exposure to moisture/light in storage ▪ Administer 15m ac.

EVALUATION: Monitor hepatic, renal, hematologic status ▪ Monitor FBS ▪ Evaluate pt closely during first wk to assess effectiveness ▪ Monitor electrolyte status, blood pH.

EDUCATION: Compliance c̄ special diet therapy ▪ Take 15m ac as directed by physician ▪ Blood/urine/glucose/ketone testing procedure ▪ Symptoms of hypoglycemia (anxiety, headache, fatigue, nausea, sweating); notify physician *immediately* ▪ Always carry lump of sugar/candy for quick use (hypoglycemia) ▪ Avoid use with alcohol ▪ Check c̄ physician before taking OTC preparations ▪ Notify physician *immediately* of symptoms of hyperglycemia (excessive hunger, thirst, urination, rapid pulse, sweet smelling breath, weight loss) ▪ Notify physician *immediately* of excessive weakness/tiredness, muscle pain, difficulty breathing, stomach discomfort, dizziness, irregular heartbeats ▪ Maintain good personal hygiene ▪ Carry medical identification (Medic/Alert) ▪ Store in tightly closed container ▪ Keep scheduled appointments c̄ physician/for blood glucose determinations ▪ Maintain optimum body weight ▪ Women: notify physician of possible pregnancy (insulin use recommended); avoid breastfeeding ▪ PO hypoglycemic needs may change c̄ ↑ stress, ↑ exercise, ↓ appetite; notify physician.

NOTES:

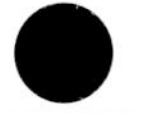

Rh_o (D) immune globulin

CATEGORY: *Immunosuppressant:* biological

Rx; Preg Cat C

BRAND NAMES

Standard dose	Microdose
Gamulin Rh (Armour)	*HypRho-D Mini-Dose*
HypRho-D (Cutter)	*MICRhoGAM*
RhoGAM (Ortho)	*Mini-Gamulin Rh*
WinRho (Nabi)	

USE: Microdose preparation: used to suppress antibody formation in women c̄ Rh^- blood after abortion/pregnancy termination up to & incl wk 12 of gestation unless father has Rh^- blood. Standard preparation: used to suppress antibody formation in women c̄ Rh^- blood after delivery, abortion/pregnancy termination, abdominal trauma during pregnancy ▪ Used to suppress antibody formation after transfusion accident. **ACTION:** Sterile solution of immunoglobulin [IgG anti-Rh_o (D)] obtained from fractionated human plasma, used to suppress immune response in nonsensitized pts c̄ Rh^- blood who receive Rh^+ blood cells because of fetomaternal hemorrhage, transfusion accident.

PHARMACOKINETICS: Not applicable.

CONTRAINDICATIONS: Hypersensitivity, previously sensitized individuals; micropreparation for genetic amniocentesis at wks 15-18, antepartum prophylaxis at wk 28. **CC:** Not intended for IV administration.

DOSAGE

OB	IM injection of total contents of single vial w/in 72h. Multiple dose required when fetomaternal hemorrhaging >30ml
Transfusion	IM injection of total contents of single vial(s) w/in ≤3d. Specific dose dependent on volume of Rh^+ blood transfused

SIDE/ADVERSE EFFECTS: CNS: lethargy ▪ MS: myalgia, localized stiffness/tenderness at injection site ▪ Other: limited allergic rxs incl anaphylaxis.

INTERACTIONS: Drug: Delay use of live vaccine for 3mo because of possible ⬇ in immune response to vaccine.

NURSING MANAGEMENT PRIORITIES

ADMINISTRATION: Assess for hx of hypersensitivity ▪ Preadministration criteria (type, cross-match, neonatal cord blood): mother must be Rh_o $(D)^-$, D^{u-}; mother should *not* have been previously sensitized to Rh_o factor: infant must be Rh_o $(D)^+$, D^{u+}, direct Coombs'; verify that lot numbers are same for cross-match solution, preparation to be administered ▪ Cross-match 5% suspension of mother's RBCs c̄ 2gtt cross-match solution ▪ Administer w/in 72h after Rh-incompatible delivery, terminated incomplete pregnancy, blood transfusions ▪ Administer IM (deltoid); do *not* administer IV ▪ Check preparation c̄ another nurse ▪ Do *not* administer to infant ▪ Do *not* administer discolored/precipitated solutions ▪ Store in refrigerator ▪ Provide emotional support.

EVALUATION: Assess for tenderness at injection site ▪ Assess for ↑ body temperature ▪ Assess for lethargy, myalgia if >1 dose administered.

EDUCATION: Explain procedure, rationale to pt, family ▪ Importance of screening both parents for Rh incompatibility.

NOTES:

rifabutin • (rif-ah-byoo-tin)

CATEGORY: *Antitubercular:* semisynthetic ansamycin antibiotic   Rx; Preg Cat B

BRAND NAME
Mycobutin (Upjohn)

DOSAGE FORM
Capsule: 150mg

USE: Prevention of disseminated *Mycobacterium avium* & *M. intracellulare* infection (*M. avium* complex [MAC]) in pts c̄ advanced AIDS. **ACTION:** Antitubercular activity not determined. Antimycobacterial activity may be related to inhibition of DNA-dependent RNA polymerase enzyme activity in susceptible strains of *M. avium* & *M. intracellulare.*

PHARMACOKINETICS

PO availability	Peak	Half-life	Protein binding	Excretion
>50%	2-4h	16-69h	85%	Via urine (50%), feces primarily as metabolites

CONTRAINDICATIONS: Hypersensitivity to drug or other rifamycins. **CC:** Not recommended for prophylaxis in pts c̄ active tuberculosis.

DOSAGE

Adult *PO*	300mg once/d or divided into 2 equal (150-mg) doses

SIDE/ADVERSE EFFECTS: CNS: headache, insomnia ▪ GI: abdominal pain, N/V/D, anorexia, dyspepsia, flatulence, taste changes ▪ HEM: neutropenia, leukopenia, ***thrombocytopenia,*** anemia ▪ HEP: ↑ AST, ALT ▪ INT: rash ▪ Other: discolored urine, myalgia.

INTERACTIONS: Drug: Use c̄ zidovudine will ↓ zidovudine blood levels.

NURSING MANAGEMENT PRIORITIES

ADMINISTRATION: Assess for hx of hypersensitivity ▪ Assess hepatic function; ↓ dosage if impaired ▪ Assess resistance to *Mycobacterium* ▪ Administer c̄ food to ↓ GI irritation; *best* on empty stomach (1h ac/2h pc); may open capsules & mix contents c̄ food ▪ Avoid exposure to heat/moisture/light in storage.

EVALUATION: Monitor VS, esp temperature ▪ Monitor respiratory status (breath sounds, sputum) ▪ Monitor CBC, UA, resistance to *Mycobacterium* ▪ May ↑ serum ALT, AST, alkaline phosphatase, bilirubin, uric acid, BUN.

EDUCATION: Drowsiness may occur; use caution in potentially hazardous activities ▪ Take as directed by physician even if symptom free; complete full course of therapy ▪ Take on empty stomach; may take c̄ food if GI irritation occurs ▪ Red-brown discoloration of body secretions (tears, urine, saliva) may occur; permanent soft contact lens discoloration ▪ Notify physician *immediately* if experiencing vomiting, ↓ appetite, lethargy, yellow eyes/skin, bleeding/bruising, chills, headache ▪ May cause mouth discomfort; changes in taste ▪ Avoid use c̄ alcohol ▪ Women: use alternative form of contraception (*not* PO estrogens) while taking drug ▪ Keep scheduled appointments c̄ physician/for blood work ▪ Store in tightly closed, light-resistant container in cool, dry area.

NOTES:

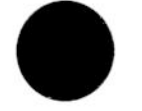

rifampin • (rif-am-pin)

CATEGORY: *Antitubercular antibiotic*

Rx; Preg Cat NA

BRAND NAMES
Rifadin (H-M-R)
Rimactane (Ciba)

DOSAGE FORMS
Capsules: 150, 300mg
Capsules: 300mg
Injection (IV): 600mg/vial

COMBINATION PRODUCT
Rifamate (H-M-R) — 300mg rifampin, 150mg INH per capsule

USE: Treatment of pulmonary tuberculosis in combination c̄ isoniazid, ethambutol, or other effective antimycobacterial agents ▪ Treatment of asymptomatic carriers of *Neisseria meningitidis* (meningococci). **ACTION:** Antimycobacterial activity due to inhibition of DNA-dependent RNA polymerase activity in susceptible organisms. Rapid emergence of resistant strains can occur. The drug is present in breast milk, colors the urine red.

PHARMACOKINETICS

PO absorption	Peak	Half-life	Protein binding	Excretion
Good	2-4h	3h	85%-91%	Via bile (60%), urine as unchanged drug, metabolites

CONTRAINDICATIONS: Hypersensitivity. **CC:** Not recommended for pts c̄ meningococcal infections due to rapid emergence of resistant strains ▪ Use c̄ caution in pts c̄ hepatic impairment.

DOSAGE: *PO/IV*

Pulmonary tuberculosis	
Pediatric	10-20mg/kg. Do *not* exceed 600mg/d
Adult	600mg in a single daily dose
Meningococcal carriers	
Pediatric	10-20mg/kg/d for 4d. Do *not* exceed 600mg/d. CDC recommends for 3mo-1y/o a dose of 5mg/kg bid for 2d & for 1-12 y/o a dose of 10mg/kg bid for 2d
Adult	600mg once/d for 3d. CDC recommends a dose of 600mg bid for 2d
Rifamate	2 capsules once/d pc

SIDE/ADVERSE EFFECTS: CNS: headache, drowsiness, dizziness, visual disturbances, inability to concentrate ▪ GI: *anorexia, N/V/D, gas, cramps,* sore mouth, heartburn, rare cases of ***pseudomembranous colitis*** ▪ HEM: ***hemolytic anemia,*** transient leukopenia, thrombocytopenia, eosinophilia ▪ INT: urticaria, rash, pruritus, ***pemphigus,*** acneform lesions ▪ Other: flulike symptoms, exudative conjunctivitis, muscular weakness, pain in the extremities, menstrual disturbances.

INTERACTIONS: Drug: PO contraceptives may lose significant activity during rifampin therapy ▪ Therapy may necessitate dosage adjustment for PO anticoagulants, corticosteroids, dapsone, dig glycosides, PO hypoglycemics, quinidine ▪ Methadone maintenance pts may experience significant withdrawal symptoms; higher doses of methadone may be required ▪ Use c̄ hepatotoxic drugs will produce additive toxicity. **Lab:** Use inhibits serum folate/vitamin B_{12} microbiologic assays.

NURSING MANAGEMENT PRIORITIES

ADMINISTRATION: Assess for hx of hypersensitivity ▪ Assess hepatic function; ↓ dosage if impaired ▪ Assess resistance to *Mycobacterium* ▪ May administer c̄ food to ↓ GI irritation; *best* on empty stomach (1h ac/2h pc); may open capsules & mix content c̄ food ▪ Avoid exposure to heat/moisture/light in storage.

EVALUATION: Monitor VS, esp temperature ▪ Monitor respiratory status (breath sounds, sputum) ▪ Monitor CBC, UA, resistance to *Mycobacterium* ▪ May ↑ serum ALT, AST, alkaline phosphatase, bilirubin, uric acid, BUN.

EDUCATION: Drowsiness may occur; use caution in potentially hazardous activities ▪ Take as ordered by physician even if symptom free; complete full course of therapy ▪ Take on empty stomach; may take c̄ food if GI irritation occurs ▪ Red-brown discoloration of body secretions (tears, urine, saliva) may occur; permanent soft contact lens discoloration ▪ Notify physician *immediately* if experiencing vomiting, ↓ appetite, lethargy, yellow eyes/skin, bleeding/bruising, chills, headache ▪ May cause mouth discomfort ▪ Avoid use c̄ alcohol ▪ Women: use alternative form of contraception (*not* oral estrogens) while taking drug ▪ Keep scheduled appointments c̄ physician/for blood work ▪ Store in tightly closed, light-resistant container in cool, dry area.

NOTES:

risperidone • (riss-pair-i-doan)

CATEGORY: *Antipsychotic*

Rx; Preg Cat C

BRAND NAME
Risperdal (Janssen)

DOSAGE FORMS
Tablet: 1, 2, 3, 4mg

USE: Management of psychotic disorders. **ACTION:** Antipsychotic mechanism not determined. May antagonize activity of dopamine & serotonin in the brain.

PHARMACOKINETICS

PO absorption	Peak	Half-life	Protein binding	Excretion
70%-94%	1-3h	3-21h	77%-90%	Via urine as metabolites, unchanged drug

CONTRAINDICATIONS: Hypersensitivity. **CC:** Extended use can produce extrapyramidal symptoms, tardive dyskinesia, possible neuroleptic malignant syndrome ▪ Use c̄ caution in pts c̄ convulsive disorders/hx of siezures ▪ Drug has a proarrhythmic effect potential.

DOSAGE

Adult *PO* Start 1mg bid, ↑ by 1-3mg bid. Further ↑ should be made at wkly intervals. Usual range is 4-16mg/d. Dosage for pts c̄ renal or hepatic impairment or the elderly is 0.5mg bid. ↑ Slowly by 0.5mg bid. Dose ↑ above 1.5mg bid should be done at wkly intervals

SIDE/ADVERSE EFFECTS: CNS: extrapyramidal symptoms, headache, insomnia, dizziness, agitation, anxiety, somnolence, aggressive behavior, ***neuroleptic malignant syndrome***, *tardive dyskinesia* ▪ CV: ***proarrhythmic effects***, orthostatic hypertension, prolonged QT cardiogram interval ▪ GI: N/V, constipation, dyspepsia ▪ Skin: rash, photosensitivity ▪ Other: ↑ salivation, rhinitis, coughing, back pain, fever.

INTERACTIONS: Drug: Use c̄ dopaminergic agonists (levodopa) may antagonize their therapeutic effects ▪ Use c̄ clozapine can ↓ risperidone levels ▪ Use c̄ carbamazepine can ↑ risperidone levels.

NURSING MANAGEMENT PRIORITIES

ADMINISTRATION: Assess for hx of hypersensitivity ▪ Assess VS, esp BP ▪ Assess hepatic, renal function; may require ↓ dosage if impaired ▪ Assess for hx of seizures; use caution ▪ Institute safety, seizure, suicide precautions ▪ Avoid abrupt withdrawal; D/C gradually ▪ Elderly/debilitated pts may require ↓ dosage.

EVALUATION: Monitor CV, hepatic, renal status ▪ Monitor BP, CBC, fluid retention (I&O, daily weight), constipation ▪ Assess for extrapyramidal rx ▪ Seizure precautions in pts c̄ hx of convulsive disorders ▪ Diabetics: monitor blood sugar (hyperglycemia).

EDUCATION: Dizziness/drowsiness may occur; use caution in potentially hazardous activities ▪ Avoid changing positions (lying/sitting/standing) rapidly ▪ Avoid use c̄ alcohol, other CNS depressants ▪ Store in tightly closed, light-resistant container ▪ Use sugarless gum/hard candy to diminish dry mouth ▪ Constipation may occur; ↑ fluids, bulk-containing foods ▪ Women: avoid breastfeeding ▪ Avoid exposure to direct sunlight, UV light; use sunscreen, protective clothing ▪ Notify physician of fever, sore throat, bruising/bleeding, tics/spasms, trembling, shuffling gait ▪ Avoid ↑ exercise, temperature extremes ▪ Check c̄ physician/pharmacist before taking OTC preparations ▪ Full drug effects may require several wks of therapy.

NOTES:

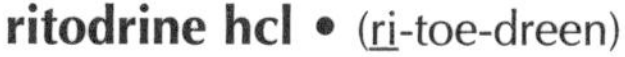

ritodrine hcl • (ri-toe-dreen)

CATEGORY: *Sympathomimetic:* β_2 adrenergic, uterine relaxant Rx; Preg Cat B

BRAND NAME	**DOSAGE FORMS**
Yutopar (Astra) (Bristol [Canada])	Injection (IV): 10mg/ml Tablet: 10mg

USE: Management of preterm labor in suitable pts. **ACTION:** Sympathomimetic activity selective for β receptors, esp β_2 adrenoreceptors of bronchial tree, peripheral vascular beds, uterus; predominant β-mimetic effect on uterine smooth muscle, which ⬇ intensity, frequency of contractions; placental drug transfer occurs, limited β_1 activity results in transitory ⬆ in maternal, fetal heart rates.

PHARMACOKINETICS

PO availability	Peak	Half-life	Protein binding	Excretion
30%	30-60m	1.3-20h	32%	Via urine as unchanged drug, metabolites

CONTRAINDICATIONS: Before wk 20 of pregnancy, conditions in which continuation of pregnancy is hazardous, incl antepartum hemorrhage requiring immediate delivery; chorioamnionitis; eclampsia, severe preeclampsia; intrauterine fetal death; maternal cardiac disease, hyperthyroidism, uncontrolled diabetes; pulmonary hypertension ▪ Preexisting maternal medical conditions seriously affected by ritodrine β-mimetic activity, incl asthma already treated c̄ β adrenergics/steroids; cardiac arrhythmias associated c̄ tachycardia/drug toxicity; hypovolemia; pheochromocytoma; ritodrine hypersensitivity; uncontrolled hypertension. **CC:** Use can result in maternal pulmonary edema/death, esp in combination c̄ corticosteroids. Persistent tachycardia >140 beats/m is indicative of impending edema ▪ Injection contains sodium metabisulfite, which can cause allergic rxs ▪ Use for preterm labor inhibition in pts c̄ membrane rupture ⬆ risk of chorioamnionitis ▪ Use before wk 20 of pregnancy not recommended.

DOSAGE

IV infusion	Usual starting dose 50-100μg/m, ⬆ q10m by 50μg/m until desired effect obtained. Usual effective range 150-350μg/m. Treatment should continue for at least 12h after uterine contractions cease
PO maintenance	10mg 30m before termination of IV therapy. Usual dosage for first 24h 10mg q2h. Usual maintenance dose 10-20mg q4-6h. Do *not* exceed 120mg/d

SIDE/ADVERSE EFFECTS: CNS: nervousness, anxiety, emotional upset, tremor, headache ▪ CV: dose-related changes in maternal BP; maternal, fetal heart rates; pulmonary edema ▪ GI: N/V/D, epigastric distress, constipation ▪ Other: rash, dyspnea, hyperventilation, lactic acidosis ▪ Fetal: hypoglycemia, ileus.

INTERACTIONS: Drug: Use c̄ corticosteroids can produce pulmonary edema ▪ Use c̄ β blockers antagonizes therapeutic effects ▪ Use c̄ anesthetics can ↑ hypotensive effects ▪ Use c̄ sympathomimetics produces additive effects.

NURSING MANAGEMENT PRIORITIES

ADMINISTRATION: Assess VS ▪ Do *not* use saline diluents unless dextrose undesirable (diabetics) ▪ Use solution w/in 48h of preparation ▪ Do *not* administer discolored/precipitated solution ▪ Place pt in left lateral position ▪ IV: use infusion-control device ▪ Restrict fluids per physician's order ▪ Store parenteral form at room temperature; do *not* freeze ▪ Provide emotional support.

EVALUATION: Monitor I&O ▪ Monitor VS, esp BP, respiratory rate (labored breathing) ▪ Monitor uterine contractions, fetal heart rate ▪ Observe for pulmonary edema; D/C drug if present ▪ Assess for ↑ serum glucose, esp diabetics.

EDUCATION: Explain procedure, rationale to pt, family ▪ Relaxation techniques ▪ Comfort measures ▪ Check c̄ physician before using OTC preparations ▪ Notify physician of contractions, rupture of membranes.

NOTES:

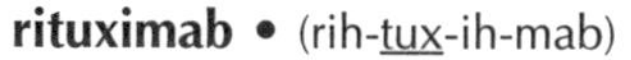

rituximab • (rih-tux-ih-mab)

CATEGORY: *Antineoplastic:* IgG immunoglobulin Rx; Preg Cat C

BRAND NAME	**DOSAGE FORM**
Rituxan (Genetech)	Injection: 10mg/ml

USE: Treatment of relapsed &/or refractory low-grade or follicular CD20 +, B-cell non-Hodgkin's lymphoma. **ACTION:** Antineoplastic effect due to specific binding of rituximab (IgG, kappa immunoglobulin) to the antigen CD20, a transmembrane protein of B-cell non-Hodgkin's lymphomas resulting in B-cell lyses.

PHARMACOKINETICS: Data is limited. After 1st infusion, serum half-life average was 59.8h & an average of 174h following the 4th infusion. Drug was detected in serum 3-6m after treatment was completed.

CONTRAINDICATIONS: Hypersensitivity to murine proteins. **CC:** Serious/life-threatening cardiac arrhythmias that develop require D/C of infusion ▪ Safety & efficacy not established for children ▪ Hypersensitivity is more prevalent c̄ IV push/bolus administration.

DOSAGE

Adult	*IV*	375mg/m^2 once/wk for doses on d1, 8, 15, 22. Infusion treatment should be administered at an initial rate of 50mg/d c̄ ↑ q30m to a maximum of 400mg/h

SIDE/ADVERSE EFFECTS: CNS: dizziness, headache, anxiety ▪ CV: hypotension/hypertension, bradycardia ▪ GI: N/V/D, abdominal pain, taste pervasion, anorexia, dyspepsia ▪ HEM: leukopenia, neutropenia, ***thrombocytopenia*** ▪ INT: pruritus, rash, urticaria ▪ RESP: bronchospasm, rhinitis, throat pain ▪ Other: asthenia, angioedema, fever, myalgia, hyperglycemia.

INTERACTIONS: None currently reported.

NURSING MANAGEMENT PRIORITIES

ADMINISTRATION: Assess for hx of hypersensitivity, incl murine proteins ▪ Obtain CBC, differential & platelet counts, electrolytes, chest x-ray before administration ▪ Assess CV, pulmonary function; notify physician if impaired ▪ Administer via IV infusion; dilute according to manufacturer's directions, use diluted solutions w/in 36h at room temperature; do *not* administer IV push/bolus; do *not* mix or dilute c̄ other drugs ▪ Have support equipment available for anaphylaxis ▪ Protect from light in storage.

EVALUATION: Monitor VS, esp BP ▪ Monitor CBC, platelets ▪ Cardiac monitoring during infusion may be necessary.

EDUCATION: Dizziness may occur; use caution c̄ ambulation ▪ Avoid exposure to infection ▪ May produce alteration in taste ▪ Notify physician *immediately* of abnormal rxs (chest pain, difficulty breathing, bleeding) ▪ Women: avoid breastfeeding ▪ Use contraception if sexually active.

NOTES:

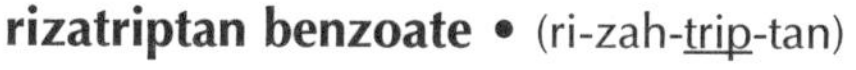

rizatriptan benzoate • (ri-zah-trip-tan)

CATEGORY: *Antimigraine:* serotonin receptor agonist Rx; Preg Cat C

BRAND NAME
Maxalt (Merck)

DOSAGE FORMS
Tablet: 5, 10mg
Tablet (disintegrating orally): 5, 10mg

USE: Treatment of acute migraine c/w/out aura. **ACTION:** Migraine is associated c̄ selective cerebral vasodilation & release of sensory neuropeptides from the trigemovascular system that incl substance P, neurokinin A, other vasoactive peptides.

Antimigraine activity of rizatriptan, a serotonin 5HT-1 receptor agonist, on selected cerebral blood vessels containing 5HT-1 receptors results in vasoconstriction & inhibition of sensory neuropeptides release from the trigemovascular system.

PHARMACOKINETICS

PO absorption	Peak serum	Half-life	Protein binding	Excretion
Good	1-1.5h	2-3h	14%	Via feces, urine primarily as metabolites

CONTRAINDICATIONS: Hypersensitivity, w/in 24h after administration of ergot-type medication, incl dihydroergotamine, ergotamine, methysergide, current or w/in 2wks of D/C MAO-I therapy, severe cardiovascular/peripheral syndrome, uncontrolled hypertension ▪ Use c̄ caution in pts on renal dialysis, hepatic insufficiency ▪ Disintegrating PO tablets contain phenylalanine ▪ Use c̄ caution in nursing mothers ▪ Not recommended for use in pts <18y/o.

DOSAGE

Adult	*PO*	Single dose of 5 or 10mg & repeated at 2 or more h intervals to a maximum of 30mg in 24h
Patients receiving propranolol		Dose is 5mg to a maximum of 15mg in 24h

SIDE/ADVERSE EFFECTS: CNS: agitation, anxiety, sleep disorders, gait abnormality, disorientation, memory impairment ▪ CV: rare angina, cold extremities, arrhythmia, facial edema ▪ GI: N/V/D, dyspepsia, excessive thirst, tongue edema, ↑ appetite ▪ GU: polyuria, rare menstruation disorders ▪ INT: pruritus, rash, urticaria, rare photosensitivity ▪ MS: arthralgia, cramps, spasm ▪ RESP: dyspnea, pharyngitis, nasal congestion, epistaxis ▪ Other: blurred vision, tinnitus, chills, fever, smell perversion.

INTERACTIONS: Drug: Use c̄ ergotlike drugs can produce additive effects.

NURSING MANAGEMENT PRIORITIES

ADMINISTRATION: Assess for hx of hypersensitivity to serotonin 5 HT-1 receptor agonists ▪ Assess CV, hepatic, renal function; use caution if impaired ▪ Assess severity of headache, associated symptoms ▪ Tablet: administer c̄ fluids at onset of attack ▪ Disintegrating PO tablet: allow to dissolve on tongue c̄ saliva; do *not* administer to children c̄ PKU (phenylalanine source) ▪ Maintain quiet environment.

EVALUATION: Monitor neurologic, CV, hepatic, renal status; notify physician if impaired ▪ Monitor severity of headache when relief is obtained.

EDUCATION: Dizziness may occur; use caution in potentially hazardous activities ▪ Avoid foods containing tyramine (aged & fermented foods) ▪ May produce visual & hearing alterations ▪ Avoid exposure to direct sunlight, UV light; use sunscreen, protective clothing ▪ Notify physician *immediately* of abnormal rxs (burning, numbness, tingling) ▪ Check with physician/pharmacist before taking any OTC preparations ▪ Women: avoid breastfeeding.

NOTES:

salmeterol • (sal-<u>met</u>-air-ol)

CATEGORY: *Sympathomimetic:* β_2 adrenergic bronchodilator — Rx; Preg Cat C

BRAND NAME	DOSAGE FORM
Serevent (A-H)	Aerosol spray: 25µg/spray

USE: Treatment of bronchial asthma ▪ Prevention of exercise-induced bronchospasm. **ACTION:** Sympathomimetic activity at β_2 receptors produces bronchodilation. Salmeterol has the longest duration of activity for a β_2 adrenergic bronchodilator.

PHARMACOKINETICS: Onset of activity within 20m after inhalation & duration is 12h.

CONTRAINDICATIONS: Hypersensitivity. **CC:** Not recommended for treatment of acute symptoms or in pts c̄ deteriorating asthma ▪ Use not intended to preclude PO or inhaled corticosteriods ▪ Use can produce paradoxic bronchospasm ▪ Salmeterol dosage should be limited to bid administration (AM, PM). Excessive use can result in significant prolongation of QT interval/ventricular arrhythmias ▪ Use c̄ caution in pts c̄ coronary insufficiency, arrhythmias, convulsive disorder, or thyrotoxicosis.

DOSAGE

Adult/Children (≥12y/o)	*Aerosol*	2 inhalations bid (q12h). For bronchospasm prophylaxis 2 inhalations 30-60m before exercising

SIDE/ADVERSE EFFECTS: CNS: headache, tremor, dizziness, nervousness ▪ CV: palpitations, tachycardia ▪ GI: N/V/D, gastric distress, viral gastroenteritis ▪ RESP: dry throat, cough, nasopharyngitis, laryngitis ▪ Other: back pain, dysmenorrhea.

INTERACTIONS: Drug: Use c̄ nonselective β blockers (eg, propranolol) will antagonize bronchodilation ▪ Use c̄ MAO-I, other sympathomimetics best avoided. **Lab:** Rare changes in glucose/potassium serum levels.

NURSING MANAGEMENT PRIORITIES

ADMINISTRATION: Assess for hx of catecholamine hypersensitivity ▪ Assess BP, pulse before administration ▪ Administer bid (AM, PM) ▪ Administer at room temperature; shake well ▪ Avoid temperature extremes, exposure to direct sunlight in storage; store c̄ nozzle end of canister down.

EVALUATION: Monitor VS, esp heart rate ▪ Monitor I&O ▪ Diabetics: closely monitor blood glucose (hyperglycemia).

EDUCATION: Take as ordered by physician; do *not* ↑ dose ▪ Do *not* use for relief of acute asthma symptoms ▪ Procedure for radial pulse determination ▪ Keep scheduled appointments c̄ physician ▪ Check c̄ physician/pharmacist before taking OTC preparations ▪ Procedure for inhalation administration (do *not* puncture/incinerate aerosol container); shake well before using.

NOTES:

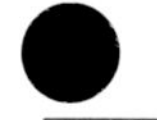

scopolamine/scopolamine hbr▲ • (skoe-pol-a-meen)

CATEGORY: *Anticholinergic:* antimuscarinic, parasympatholytic — Rx; Preg Cat C

BRAND NAMES	DOSAGE FORMS
Scopolamine HBr (various)	Capsule, injection▲
Transderm-Scop (C-G)	Transdermal disc (1.5mg)

USE: Prevention of N/V from motion sickness (transdermal disc should be applied to skin in postauricular area) ▪ Preanesthetic medication; induction of obstetric amnesia, in conjunction c̄ barbiturate/ sedative analgesic ▪ May be used (obsolete) as antispasmodic, antiparkinsonian, cycloplegic, mydriatic, sedative. **ACTION:** Anticholinergic activity due to competition c̄ acetylcholine for muscarinic receptors at postganglionic fiber of parasympathetic nervous system; sedative/tranquilizing effect on CNS.

PHARMACOKINETICS

Route	Peak	Excretion
PO	1-2h	Liver metabolites via urine
IM	1-2h	Liver metabolites via urine

CONTRAINDICATIONS: Hypersensitivity, narrow-angle glaucoma, prostatic hypertrophy/pyloric obstruction, impaired hepatic/renal function. **CC:** Use c̄ caution in presence of impaired liver/kidney function, intestinal obstruction, pyloric/urinary bladder obstruction ▪ Rare episodes of adverse effects, including N/V, equilibrium disturbance, headache c̄ D/C of transdermal disc.

DOSAGE

Pediatric	*IM/IV/SC*	0.006mg/kg
Adult	*PO*	0.4-0.8mg
	IM/IV/SC	0.32-0.65mg
	Disc	1 q3d (delivers 0.5mg drug at constant rate over 3d)

SIDE/ADVERSE EFFECTS: CNS: mental confusion, psychotic signs, somnolence ▪ CV: tachycardia ▪ EENT: blurred vision, cycloplegia, mydriasis, ↑ ocular tension, photophobia ▪ GU: urinary retention ▪ INT: skin rash.

INTERACTIONS: Drug: Use c̄ antihistamines, phenothiazines, TCAs produces ↑ anticholinergic effects ▪ MAO-I ↑ activity by ↓ anticholinergic biotransformation.

NURSING MANAGEMENT PRIORITIES

ADMINISTRATION: Assess for hx of belladonna alkaloid hypersensitivity ▪ Administer tablets 1h before motion-producing event ▪ Avoid exposure to moisture/light in storage ▪ Wash hands after application of transdermal disc; apply to dry area behind ear ▪ Elderly pts may require ↓ dosage.

EVALUATION: Monitor VS, esp heart rate ▪ Observe for exaggerated anticholinergic effects ▪ Monitor neurologic status (amnesia, confusion) ▪ Monitor I&O; assess for urinary retention.

EDUCATION: Advise pt of expected anticholinergic side effects (dry mouth, photophobia, constipation) ▪ D/C drug, notify physician *immediately* on appearance of skin rash, flushing of skin, eye pain ▪ Avoid concurrent antacid administration ▪ Avoid strenuous work/exercise during hot, humid weather ▪ Use sugarless gum/hard candy to diminish dry mouth ▪ Avoid OTC cough/ cold/allergy preparations ▪ Drowsiness, blurred vision may occur; avoid potentially hazardous activities ▪ Store in original, tightly closed, light-resistant container ▪ Frequent oral hygiene ▪ Take capsules 1h before motion-producing event ▪ Procedure for application of transdermal disc; wash hands after applying transdermal disc.

NOTES:

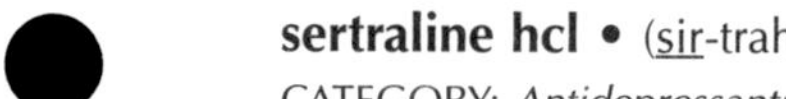

sertraline hcl • (sir-trah-leen)

CATEGORY: *Antidepressant:* selective serotonin reuptake inhibitor (SSRI) Rx; Preg Cat B

BRAND NAME
Zoloft (Roerig)

DOSAGE FORMS
Tablet: 50, 100mg

USE: Treatment of depression. Use for >16wks not currently evaluated. **ACTION:** Antidepressant activity appears related to selective inhibition of serotonin (5-hydroxytryptamine) reuptake c̄ little effect on norepinephrine & dopamine reuptake in CNS.

PHARMACOKINETICS

PO absorption	Peak	Half-life	Protein binding	Excretion
Good	4-5-8.4h	26h	98%	Via urine, feces primarily as metabolites

CONTRAINDICATIONS: Concurrent use c̄ MAO-I. **CC:** Use can result in rare cases of mania/hypomania ▪ Use can result in significant weight loss ▪ Use c̄ caution in pts c̄ convulsive disorders, suicidal tendencies ▪ Use associated c̄ hyponatremia, altered platelet function.

DOSAGE

Adult *PO* — Initial dose of 50mg c̄ range of 50-200mg/d taken once/d

SIDE/ADVERSE EFFECTS: CNS: headache (20.3%), insomnia (61.4%), somnolence (13.4%), dizziness (11.7%), tremor (10.7%), paresthesia (2%) ▪ CV: palpitations (3.5%), chest pain ▪ EENT: abnormal vision (4.2%), tinnitus, pharyngitis ▪ GI: nausea (26.1%), diarrhea (17.7%), dry mouth (16.3%), constipation (8.4%), dyspepsia (6%), vomiting (3.0%), flatulence (3.3%), anorexia, abdominal pain ▪ GU: Male (15.5%) & female (1.7%) dysfunction, menstrual disorders, urinary disorders ▪ INT: skin rash ▪ Other: fatigue (10.6%), sweating (8.4%), hot flashes, back pain, fever.

INTERACTIONS: Drug: Use c̄ other highly protein-bound drugs such as digitoxin, warfarin may ↑ their activity by protein displacement ▪ Use c̄ MAO-I or w/in 1d of D/C MAO-I use not recommended ▪ Use c̄ PO hypoglycemics may ↑ their effects ▪ Use c̄ diazepam can ↓ its excretion ▪ Use c̄ alcohol not recommended.

NURSING MANAGEMENT PRIORITIES

ADMINISTRATION: Assess for hx of hypersensitivity ▪ Assess for hx of seizures; use caution ▪ Assess hepatic, renal status; ↓ dosage if impaired ▪ Administer consistently c̄ or w/out food in AM or PM ▪ Institute safety, seizure precautions ▪ Institute suicide precautions ▪ Avoid abrupt withdrawal; D/C gradually ▪ Avoid moisture/heat/direct light in storage ▪ Elderly pts may require ↓ dosage.

EVALUATION: Monitor CV, hepatic, renal status ▪ Monitor fluid retention (I&O, daily weight), constipation ▪ Assess for weight loss (anorectic effect) ▪ Assess for symptoms of abrupt withdrawal (nausea, headache, malaise) ▪ Assess for actual swallowing of PO forms ▪ Assess for skin rash, hives; notify physician, D/C drug ▪ Diabetics: monitor blood glucose (hypoglycemia).

EDUCATION: Dizziness/drowsiness may occur; use caution in potentially hazardous activities ▪ Avoid changing positions (lying/sitting/standing) rapidly ▪ Diarrhea may occur ▪ Avoid use c̄ alcohol, other CNS depressants for up to 1wk after end of therapy ▪ Take consistently c̄ or w/out food ▪ Take as directed by physician ▪ Use sugarless gum/hard candy to diminish dry mouth ▪ Constipation may occur; ↑ fluids, bulk-containing foods ▪ Notify physician of skin rash, hives; D/C drug ▪ Check c̄ physician/pharmacist before taking OTC/Rx preparations ▪ Notify physician/dentist of use before treatment ▪ Store in tightly closed, light-resistant container ▪ Encourage recreational/diversional interests ▪ Notify physician of weight loss, fever, sore throat, malaise ▪ Keep scheduled appointments c̄ physician ▪ Women: notify physician of possibility of pregnancy; avoid breastfeeding ▪ Full drug effects may require several wks of therapy.

NOTES:

sodium bicarbonate

CATEGORY: *Alkalinizing agent* OTC/Rx*; Preg Cat C

DOSAGE FORMS
Injection (IV)*, PO powder, tablet

USE: Treatment of metabolic acidosis ▪ Antacid ▪ Urinary alkalinizer for selected drug OD management ▪ Prophylaxis of renal calculi. **ACTION:** Chemical correction of acidic conditions; 1g sodium bicarbonate provides 11.9mEq sodium, 11.9mEq bicarbonate.

PHARMACOKINETICS: Not applicable.

CONTRAINDICATIONS: Alkalosis, chloride loss, hypocalcemia. **CC:** Excessive use can produce hypokalemia, predispose to cardiac arrhythmias. Administer in repeated small doses ▪ Rapid administration can result in alkalosis. In cardiac failure, risk of rapid IV infusion must be balanced against risk of fatality due to acidosis ▪ Use c̄ caution in pts c̄ CHF, renal impairment, the elderly ▪ Severe alkalosis can be treated c̄ calcium gluconate injection.

DOSAGE

Pediatric	*PO*	6-12y/o: Usual dose 520mg repeated once in 30m as antacid
	IV	Same as for adults
Adult	*PO*	0.3-2g 1-4 times/d as antacid. Usual dose for alkalinization of urine, 4g followed by 1-2g q4h. Do *not* exceed total 16g/d
	IV	Cardiac arrest: 1mEq/kg followed by 0.5mEq/kg, repeated q10m of continued arrest. Less urgent metabolic acidosis/urinary alkalinizer: 2-5mEq/kg over 4-8h

SIDE/ADVERSE EFFECTS: CNS: nervousness, headache ▪ CV: ***irregular heartbeat,*** edema ▪ GI: N/V, loss of appetite ▪ MET: alkalosis.

INTERACTIONS: Drug: Use c̄ methenamine best avoided ▪ Use c̄ corticosteroids can produce hypernatremia ▪ Use c̄ *basic* drugs will ↑ their effects by ↓ urinary excretion.

NURSING MANAGEMENT PRIORITIES

ADMINISTRATION: Assess ABGs ▪ PO: chew thoroughly; take c̄ full glass H_2O; do *not* administer w/in 2h of milk, other PO drugs ▪ Effervescent tablet: dissolve completely before administering ▪ IV: dilute according to manufacturer's directions; flush lines before, after use ▪ Do *not* administer discolored/precipitated solutions ▪ Do *not* mix c̄ catecholamines in solution.

EVALUATION: Monitor VS, esp BP ▪ Monitor ABGs, F/E status (hypokalemia, hypernatremia) ▪ Cardiac monitoring (parenteral) ▪ Check IV site closely; avoid extravasation.

EDUCATION: Notify physician *immediately* of "skipped" heartbeats, tremors, muscle cramps, lethargy; D/C drug ▪ Effervescent tablet: wait until bubbling stops before taking ▪ Do *not* take for >2wks w/out checking c̄ physician ▪ Avoid taking c̄ milk products/enteric-coated preparations ▪ Check c̄ physician/pharmacist before taking OTC preparations.

NOTES:

spectinomycin hcl • (spek-tin-oh-mye-sin)

CATEGORY: *Antibiotic* Rx; Preg Cat NA

BRAND NAME
Trobicin (Upjohn)

DOSAGE FORMS
Powder for IM injection:
2-g vial c̄ 3.2ml of diluent,
4-g vial c̄ 6.2ml of diluent

USE: Treatment of gonorrhea. However, the drug is usually used only in cases that are resistant (penicillinase-producing *Neisseria gonorrhoeae*) to the penicillins or in pts who are hypersensitive to the penicillins, cephalosporins, or other suitable drugs. **ACTION:** Bacteriostatic activity due to inhibition of ribosomal protein synthesis in susceptible organisms.

PHARMACOKINETICS

IM peak	Half-life	Protein binding	Excretion
1-2h	1.2-2.8h	Very low	70%-100% in 48h via urine

CONTRAINDICATIONS: Hypersensitivity. **CC:** Not intended for treating syphilis ▪ All pts should be tested for syphilis before treatment ▪ Resistance to spectinomycin can develop.

DOSAGE: *IM*

Pediatric	CDC recommends 40mg/kg as a single dose
Adult	2g as a single dose or 4g as a single dose for cases occurring or pts living in geographic areas where penicillin resistance is prevalent For disseminated gonococcal infection: 2g/12h

SIDE/ADVERSE EFFECTS: Local: *soreness at injection site* ▪ MET: ↑ in alkaline phosphatase, BUN, ALT (serum glutamate pyruvate transaminase) ▪ Other: anaphylaxis, chills, dizziness, fever, insomnia, urticaria, N/V, rash.

INTERACTIONS: Drug: No significant interactions reported.

NURSING MANAGEMENT PRIORITIES

ADMINISTRATION: Assess for hx of hypersensitivity ▪ Obtain C&S before therapy ▪ Administer deep IM injection ▪ Maintain hydration.

EVALUATION: Monitor VS, esp temperature ▪ Monitor renal function (nephrotoxicity); notify physician.

EDUCATION: Dizziness may occur; use caution in potentially hazardous activities ▪ May experience pain at injection site ▪ ↑ Fluid intake (8-10 glasses/d) ▪ Notify physician *immediately* of fever, chills, difficult breathing, ↓ urination, rash ▪ Identify all sexual contacts for treatment; maintain good perineal hygiene.

NOTES:

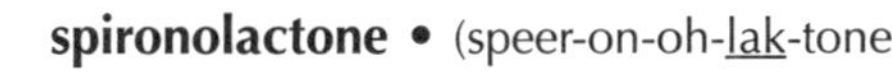

spironolactone • (speer-on-oh-lak-tone)

CATEGORY: *Diuretic:* aldosterone antagonist, potassium-sparing diuretic Rx; Preg Cat NA

BRAND NAME
Aldactone (Searle)

DOSAGE FORMS
Tablet: 25, 50, 100mg

COMBINATION PRODUCTS
Aldactazide 25/25; 50/50 (Searle) spironolactone/hydrochlorothiazide per tablet: 25mg/25mg; 50mg/50mg

USE: Diagnosis of 1° hyperaldosteronism ▪ Short-term preop treatment of 1° hyperaldosteronism ▪ Maintenance in pts c̄ discrete aldosterone-producing adrenal adenomas, bilateral micronodular/macronodular adrenal hyperplasia (idiopathic hyperaldosteronism) ▪ Treatment/prevention of hypokalemia when other methods are inadequate ▪ Treatment of nephrosis in pts not suitable to other methods ▪ Adjunct in treating hypertension, edema due to CHF/cirrhosis of liver. **ACTION:** Spironolactone is a competitive antagonist of aldosterone; displaces it from sodium-potassium exchange receptors in distal convoluted tubules, resulting in potassium retention, excretion of H_2O, sodium; drug also exhibits antihypertensive activity.

PHARMACOKINETICS

PO absorption	Peak	Half-life	Protein binding	Excretion
90%	2-4h as metabolites	13-24h as metabolites	90%	Via urine as metabolites

CONTRAINDICATIONS: Hypersensitivity, anuria, significant renal insufficiency, hyperkalemia. **CC:** Avoid unnecessary use due to possible tumorigenic activity ▪ Dietary/dosage formulations of potassium supplementation is usually not required.

DOSAGE

Pediatric	*PO*	1.5mg/lb/d divided for edema
Adult	*PO*	
Edema		100mg/d for at least 5d. Adjust according to response
Hyperaldosteronism		
Short diagnostic test		400mg/d for 4d
Long diagnostic test		400mg/d for 3-4wks
Maintenance		Lowest effective dose
Preop preparation		100-400mg/d

Hypertension	50-100mg/d divided for at least 2wks. Adjust according to response
Hypokalemia	Aldactazide 25/25, 50/50 Usual maintenance dose is 1-4 tablets for edema, 2-4 tablets/d for hypertension

SIDE/ADVERSE EFFFECTS: CNS: drowsiness, headache, lethargy, confusion ▪ GI: *cramps,* diarrhea ▪ GU: amenorrhea/irregular menses, postmenopausal bleeding, impotence ▪ INT: urticaria, drug fever, skin rash, hirsutism ▪ MET: hyperkalemia ▪ Other: gynecomastia, carcinoma of breast (no cause/effect relationship established), deepening of voice.

INTERACTIONS: Drug: Use c̄ digoxin/lithium may ↑ toxicity ▪ Use c̄ ganglionic blocking agents ↑ their activity; ↓ dosage may be required ▪ Use c̄ ACE-I, indomethacin can produce severe hyperkalemia.

NURSING MANAGEMENT PRIORITIES

ADMINISTRATION: Assess for hx of hypersensitivity, F/E balance; serum K^+ level (normal: 3.5-5mEq/L); do *not* administer if hyperkalemic; notify physician ▪ Assess renal function; do *not* administer if impaired ▪ Administer c̄ food/milk on arising; may crush tablets ▪ Avoid exposure to moisture/light in storage ▪ Elderly pts may require ↓ dosage.

EVALUATION: Monitor F/E, hepatic, renal status ▪ Monitor VS, esp BP, pulse; serum for ↑ BUN, creatinine, uric acid ▪ Assess for hyperkalemia; notify physician ▪ Monitor fluid retention.

EDUCATION: Expect ↑ urine output ▪ May cause weakness, lethargy ▪ Take c̄ food/milk on rising, at same time qd, even if symptom free; may crush tablets ▪ Take as directed; do *not* skip doses ▪ Notify physician of signs of hyperkalemia (weakness, tingling/numbness, irregular heartbeat) ▪ Avoid changing positions (lying/sitting/standing) rapidly ▪ Avoid high-Na^+/K^+ foods ▪ Check c̄ physician before using salt substitutes ▪ Check c̄ physician before taking OTC preparations ▪ Store in tightly closed, light-resistant container ▪ Keep appointments c̄ physician; have BP checked regularly ▪ Full drug effect may require several wks of therapy.

NOTES:

stavudine • (stay-view-deen) 288

CATEGORY: *Antiviral* Rx; Preg Cat C

BRAND NAME
Zerit (B-MS)

DOSAGE FORMS
Capsule: 15, 20, 30, 40mg

USE: Treatment of advanced HIV infections. **ACTION:** Antiviral activity due to inhibition of HIV replication. Drug is a synthetic thymidine nucleoside analog that inhibits HIV reverse transcriptase enzyme & ⬇ viral DNA synthesis by causing DNA chain termination.

PHARMACOKINETICS

PO absorption	Peak	Half-life	Protein binding	Excretion
86%	1h	1-1.5h	Negligible	Via urine as metabolites, unchanged drug

CONTRAINDICATIONS: Hypersensitivity. **CC:** Drug is intended for advanced HIV infections in pts intolerant to or c̄ significant immunologic deterioration c̄ standard HIV treatment modalities ▪ Use c̄ extreme caution in pts c̄ hx of neuropathy.

DOSAGE
Adult *PO* <60kg: 30mg bid. Dosage for resumption of treatment (after recovery from peripheral neuropathy) is 15mg bid
>60kg: 40mg bid; resumption of treatment is 20mg bid

SIDE/ADVERSE EFFECTS: Peripheral neuropathy is the most significant adverse effect & is characterized by pain, numbness/tingling of hands or feet. CNS: ***peripheral neuropathy***, insomnia, anxiety, depression, nervousness, dizziness ▪ CV: chest pain, vasodilation ▪ GI: N/V, anorexia, dyspepsia ▪ INT: rash, pruritus, maculopapular rash ▪ RESP: dyspnea ▪ Other: myalgia, arthralgia, conjunctivitis, dysuria, genital pain.

INTERACTIONS: Drug: Use c̄ neurotoxic drugs can produce additive effects.

NURSING MANAGEMENT PRIORITIES
ADMINISTRATION: Assess for hx of hypersensitivity ▪ May be administered w/out regard to meals.

EVALUATION: Monitor VS, esp temperature ▪ Assess for development of neuropathy (numbness, tingling, pain in distal extremities) ▪ Monitor hepatic, renal status.

EDUCATION: Take as ordered by physician at equal intervals around clock to maintain blood levels; do *not* ↑ dose ▪ Do *not* share drug ▪ Report numbness, tingling, pain in arms/legs to physician *immediately* ▪ Women: avoid breastfeeding ▪ Used to control, *not* cure, HIV infections ▪ Check c̄ physician/pharmacist before taking OTC preparations ▪ Avoid sexual contact, blood donation (risk of HIV transmission) ▪ Keep scheduled appointments c̄ physician/for blood work.

NOTES:

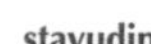

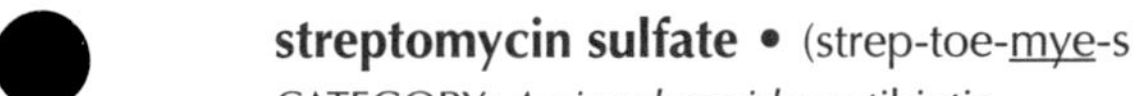

streptomycin sulfate • (strep-toe-mye-sin)

CATEGORY: *Aminoglycoside:* antibiotic

Rx; Preg Cat NA

BRAND NAME
Streptomycin Sulfate (various)

DOSAGE FORMS
Injection (IM), powder for injection (IM)

USE: Indicated in treatment of infections caused by *Calymmatobacterium granulomatis* (granuloma inguinale), *Francisella tularensis* (tularemia), *Yersinia pestis* (plague) ▪ In combined therapy for tuberculosis ▪ In combined therapy ($\bar{c}$ penicillin) for enterococcal, α-, nonhemolytic streptococcal endocarditis. **ACTION:** Bactericidal activity due to inhibition of ribosomal protein synthesis in susceptible organisms.

PHARMACOKINETICS

IM peak	Half-life	Protein binding	Excretion
1h	2-3h	35%	29%-89% unchanged in urine in 24h

CONTRAINDICATIONS: Hypersensitivity, hx of serious aminoglycoside toxicity. **CC:** Use of aminoglycosides during pregnancy can result in bilateral congenital deafness ▪ Use can produce serious ototoxicity, nephrotoxicity ▪ Injection contains sodium metabisulfite, which can cause allergic rxs.

DOSAGE: For pts $\bar{c}$ normal renal function

Pediatric	*IM*	Neonates: 20-30mg/kg/d in 2 doses Children: 40mg/kg/d in 2 doses
Adult	*IM*	
Tularemia		1-2g/d divided for 7-10d until pt is afebrile for 5-7d
Plague		2-4g/d divided until pt is afebrile 3d
Tuberculosis		1g/d $\bar{c}$ 200-300mg isoniazid, 5g paraaminosalicylic acid tid
Enterococcal endocarditis		0.5-1g bid for 4wks in combination $\bar{c}$ penicillin
α-, nonhemolytic strep endocarditis		1g bid for 1wk, 0.5g bid for 2nd wk, in combination $\bar{c}$ penicillin

SIDE/ADVERSE EFFECTS: CNS: peripheral paresthesia, amblyopia ▪ CV: myocarditis ▪ EENT: ***ototoxicity*** (auditory, vestibular damage), dizziness, vertigo, tinnitus, roaring in ears, hearing loss ▪ HEM: ***agranulocytosis, aplastic ane-***

mia, eosinophilia, leukopenia, pancytopenia, ***thrombocytopenia*** ▪ HEP: hepatic necrosis ▪ INT: ***exfoliative dermatitis*** ▪ Other: neuromuscular blockade c̄ high doses, esp in young children.

INTERACTIONS: Drug: Avoid use c̄ neurotoxic/nephrotoxic drugs such as other aminoglycosides, colistin, ethacrynic acid, furosemide, polymyxin B, vancomycin ▪ Dimenhydrinate can mask aminoglycoside ototoxicity ▪ Use c̄ succinylcholine/tubocurarine ↑ their activity; Ca salts can reverse blockade ▪ PO anticoagulant activity may ↑ due to ↓ intestinal vitamin K synthesis.

NURSING MANAGEMENT PRIORITIES

ADMINISTRATION: Assess for hx of aminoglycoside hypersensitivity ▪ Obtain C&S before therapy ▪ Obtain pt weight for dosage calculation ▪ Determine creatinine clearance before administration ▪ Dissolve sterile powder in sterile H_2O for injection or normal saline solution according to manufacturer's directions; avoid contact c̄ solution ▪ Use reconstituted solution w/in 2d at room temperature, w/in 14d refrigerated ▪ Store in original container; darkened vial does *not* affect potency ▪ Administer slowly by *deep* IM injection; rotate sites; avoid inflamed areas ▪ Avoid solutions stronger than 500mg/ml ▪ Do *not* add preservatives to intrathecal preparations ▪ Avoid topical/inhalation administration (↑ risk of sensitization) ▪ Maintain hydration ▪ Elderly pts may require ↓ dosage.

EVALUATION: Assess for hearing dysfunction ▪ Monitor hepatic, renal, VIII CN function ▪ Monitor VS, esp temperature ▪ Assess for edema in extremities ▪ Assess for neuromuscular blockade, respiratory paralysis, nephrotoxicity ▪ Observe for signs of superinfection (diarrhea, URI, coated tongue) ▪ Assess for hypersensitivity rx (fever, difficult breathing, rash) ▪ Monitor tuberculosis pts for changes in sputum.

EDUCATION: Report hearing, balance difficulties to physician at once ▪ ↑ Fluid intake (10-12 glasses/d).

NOTES:

sucralfate • (soo-kral-fate)

CATEGORY: *Antiulcer agent* Rx; Preg Cat B

BRAND NAME
Carafate (MMD)

DOSAGE FORMS
Suspension: 1g/10ml
Tablet: 1g

USE: Short-term treatment of duodenal ulcers. **ACTION:** Antiulcer activity due to formulation of drug-secretion complex that covers ulcer; protects from acid, pepsin, bile; facilitates healing process at ulcer site. Ulcer-adherent complex formed between drug, proteinaceous exudates from ulcer site; drug minimally absorbed.

PHARMACOKINETICS: Not applicable.

CONTRAINDICATIONS: None currently known. **CC:** Successful treatment (healing) of duodenal ulcers does not preclude posttreatment development ▪ Use c̄ caution in presence of impaired renal function.

DOSAGE

Adult *PO*	1g qid ac, at hs. Usual maintenance dose 1g bid

SIDE/ADVERSE EFFECTS: CNS: dizziness, sleepiness ▪ GI: *constipation*, N/D, gastric upset, dry mouth ▪ INT: rash.

INTERACTIONS: Drug: Use c̄ cimetidine, phenytoin, tetracycline ⬇ PO absorption; give 2h before/after sucralfate ▪ Use c̄ aluminum-containing antacids can ⬆ aluminum body levels.

NURSING MANAGEMENT PRIORITIES

ADMINISTRATION: Administer 1h ac, at hs c̄ full glass H_2O; do *not* chew tablets ▪ Do *not* administer antacids w/in ½h of drug ▪ Have pharmacist prepare solution for NG tube administration ▪ For short-term use only (<8wks).

EVALUATION: Monitor GI status (constipation).

EDUCATION: Take on empty stomach ▪ Take as ordered by physician; do *not* change dose ▪ Constipation may occur; ⬆ fluid intake (8-10 glasses/d), bulk in diet ▪ Avoid use c̄ smoking.

NOTES:

sulfamethoxazole/sulfisoxazole • (sul-fa-meth-ox-a-zole/sul-fi-sox-a-zole)

CATEGORY: *Sulfonamide:* antibacterial, antiinfective — Rx; Preg Cat C

BRAND NAMES	DOSAGE FORMS
sulfamethoxale	
Gantanol (Roche)	PO suspension: 500mg/5ml Tablet: 500mg
sulfisoxazole	
Gantrisin (Roche)	Tablet: 500mg
sulfisoxazole acetyl	
Gantrisin (Roche)	Pediatric suspension: 500mg/ml Syrup: 500mg/5ml

COMBINATION PRODUCTS

Bactrim (G-W), Septra (Roche)	trimethoprim/sulfamethoxazole: see co-trimoxazole

USE: Treatment of UTIs caused by susceptible strains of *Enterobacter* spp, *Escherichia coli, Klebsiella* spp, *Proteus mirabilis, P. vulgaris, Staphylococcus aureus* ▪ Drug of choice for nocardiosis ▪ Adjunct in treatment of malaria, toxoplasmosis. **ACTION:** Bacteriostatic activity due to inhibition of folic acid synthesis in susceptible microorganisms; addition of phenazopyridine (urinary analgesic) helps ⬇ dysuria.

PHARMACOKINETICS

PO absorption	Peak	Half-life	Protein binding	Excretion
sulfamethoxazole				
Incomplete	3-4h	7-12h	50%-70%	25%-70% via urine in 24h
sulfisoxazole				
Rapid	2-4h	4-8h	85%	95% via urine in 24h

CONTRAINDICATIONS: Hypersensitivity, pregnancy at term, nursing mothers, infants <2mo (except in treatment of congenital toxoplasmosis). **CC:** Not recommended for pts c̄ β-hemolytic group A streptococcal infections ▪ Use c̄ caution in pts c̄ bronchial asthma, impaired hepatic/renal function, severe allergies.

DOSAGE: *PO*

sulfamethoxazole

Neonatal (>2mo)/Pediatric	50-60mg/kg loading dose followed by 25-30mg/kg q12h. Do *not* exceed 75mg/kg/d
Adult	2g loading dose followed by 1-2g 2-3 times/d

sulfisoxazole

Neonatal (>2mo)/ Pediatric	75mg/kg loading dose followed by 150mg/kg/d in 4-6 doses. Emulsion dosage 60-75mg/kg loading dose followed by 60-75mg/kg bid. Do *not* exceed 6g/d
Adult	2-4g loading dose followed by 4-8g/d in 4-6 doses. Emulsion dosage 4-5g q12h

SIDE/ADVERSE EFFECTS: CNS: headache, peripheral neuritis, depression, ataxis, ***convulsions*** ▪ GI: N/V/D, anorexia, abdominal pain, ***pancreatitis,*** stomatitis ▪ GU: crystalluria, toxic nephrosis ▪ HEM: ***agranulocytosis, aplastic anemia, hemolytic anemia, thrombocytopenia,*** purpura, methemoglobinemia, hypoprothrombinemia, leukopenia ▪ INT: maculopapular/bullous eruptions, ***Stevens-Johnson syndrome, epidermal necrolysis, exfoliative dermatitis,*** urticaria, photosensitization ▪ MS: arthralgia ▪ Other: serum sickness, allergic myocarditis, periorbital edema.

INTERACTIONS: Drug: Use c̄ urinary acidifiers absolutely contraindicated because of high probability of crystalluria ▪ Avoid p-aminobenzoic preparations during therapy ▪ Use c̄ PO anticoagulant may require dosage adjustment due to ↓ vitamin K synthesis in GI tract ▪ Sulfonamides can enhance activity of PO hypoglycemics, methotrexate.

NURSING MANAGEMENT PRIORITIES

ADMINISTRATION: Assess for hx of sulfonamide hypersensitivity; furosemide, thiazide diuretics ▪ Obtain C&S before therapy ▪ Administer 1h ac/2h pc c̄ full glass H_2O ▪ PO suspension: shake well before using ▪ Avoid use in group A β-hemolytic streptococcal infections ▪ Maintain hydration ▪ Avoid exposure to moisture/light in storage.

EVALUATION: Monitor VS, esp temperature; CBC, UA; I&O, hepatic, renal status.

EDUCATION: Complete full course of therapy (usually 10d) even if symptoms subside ▪ Take on empty stomach c̄ full glass H_2O ▪ Take at equal intervals to maintain blood levels ▪ Store in tightly closed, light-resistant container ▪ Maintain good personal hygiene (esp perineal, oral) ▪ Maintain fluid intake (6-8 glasses/d) ▪ Avoid exposure to direct sunlight, UV light (sunlamps); use sunscreen, protective clothing ▪ Use calibrated measuring device for PO liquid forms ▪ Women: avoid breastfeeding ▪ Notify physician/dentist of sulfonamide use before general anesthesia ▪ Notify physician of fever, sore throat, difficult breathing, rash, bruising/bleeding.

NOTES:

sumatriptan succinate •(sue-ma-trip-tan)

CATEGORY: *Antimigraine agent:* serotonin receptor agonist   Rx; Preg Cat C

BRAND NAME

Imitrex (G-W)

DOSAGE FORMS

Injection (SC): 12mg/ml
Nasal spray: 5-, 20-mg dose spray devices
Tablet: 25, 50mg

USE: Treatment of acute migraine c̄/w/out aura & cluster headache (SC injection). **ACTION:** Migraine is associated c̄ selective cerebral vasodilation, release of sensory neuropeptides from the trigemovascular system that incl substance P, neurokinin A, other vasoactive peptides.

Antimigraine activity of sumatriptan, a serotonin 5HT-1 receptor agonist, appears related to specific agonist activity on selected cerebral blood vessels containing 5HT-1 receptors, resulting in vasoconstriction & inhibition of sensory neuropeptide release from the trigemovascular system.

PHARMACOKINETICS

PO absorption	Peak serum	Half-life	Protein binding	Excretion
Low	2-2.5h	2.5h	14%-21%	Via feces, urine primarily as metabolites

CONTRAINDICATIONS: Hypersensitivity w/in 24h after administration of ergot-type medication, incl dihydroergotamine, ergotamine, methysergide, current &/or w/in 2wks of D/C MAO-I therapy, severe cardiovascular/peripheral syndromes. **CC:** Use of 5HT-1 agonists requires a + diagnosis of migraine ▪ Use can produce significant cardiovascular events incl MI, ventricular tachycardia/fibrillation, cardiac arrest, death ▪ Use may cause corneal opacities ▪ Safety & efficacy in pediatric pts not established.

DOSAGE

Adult	*PO*	25mg to maximum 100mg as single dose & repeated once ≥q2h to a maximum of 300mg in 24h

Spray	5, 10, or 20mg administered into 1 nostril & repeated if needed once q2h to a maximum of 24mg in 24h
SC injection	6mg & repeated if needed once in ≥1h. Do *not* exceed 12mg/24h

SIDE/ADVERSE EFFECTS: CNS: confusion, headache, dizziness, sedation ▪ CV: ***abnormal EKG, atrial/ventricular arrhythmias,*** hypotension ▪ GI: N/V/D, taste disturbances, gastroesophageal reflux ▪ GU: dysmenorrhea, ↑ urination, intermenstrual bleeding ▪ HEM: rare anemia ▪ INT: erythema, pruritus, rash ▪ Local: neck stiffness, back/neck pain (spray) ▪ RESP: dyspnea, asthma ▪ Other: hearing/ visual disturbances, tender breasts.

INTERACTIONS: Drug: Use c̄ MAO-I contraindicated ▪ Use c̄ ergot-type drugs will cause additive vasospastic rx.

NURSING MANAGEMENT PRIORITIES

ADMINISTRATION: Assess for hx of hypersensitivity to serotonin 5HT-1 receptor agonists ▪ Assess CV function; use caution if impaired ▪ Assess severity of headache, associated symptoms ▪ PO: administer c̄ fluids at onset of attack ▪ Parenteral: administer SC only; avoid IM, IV ▪ Protect from light in storage ▪ Maintain quiet environment.

EVALUATION: Monitor neurologic, CV status; notify physician if impaired ▪ Monitor severity of headache, when relief is obtained ▪ Monitor injection site for local rx (redness, burning); notify physician.

EDUCATION: Dizziness/drowsiness may occur; use caution in potentially hazardous activities ▪ Procedure for SC self-dosing (<12mg/24h), nasal spray administration ▪ Avoid foods containing tyramine (aged & fermented foods) ▪ May produce visual & hearing alterations ▪ Notify physician *immediately* of abnormal rx (burning, numbness, tingling) ▪ Check c̄ physician/pharmacist before taking any OTC preparations ▪ Women: avoid breastfeeding.

NOTES:

tacrine hcl • (<u>tack</u>-reen)

CATEGORY: *Centrally acting cholinesterase inhibitors:* antidementia agent Rx; Preg Cat C

BRAND NAME	**DOSAGE FORMS**
Cognex (P-D)	Capsule: 10, 20, 30, 40mg

USE: Palliative treatment of mild to moderate symptoms of dementia of Alzheimer's disease. **ACTION:** Alzheimer's disease is associated c̄ ↓ in cholinergic neurons in the brain resulting in a deficiency of acetylcholine. The anticholinesterase activity of tacrine in the brain results in ↑ acetylcholine levels, which help ↓ early symptoms of dementia associated c̄ Alzheimer's disease.

PHARMACOKINETICS

PO absorption	Peak	Half-life	Protein binding	Excretion
Rapid	1-2h	2-4h	77%-90%	Via urine primarily as metabolites

CONTRAINDICATIONS: Hypersensitivity to drug or acridine derivatives in pts who develop confirmed drug-associated jaundice (bilirubin >3mg/dl) c̄ previous treatment. **CC:** Use c̄ caution in pts c̄ conduction dysfunction due to possible vagotonic activity, liver dysfunction, hx of ulcer diseases due to ↑ acid secretion ▪ Monitor transaminase serum levels esp ALT ≥16wks after initiation of therapy, then once a month for 2mo & q3mo thereafter.

DOSAGE: Dosage must be based on wkly serum transaminase levels for at least 18wks following the start of treatment. Also, females average approximately 50% higher serum concentrations than males, & administration c̄ food will ↓ drug bioavailability by 30%-50%.

Adult *PO* Initiate c̄ 10mg qid for at least 6wks. ↑ To 20mg qid for ≥4wks c̄ acceptable transaminase levels & pt tolerance. Further ↑ of 40mg/d can be made at 4-wk intervals to a maximum dose of 160mg/d divided into 4 equal doses.

SIDE/ADVERSE EFFECTS: CNS: headache, agitation, depression, anxiety, hallucination, hostility, confusion, dizziness, insomnia, tremor, ***rare convulsions*** ▪ CV: hypertension, angina, ***ECG abnormalties*** (eg, fibrillation, AV block, etc.) ▪ GI: N/V/D (most frequent), anorexia, dyspepsia, constipation, flatulence ▪ GU: urinary frequency, infection ▪ HEP: ↑ serum transaminase levels ▪ RESP: rhinitis, coughing, infection ▪ Other: back pain, ↓ weight, fatigue.

INTERACTIONS: Drug: Use c̄ anticholinergics can produce mutual antagonism ▪ Smoking can ↓ drug blood levels by up to 33% ▪ Use c̄ other parasympathomimetics (cholinergics) can produce additive results ▪ Use c̄ cimetidine can ↑ tacrine blood levels ▪ Use c̄ theophylline will ↑ its effects ▪ Use c̄ succinylcholine-type muscle relaxants will produce ↑ muscular relaxation.

NURSING MANAGEMENT PRIORITIES

ADMINISTRATION: Assess for hx of hypersensitivity ▪ Administer 1h ac at equal intervals around clock ▪ Assess for hx of seizures; use caution ▪ Institute safety, seizure precautions ▪ Avoid abrupt withdrawal; D/C gradually (cognitive deterioration) ▪ Avoid moisture; store at room temperature.

EVALUATION: Monitor VS, IOP ▪ Monitor I&O, fluid retention, CHF ▪ Monitor ALT (hepatotoxicity) ▪ Monitor for active or occult GI bleeding in high-risk pts (ulcer development) ▪ Diabetics: monitor blood sugar (hyperglycemia).

EDUCATION: Dizziness/drowsiness may occur; use caution in potentially hazardous activities ▪ Take 1h ac at equal intervals around clock to maintain blood levels ▪ Notify physician of clinical improvement (↑ mental function); abnormal rxs (diarrhea, rash, jaundice) ▪ Used to control, *not* cure, symptoms of Alzheimer's disease ▪ Keep scheduled appointments c̄ physician/for blood work (liver function tests) ▪ Store in tightly closed container ▪ Full drug effects may require several wks of therapy.

NOTES:

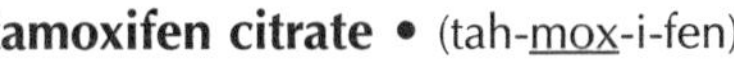

tamoxifen citrate • (tah-mox-i-fen)

CATEGORY: *Antineoplastic:* nonsteroidal antiestrogenic agent — Rx; Preg Cat D

BRAND NAME	DOSAGE FORM
Nolvadex (Zeneca)	Tablet: 10, 20mg

USE: Treatment of node negative breast cancer following surgical intervention or irradiation therapy ▪ Treatment of node positive breast cancer following surgery or irradiation therapy ▪ Treatment of metastatic breast cancer in women & men. **ACTION:** Antineoplastic effect related to potent antiestrogenic effects in the breast. Drug competes c̄ & blocks estrogen at estrogen receptor sites in tumors that contain high concentrations of estrogen receptors, resulting in inhibition of estrogen growth stimulation in the tumor(s). Tamoxifen has little or no activity, esp in breast tumors c̄ ↓ cytoplasmic estrogen receptor sites. In addition, drug exhibits some indigenous estrogenic activity in bone & endometrium tissue.

PHARMACOKINETICS

PO absorption	Peak	Half-life	Excretion
Slow	5 hr	5-7 d	Via feces primarily as metabolites

CONTRAINDICATIONS: Hypersensitivity **CC:** Use may induce cataracts, corneal changes, endometrial cancer, hypercalcemia, menstrual irregularities, retinopathy, fatty liver, hepatitis, hepatic necrosis.

DOSAGE

Adult	*PO*	20-40mg/d Doses >20mg/d should be divided (AM, PM)

SIDE/ADVERSE EFFECTS: GI: N/V/D, taste changes ▪ GU: amenorrhea, oligomenorrhea, ovarian cysts, vaginal bleeding, endometriosis, uterine fibroids ▪ HEM: rare cases of ***thrombocytopenia,*** hyperlipidemias ▪ HEP: liver irregularities ▪ INT: pruritus vulvae, skin rash ▪ Other: flushing, bone pain, edema.

INTERACTIONS: Drug: Use c̄ warfarin can ↑ hypoprothrombinemic effect. **Lab:** ↑ T_4 level w/out clinical symptoms.

NURSING MANAGEMENT PRIORITIES

ADMINISTRATION: Check pt hx for recent course of radiation/antineoplastic agents ▪ Assess PO cavity for ulceration; notify physician ▪ Assess renal function; may require ⬇ dosage if impaired ▪ Administer antiemetic before therapy ▪ Administer in AM & PM ▪ Provide emotional support ▪ Avoid exposure to moisture/light in storage.

EVALUATION: Monitor hepatic, renal function; CBC, esp WBCs, platelets throughout therapy; notify physician if ⬇ ▪ Assess for infection, bleeding, anemia ▪ Assess hydration status (I&O, daily weight) ▪ Monitor vision; notify physician if ⬇.

EDUCATION: Store in dry, tightly closed, light-resistant container ▪ ⬆ Fluid intake (8-10 glasses/d) ▪ Avoid exposure to infection ▪ Check c̄ physician before immunization (pt, family) ▪ Diet as tolerated; avoid spicy foods ▪ Maintain good oral hygiene; use soft-bristled toothbrush ▪ Notify physician of symptoms of bone marrow depression (fever, sore throat, bruising, bleeding, lethargy) ▪ Avoid exposure to direct sunlight, UV light ▪ Loss of hair may occur (reversible) ▪ May alter taste sensation ▪ Compliance c̄ prescribed dosage regimen ▪ Women: avoid breastfeeding ▪ Check c̄ physician/pharmacist before taking OTC preparations ▪ Use contraception if sexually active.

NOTES:

temazepam/triazolam • (tem-az-e-pam/trye-ay-zoe-lam)

CATEGORY: *Benzodiazepine:* hypnotic

Rx C-IV; Preg Cat X

BRAND NAMES	DOSAGE FORMS
temazepam	
Restoril (Novartis)	Capsule: 15, 30mg
triazolam	
Halcion (Upjohn)	Tablet: 0.125, 0.25mg

USE: Short-term treatment of insomnia associated c difficulty in falling asleep, frequent awakenings, or early morning awakening. **ACTION:** Hypnotic activity extends to all stages (0-4) of sleep; improves total sleep time, ↓ number of nocturnal awakenings; REM sleep not affected

CONTRAINDICATIONS: Hypersensitivity, narrow-angle glaucoma, pregnancy. **CC:** Use can produce dependence, withdrawal symptoms when D/C ▪ Insomnia that does not respond after 7-10d of retreatment requires reevaluation before reuse.

DOSAGE: *PO*

temazepam	
Adult	15-30mg 30m before hs
Geriatric	7.5mg at hs, then adjusted
triazolam	
Adult	0.25-0.5mg at hs
Geriatric	0.125-0.25mg at hs

SIDE/ADVERSE EFFECTS: CNS: ataxia, *dizziness, drowsiness,* fatigue, hangover, hallucinations, *headache,* hyperexcited states, paradoxic anxiety ▪ GI: N/V ▪ HEM: rare WBC count irregularities ▪ Other: memory impairment, anterograde amnesia.

INTERACTIONS: Drug: Use c̄ other CNS depressants produces additive effects ▪ Use of triazolam c̄ erythromycin can result in ↑ hypnotic effects.

PHARMACOKINETICS

	PO absorption	Onset	Peak	Half-life	Protein binding	Excretion
temazepam	Very good	30-40m	2-3h	10h	96%	Via urine as metabolites
triazolam	Readily	—	1.3h	1.6-5.1h	—	Via urine as metabolites, unchanged drug

NURSING MANAGEMENT PRIORITIES

ADMINISTRATION: Assess for hx of benzodiazepine hypersensitivity ▪ Use c̄ caution in hepatic disease ▪ Avoid exposure to heat/moisture/light in storage ▪ Avoid abrupt withdrawal ▪ Elderly pts may require ↓ dosage ▪ ↓ Environmental stimuli.

EVALUATION: Monitor renal, hepatic status ▪ Assess for symptoms of abrupt withdrawal (tremors, abdominal/muscle cramps, convulsions) c̄ prolonged use ▪ Check for signs of dependence (↑ drug request) ▪ Monitor activity status (safety precautions) ▪ Assess for tolerance to therapeutic dose ▪ Assess for paradoxic rxs (CNS stimulation), esp elderly ▪ Check for depression; suicide precautions prn ▪ Assess pt sleep patterns.

EDUCATION: Drowsiness may occur; use caution in potentially hazardous activities ▪ Avoid use c̄ alcohol, other CNS depressants ▪ Indiscriminate use may lead to dependence ▪ Do *not* smoke after taking drug ▪ Do *not* keep at bedside ▪ Take as ordered by physician; do *not* ↑ dose ▪ Women: avoid breastfeeding, do not use if pregnant ▪ Check c̄ physician/pharmacist before taking OTC preparations ▪ Practice relaxation exercises, ventilation of feelings ▪ Utilize sleep producers (reading, warm milk, soft music).

NOTES:

terbinafine hcl • (ter-bin-ah-feen)

CATEGORY: *Antifungal* Rx; Preg Cat B

BRAND NAME
Lamisil (Novartin)

DOSAGE FORMS
Cream: 1%
Tablet: 250mg

USE: Systemic treatment of fingernail/toenail onychomycosis due to susceptible dermatophytes ▪ Topical treatment of susceptible dermatophyte infections of the skin incl athlete's foot (tinea pedis), ringworm (tinea corporis), jock itch (tinea cruris), plantar tinea pedis (moccasin type). **ACTION:** Antifungal activity due to inhibition of the enzyme squalene epoxidase, which is required for synthesis of ergosterol, an essential component of the fungal cell membrane. In addition, there is an ↑ of sequalene w/in the mycotic cell.

PHARMACOKINETICS

PO absorption	Peak	Half-life	Protein binding	Excretion
>70%	2h	36h	99%	70% via urine primarily as metabolites

CONTRAINDICATIONS: Hypersensitivity. **CC:** Use can result in rare cases of hepatobiliary dysfunction, incl cholestatic hepatitis ▪ Liver function tests are required for treatment ≥6wks ▪ Ocular lens & retinal changes have been reported ▪ Drug is excreted in breast milk, & use in nursing mothers Is not recommended ▪ Topical cream is for dermatologic use only ▪ Safety in pediatric pts is not established ▪ Rare cases of neutropenia ▪ Use c̄ caution in pts c̄ hepatic renal impairment.

DOSAGE

Adult	*PO*	250mg once/d for 6wks for fingernail infections & 12wks for toenail infections.

SIDE/ADVERSE EFFECTS: CNS: headache ▪ GI: N/V/D, dyspepsia, abdominal pain, flatulence, taste disturbances ▪ HEM: ***severe neutropenia, thrombocytopenia*** ▪ INT: rash, pruritus, urticaria, ***toxic epidermal necrolysis, Stevens-Johnson syndrome*** ▪ Other: hepatobiliary dysfunction, visual changes, alopecia.

Note: Side/adverse effects: common in *italic*; serious in ***boldface italic***.

*Available in Canada only.

INTERACTIONS: Drug: Use c̄ cyclosporine will ↑ its clearance by 15% ▪ Terbinafine clearance is ↑ 100% when used c̄ rifampin & ↓ 33% when used c̄ cimetidine. **Lab:** Transient ↓ in absolute lymphocyte counts.

NURSING MANAGEMENT PRIORITIES

ADMINISTRATION: Assess for hx of hypersensitivity ▪ Obtain C&S before therapy ▪ Assess hepatic function; ↓ dosage if impaired ▪ Administer c̄ food.

EVALUATION: Monitor VS, esp temperature, BP ▪ Monitor hepatic function.

EDUCATION: Dizziness/drowsiness may occur, use caution in potentially hazardous activities ▪ Take as directed by physician at same time qd; do *not* change dose ▪ Take c̄ food ▪ May produce alteration in taste ▪ Notify physician of visual changes ▪ Check c̄ physician/pharmacist before taking OTC preparations ▪ Store in tightly closed container ▪ Women: avoid breastfeeding ▪ Avoid use c̄ alcohol.

NOTES:

tetracycline hcl • (te-tra-sye-kleen)

CATEGORY: *Tetracycline:* broad-spectrum antibiotic Rx; Preg Cat NA

BRAND NAMES
Achromycin V (Lederle)
Panmycin (Upjohn)
Sumycin (Apothecon)

DOSAGE FORMS: Capsule, IM injection, IV injection, syrup, tablets.

USE: Tetracyclines are the drug(s) of choice for chlamydial, mycoplasmal, rickettsial infections; acne control, balantidiasis, brucellosis, chancroid, cholera, granuloma inguinale, shigellosis, spirochetal relapsing fever ▪ Alternative in penicillin allergy/infections when bacteriologic testing indicates good activity ▪ Treatment of *Helicobacter pylori* infection (ulcers) c̄ other suitable agents & Lyme's disease. **ACTION:** Bacteriostatic effect due to inhibition of ribosomal protein synthesis.

CONTRAINDICATIONS: Hypersensitivity, pregnancy, nursing mothers, children <8y/o. **CC:** Use in children <8y/o or during last half of pregnancy may cause yellow-gray-brown discoloration of teeth & fetal skeletal growth retardation.

DOSAGE

Pediatric	*PO*	20-50mg/kg/d divided
	IM	15-25mg/kg/d divided
	IV	10-20mg/kg/d divided
Adult	*PO*	250-500mg qid
	IM	250-300mg qd
	IV	250-500mg bid
Gonorrhea	*PO*	1.5g then 500mg qid for 4d
Syphillis	*PO*	30-40g in equal doses over 10-15d

PHARMACOKINETICS

PO absorption		Peak			
No food	Food	No food	Half-life	Protein binding	Excretion
60%-80%	10%-30%	2-4h	6-12h	20%-65%	60% excreted unchanged in urine

SIDE/ADVERSE EFFECTS: GI: *gastric upset, diarrhea,* bleeding, enterocolitis ▪ GU: dose-related ⬆ BUN ▪ HEM: *hemolytic anemia, thrombocytopenia* ▪ INT: *monilial overgrowth*, maculopapular rashes, exacerbation of systemic LE, photosensitivity ▪ MS: bulging fontanels in neonates (reversible), fetal skeletal retardation.

INTERACTIONS: Drug: Do *not* use c̄ antacids, antidiarrheals, bactericidal antibiotics, dairy products, methoxyflurane ▪ PO anticoagulants may require ⬇ dose, esp during extended antibiotic therapy.

NURSING MANAGEMENT PRIORITIES

ADMINISTRATION: Assess for allergy before administration ▪ Obtain C&S before therapy ▪ Administer PO dose 1h ac/2h pc ▪ Avoid PO administration c̄ milk, dairy products, antacids ▪ Shake PO suspensions well before pouring ▪ IM: inject *deeply* into muscle; contains local anesthetic, can lead to CV collapse if injected into vasculature ▪ IV: dilute; administer *slowly* ▪ Discard parenteral preparations after 24h ▪ Avoid exposure to heat/moisture/light in storage ▪ Do *not* administer to pregnant women, neonates, children <8y/o (may cause permanent discoloration of teeth).

EVALUATION: Monitor pts receiving anticoagulant therapy; may potentiate bleeding ▪ Assess renal, hepatic status ▪ Monitor VS, esp temperature ▪ Observe for signs of superinfection (diarrhea, perineal itching, oral ulcers) ▪ Urine glucose: false + c̄ Clinitest; false − c̄ Clinistix/Tes-Tape.

EDUCATION: Complete full course of therapy (usually 10d) even if symptoms subside ▪ Avoid prolonged exposure to direct sunlight, UV light (sunlamps); use sunscreen, protective clothing ▪ Take c̄ full glass H_2O on empty stomach; do *not* take w/in 1h of hs ▪ Diarrhea may occur ▪ Store in dry, opaque container ▪ Avoid products containing Al^{+++}, Mg^{++}, Ca^{++}, Fe^{++}, Zn^{++} ▪ Discard outdated, unused preparations.

NOTES:

theophylline • (thee-off-i-lin)

CATEGORY: *Bronchodilator:* xanthine drug

Rx; Preg Cat C

BRAND NAMES

Bronkodyl (Winthrop)
Elixophyllin (Forest)
(Pentagone [Canada])
**Pulmophylline (Riva)*
Quibron-T (Bristol)
**Quibron-T/SR (Bristol)*
Respbid (B-I)
Slo-Bid Gyrocaps (RPR)
Slo-Phyllin Gyrocaps (RPR)
Sustaire (Pfizer)
Theo-24 (Searle)
Theobid Duracaps (Russ)
Theo-Dur (Key)
(Astra [Canada])
Theolair (3M Riker)

DOSAGE FORMS: Capsule (regular, extended release), elixir, syrup, tablet (regular, extended release).

USE: Treatment of asthma, reversible bronchospasm associated c̄ chronic bronchitis, emphysema. **ACTION:** Bronchodilation due to direct relaxation of respiratory smooth muscle; drug stimulates CNS, produces diuresis, has positive chronotropic/inotropic cardiac effect.

PHARMACOKINETICS

PO absorption	Peak	Half-life	Protein binding	Excretion
Usually complete	1-2h	7-9h	56%	Via urine as metabolites, unchanged drug

CONTRAINDICATIONS: Hypersensitivity, active peptic ulcers, untreated seizure disorders. **CC:** Use can induce/worsen arrhythmias ▪ Toxicity c̄ plasma levels >20-25μg/ml ▪ Use c̄ caution in presence of impaired liver function, pts >55y/o, esp males c̄ chronic lung disease, cardiovascular disease.

DOSAGE: Must be individualized.

Pediatric	*PO*	Usual dose 2.5mg/kg q6h
Adult	*PO*	Usual dose 160mg q6h

SIDE/ADVERSE EFFECTS: CNS: *headache*, reflex hyperexcitability, ***clonic/tonic generalized convulsions***, insomnia, *nervousness* ▪ CV: hypotension, tachycardia, ***ventricular arrhythmias,*** palpitations ▪ GI: N/V/D, epigastric pain ▪ GU: albuminuria, diuresis ▪ RESP: tachypnea.

Note: Side/adverse effects: common in *italic;* serious in ***boldface italic***

*Available in Canada only.

INTERACTIONS: Drug: ↑ Serum levels c̄ cimetidine, allopurinol, erythromycin, PO contraceptives, flu vaccine, ↓ c̄ rifampin ▪ ↑ Excretion of lithium, ↓ propranolol effects ▪ Use c̄ adrenergic drugs ↑ CNS stimulation ▪ Use c̄ sucralfate ↓ PO absorption ▪ Use c̄ ciprofloxacin can produce fatal rxs incl cardiac arrest, seizures, respiratory failure. **Food:** Meals inhibit PO absorption c̄ extended action formulations.

NURSING MANAGEMENT PRIORITIES

ADMINISTRATION: Assess for hx of xanthine hypersensitivity ▪ PO: may administer pc c̄ full glass H_2O; *best* on empty stomach; do *not* crush enteric-coated SR preparations, administer whole ▪ PO suspension: shake well before pouring ▪ Parenteral: use cardiac monitoring ▪ Do *not* administer discolored/precipitated solutions ▪ Check compatibility chart for IV administration ▪ Maintain hydration (2000ml/d) ▪ Elderly pts may require ↓ dosage.

EVALUATION: Monitor VS, esp heart rate ▪ Monitor I&O ▪ Monitor respiratory status (breath sounds, sputum) ▪ Parenteral: monitor ABGs, electrolytes ▪ Therapeutic blood levels: 10-20μg/ml.

EDUCATION: Dizziness may occur; use caution in potentially hazardous activities ▪ Take c̄ meals/full glass H_2O to ↓ GI irritation ▪ Swallow enteric-coated/SR preparations whole; do *not* break, crush, chew ▪ Take as ordered by physician; do *not* ↑ dose ▪ Notify physician of irritability, GI distress, palpitations; D/C drug ▪ ↑ Fluid intake (8-10 glasses/d) ▪ Avoid smoking, caffeine-containing substances ▪ Women: avoid breastfeeding ▪ Do *not* substitute brand-name preparations ▪ Check c̄ physician/pharmacist before taking OTC preparations.

OVERDOSE MANAGEMENT: Symptoms incl anorexia, nausea, restlessness, hyperthermia, convulsions, cardiac arrhythmias ▪ Emergency treatment: maintain respiration c̄ oxygen; give 5% dextrose for dehydration; control convulsions c̄ IV diazepam/short-acting barbiturates.

NOTES:

thiopental sodium • (thye-oh-pen-tal)

CATEGORY: *Barbiturate:* anesthetic

Rx C-III; Preg Cat C

BRAND NAME
Pentothal (Abbott)

DOSAGE FORMS
Injection (IV)
Rectal suspension

USE: Anesthetic agent for short surgical procedures ▪ Anesthesia induction, supplement for regional anesthesia ▪ Narcoanalysis, narcosynthesis, treatment of acute convulsive conditions ▪ Neurosurgical pts c̄ ↑ ICP c̄ adequate ventilation. **ACTION:** Hypnotic activity due to depression of midbrain reticular formation.

PHARMACOKINETICS: Produces hypnosis in 30-40s IV; half-life 3-8h; protein binding 80%.

CONTRAINDICATIONS: Hypersensitivity to drug, other barbiturates; status asthmaticus, porphyria; relative contraindications incl severe cardiovascular disease, hypotension, shock, conditions in which hypnotic effect may be prolonged/potentiated. **CC:** Use c̄ caution in pts c̄ Addison's disease, cardiovascular disorders, liver impairment, myasthenia gravis, respiratory dysfunction ▪ Rectal administration not recommended in presence of lower bowel bleeding, inflammation, ulcers, or neoplastic lesions.

DOSAGE: Dose required must be titrated according to surgical requirement, pt age, sex, weight.

Anesthesia	50-75mg at 20-40s intervals. After anesthesia obtained, additional dose 25-50mg can be given whenever pt moves
Convulsions	75-125mg. Convulsions due to local anesthetics may require 125-250mg
Neurosurgical	1.5-2.5mg/kg
Psychiatric	100mg/m. D/C when pt becomes confused (usually indicated by failure to correctly count backward), before sleep produced

SIDE/ADVERSE EFFECTS: CV: myocardial depression ▪ RESP: respiratory depression, bronchospasm ▪ Other: laryngospasm.

INTERACTIONS: Drug: Use c̄ CNS depressants may ↑ effect of ultra–short-acting barbiturates.

NURSING MANAGEMENT PRIORITIES

ADMINISTRATION: Assess for hx of barbiturate hypersensitivity ▪ Do *not* mix any drugs into infusion solutions ▪ Follow manufacturer's directions for specific mg/ml dilutions ▪ Discard unused dilutions after 24h ▪ Do *not* administer discolored/precipitated solution ▪ Have emergency support equipment available ▪ IV: inject test dose (25-75mg), observe pt for 1m; inject *slowly* ▪ Rectal: administer cleansing enema only in cases of fecal impaction.

EVALUATION: Monitor hepatic, renal, cardiac, respiratory status ▪ Assess for paradoxic rxs (CNS stimulation), esp in elderly ▪ Monitor VS, esp BP, q5m.

EDUCATION: Safety precautions may be instituted (bedrails, restraints).

OVERDOSE MANAGEMENT: Principal symptom: exaggerated CNS depression ▪ Respiration depressed, pupils may be constricted, shock, coma ▪ Emergency medical treatment: administer IV fluids, vasopressor to maintain BP; force renal excretion c̄ osmotic diuretics.

NOTES:

thyroid extract • (thye-roid)

CATEGORY: *Thyroid hormone:* desiccated thyroid — Rx; Preg Cat A

BRAND NAME	DOSAGE FORMS
Thyroid (various)	Capsule (in oil): 65, 130, 195, 325mg Tablet: 16, 32, 65, 98, 130, 195, 260, 325mg

USE: Treatment of hypothyroidism. **ACTION:** Thyroid hormones regulate general body metabolism by controlling cellular oxidative process; influence growth, tissue differentiation, maturation.

PHARMACOKINETICS: Natural thyroid preparations exhibit adequate (but variable) PO absorption, full therapeutic effect usually requires 1-3wks, excretion via feces & urine.

CONTRAINDICATIONS: Thyrotoxicosis, uncorrected adrenocortical deficiency, acute MI. **CC:** Use in obese pts as a sole agent/in combination c̄ an anorexiant adrenergic can produce serious toxicity, which can be life threatening.

DOSAGE FORMS: Must be individualized.

Pediatric/Adult *PO*	Usual maintenance dose 65-195mg/d

SIDE/ADVERSE EFFECTS: Usually limited to OD ▪ CNS: headache, insomnia, nervousness, tremors ▪ CV: angina, ***cardiac arrhythmias,*** palpitations, tachycardia ▪ GI: diarrhea ▪ Other: intolerance to heat; sweating, weight loss.

INTERACTIONS: Drug: Use c̄ epinephrine in pts c̄ coronary disease may induce coronary insufficiency ▪ Use c̄ PO anticoagulants ↑ their activity, requires ↓ anticoagulant doses ▪ Use c̄ cholestyramine ↓ PO absorption of thyroid preparations ▪ Use in diabetic pts may require ↑ dosage of hypoglycemic agents.

NURSING MANAGEMENT PRIORITIES

ADMINISTRATION: Assess for hx of hypersensitivity ▪ Administer daily dose before breakfast ▪ Avoid exposure to moisture in storage ▪ Elderly pts may require ↓ dosage.

EVALUATION: Monitor VS, esp heart rate ▪ Observe for signs of OD (chest pain, fever, nervousness, rapid/irregular heartbeat) ▪ Monitor thyroid function tests (T_3, T_4, TSH); evaluate pt use of iodine-containing substances before exam ▪ Diabetics: closely monitor blood glucose (hyperglycemia) ▪ May potentiate anticoagulant effect; assess for bleeding/bruising.

EDUCATION: Take as ordered by physician; do *not* change dose ▪ Avoid high-iodine foods (soybeans, cabbage, shellfish) ▪ Procedure for checking radial pulse ▪ Take pulse on arising qd; notify physician if ↑ or irregular, D/C drug ▪ Keep scheduled appointments c̄ physician/for lab work ▪ Do *not* change brand-name preparations ▪ Notify physician *immediately* of difficult breathing, chest pain, rapid/irregular heartbeat; D/C drug ▪ Check c̄ physician/pharmacist before taking OTC preparations ▪ Notify physician/dentist of use before therapy.

NOTES:

ticarcillin disodium • (tye-kar-sill-in)

CATEGORY: *Extended-spectrum penicillin* Rx; Preg Cat C

BRAND NAME	DOSAGE FORMS
Ticar (SKB)	Powder for injection (IM/IV): 1-, 3-, 6-g vial; 3g IVPB; 20, 30g bulk

COMBINATION PRODUCT

Timentin (SKB)	ticarcillin disodium/clavulanic acid per vial: 3g/100mg, 3g/200mg

USE: Treatment of infections due to susceptible strains of *Enterobacter* spp, *Escherichia coli, Morganella morganii, Proteus* spp, *Pseudomonas aeruginosa* ▪ In combination c̄ aminoglycoside (eg, gentamicin sulfate) in treatment of selected strains of *P. aeruginosa.* **ACTION:** Bactericidal activity due to inhibition of mucopeptide cell wall synthesis in susceptible organisms; addition of clavulanic acid helps protect ticarcillin from action of penicillinase, if present.

PHARMACOKINETICS

IM absorption	Peak	Protein binding	Excretion
Rapid	30-75m	45%-65%	80%-93% via tubular secretion, glomerular filtration w/in 24h

CONTRAINDICATIONS: Hypersensitivity to any penicillin. **CC:** Penicillins can produce serious, occasionally fatal (anaphylaxis) hypersensitivity rxs ▪ Possible cross-allergenicity c̄ cephalosporins, other β-lactam antibiotics ▪ Use can produce pseudomembranous colitis.

DOSAGE

Neonatal	*IM/IV*	<2000g: 75mg/kg/12h for first 7d. After 7d of age, 75mg/kg/8h >2000g: 75mg/kg/8h for first 7d. After 7d of age, 100mg/kg/8h
Pediatric	*IM/IV*	>40kg: same as adult
Adult	*IM/IV*	150-300mg/kg/d divided, q3h, 4h, or 6h

Timentin		
Pediatric		
≥3mo	*IV*	<60kg: 50mg/kg/dose q4-6h based on ticarcillin content >60kg: 3.1g q4-6h
Adult	*IV*	3.1g q4-6h & 3.2g q8h for UTI For gynecolic infections: 200-300mg/kg q4-6h

SIDE/ADVERSE EFFECTS: CNS: possible ***convulsions,*** neuromuscular irritability c̄ extremely high doses ▪ GI: N/V/D ▪ HEM: anemia, eosinophilia, leukopenia, neutropenia, ***thrombocytopenia*** ▪ HEP: ↑ serum AST, ALT ▪ INT: rash, pruritus, urticaria ▪ Other: local discomfort at site of injection; induration usually not present; fever, ***anaphylaxis.***

INTERACTIONS: Drug: Bacteriostatic antibiotics c̄ any penicillin can lead to antibiotic antagonism ▪ PO anticoagulant therapy may require dose adjustment.

NURSING MANAGEMENT PRIORITIES

ADMINISTRATION: Assess for hx of penicillin hypersensitivity ▪ Obtain C&S before therapy ▪ IM: reconstitute 1g/2ml sterile H_2O for injection (1-g dose equals 2.5ml solution); inject in UOQ of buttock or midlateral thigh (children); do *not* exceed 2g/injection site ▪ IV: reconstitute 1g/4ml sterile H_2O for injection; administer *slowly*; may be added to 5% dextrose, 10% invert sugar, normal saline, Ringer/lactated Ringer injection; rotate sites q48h ▪ IVPB: use at least 1g/10ml diluent ▪ Have support equipment available for anaphylaxis ▪ Reconstituted solutions are stable for 24h at room temperature, 72h refrigerated.

EVALUATION: Monitor hepatic, neuromuscular, renal status ▪ Monitor VS, esp temperature ▪ Monitor bleeding time, serum K^+, Na^+ ▪ Monitor I&O ▪ Monitor CBC ▪ Observe for signs of superinfection (diarrhea, perineal itching, oral ulcers) ▪ Assess for hypersensitivity rx (fever, difficult breathing, rash) ▪ Check IV insertion site carefully (phlebitis).

EDUCATION: Diarrhea may occur ▪ Maintain good personal hygiene (esp perineal, oral) ▪ Maintain fluid intake (6-8 glasses/d) ▪ Notify physician of symptoms of allergic rx (fever, difficult breathing, rash) ▪ Carry identification (MedicAlert) if penicillin allergic.

NOTES:

ticlopidine hcl • (tye-kloe-pih-deen)

CATEGORY: *Antiplatelet:* platelet aggregation inhibitor Rx; Preg Cat B

BRAND NAME	**DOSAGE FORM**
Ticlid (Syntex)	Tablet: 250mg

USE: To ⬇ thrombotic stroke in at-risk pts or in pts who have experienced thrombotic stroke. Use should be limited to pts who are intolerant to aspirin therapy. **ACTION:** Produces time- and dose-dependent inhibition in platelet aggregation, release of platelet aggregation products by interfering c̄ platelet membrane function. Effect on individual platelets is nonreversible; ⬆ in platelet life span.

PHARMACOKINETICS

PO absorption	Peak	Half-life	Protein binding	Excretion
Rapid	2h	12.6h then 4-5d	98%	Via urine, feces primarily as metabolites

CONTRAINDICATIONS: Hypersensitivity, severe liver impairment, active bleeding, neutropenia, thrombocytopenia. **CC:** Use can produce mild to severe neutropenia, which usually occurs between 3wks & 3mos after initiation of treatment ▪ Use c̄ caution in pts c̄ liver/renal impairment, ulcers, other bleeding tendencies.

DOSAGE

Adult *PO*	250mg bid c̄ food

SIDE/ADVERSE EFFECTS: CNS: dizziness, headache, *intracerebral bleeding* ▪ GI: N/V/D, dyspepsia, anorexia, abdominal pain, flatulence, *bleeding* ▪ HEM: ***neutropenia, thrombocytopenia,*** anemia ▪ INT: urticaria, pruritus ▪ Other: tinnitus, asthenia, epistaxis, pain.

INTERACTIONS: Drug: Use c̄ antacids will ⬇ PO absorption ▪ Use c̄ aspirin not recommended ▪ Use c̄ theophylline may ⬆ its activity. **Lab:** ⬆ In serum cholesterol.

NURSING MANAGEMENT PRIORITIES

ADMINISTRATION: Assess for hx of hypersensitivity ▪ Assess hepatic, renal function; use caution if impaired ▪ Administer c̄ food to ⬇ GI irritation ▪ Delay antacid administration for 2h after dose.

EVALUATION: Monitor CBC ▪ Monitor hepatic, renal status ▪ May ↑ serum cholesterol, triglycerides ▪ Assess for hearing disturbances; D/C drug, notify physician ▪ Observe pt for signs of ↑ bleeding, incl abdominal/lumbar pain.

EDUCATION: Dizziness may occur; use caution in potentially hazardous activities ▪ Notify physician *immediately* of fever, sore throat, unusual bleeding/bruising, blood detected in urine/stool, hearing disturbances ▪ Take c̄ food ▪ Use soft-bristled toothbrush; electric razor/depilatory for hair removal ▪ Diarrhea may occur ▪ Avoid exposure to infection-producing situations ▪ Notify physician/dentist of drug use before treatment ▪ Women: avoid breastfeeding ▪ Check c̄ physician/pharmacist before taking OTC preparations.

NOTES:

timolol maleate • (tim-oh-lole)

CATEGORY: *β–adrenergic blocker*

Rx; Preg Cat C

BRAND NAMES

Blocadren (Merck)
Timoptic (Merck)

DOSAGE FORMS

Tablet: 5, 10, 20mg
Ophthalmic solution: 0.25%, 0.5%
Occudose (unit dose container): 0.25%, 0.5%

COMBINATION PRODUCT

Timolide 10-25 (MSD) timolol maleate/hydrochlorothiazide per tablet: 10mg/25mg

USE: Treatment of hypertension as sole agent/in combination c̄ other antihypertensive drugs, esp thiazide diuretic ▪ To ⬇ mortality in stable pts after MI ▪ Treatment of chronic open-angle glaucoma, aphakic glaucoma, 2° glaucoma ▪ Migraine prophylaxis. **ACTION:** Blocks access of catecholamines to β_1, β_2 receptors, resulting in bronchial constriction, ⬇ heart rate, myocardial contractility; antihypertensive effect not determined; drug applied topically to treat glaucoma.

PHARMACOKINETICS

PO absorption	Peak	Half-life	Protein binding	Excretion
90%	1-2h	4h	10%	Via urine, feces

CONTRAINDICATIONS: Hypersensitivity, bronchial asthma, cardiogenic shock, sinus bradycardia, heart block >1°, cardiac failure. **CC:** Abrupt D/C can ⬆ ischemic heart disease ▪ Possible cardiac failure c̄ ⬇ myocardial contractility ▪ Tachycardia of hyperthyroidism may be masked, abrupt D/C may induce thyrotoxicosis ▪ Use c̄ caution in pts c̄ bronchospastic disorders, peripheral vascular disease.

DOSAGE

Adult *PO*

Hypertension	Initial dose 10mg bid. Usual range 20-40mg divided, to maximum 60mg/d
MI prevention	10mg bid
Glaucoma	Initial dose 1gtt 0.25% or 0.5% solution bid
Migraine	10-30mg/d
Timolide	Initial dose 1 tablet/d, then adjust

SIDE/ADVERSE EFFECTS: CNS: *dizziness*, mental depression, fatigue, hallucinations ■ CV: *bradycardia,* CHF, hypotension, peripheral vascular insufficiency, ***exacerbation of AV block*** ■ EENT: dry mouth/eyes, visual disturbances ■ GI: *N/V/D*, cramps, constipation, ischemic colitis ■ GU: impotence ■ HEM: ***agranulocytosis, thrombocytopenia,*** purpura ■ INT: alopecia ■ RESP: bronchospasm.

INTERACTIONS: Drug: Use c̄ reserpine, other catecholamine-depleting drugs can result in serious adrenergic blockage ■ Nonselective β adrenergics antagonize therapeutic effects ■ Usually contraindicated c̄ furazolidone, general anesthetics, MAO-I.

NURSING MANAGEMENT PRIORITIES

ADMINISTRATION: Assess for hx of hypersensitivity; apical pulse (if <60/m, hold drug, notify physician); respiratory function (do *not* administer if impaired) ■ PO: may crush, administer c̄ liquid ■ Ophthalmic: place pressure on lacrimal sacs for 1m ■ Avoid abrupt withdrawal ■ Elderly pts may require ↓ dosage.

EVALUATION: Monitor VS, esp BP, heart rate; I&O; IOP ■ Diabetics: closely monitor blood glucose levels (hypoglycemia) ■ Assess for edema in extremities; peripheral circulation ■ Monitor hepatic, CV, renal, hemopoietic status c̄ long-term use.

EDUCATION: Dizziness may occur; use caution in potentially hazardous activities ■ Avoid changing positions (lying/sitting/standing) rapidly ■ Take as ordered by physician; do *not* change dose ■ Procedure for checking radial pulse ■ Check pulse before taking; if <60/m, do *not* take drug; notify physician ■ Do *not* abstain from food for >12h (low blood sugar) ■ Used to control, *not* cure, hypertension ■ Avoid ↑ exercise, temperature extremes, smoking, use c̄ alcohol ■ Maintain optimum weight ■ Avoid high-Na^+ foods ■ Check c̄ physician/pharmacist before taking OTC preparations ■ Notify physician/dentist of use before treatment ■ Do *not* D/C drug w/out checking c̄ physician ■ Carry identification (MedicAlert) if taking timolol ■ Diabetics: carefully monitor blood/urine glucose levels; observe for symptoms of hypoglycemia ■ Keep scheduled appointments for eye exams ■ Procedure for ophthalmic administration.

NOTES:

tobramycin sulfate • (toe-bra-mye-sin)

CATEGORY: *Aminoglycoside:* antibiotic — Rx; Preg Cat D

BRAND NAME	DOSAGE FORMS
Nebcin (Lilly)	Injection (IM/IV): 60mg/1.5ml, 60mg/6ml, 80mg/2ml, 80mg/8ml, 1.2g/30ml; Pediatric: 20mg/2ml
Tobi (Patho Genesis)	Nebulizer solution: 300mg/ampule

USE: Indicated for infections caused by susceptible strains of *Citrobacter* spp, *Enterobacter* spp, *Escherichia coli, Klebsiella-Enterobacter* grp, *Proteus* spp (indole +/−), *Providencia* spp, *Pseudomonas aeruginosa, Serratia* spp ▪ Alternative for penicillin-resistant staphylococcal infections ▪ Management of cystic fibrosis pts c̄ *Pseudomonas aeruginosa* (Nebulizer solution). **ACTION:** Bactericidal activity due to inhibition of ribosomal protein synthesis in susceptible organisms.

PHARMACOKINETICS

IM peak	Half-life	Excretion
0.5-1.5h	2h	85% unchanged in urine in 8h

CONTRAINDICATIONS: Hypersensitivity, hx of serious aminoglycoside toxicity. **CC:** Use of an aminoglycoside during pregnancy can result in bilateral congenital deafness ▪ Use can produce serious ototoxicity, nephrotoxicity ▪ Use c̄ caution in newborns ▪ Injection contains sodium bisulfite, which can cause allergic rxs.

DOSAGE: For pts c̄ normal renal function. Treatment usually 7-10d.

Pediatric	*IM/IV*	<1wk old: Up to 4mg/kg/d in 2 equal doses, q12h Children: 6-7.5mg/kg/d in 3-4 equal doses. More serious infections may require 5mg/kg/d in 3-4 equal doses
Adult	*IM/IV*	3mg/kg/d in 3 equal doses, q8h. ⬇ Dosage as soon as clinically indicated. Life-threatening infections: 5mg/kg/d in 3-4 equal doses
Nebulizer solution		
Adult/Children≥6y/o		300mg bid for 28d

SIDE/ADVERSE EFFECTS: CNS: headache, paresthesia ▪ EENT: ***ototoxicity*** (auditory, vestibular damage), dizziness, vertigo, tinnitus, roaring in ears, hearing loss ▪ GU: ***nephrotoxicity:*** casts, proteinuria, ↑ BUN, NPN, serum creatinine ▪ INT: rash ▪ Other: fever.

INTERACTIONS: Drug: Avoid use c̄ neurotoxic/nephrotoxic drugs such as other aminoglycosides, colistin, ethacrynic acid, furosemide, polymyxin B, vancomycin ▪ Dimenhydrinate can mask aminoglycoside ototoxicity ▪ Use c̄ succinylcholine/tubocurarine ↑ their activity; Ca salts can reverse blockade ▪ PO anticoagulant activity may ↑ due to ↓ intestinal vitamin K synthesis.

NURSING MANAGEMENT PRIORITIES

ADMINISTRATION: Assess for hx of aminoglycoside hypersensitivity ▪ Obtain C&S before therapy ▪ Obtain pt weight for dosage calculation ▪ Determine creatinine clearance before administration ▪ IV: single dose may be diluted in 50-100ml sterile normal saline, 5% dextrose; infuse over 20-60m; use less diluent for pediatric IV; may mix c̄ dextrose, Ringer/lactated Ringer injection, normal saline solution ▪ Do *not* mix c̄ other drugs, incl penicillin ▪ Store in original container; avoid exposure to heat ▪ IM: administer by *deep, slow* injection; rotate sites; avoid inflamed areas ▪ Maintain hydration ▪ Elderly pts may require ↓ dosage.

EVALUATION: Assess for hearing dysfunction ▪ Monitor hepatic, renal, VIII CN function ▪ Monitor VS, esp temperature ▪ Assess for edema in extremities ▪ Assess for neuromuscular blockade, respiratory paralysis, nephrotoxicity ▪ Observe for signs of superinfection (diarrhea, URI, coated tongue) ▪ Assess for hypersensitivity rx (fever, difficult breathing, rash) ▪ Assess peak (<12μg/ml), trough (<2μg/ml) serum concentrations.

EDUCATION: Report hearing, balance difficulties to physician at once ▪ ↑ Fluid intake (10-12 glasses/d).

NOTES:

tocainide hcl • (toe-kay-nide)

CATEGORY: *Antiarrhythmic* Rx; Preg Cat C

BRAND NAME
Tonocard (MSD)
(Astra [Canada])

DOSAGE FORMS
Tablet: 400, 600mg

USE: Treatment of life-threatening ventricular arrhythmias incl PVCs, unimultifocal couplets, ventricular tachycardia. **ACTION:** Antiarrhythmic effect due to depression of ventricular automaticity, depolarization during diastole; drug has no appreciable effect on atrial arrhythmias, produces effects similar to lidocaine (group IB antiarrhythmic).

PHARMACOKINETICS

PO absorption	Peak	Half-life	Protein binding	Excretion
Almost complete	0.5-2h	15h	10%-20%	80% via urine in 72h primarily as metabolites

CONTRAINDICATIONS: Hypersensitivity to drug/local anesthetics of amide type, 2°/3° atrioventricular block w/out pacemaker. **CC:** Use associated c̄ accelerated ventricular rates, blood dyscrasias, fibrosing alveolitis, pneumonia, pulmonary edema/fibrosis, interstitial pneumonitis ▪ Use c̄ caution in pts c̄ liver/kidney disease.

DOSAGE

Adult *PO*	Initial dose 400mg q8h, c̄ daily range 1200-1800mg in 3 doses; higher doses may be required

SIDE/ADVERSE EFFECTS: CNS: *dizziness*, paresthesia, tremor, confusion, restlessness ▪ CV: hypotension, bradycardia, palpitations, chest pain, ***left ventricular failure*** ▪ EENT: blurred vision, nystagmus, tinnitus, hearing loss ▪ GI: *nausea,* V/D, anorexia ▪ HEM: ***agranulocytosis,*** leukopenia, ***thrombocytopenia,*** hypoplastic anemia ▪ INT: lupus, rash ▪ MS: arthralgia ▪ RESP: ***pulmonary fibrosis, interstitial pneumonitis***, edema ▪ Other: night sweats, ***LE syndrome.***

INTERACTIONS: Drug: Use c̄ metoprolol may produce additive effects.

NURSING MANAGEMENT PRIORITIES

ADMINISTRATION: Assess for hx of hypersensitivity (incl amide-type local anesthetics) ▪ Assess hepatic, renal function; may require ⬇ dosage if impaired ▪ Administer c̄ food ▪ Assess serum K^+ levels (normal range: 3.5-5mEq/L); correct imbalances before administration ▪ Maintain blood levels; administer at equal intervals around clock ▪ If switching from lidocaine, administer tocainide 6h *before* stopping lidocaine ▪ Elderly pts may require ⬇ dosage.

EVALUATION: Monitor VS, esp heart rate, BP ▪ Assess for CHF (dyspnea, peripheral edema, ⬆ weight); notify physician ▪ Monitor serum for ⬆ alkaline phosphatase c̄ prolonged use ▪ Monitor ECG, CBC, blood levels throughout therapy ▪ Assess for tremors (signifies maximum dose) ▪ Therapeutic blood levels: 3.5-10μg/ml.

EDUCATION: Dizziness may occur; use caution in potentially hazardous activities ▪ Avoid changing positions (lying/sitting/standing) rapidly ▪ Take as ordered by physician; do *not* skip doses ▪ Take at equal intervals around clock, c̄ food to ⬇ GI irritation ▪ Procedure for checking radial pulse ▪ Notify physician *immediately* of irregular pulse, lethargy, fever, sore throat, bruising/bleeding ▪ Keep scheduled appointments c̄ physician ▪ Notify physician/dentist of use before treatment ▪ Full drug effect may require several days of therapy.

NOTES:

tolazamide/tolbutamide/tolbutamide sodium▲ •

(tole-az-ah-mide/tole-byoo-ta-mide)

CATEGORY: *Oral hypoglycemic:* antidiabetic, 1st-generation sulfonylurea Rx; Preg Cat C

BRAND NAMES	DOSAGE FORMS
tolazamide	
Tolinase (Upjohn)	Tablet: 100, 250, 500mg
tolbutamide	
**Mobanol (Horner)*	Tablet: 500mg
**Novobutamide (Novopharm)*	
Orinase (Upjohn)	Powder for diagnostic injection (IV)▲: 1-g vial c̄ diluent Tablet: 250, 500mg

USE: Management of type II (noninsulin-dependent) diabetes that cannot be controlled by diet alone. **ACTION:** Antidiabetic activity due to stimulation of insulin release from functioning β cells of pancreas.

CONTRAINDICATIONS: Hypersensitivity, diabetic ketoacidosis c̄, w/out coma. **CC:** Use can ↑ risk of cardiovascular mortality in contrast to diet or insulin treatment.

DOSAGE

Adult	*PO*	Must be individualized
tolazamide		Usual maintenance dose 100mg-1g/d
tolbutamide		Usual maintenance dose 0.2-2g/d
	IV	Usual IV diagnostic test dose 1g as single dose

SIDE/ADVERSE EFFECTS: GI: *nausea, epigastric fullness,* heartburn ▪ HEM: ***aplastic anemia, agranulocytosis,*** leukopenia, ***hemolytic anemia,*** pancytopenia, ***thrombocytopenia*** ▪ INT: erythema, morbilliform/maculopapular eruptions, photosensitivity ▪ MET: hypoglycemia.

PHARMACOKINETICS

PO absorption	Onset	Peak	Duration	Half-life	Excretion
tolbutamide					
Rapid	1h	3-5h	6-12h	4-7h	75% via urine
tolazamide					
Rapid	2-4h	2-6h	10h	7h	85% via urine

Note: Side/adverse effects: common in *italic;* serious in ***boldface italic.***

*Available in Canada only.

INTERACTIONS: Drug: Use c̄ alcohol, MAO-I, phenylbutazones, β blockers can significantly ↑ hypoglycemic effects ▪ Use c̄ anabolic steroids, chloramphenicol, guanethidine, PO anticoagulants, probenecid, salicylates, sulfinpyrazone, sulfonamides ↑ hypoglycemic effects ▪ Use c̄ adrenergics, corticosteroids, phenytoin, thiazides, thyroid preparations ↓ hypoglycemic effects ▪ Use c̄ NSAIAs can ↑ hypoglycemic effects.

NURSING MANAGEMENT PRIORITIES

ADMINISTRATION: Assess for hx of hypersensitivity ▪ Administer as single AM dose/d c̄ breakfast/divided doses c̄ meals ▪ Avoid exposure to moisture in storage ▪ Elderly pts may require ↓ dosage.

EVALUATION: Monitor hepatic, renal, hematologic status ▪ Monitor FBS ▪ Evaluate pt closely during first wk to assess effectiveness ▪ Monitor for signs of hypoglycemia/ hyperglycemia.

EDUCATION: Compliance c̄ special diet therapy ▪ Blood/ urine glucose/ketone testing procedure ▪ Symptoms of hypoglycemia (anxiety, headache, fatigue, nausea, sweating); notify physician immediately ▪ Always carry lump of sugar/candy for quick use c̄ hypoglycemia ▪ Avoid alcohol ▪ Check c̄ physician before taking OTC preparations ▪ Symptoms of hyperglycemia (excessive hunger, thirst, urination; rapid pulse, sweet-smelling breath, weight loss); notify physician immediately ▪ Need for good personal hygiene ▪ Carry identification (MedicAlert) ▪ Store in tightly closed container ▪ Keep scheduled appointments c̄ physician/for blood glucose determinations ▪ Schedule periodic eye exams ▪ Maintain optimum body weight ▪ Avoid prolonged exposure to direct sunlight; use sunscreen, protective clothing ▪ Women: avoid breastfeeding ▪ PO hypoglycemic needs may change c̄ ↑ stress, ↑ exercise, ↓ appetite; notify physician.

NOTES:

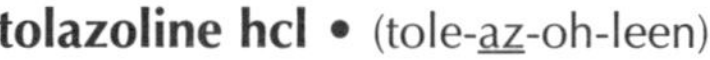

tolazoline hcl • (tole-az-oh-leen)

CATEGORY: *α–-adrenergic blocker:* pulmonary antihypertensive, sympatholytic Rx; Preg Cat C

BRAND NAME	DOSAGE FORM
Priscoline (C-G)	Injection (IV): 25mg/ml

USE: Treatment of persistent neonatal pulmonary hypertension when systemic arterial oxygenation cannot be maintained by usual supportive care. **ACTION:** Antihypertensive effect due to direct peripheral activity & moderate competitive blocking of α adrenoreceptors ↓ pulmonary arterial BP, vascular resistance.

PHARMACOKINETICS

Half-life	Onset	Excretion
3-10h	≤30m	Rapidly in urine as unchanged drug

CONTRAINDICATIONS: Hypersensitivity. **CC:** Drug stimulates gastric secretions, which can result in 2° hypochloremic alkalosis ▪ Use of antacids in infants may prevent GI bleeding ▪ Acidosis may ↓ therapeutic effectiveness.

DOSAGE

Neonatal *IV*	1-2mg/kg via scalp vein, followed by infusion 1-2mg/kg/h

SIDE/ADVERSE EFFECTS: CV: hypertension, hypotension, tachycardia, ***cardiac arrhythmias, pulmonary hemorrhage,*** edema ▪ GI: hemorrhage, N/V/D ▪ GU: oliguria, hematuria ▪ HEM: ***thrombocytopenia,*** leukopenia.

INTERACTIONS: Drug: Use $\bar{c}$ alcohol can cause toxic disulfiram rx, an interaction not possible $\bar{c}$ neonate ▪ Use $\bar{c}$ norepinephrine/epinephrine may cause severe hypotension followed by sudden rebound in BP.

NURSING MANAGEMENT PRIORITIES

ADMINISTRATION: Assess for hx of hypersensitivity ▪ Assess BP; do *not* administer if systolic BP <40mmHg ▪ Have support equipment available.

EVALUATION: Monitor BP; observe for hypotension ▪ Assess peripheral circulation (skin color, temperature, pulses) ▪ Monitor for ↑ gastric juice acidity, pepsin; ↓ RBC, WBC, platelet count ▪ Monitor fluid/electrolyte, acid-base status ▪ Monitor VS, ABGs.

EDUCATION: Avoid changing positions (horizontal/vertical) rapidly ▪ Avoid use of alcohol-containing substances ▪ Keep pt warm; avoid extremely hot objects ▪ Avoid positions that may impair peripheral circulation.

NOTES:

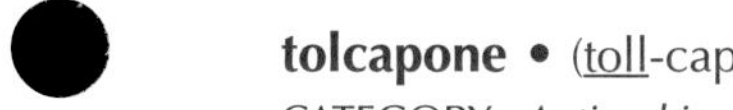

tolcapone • (toll-cap-own)

CATEGORY: *Antiparkinsonian agent*

Rx; Preg Cat C

BRAND NAME
Tasmar (Roche)

DOSAGE FORM
Tablet: 100, 200mg

USE: Adjunct to levodopa/carbidopa in treatment of idiopathic Parkinson's disease. **ACTION:** Parkinson's disease is related to ↓ levels of dopamine in the corpus striatum. Administered levodopa enters the CNS, is converted into dopamine in the basal ganglia; concentration of dopamine ↑, symptoms of Parkinson's disease ↓. Tolcapone inhibits catechol-ortho-methyl transferase (COMT) enzyme from metabolizing circulating levodopa, resulting in ↑ blood levels of levodopa for transport to brain. Accordingly, tolcapone is an indirect dopaminergic agent.

PHARMACOKINETICS

PO absorption	Half-life	Protein binding	Excretion
65%	2-3h	99.9%	Via urine (60%), feces (40%) as metabolites

CONTRAINDICATIONS: Hypersensitivity. **CC:** Use c̄ nonselective MAO-I is not recommended due to inhibition of catecholamine metabolism ▪ Use in pts c̄ liver/renal impairment requires caution ▪ Use can cause ↑ orthostatic hypotension, dyskinesia, hallucinations.

DOSAGE

Adult	*PO*	Initial dose of 100 or 200mg tid as an adjunct to levodopa/carbidopa therapy. Do *not* exceed 600mg/d

SIDE/ADVERSE EFFECTS: CNS: dyskinesia (most common), dystonia, dreaming/hallucinations, confusion, dizziness, somnolence ▪ CV: orthostatic hypotension, chest pain ▪ GI: N/V/D, anorexia, constipation, dyspepsia ▪ GU: UTI ▪ MS: muscle cramps, falling ▪ RESP: URI, dyspnea, influenza.

INTERACTIONS: Drug: Use c̄ warfarin requires caution ▪ COMT metabolized drugs, such as catecholamines (epinephrine, etc.) may require ↓ doses. **Food:** ↓ Bioavailability when administered 1h ac or 2h pc.

NURSING MANAGEMENT PRIORITIES

ADMINISTRATION: Assess for hx of hypersensitivity ▪ Administer c̄ food ▪ Avoid abrupt withdrawal ▪ Elderly may require ↓ dosage.

EVALUATION: Monitor VS, esp BP ▪ Monitor CV, pulmonary, hepatic, renal status; notify physician if impaired ▪ Observe pt for dyskinesic/dystonic rxs; notify physician.

EDUCATION: Dizziness/drowsiness may occur; use caution in potentially hazardous activities ▪ Take c̄ food ▪ Avoid changing positions (lying/sitting/standing) rapidly ▪ May produce hallucinations ▪ Notify physician *immediately* of abnormal rxs (chest pain, abnormal muscle movements, difficulty breathing) ▪ Safety precautions c̄ ↑ activity.

NOTES:

tolmetin sodium • (tole-met-in)

CATEGORY: *Antiinflammatory:* NSAIA

Rx; Preg Cat C

BRAND NAMES

Tolectin (McNeil)
Tolectin DS (McNeil)

DOSAGE FORMS

Tablet: 200, 600mg
DS capsule: 400mg

USE: Treatment of rheumatoid/juvenile/osteoarthritis. **ACTION:** Antiinflammatory activity appears related to inhibition of prostaglandin synthesis.

PHARMACOKINETICS

PO absorption	Peak	Half-life	Protein binding	Excretion
Complete	30-60m	1h	99%	Via urine in 24h primarily as metabolites

CONTRAINDICATIONS: Hypersensitivity, aspirin/other NSAIA hypersensitivity. **CC:** Use ↑ risk of GI bleeding, ulcers, perforation.

DOSAGE FORMS

Pediatric	*PO*	20mg/kg/d divided. Usual range 15-30mg/kg/d. Do *not* exceed 30mg/kg/d
Adult	*PO*	400mg tid, then adjust. Usual range 600-1800mg/d in 3-4 equal doses, c̄ maximum 2g/d

SIDE/ADVERSE EFFECTS: CNS: *headache, dizziness,* drowsiness ▪ CV: edema, CHF, ↑ BP ▪ EENT: tinnitus, blurred vision, retinal/macular changes ▪ GI: *abdominal pain, nausea,* constipation, flatulence, vomiting, stomatitis ▪ GU: hematuria, proteinuria, dysuria ▪ HEM: ***agranulocytosis*** (rare), ***hemolytic anemia,*** granulocytopenia ▪ HEP: ***severe/fatal hepatitis*** ▪ INT: purpura, urticaria, skin irritation, ***erythema multiforme*** ▪ Other: weight gain/loss, fever, ***anaphylactoid rxs.***

INTERACTIONS: Drug: Use c̄ ulcerogenic drugs produces additive effects ▪ Use c̄ PO anticoagulants may ↑ their activity ▪ Aspirin ↓ tolmetin plasma levels.

NURSING MANAGEMENT PRIORITIES

ADMINISTRATION: Assess for hx of NSAIA hypersensitivity ▪ Avoid administration in pts c̄ hx of asthma, bleeding disorders, salicylate hypersensitivity ▪ Assess for hx of peptic ulcer; use c̄ caution ▪ Assess renal function; may require ⬇ dosage if impaired ▪ Administer on arising & at hs, c̄ food/milk/antacids to ⬇ GI irritation; tablets may be crushed/capsules opened; encourage upright position for 15-30m ▪ Avoid exposure to moisture in storage ▪ Elderly pts may require ⬇ dosage.

EVALUATION: Monitor renal status c̄ prolonged use ▪ Monitor I&O, daily weight c̄ prolonged use ▪ Assess for edema in extremities ▪ Assess for visual/hearing disturbances; D/C drug, notify physician.

EDUCATION: Dizziness/drowsiness may occur; use caution in potentially hazardous activities ▪ Take c̄ food/milk/antacid to ⬇ GI distress; maintain upright position for 15-30m ▪ Take as ordered by physician; do *not* ⬆ dose ▪ Notify physician *immediately* of bleeding, ⬇ urine output, swelling of feet/legs, lethargy, GI distress, jaundice, visual disturbances ▪ Avoid taking c̄ aspirin/other NSAIAs ▪ Avoid use c̄ alcohol ▪ Check c̄ physician/pharmacist before taking OTC preparations ▪ Notify physician/dentist of use before treatment ▪ Store in tightly closed container ▪ Avoid exposure to direct sunlight, UV light (sunlamps); use sunscreen, protective clothing ▪ Full drug effects may require several wks of therapy.

NOTES:

tolterodine tartrate • (toll-tear-oh-deen)

CATEGORY: *Antimuscarinic:* urinary bladder stabilizer Rx; Preg Cat C

BRAND NAME	DOSAGE FORMS
Detrol (Upjohn)	Tablet: 1, 2mg

USE: Treatment of urinary frequency as a result of overactive bladder. **ACTION:** Reduction of bladder instability & urinary incontinence caused by competitive inhibition (antagonism) of bladder cholinergic muscarinic receptors to cholinergic innervation resulting in ↓ in residual bladder urine. Antimuscarinic (anticholinergic) activity of the drug is not limited to the bladder.

PHARMACOKINETICS

PO absorption	Peak	Half-life	Protein binding	Excretion
Rapid & high	1-2h	1.9-3.7h	96%	Via urine (77%), feces (17%) as metabolites

CONTRAINDICATIONS: Hypersensitivity, gastric/urinary retention, uncontrolled narrow-angle glaucoma. **CC:** Use c̄ caution in pts c̄ pyloric stenosis/other obstructive GI conditions ▪ Pts c̄ hepatic impairment require a dosage adjustment of >1mg bid ▪ Use c̄ caution in pts c̄ treated-narrow-angle glaucoma ▪ Use in nursing mothers not currently recommended ▪ Drug is present in rodent breastmilk ▪ Safety & efficacy not established for children.

DOSAGE

Adult	*PO*	2mg bid

SIDE/ADVERSE EFFECTS: CNS: dizziness, headache, somnolence, nervousness ▪ EENT: abnormal vision, xerophthalmia ▪ GI: N/V/D, constipation, dry mouth, abdominal pain ▪ GU: dysuria, UTI, urinary retention ▪ INT: dry skin, erythema, pruritus, rash ▪ RESP: bronchitis, chest pain, URI, coughing, rhinitis, sinusitis ▪ Other: fatigue, arthralgia, hypertension, weight gain.

INTERACTIONS: Drug: Use c̄ macrolide antibiotics, conazole, antifungals requires a dose of >1mg bid because of enzyme inhibition. **Food:** Food ⬆ tolterodine bioavailability.

NURSING MANAGEMENT PRIORITIES

ADMINISTRATION: Assess for hx of hypersensitivity ▪ Assess degree of bladder dysfunction ▪ Assess GI, hepatic, renal function; use caution if impaired ▪ Assess for hx of narrow-angle glaucoma; notify physician ▪ Administer c̄ food.

EVALUATION: Monitor VS, esp BP ▪ Monitor hepatic status; notify physician if impaired ▪ Monitor bladder control, noting signs of improvement (⬇ urinary frequency, ⬇ urge incontinence).

EDUCATION: Dizziness may occur; use caution in potentially hazardous activities ▪ Take c̄ food ▪ Use sugarless gum/hard candy to diminish dry mouth ▪ May produce visual alterations ▪ Notify physician *immediately* of abnormal rxs (chest pain, difficulty breathing) ▪ Women: avoid breastfeeding.

NOTES:

toremifene citrate • (tore-rem-ih-feen)

CATEGORY: *Antineoplastic:* nonsteroidal antiestrogen agent Rx; Preg Cat D

BRAND NAME	**DOSAGE FORM**
Fareston (Schering)	Tablet: 60mg

USE: Treatment of metastatic breast cancer in postmenopausal women who are estrogen-receptor (ER) + or c̄ unknown ER tumors. **ACTION:** Toremifene is extremely similar to tamoxifen in chemical structure & only differs by an additional chlorine atom.

Antineoplastic effect related to potent antiestrogenic effects in breasts. Drug competes c̄/blocks estrogen at ER sites in tumors that contain high concentrations of ERs, resulting in inhibition of estrogen growth stimulation in the tumor(s). Drug exhibits enterohepatic recirculation & has an elimination half-life of about 5d.

PHARMACOKINETICS

PO absorption	Peak	Half-life	Protein binding	Excretion
Good	3h	4h	99.5%	Via feces primarily as metabolites

CONTRAINDICATIONS: Hypersensitivity. **CC:** Use c̄ caution in pts c̄ hepatic impairment due to ↑ in elimination half-life ▪ Use may induce hypercalcemia, tumor flare up (transient ↑ in tumor size), musculoskeletal pain, erythema, cataracts, other ocular toxicities ▪ Treatment requires monitoring blood counts, hepatic function, pts c̄ bone metastases for hypercalcemia ▪ Thromboembolic disease generally precludes these pts from toremifene therapy ▪ No clinical indications for use in pediatric pts.

DOSAGE

Adult	*PO*	60mg once/d

SIDE/ADVERSE EFFECTS: CV: edema, ***cardiac failure*** ▪ EENT: abnormal vision, cataracts, corneal keratopathy, glaucoma ▪ GI: N/V, anorexia ▪ HEM: ***pulmonary embolsim*** ▪ Other: dizziness, hot flashes, sweating, vaginal bleeding/discharge.

INTERACTIONS: Drug: Use c̄ PO anticoagulants requires caution due to ↑ changes in PT ■ Use c̄ enzyme inducers, incl carbamazepine, phenobarbital, phenytoin, ↑ metabolism of toremifene & ↓ metabolism c̄ conazole antifungals, macrolide antibiotics (eg, erythromycin). **Lab:** ↑ Serum levels of AST, alkaline phosphatase, bilirubin.

NURSING MANAGEMENT PRIORITIES

ADMINISTRATION: Check pt hx for recent course of radiation/antineoplastic agents ■ Assess renal function; may require ↓ dosage if impaired ■ Administer antiemetic before therapy ■ Provide emotional support ■ Avoid exposure to moisture/light in storage.

EVALUATION: Monitor hepatic, renal function; CBC, esp WBCs, platelets throughout therapy; notify physician if ↓ ■ Assess for infection, bleeding, anemia ■ Assess hydration status (I&O, daily weight) ■ Monitor vision; notify physician if ↓.

EDUCATION: Store in dry, tightly closed, light-resistant container ■ ↑ Fluid intake (8-10 glasses/d) ■ Avoid exposure to infection ■ Check c̄ physician before immunization (pt, family) ■ Diet as tolerated; avoid spicy foods ■ Maintain good oral hygiene; use soft-bristled toothbrush ■ Notify physician of symptoms of bone marrow depression (fever, sore throat, bruising, bleeding, lethargy) ■ Compliance c̄ prescribed dosage regimen ■ Women: avoid breastfeeding ■ Check c̄ physician/pharmacist before taking OTC preparations ■ Use contraception if sexually active ■ Notify physician of visual changes, chest pain, difficulty breathing.

NOTES:

tramadol hcl • (trah-ma-dole)

CATEGORY: *Central-acting analgesic* Rx; Preg Cat C

BRAND NAME	DOSAGE FORM
Ultram (Ortho-McNeil)	Tablet: 50mg

USE: Analgesic for moderate to moderately severe pain. **ACTION:** Analgesic activity appears related to CNS inhibition of norepinephrine, serotonin reuptake, drug binding to mu (μ) opioid receptors.

PHARMACOKINETICS

PO absorption	Peak	Half-life	Excretion
Almost complete	2-3h	6-7h	Via urine primarily as metabolites (60%)

CONTRAINDICATIONS: Hypersensitivity, intoxication c̄ alcohol, centrally acting analgesics, hypnotic opioids, psychotropic drugs. **CC:** ↑ Seizure risk when administered c̄ other drugs that ↓ seizure threshold (MAO-I, neuroleptics) ▪ Use c̄ caution c̄ CNS depressants ▪ Hepatic, renal impairment may require ↓ doses.

DOSAGE

Adult	*PO*	50-100mg q4-6h prn. Do *not* exceed 400mg/d. Dosage c̄ renal impairment requires a dosage interval of 12h & total daily maximum dose of 200mg. Dosage c̄ cirrhosis is 50mg q12h.

SIDE/ADVERSE EFFECTS: CNS: dizziness, headache, somnolence, agitation, ***possible seizures*** ▪ CV: orthostatic hypotension, palpitations, vasodilation ▪ GI: N/V/D, dry mouth, constipation, anorexia, dyspepsia, ***bleeding*** ▪ GU: menopausal symptoms, urinary frequency/retention ▪ INT: pruritus, rash, urticaria ▪ Other: visual disturbances, ***cataracts,*** hypotonia.

INTERACTIONS: Drug: Use c̄ carbamazepine will ↑ tramadol metabolism, may require ↑ in dosage ▪ Use c̄ MAO-I requires caution. **Lab:** ↑ In liver enzymes, creatinine, proteinuria. **Food:** Meals do not affect PO absorption.

NURSING MANAGEMENT PRIORITIES

ADMINISTRATION: Assess for hx of hypersensitivity ▪ Assess renal, hepatic function; may require ↓ dosage if impaired ▪ Assess quality, intensity, location of pain ▪ Have narcotic antagonist, support measures available ▪ Administer c̄/w/out food ▪ Avoid administration in pts c̄ suspected head injury ▪ Assess for alcohol, opioid intoxication; do *not* administer ▪ Administer before pt has intense pain ▪ Institute safety, seizure precautions ▪ Utilize + power of suggestion ▪ Elderly pts may require ↓ dosage.

EVALUATION: Monitor CV, hepatic function ▪ Assess renal function, urinary retention ▪ Assess bowel function, abdominal distention ▪ Check for signs of dependence (↑ drug request) ▪ Assess for relief of pain.

EDUCATION: Dizziness may occur; use caution in potentially hazardous activities ▪ Avoid changing positions (lying/sitting/standing) rapidly ▪ Avoid excessive sensory stimulation ▪ Take c̄/w/out food ▪ Constipation may occur; ↑ fluid, bulk-containing foods ▪ Avoid use c̄ alcohol, CNS depressants ▪ Women: notify physician of possible pregnancy; avoid breastfeeding.

NOTES:

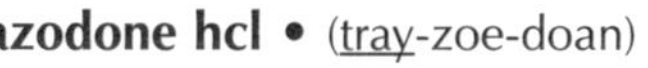

trazodone hcl • (tray-zoe-doan)

CATEGORY: *Antidepressant*　　Rx; Preg Cat C

BRAND NAME
Desyrel (MJP)

DOSAGE FORMS
Tablet: 50, 100, 150mg

USE: Treatment of depression. **ACTION:** Antidepressant activity appears related to inhibition of serotonin reuptake in CNS.

PHARMACOKINETICS

PO absorption	Peak	Half-life	Excretion
Good	1-2h	3-9h	Via urine, feces as metabolites

CONTRAINDICATIONS: Hypersensitivity. **CC:** Use associated c̄ priapism, which may require surgical correction ▪ Not recommended during initial recovery of MI.

DOSAGE

Adult *PO* Initial dose of 150mg/d in divided doses, ↑ by 50mg/d q3-4d. Do *not* exceed 400mg/d for outpts, 600mg/d for inpts

SIDE/ADVERSE EFFECTS: CNS: drowsiness, dizziness, nervousness, headache, insomnia, incoordination, confusion, anger, hostility, impaired memory ▪ CV: hypotension, hypertension, palpitations, edema ▪ EENT: blurred vision, tinnitus, nasal congestion, red eyes ▪ GI: dry mouth, constipation, N/V/D, pain, ↓ appetite ▪ Other: muscle pain, malaise, sweating.

INTERACTIONS: Drug: Use c̄ CNS depressants produces additive drowsiness ▪ Use c̄ digoxin, phenytoin ↑ their effects.

NURSING MANAGEMENT PRIORITIES

ADMINISTRATION: Assess for hx of hypersensitivity ▪ Assess for hx of seizures; use caution ▪ Assess hepatic, renal status; ↓ dosage if impaired ▪ Administer pc ▪ Institute safety, seizure precautions ▪ Institute suicide precautions ▪ Avoid abrupt withdrawal; D/C gradually ▪ Avoid moisture/heat/direct light in storage ▪ Elderly pts may require ↓ dosage.

EVALUATION: Monitor BP (hypertension c̄ antihypertensive therapy) ▪ Monitor CV, hepatic, renal status ▪ Monitor fluid retention (I&O, daily weight), constipation ▪ Assess for weight loss (anorectic effect) ▪ Assess for symptoms of abrupt withdrawal (nausea, headache, malaise) ▪ Assess for actual swallowing of PO forms ▪ Assess for skin rash, hives; notify physician, D/C drug.

EDUCATION: Dizziness/drowsiness may occur; use caution in potentially hazardous activities ▪ Avoid changing positions (lying/sitting/standing) rapidly ▪ Avoid use c̄ alcohol, other CNS depressants for up to 1wk after end of therapy ▪ Take shortly pc ▪ Take as directed by physician ▪ Use sugarless gum/hard candy to diminish dry mouth ▪ Constipation may occur; ↑ fluids, bulk-containing foods ▪ Notify physician of skin rash, hives; D/C drug ▪ Check c̄ physician/pharmacist before taking OTC/Rx preparations ▪ Notify physician/dentist of use before treatment ▪ Store in tightly closed, light-resistant container ▪ Encourage recreational/diversional interests ▪ Notify physician of weight loss, fever, sore throat, malaise ▪ Keep scheduled appointments c̄ physician ▪ Women: notify physician of pregnancy possibility; avoid breastfeeding ▪ Full drug effects may require several wks of therapy.

NOTES:

triamcinolone/triamcinolone acetonide▲/ triamcinolone diacetate△ • (trye-am-sin-oh-lone)

CATEGORY: *Glucosteroid:* corticosteroid Rx; Preg Cat NA

BRAND NAMES
Aristocort (Fujisawa)
Kenacort (Apothecon)
Kenalog (Squibb)▲

AVAILABLE PREPARATIONS
Injection suspension,△ syrup,△ tablets, various topical preparations

USE: Treatment of adrenocortical deficiency, adrenogenital syndrome, other endocrine disorders; allergic states, collagen diseases, dermatologic diseases, GI diseases, hematologic disorders, ophthalmologic diseases, respiratory diseases, rheumatic disorders ▪ Treatment of tuberculous meningitis; neurologic/myocardial involvement associated c̄ trichinosis ▪ Remission of proteinuria in nephrotic syndrome, acute exacerbation of multiple sclerosis ▪ Palliative management of leukemias/lymphomas. **ACTION:** Glucosteroids cause wide variety of pharmacologic activity; two major effects are potent antiinflammatory effect, inhibition of immune response.

PHARMACOKINETICS: PO administration usually produces peak effect in 1-2h, c̄ duration about 2.25d.

CONTRAINDICATIONS: Hypersensitivity, administration of live viral vaccines c̄ immunosuppressant doses. Systemic fungal infections. **CC: Food:** *See* cortisone acetate.

DOSAGE

Adult *PO*	6-60mg/d
Diacetate injection	40mg/wk IM; 5-40mg intra-articular/intrasynovial. Intralesional/sublesional 5-48mg, c̄ maximum 12.5mg/injection site
Acetonide injection	40-80mg IM; 2.5-60mg intra-articular/intrabursal

SIDE/ADVERSE EFFECTS: CNS: ***convulsions,*** headache, psychic impairment, vertigo, mood swings; pseudotumor cerebri may develop after treatment ▪ CV: edema due to Na^+ retention, CHF, hypertension ▪ EENT: ↑ IOP, glaucoma, posterior subcapsular cataracts, exophthalmos ▪ END: cushingoid states, growth suppression in children, menstrual irregularities, 2° adrenocortical/pituitary unresponsiveness, hyperglycemia, carbohydrate intolerance ▪ GI: peptic ulcer/***possible perforation, pancreatitis,***

Note: Side/adverse effects: common in *italic;* serious in ***boldface italic.***

▲Available in Canada only.

abdominal distention, ulcerative esophagitis ▪ INT: poor wound healing, fragile skin, petechiae/ecchymoses, facial erythema, ↑ sweating, urticaria, hirsutism ▪ MET: negative nitrogen balance, hypokalemic alkalosis ▪ MS: muscle weakness/loss of mass, fracture of long bones, osteoporosis.

INTERACTIONS: Drug: Severe hypokalemia can occur c̄ diuretics (nonpotassium sparing) ▪ Use c̄ ulcerogenic drugs (eg, aspirin, indomethacin) can produce additive effects ▪ Use c̄ antidiabetic agents may require higher doses of antidiabetic drugs.

NURSING MANAGEMENT PRIORITIES

ADMINISTRATION: Assess for hx of hypersensitivity ▪ Administer single daily dose *before* 9AM; multiple doses at equal intervals ▪ PO: administer c̄ food/milk/antacids ▪ Do *not* administer IV ▪ IM: shake well; do *not* mix, dilute, freeze; inject *deeply* into gluteal UOQ (avoid deltoid); rotate sites ▪ Avoid abrupt withdrawal; ↓ dose gradually ▪ Avoid exposure to heat/light in storage ▪ Elderly pts may require ↓ dosage; monitor BP.

EVALUATION: Monitor VS, esp BP; hydration status (I&O, daily weight) ▪ Diabetics: closely monitor blood/urine glucose levels (hyperglycemia) ▪ Assess mental/emotional status; avoid use c̄ TCAs if depression is induced ▪ Monitor serum electrolytes (esp K^+, Na^+), vision/IOP, stools for occult blood c̄ prolonged use ▪ Assess for ↓ appetite.

EDUCATION: Avoid changing positions (lying/sitting/standing) rapidly ▪ Take c̄ food/milk (single dose *before* 9AM; multiple doses at equal intervals) ▪ Take as ordered by physician; do *not* ↑ dose/D/C ▪ Eat foods high in K^+, high in protein; avoid black licorice ▪ Follow diet low in Na^+ ▪ Check c̄ physician before immunization (pt, family) ▪ Avoid exposure to infection ▪ Report following symptoms *immediately* to physician: anorexia, difficult breathing, weakness, dizziness; may appear during periods of ↑ stress/trauma ▪ Notify physician of black/tarry stools, slow wound healing, blurred vision, bruising/ bleeding, weight gain, emotional changes ▪ Diabetics: closely monitor blood/urine glucose levels ▪ Store in tightly closed, light-resistant container ▪ Keep scheduled appointments c̄ physician/for blood work/for eye exams ▪ Women: avoid breastfeeding ▪ Body image changes may occur c̄ prolonged therapy (reversible).

NOTES:

triamterene • (trye-am-ter-een)

CATEGORY: *Diuretic:* potassium-sparing diuretic — Rx; Preg Cat B

BRAND NAME	**DOSAGE FORMS**
Dyrenium (SKB)	Capsule: 50, 100mg

COMBINATION PRODUCTS

Dyazide (SKB)	triamterene/hydrochlorothiazide per capsule: 50mg/25mg
Maxzide (Lederle)	triamterene/hydrochlorothiazide per tablet: 75mg/50mg
Maxzide-25MG	triamterene/hydrochlorothiazide per tablet: 37.5mg/25mg
**Novotriamide (Novopharm)*	triamterene/hydrochlorothiazide per tablet: 50mg/25mg

USE: Edema associated c̄ CHF, cirrhosis of liver, nephrotic syndrome ▪ Steroid-induced edema, idiopathic edema, edema due to 2° hyperaldosteronism ▪ Combination products are employed as antihypertensives (due to hydrochlorothiazide content). **ACTION:** Triamterene acts directly at portion of distal tubule under control of mineralosteroids (esp aldosterone) to inhibit reabsorption of sodium ions in exchange for potassium, hydrogen ions; drug has no appreciable antihypertensive activity.

PHARMACOKINETICS

PO absorption	Onset	Duration	Protein binding	Excretion
Good	2-4h	7-9h	67%	Via urine as metabolites, unchanged drug

CONTRAINDICATIONS: Hypersensitivity, anuria, significant renal insufficiency, hyperkalemia. **CC:** Use associated c̄ hyperkalemia, possible arrhythmias ▪ Use c̄ caution in pts c̄ diabetes, renal dysfunction, the elderly.

DOSAGE

Adult *PO*	Usual dose 100mg bid pc. Do *not* exceed 300mg/d
Dyazide	Usual adult dose 1-2 capsules bid pc
Maxzide	Usual adult dose 1 tablet/d
Maxzide-25MG	Usual adult dose 1-2 tablets/d as single dose

*Available in Canada only.

SIDE/ADVERSE EFFECTS: CNS: headache, weakness, dizziness ▪ GI: N/V/D, dry mouth ▪ HEM: ***megaloblastic anemia*** (rare) ▪ INT: *photosensitivity, rash* ▪ MET: hyperkalemia ▪ Other: ***anaphylaxis.***

INTERACTIONS: Drug: Use c̄ lithium best avoided because of ↑ in lithium serum levels ▪ Use c̄ dig glycosides may ↑ their activity.

NURSING MANAGEMENT PRIORITIES

ADMINISTRATION: Assess for hx of hypersensitivity ▪ Assess F/E balance; serum K^+ level (normal: 3.5-5mEq/L); do *not* administer if hyperkalemic; notify physician ▪ Assess renal function; do *not* administer if impaired ▪ Administer pc ▪ Avoid exposure to moisture/light in storage ▪ Elderly pts may require ↓ dosage.

EVALUATION: Monitor F/E, hepatic, renal status ▪ Monitor VS, esp BP, pulse ▪ Monitor serum for ↑ BUN, creatinine, uric acid ▪ Assess for hyperkalemia; D/C drug, notify physician ▪ Monitor fluid retention (I&O, daily weight).

EDUCATION: Expect ↑ urine output; have bathroom facilities easily accessible ▪ May cause weakness, lethargy ▪ Take c̄ food/milk on waking, at same time qd, even if symptom free; take second dose (if ordered) after dinner ▪ Used to control, *not* cure, hypertension ▪ Notify physician of signs of hyperkalemia (weakness, tingling/numbness, irregular heartbeat) ▪ Avoid changing positions (lying/sitting/standing) rapidly ▪ Take as directed by physician; do *not* skip doses ▪ Avoid high-Na^+ foods (canned soups, lunch meats, cheese) ▪ Avoid high-K^+ foods (bananas, citrus juices, raisins) ▪ Check c̄ physician before using salt substitutes ▪ Maintain optimum weight ▪ Avoid exposure to direct sunlight, UV light (sunlamps); use sunscreen, protective clothing ▪ Check c̄ physician/ pharmacist before taking OTC preparations ▪ Store in tightly closed, light-resistant container ▪ Keep scheduled appointments c̄ physician; have BP checked regularly ▪ Full drug effect may require several wks of therapy.

NOTES:

trimethobenzamide hcl • (trye-meth-oh-ben-za-mide)

CATEGORY: *Antiemetic*

Rx; Preg Cat NA

BRAND NAME

Tigan (Roberts)

DOSAGE FORMS

Capsule: 100, 250mg
Injection (IM): 100mg/ml
Pediatric suppository: 100mg
Suppository: 200mg

USE: Control of N/V. **ACTION:** Antiemetic activity due to inhibition of chemoreceptor trigger zone in medulla.

PHARMACOKINETICS

Route	Onset	Duration	Excretion
PO	10-45m	3-4h	Via urine, feces as unchanged drug, metabolites
IM	15-40m	2-3h	

CONTRAINDICATIONS: Hypersensitivity, injection in children, suppositories in newborn infants, suppositories in pts hypersensitive to benzocaine. **CC:** Use in children c̄ viral diseases associated c̄ Reye's syndrome ▪ Not recommended for uncomplicated vomiting of children; use should be restricted to prolonged vomiting of known cause ▪ Use can produce extrapyramidal symptoms, hepatotoxicity.

DOSAGE

Pediatric	*PO*	
30-90 lb		100-200mg 3-4 times/d
	Rectal	
<30lb		100mg 3-4 times/d
30-90lb		100-200mg 3-4 times/d
Adult	*PO*	250mg 3-5 times/d
	IM	200mg 3-5 times/d
	Rectal	200mg 3-5 times/d

SIDE/ADVERSE EFFECTS: CNS: ***Parkinson-like symptoms, coma, convulsions,*** headache, drowsiness, dizziness, disorientation, mood depression ▪ EENT: blurred vision ▪ GI: diarrhea ▪ HEP: ***jaundice*** ▪ MS: muscle cramps, opisthotonos.

INTERACTIONS: Drug: Use c̄ CNS depressants can produce additive depression ▪ Use c̄ ototoxic drugs can mask their toxic effects ▪ Sequential use of antiemetic agents in pts recently given barbiturates, belladonna alkaloids, phenothiazines can result in opisthotonos, convulsions, coma, extrapyramidal symptoms.

NURSING MANAGEMENT PRIORITIES

ADMINISTRATION: Assess for hx of hypersensitivity ▪ PO: take c̄ H_2O; may empty capsule ▪ IM: administer via Z-track ▪ Do *not* administer IV ▪ Avoid exposure to light in storage ▪ Store suppositories in refrigerator.

EVALUATION: Monitor VS, esp BP ▪ Monitor F/E status ▪ Assess for potentiation of CNS depressants.

EDUCATION: Dizziness/drowsiness may occur; use caution in potentially hazardous activities ▪ Notify physician *immediately* of rash, lethargy, tremors; D/C drug ▪ Take 15-30m before activity that may precipitate vomiting ▪ Avoid use c̄ alcohol, other CNS depressants ▪ Use sugarless gum/hard candy to diminish dry mouth ▪ *Not* used to prevent motion sickness ▪ Procedure for suppository insertion.

NOTES:

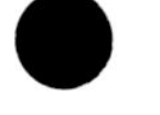

trimethoprim • (trye-meth-oh-prim)

CATEGORY: *Antiinfective:* urinary tract antimicrobial Rx; Preg Cat C

BRAND NAMES
Proloprim (G-W)
Trimpex (Roche)

DOSAGE FORMS
Tablet: 100, 200mg
Tablet: 100mg

DOSAGE
Adult *PO* 100mg q12h for 10d; use one-half dosage in pts c̄ creatinine clearance 15-30ml/m

USE: Treatment of initial episodes of uncomplicated UTIs caused by susceptible strains of *Enterobacter* spp, *Escherichia coli, Klebsiella* spp, *Proteus mirabilis, Staphylococcus,* coagulase-negative organisms. **ACTION:** Bacteriostatic activity due to inhibition of folic acid synthesis.

PHARMACOKINETICS

PO absorption	Peak	Half-life	Protein binding	Excretion
Rapid	1-4h	8-10h	44%	50%-60% via urine as unmetabolized drug (80%) in 24h

CONTRAINDICATIONS: Hypersensitivity, folate-deficient megaloblastic anemia. **CC:** Large doses of drug have been associated c̄ ⬇ hematopoiesis ▪ Use c̄ caution in pts c̄ known or suspected folate deficiency, impaired hepatic/ renal function.

SIDE/ADVERSE EFFECTS: GI: epigastric distress, N/V, glossitis ▪ HEM: ***thrombocytopenia,*** leukopenia, neutropenia, ***megaloblastic anemia,*** methemoglobinemia ▪ INT: *rash*, pruritus, ***exfoliative dermatitis*** ▪ MET: ⬆ serum transaminase, creatinine, BUN.

INTERACTIONS: Drug: Use c̄ phenytoin can ⬆ its activity.

NURSING MANAGEMENT PRIORITIES
ADMINISTRATION: Assess for hx of hypersensitivity ▪ Obtain C&S before therapy ▪ Assess renal function; may require ⬇ dosage if impaired ▪ Administer 1h ac/2h pc (c̄ food if GI irritation occurs) ▪ Administer folic acid concurrently if megaloblastic anemia is present ▪ Maintain hydration ▪ Avoid exposure to moisture in storage.

EVALUATION: Monitor hepatic, renal status ▪ Monitor VS, esp temperature ▪ Monitor CBC, UA ▪ Monitor I&O.

EDUCATION: Complete full course of therapy (usually 10d) even if symptoms subside ▪ Take on empty stomach c̄ full glass of H_2O; if upset stomach occurs, take c̄ food ▪ Take at equal intervals around clock to maintain blood levels ▪ Store in tightly closed, light-resistant container ▪ Discard unused, outdated preparations ▪ Maintain good personal hygiene (esp perineal, oral) ▪ ↑ Fluid intake (8-10 glasses/d) ▪ Notify physician of fever, sore throat, difficult breathing, rash, bruising/bleeding ▪ Women: avoid pregnancy, breastfeeding ▪ Do *not* give to infants or children.

NOTES:

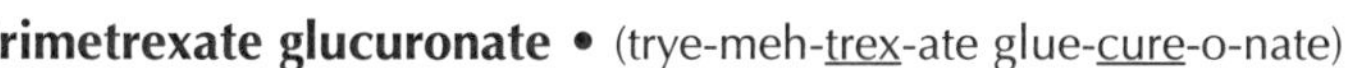

trimetrexate glucuronate • (trye-meh-trex-ate glue-cure-o-nate)

CATEGORY: *Antiprotozoan agent:* folic acid antagonist — Rx; Preg Cat D

BRAND NAME	DOSAGE FORM
Neutrexin (US Bioscience)	IV powder for injection: 25mg/vial

USE: Alternative treatment of moderate to severe *Pneumocystitis carinii* pneumonia in immunocompromised pts. **ACTION:** Antiprotozoan activity due to folic acid antagonism resulting in inhibition of nucleic acid (DNA, RNA) & protein synthesis in susceptible organisms producing cell death. Trimetrexate is also highly toxic to host cells (bone marrow suppression). To ⬇ this possibility, leucovorin (folic acid derivative) must be coadministered c̄ trimetrexate. However, leucovorin does not protect the pathogenic protozoan because it cannot penetrate into the protozoan cell.

PHARMACOKINETICS: Very limited studies have been done. A dose regimen of 30mg/m^2/d over 21d produces a biphasic plasma decline over 24h c̄ a terminal half-life of 7-15h. Protein binding is reported to be 95%-98%.

CONTRAINDICATIONS: Significant hypersensitivity to drug, leucovorin, or methotrexate. **CC:** Drug therapy must include concurrent use of leucovorin to preclude serious/fatal toxicities that include bone marrow depression, PO/GI ulceration, hepatic/renal dysfunction.

DOSAGE

Adult	*IV*	45mg/m^2/d infused over 60-90m for 21d c̄ leucovorin dose of 20mg/m^2 IV over 5-10m q6h or as a PO dose for 24d

SIDE/ADVERSE EFFECTS: CNS: confusion ▪ GI: N/V, ulcers ▪ HEM: anemia, *neutropenia*, ***thrombocytopenia*** ▪ HEP: ⬆ ALT, AST, alkaline phophatase, bilirubin ▪ INT: rash, pruritus ▪ MET: hypocalcemia, hyponatremia ▪ REN: ⬆ serum creatinine ▪ Other: fatigue, fever.

INTERACTIONS: Drug: Use c̄ acetaminophen, erythromycin, fluconazole, ketoconazole, miconazole, rifabutin, rifampin can alter trimetrexate activity & requires close monitoring.

NURSING MANAGEMENT PRIORITIES

ADMINISTRATION: Assess for hx of hypersensitivity ▪ Obtain C&S before therapy ▪ Assess renal function; may require ⬇ dosage if impaired ▪ Dilute according to manufacturer's directions; administer over 60-m period; flush IV line $\bar{c}$ 5% dextrose before, after administration ▪ Avoid contact $\bar{c}$ skin; wash thoroughly $\bar{c}$ soap & water ▪ Avoid exposure to heat/light in storage.

EVALUATION: Monitor VS, CBC ▪ Monitor hematologic, renal, hepatic function ▪ Avoid extravasation; assess for pain, redness at site ▪ Monitor renal function (nephrotoxicity); notify physician.

EDUCATION: Notify nurse/physician of pain, redness at IV injection site ▪ Notify physician *immediately* of bleeding/bruising, difficult breathing, rash.

NOTES:

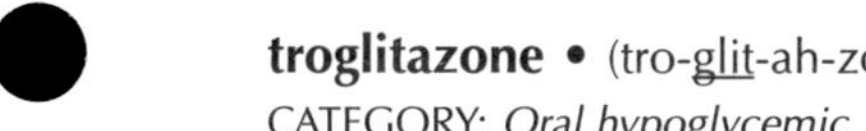

troglitazone • (tro-glit-ah-zone)

CATEGORY: *Oral hypoglycemic* Rx; Preg Cat B

BRAND NAME	**DOSAGE FORMS**
Rezulin (P-O)	Tablet: 200, 400mg

USE: Management of type II diabetes in pts c̄ insulin treatment (>30u/d) who exhibit inadequate control of hypoglycemia. **ACTION:** Antidiabetic activity due to improving target cell response to insulin resulting in ⬇ blood glucose levels. Drug ⬇ output of hepatic glucose (gluconeogenesis), ⬆ insulin-dependent glucose disposal in skeletal muscle, does not influence insulin secretion. Troglitazone is only active in presence of insulin.

PHARMACOKINETICS

PO absorption	Peak	Half-life	Protein binding	Excretion
Rapid	2-3h	16-34h	99%	Primarily via feces as metabolites

CONTRAINDICATIONS: Hypersensitivity. CC: Safety in nursing mothers, pediatric pts not established ▪ Use has resulted in extremely rare liver function test abnormalities ▪ Prior to troglitazone therapy, possible 2° causes (infection, poor insulin injection administration) or hyperglycemia should be investigated, ruled out.

DOSAGE

Adult	*PO*	Must be individualized. Start c̄ 200mg once/d c̄ current daily insulin injection. May be ⬆ after 2-4wks in responsive pts. Ususal dose is 400mg c̄ a daily maximum dose of 600mg. Adjustment in insulin dosage should be individualized based on glucose lowering response

SIDE/ADVERSE EFFECTS: CNS: headache (frequent), dizziness ▪ GI: N/D ▪ Other: infection (most frequent effect), pain, accidental injury, asthenia, rhinitis, peripheral edema, pharyngitis.

INTERACTIONS: Drug: Use c̄ PO contraceptives ⬇ plasma levels (≥30%) & may require an ⬆ in dosage ▪ Use c̄ terfenadine will ⬇ its therapeutic effect ▪ Use c̄ cholestyramine ⬇ troglitazone PO absorption by 70% & is not recommended for concurrent use. **Lab:** reversible elevations in AST, ALT ▪ Small ↑ in hemoglobin, hematocrit, neutrophil counts.

NURSING MANAGEMENT PRIORITIES

ADMINISTRATION: Assess for hx of hypersensitivity ▪ Assess for renal, hepatic function; may require ↓ dosage if impaired, use caution ▪ Administer c̄ meals.

EVALUATION: Monitor hepatic (liver function studies), renal, hematologic status ▪ Monitor FBS ▪ Evaluate pt closely during first few wks to assess effectiveness ▪ Monitor for signs of hypoglycemia/hyperglycemia ▪ Monitor for signs of infection; notify physician.

EDUCATION: Compliance c̄ special diet therapy ▪ Take meals as directed by physician ▪ Blood/urine glucose/ketone testing procedure ▪ Symptoms of hypoglycemia (anxiety, headache, fatigue, nausea, sweating); notify physician *immediately* ▪ Always carry lump of sugar/candy for quick use (hypoglycemia) ▪ Avoid use c̄ alcohol ▪ Notify physician *immediately* of symptoms of hyperglycemia (excessive hunger, thirst, urination, rapid pulse, sweet smelling breath, weight loss) ▪ Notify physician *immediately* of excessive weakness/tiredness, muscle pain difficulty breathing, stomach discomfort, dizziness, irregular heartbeats ▪ Maintain good personal hygiene ▪ Carry medical identification (MedicAlert) ▪ Store in tightly closed container ▪ Keep scheduled appointments for liver function studies/c̄ physician ▪ Notify physician of signs of infection (fever, sore throat) ▪ Maintain optimum body weight ▪ Women: notify physician of possible pregnancy; avoid breastfeeding ▪ PO hypoglycemic needs may change c̄ ↑ stress, ↑ exercise, ↑ appetite; notify physician.

NOTES:

valproic acid/valproate sodium▲ • (val-proe-ic)

CATEGORY: *Anticonvulsant* Rx; Preg Cat D

BRAND NAME
Depacon▲ (Abbott)
Depakene (Abbott)

DOSAGE FORMS
IV injection: 100mg/ml
Capsule: 250mg
Syrup▲: 250mg/5ml

USE: Treatment of simple/complex absence seizures incl petit mal ▪ Adjunct in treatment of multiple seizure types incl absence seizures. **ACTION:** Anticonvulsant mechanism not determined; studies indicate valproic acid may ↑ brain levels of γ-aminobutyric acid (GABA), an inhibitory neurotransmitter.

PHARMACOKINETICS

PO absorption	Peak	Half-life	Protein binding	Excretion
Rapid	1-4h	6-16h	90%	Via urine as unchanged drug, metabolites

CONTRAINDICATIONS: Hypersensitivity, hepatic disease, significant hepatic dysfunction. **CC:** Use associated c̄ severe/fatal hepatic failure usually w/in first 6mos of treatment ▪ Use during pregnancy may produce teratogenic effects ▪ Drugs are excreted in breast milk.

DOSAGE

Pediatric/Adult *PO*	Initial dose 15mg/kg/d, ↑ at 1-wk intervals by 5-10mg/kg/d until seizures controlled or adverse effects preclude further ↑; maximum daily dose 60mg/kg/d
IV	20mg/m infusion over 60m. Do *not* use for more than 14d

SIDE/ADVERSE EFFECTS: CNS: sedation, ataxia, headache, nystagmus, diplopia, asterixis, dysarthria, dizziness, incoordination ▪ END: irregular menses, secondary amenorrhea, breast enlargement (rare), galactorrhea, abnormal thyroid tests ▪ GI: *N/V/D, gastric distress,* abdominal cramps, ***pancreatitis*** ▪ HEM: ***thrombocytopenia,*** leukopenia, eosinophilia ▪ HEP: dose-related ↑ AST, ALT, LDH; severe behavioral deterioration.

INTERACTIONS: Drug: Use c̄ CNS depressants can produce additive depression ▪ Use c̄ barbiturates may produce ↑ serum levels of barbiturates ▪ Use c̄ clonazepam may produce absence status ▪ Use c̄ drugs affecting coagulation best avoided ▪ Use c̄ phenytoin may produce breakthrough seizures.

NURSING MANAGEMENT PRIORITIES

ADMINISTRATION: Assess for hx of hypersensitivity ▪ Assess hepatic function; do *not* administer if impaired ▪ Administer capsules whole; do *not* crush/chew ▪ Avoid abrupt withdrawal; D/C gradually; institute strict seizure precautions if drug abruptly withdrawn ▪ Avoid exposure to moisture/light in storage; do *not* refrigerate.

EVALUATION: Monitor hepatic, renal, cardiac, respiratory status ▪ Monitor occurrence/characteristics of seizures ▪ Monitor activity status (safety precautions) ▪ May produce false + urine ketones ▪ Therapeutic blood levels: 50-100μg/ml.

EDUCATION: Drowsiness may occur; use caution in potentially hazardous activities ▪ Avoid use c̄ alcohol, other CNS depressants ▪ Take as ordered by physician; do *not* ↑ dose ▪ Take c̄ food to ↓ GI distress; swallow capsules whole ▪ Dietary protein restrictions (hyperammonemia) ▪ Notify physician/dentist of use before treatment ▪ Notify physician *immediately* of bruising/bleeding ▪ Check c̄ physician/pharmacist before taking OTC preparations ▪ Store in tightly closed, light-resistant container ▪ Carry identification (MedicAlert) ▪ Do *not* omit daily dose.

NOTES:

vancomycin hcl • (van-koe-mye-sin)

CATEGORY: *Antibiotic*

Rx; Preg Cat C

BRAND NAMES	DOSAGE FORMS
Vancocin HCl (Lilly)	Capsule: 125, 250mg Powder for injection (IV): 500mg, 1g/vial Powder for PO solution: 1-, 10-g container
Vancoled (Lederle)	Powder for injection (IV): 500mg/vial

USE: Treatment of severe infections due to susceptible methicillin-resistant strains of staphylococci ▪ Endocarditis caused by staphylococci, *Streptococcus* spp, diphtheroids ▪ In combination c̄ an aminoglycoside for enterococcal endocarditis ▪ In combination c̄ rifampin for endocarditis ▪ Alternative in penicillin-allergic pts c̄ heart damage who require dental procedures ▪ Life-threatening infections that are resistant to less toxic antibiotics ▪ PO treatment (drug not absorbed) of staphylococcal enterocolitis & antibiotic-induced pseudomembranous colitis produced by *Clostridium difficile*. **ACTION:** Antibacterial activity due to inhibition of cell wall synthesis in susceptible organisms. The drug also affects cell membrane permeability, RNA synthesis.

PHARMACOKINETICS

IV peak	Half-life	Protein binding	Excretion
5m	4-6h	55%	80% of a single dose via urine after 24h as unchanged drug

CONTRAINDICATIONS: Hypersensitivity. **CC:** Rapid IV bolus administration has been associated c̄ hypotension, rare cases of cardiac arrest ▪ PO formulations have poor PO absorption, are intended for treatment of colitis.

DOSAGE

IV: For normal renal function, c̄ each dose administered over a 60-m period

Neonate	Initial dose of 15mg/kg, followed by 10mg/kg q12h for first week of life & q8h thereafter up to age of 1mo
Pediatric	40mg/kg/24h in divided doses
Adult	2g/d divided (500mg q6h or 1g q12h)

PO

Pediatric	40mg/kg/d in 3-4 divided doses for 7-10d. Do *not* exceed 2g/d
Adult	0.5-2g/d in 3-4 divided doses for 7-10d

SIDE/ADVERSE EFFECTS: EENT: ***autotoxicity c̄ hearing loss*** ▪ GU: ***nephrotoxicity*** c̄ rare renal failure ▪ HEM: reversible neutropenia, ***rare thrombocytopenia*** ▪ INT: rash, ***rare Stevens-Johnson syndrome***, ***toxic epidermal necrolysis*** ▪ Other: ***infrequent pseudomembranous colitis***, tissue irritation at IV site.

INTERACTIONS: Drug: Use c̄ autotoxic & nephrotoxic drugs produces additive effects.

NURSING MANAGEMENT PRIORITIES

ADMINISTRATION: Assess for hx of hypersensitivity ▪ Obtain C&S before therapy ▪ Obtain pt weight for dose calculation ▪ Determine creatinine clearance before administration ▪ PO: used to treat local intestinal infections; reconstitute powder according to manufacturer's directions c̄ distilled/deionized H_2O, stable for 14d (refrigerated) ▪ IV: administer via IV infusion only, over 60-m period; prepare according to manufacturer's directions, stable for 96h (refrigerated) ▪ Maintain hydration ▪ Elderly pts may require ↓ dosage.

EVALUATION: Monitor VS, esp temperature ▪ Assess hearing (ototoxicity), UA (nephrotoxicity); notify physician ▪ Monitor CBC (leukopenia, neutropenia); notify physician ▪ Assess for "red neck" syndrome (hypotension, erythema of face, neck, upper body) ▪ IV: avoid extravasation; assess for pain, edema, redness at insertion site ▪ May ↑ BUN.

EDUCATION: Drowsiness may occur; use caution in potentially hazardous activities ▪ Notify nurse/physician *immediately* of hearing disturbances, difficult breathing, blood in urine ▪ May cause unpleasant taste.

NOTES:

vasopressin • (vay-soe-press-in)

CATEGORY: *Posterior pituitary hormone:* antidiuretic

Rx; Preg Cat NA

BRAND NAME
Pitressin (P-D)

DOSAGE FORMS
Injection (aqueous) (IM/SC): 20 pressor U/ml

USE: Treatment of abdominal distention, diabetes insipidus ▪ Abdominal roentgenography. **ACTION:** Vasopressin causes contraction of smooth muscle of GI tract, vascular beds; antidiuretic activity due to H_2O reabsorption in renal tubule. **USE:** Treatment of abdominal distention, diabetes insipidus ▪ Abdominal roentgenography.

PHARMACOKINETICS: Aqueous injection has duration of antidiuretic activity 2-8h, oil-based injection 48-72h.

CONTRAINDICATIONS: Hypersensitivity. **CC:** Use can produce H_2O intoxication ▪ Extravasation will produce severe local neurosis, vasoconstriction ▪ Use c̄ caution in pts c̄ coronary artery disease, other vascular disorders.

DOSAGE: *IM* is preferred route

Adult

Abdominal distention	Usual postop dose 5U initially, ⬆ to 10U prn for subsequent administration IM/SC
Abdominal roentgenography	10U injection given 2h & ½h, respectively, before procedure
Diabetes insipidus	5-10U repeated 2-3 times/d prn. Aqueous injection: can be administered by nasal spray/on pledgets inserted into nose. Dosage must be individualized. Oil injection: 0.3-1ml IM, repeat prn

SIDE/ADVERSE EFFECTS: CNS: tremor, vertigo, head pain, sweating ▪ GI: cramps, flatulence, N/V ▪ INT: urticaria ▪ RESP: bronchial constriction ▪ Other: ***anaphylaxis,*** pallor.

INTERACTIONS: Drug: Use c̄ chlorpropamide/clofibrate may enhance antidiuretic effect ▪ Use c̄ lithium, alcohol, demeclocycline may block antidiuretic effect.

NURSING MANAGEMENT PRIORITIES

ADMINISTRATION: Assess for hx of hypersensitivity ▪ Assess bowel sounds, measure abdominal girth before administration ▪ Administer 1-2 glasses H_2O immediately after injection (⬆ effectiveness).

EVALUATION: Monitor VS, esp BP ▪ Monitor F/E status (I&O, specific gravity, daily weight) esp in children ▪ Assess for H_2O intoxication (lethargy, confusion, headache) ▪ Assess for urinary retention, abdominal distention (use rectal tube to expel flatus) ▪ Monitor IV site closely; prevent extravasation.

EDUCATION: Notify physician of ↑ thirst, ↑ urination ▪ Rectal tube will be inserted to relieve gas/fullness in abdomen ▪ Avoid ingestion of concentrated fluids, excessive use of alcohol, acetaminophen (Tylenol) ▪ IM injection may be painful ▪ Procedure for specific gravity determination.

NOTES:

venlafaxine • (ven-lah-<u>fax</u>-een)

CATEGORY: *Antidepressant* Rx; Preg Cat C

BRAND NAME
Effexor (W-A)

DOSAGE FORMS
Tablet: 25, 37.5, 50, 75, 100mg

USE: Treatment of depression. **ACTION:** Antidepressant activity appears related to inhibition of serotonin (5-hydroxytryptamine) & norepinephrine reuptake in cranial neurons. Also, drug exhibits weak inhibition of dopamine reuptake. Avoid abrupt withdrawal of drug.

PHARMACOKINETICS

PO absorption	Half-life	Protein binding	Excretion
>90%	5-11h	25%-29%	87% of PO dose via urine as unchanged drug, metabolites in 48h

CONTRAINDICATIONS: Hypersensitivity, MAO-I. **CC:** Use associated c̄ sustained hypertension, rare cases of seizures ▪ Use can result in possible activation of mania/hypomania, treatment emergence anxiety ▪ Use c̄ caution in pts c̄ hepatic/renal disease.

DOSAGE

Adult	*PO*	For normal, hepatic, renal function, initiate c̄ 75mg/d in 2-3 divided doses c̄ meals. If required, ↑ dose in increments of 75mg/d about q5d to maximum of 350mg/d in 3 divided doses

SIDE/ADVERSE EFFECTS: CNS: anxiety, dizziness, nervousness, headache, insomnia/somnolence, tremor, abnormal dreams ▪ CV: hypertension, vasodilation ▪ EENT: blurred vision, tinnitus ▪ GI: N/V/D, anorexia, constipation, dyspepsia, flatulence ▪ GU: impotence, orgasm/ejaculation irregularities ▪ INT: pruritus, rash, sweating ▪ Other: asthenia, yawning, urinary frequency.

INTERACTIONS: Drug: Use c̄ MAO-I best avoided ▪ Use c̄ cimetidine can result in slight ↑ of venlafaxine activity.

NURSING MANAGEMENT PRIORITIES

ADMINISTRATION: Assess for hx of hypersensitivity ▪ Assess hepatic, renal function; may require ↓ dosage if impaired ▪ Assess for hx of seizures; use caution ▪ Administer c̄ food to ↓ GI distress ▪ Institute safety, seizure precautions ▪ Institute suicide precautions ▪ Avoid abrupt withdrawal; D/C gradually ▪ Avoid moisture/heat/direct light in storage ▪ Elderly pts may require ↓ dosage.

EVALUATION: Monitor CV, hepatic, renal status ▪ Monitor fluid retention (I&O, daily weight), constipation ▪ Assess for weight loss (anorectic effect) ▪ Assess for symptoms of abrupt withdrawal (nausea, headache, malaise) ▪ Assess for actual swallowing of PO forms ▪ Assess for skin rash, hives; notify physician, D/C drug ▪ Diabetics: monitor blood glucose (hypoglycemia).

EDUCATION: Dizziness may occur; use caution in potentially hazardous activities ▪ Avoid changing positions (lying/sitting/standing) rapidly ▪ Avoid use c̄ alcohol, other CNS depressants for up to 1wk after end of therapy ▪ Take c̄ food ▪ Take as directed by physician ▪ Use sugarless gum/hard candy to diminish dry mouth ▪ Constipation may occur; ↑ fluids, bulk-containing foods ▪ Notify physician/dentist of use before treatment ▪ Notify physician of skin rash, hives; D/C drug ▪ Check c̄ physician/pharmacist before taking OTC/Rx preparations ▪ Store in tightly closed, light-resistant container ▪ Encourage recreational/diversional interests ▪ Notify physician of weight loss, fever, sore throat, malaise ▪ Keep scheduled appointments c̄ physician ▪ Women: notify physician of possibility of pregnancy; avoid breastfeeding ▪ Full drug effects may require several wks of therapy.

NOTES:

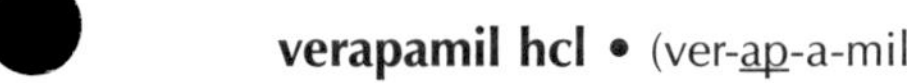

verapamil hcl • (ver-ap-a-mill) 324

CATEGORY: *Calcium blocker:* antianginal, antiarrhythmic, slow channel blocker Rx; Preg Cat C

BRAND NAMES	**DOSAGE FORMS**
Calan (Searle)	SR caplets: 120, 180, 240mg
	Tablet: 40, 80, 120mg
Isoptin (Knoll)	Injection (IV): 5mg/2ml
	Tablet: 40, 80, 120mg
**Isoptin Oral (Searle)*	Tablet: 80, 120mg
Verelan (Lederle)	SR capsule: 120, 180, 240mg

USE: Treatment of chronic stable, vasospastic, unstable angina pectoris (PO) ▪ Treatment of paroxysmal supraventricular tachycardia (IV) ▪ Prophylaxis of paroxysmal supraventricular tachycardia ▪ Temporary control of rapid ventricular rate in atrial flutter/atrial fibrillation (IV) ▪ Treatment of essential hypertension (SR only). **ACTION:** Antianginal effect due to inhibition of extracellular calcium-ion transmembrane migration in cardiac, vascular smooth muscle via slow channel passageway, resulting in coronary dilation; ↑ myocardial oxygen supply, ↓ oxygen-consumption. Antiarrhythmic effect due to sinus arrest in sick sinus syndrome; slowing of conduction, lengthening of refractory period in atrioventricular node.

CONTRAINDICATIONS: Hypersensitivity, severe hypotension/cardiogenic shock, 2°/3° atrioventricular block, sick sinus syndrome (except $\bar{c}$ pacemaker), CHF (unless 2° to supraventricular tachycardia amenable to verapamil IV), IV β-adrenergic administration, atrial flutter $\bar{c}$ hx of accessory bypass tracts (IV), severe left ventricular dysfunction (PO). **CC:** IV administration must be given over a ≥2-m period.

PHARMACOKINETICS

	PO absorption	Onset	Peak	Half-life	Protein binding	Excretion
PO	90%	30m	1-2h	2-5h	90%	70% via urine, 16% in feces in 5d as metabolites
IV	—	3-5m	5m	4.5-12h	90%	

Note: Side/adverse effects: common in *italic;* serious in ***boldface italic.*** *Available in Canada only.

DOSAGE

Pediatric	*IV*	≤1y/o: 0.1-0.2mg/kg as bolus over 2m. Repeat dose may be given after 30m. 1-15y/o: 0.1-0.3mg/kg as bolus over 2m. Do *not* exceed 5mg/dose. Repeat dose (not exceeding 10mg) may be given after 30m
Adult	*PO*	Starting dose 80mg 3-4 times/d, c̄ daily range 240-480mg. Optimum dose range usually 320-480mg/d. Daily dose >480mg not currently established
	IV	5-10mg as bolus over 2m. Repeat dose ≤10mg may be given after 30m
Geriatric	*IV*	5-10mg as bolus over 3m. Repeat dose ≤10mg may be given after 30m

SIDE/ADVERSE EFFECTS: CNS: *dizziness*, headache, insomnia, confusion ▪ CV: *hypotension*, peripheral edema, ***AV block,*** bradycardia, CHF ▪ EENT: blurred vision ▪ GI: *constipation,* nausea ▪ GU: gynecomastia, spotty menstruation ▪ INT: alopecia ▪ MS: muscle cramps.

INTERACTIONS: Drug: Use c̄ dig may ⬆ dig body levels ▪ Use c̄ disopyramide best avoided ▪ Use c̄ antihypertensives may ⬆ hypotensive effects.

NURSING MANAGEMENT PRIORITIES

ADMINISTRATION: Assess for hx of hypersensitivity, heart failure (use c̄ caution) ▪ Assess BP, heart rate; if apical pulse <60, hold dose, notify physician ▪ IV: cardiac monitor; administer IV, over 2m (3m for elderly); maintain supine position 1h after administration ▪ Avoid exposure to light/freezing ▪ Do *not* administer discolored/precipitated solutions ▪ Have emergency support equipment available ▪ Elderly pts may require ⬇ dosage.

EVALUATION: Monitor VS, esp BP (IV: q5-10m), heart rate; I&O; hepatic, renal status ▪ Assess for CHF, notify physician ▪ Digitalized pts: assess for dig toxicity (bradycardia, anorexia, palpitations).

EDUCATION: Dizziness may occur; use caution in potentially hazardous activities ▪ Avoid changing positions (lying/sitting/standing) rapidly ▪ Procedure for checking radial pulse ▪ If pulse slow (<60)/irregular, do *not* take dose, notify physician ▪ Avoid use c̄ caffeine, alcohol ▪ Check c̄ physician/ pharmacist before taking OTC preparations ▪ Take as ordered by physician; do *not* change dose ▪ Notify physician of difficult breathing, chest pain, swelling of hands or legs; D/C drug ▪ Keep appointments c̄ physician ▪ Continue to use sublingual nitroglycerin (if ordered) to relieve sudden chest pain or for prophylaxis before exertion.

NOTES:

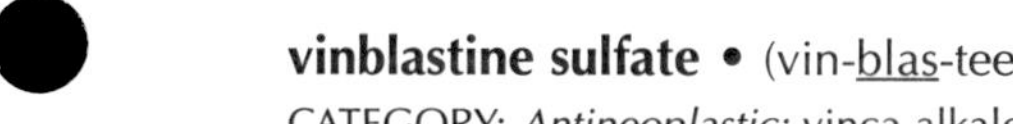

vinblastine sulfate • (vin-blas-teen)

CATEGORY: *Antineoplastic:* vinca alkaloid

Rx; Preg Cat D

BRAND NAMES	DOSAGE FORMS
Velban (Lilly)	Powder for injection (IV): 10-mg vial
**Velbe (Lilly)*	Powder for injection (IV): 10-mg vial

USE: Palliation of advanced carcinoma of testes, generalized Hodgkin's disease, histiocytic lymphoma, Kaposi's sarcoma, Letterer-Siwe disease, lymphocytic lymphoma, mycosis fungoides ▪ Breast cancer, choriocarcinoma unresponsive to other treatment. **ACTION:** Antineoplastic activity due to microtubular protein binding, resulting in mitotic arrest during metaphase; drug also interferes c̄ glutamic acid, aspartate metabolism, nucleic acid synthesis; vinblastine also exerts immunosuppressive activity.

PHARMACOKINETICS: Limited studies indicate rapid distribution from blood into body tissue; drug metabolized in liver, excreted via urine, feces.

CONTRAINDICATIONS: Leukopenia, bacterial infection. **CC:** For IV use only. Fatal if administered intrathecally.

DOSAGE: *(IV)* Leukopenic response to drug usually restricts administration to single weekly doses; recommended weekly schedule:

	Pediatric	Adult
Dose 1	2.5mg/m^2	3.7mg/m^2
Dose 2	3.75mg/m^2	5.5mg/m^2
Dose 3	5mg/m^2	7.4mg/m^2
Dose 4	6.25mg/m^2	9.25mg/m^2
Dose 5	7.5mg/m^2	11.1mg/m^2

Dose should not be ↑ after dose that ↓ WBC to 3000 cells/mm^3. Maintenance dose should be 1 increment lower than dose that will produce leukopenia count of 3000. Do *not* administer weekly dose, even though 7d may have elapsed, until WBC ≥ 4000. Duration of maintenance varies c̄ disease, combination of drugs used.

SIDE/ADVERSE EFFECTS: CNS: numbness, peripheral neuritis, paresthesias, headache, loss of deep tendon reflexes, ***convulsions***, depression ▪ GI: N/V, anorexia, PO vesiculation, pharyngitis, ***rectal bleeding, peptic ulcer hemorrhage, hemorrhagic enterocolitis*** ▪ HEM: *leukopenia* ▪ INT: local rxs (cellulitis, phlebitis, sloughing at IV site) ▪ Other: weakness, vesiculation of skin, pain at tumor site.

Note: Side/adverse effects: common in *italic;* serious in ***boldface italic.***

*Available in Canada only.

INTERACTIONS: Drug: Use of live vaccines contraindicated during therapy ■ Radiation therapy, bone marrow depressants produce additive bone marrow depression.

NURSING MANAGEMENT PRIORITIES

ADMINSTRATION: Check pt hx for recent course of radiation or antineoplastic agents; report to physician ■ Assess hepatic function; ↓ dosage if impaired ■ Avoid exposure to moisture/light in storage ■ Avoid contact c̄ eyes during preparation ■ Administer antiemetic before therapy ■ Avoid IM injections during therapy ■ Provide emotional support ■ Reconstitute c̄ 10ml NaCl injection; may administer IVPB, direct IV (over 1m); may refrigerate for 30d w/out loss of potency ■ Rinse needle, syringe c̄ venous blood before withdrawal.

EVALUATION: Monitor VS (avoid rectal temperature) ■ Monitor CBC throughout therapy; if WBC <4000, platelets <100,000/mm^3, do not administer ■ Assess for infection, bleeding, anemia ■ May produce ↑ serum uric acid level ■ Monitor hepatic function ■ Assess abdominal distention, bowel sounds; administer laxative as ordered for constipation ■ Monitor IV site closely; avoid extravasation ■ Assess hydration status (I&O, daily weight) ■ Assess for neurotoxicity, skin breakdown ■ Assess for mental depression.

EDUCATION: Store in tightly closed, light-resistant container ■ ↑ Fluid intake (8-10 glasses/d) ■ Avoid exposure to infection ■ Check c̄ physician before immunization (pt, family) ■ Diet as tolerated; avoid spicy foods ■ Maintain good oral hygiene; use soft-bristled toothbrush ■ Notify physician of symptoms of bone marrow depression (fever, sore throat, bruising, bleeding, lethargy) ■ Women: avoid breastfeeding ■ Avoid exposure to direct sunlight, UV light (sunlamps); use sunscreen, protective clothing ■ Encourage ventilation of feelings ■ Use contraception if sexually active.

NOTES:

vincristine sulfate • (vin-kris-teen)

CATEGORY: *Antineoplastic:* vinca alkaloid

Rx; Preg Cat D

BRAND NAME	DOSAGE FORM
Oncovin (Lilly)	Injection (IV): 1mg/ml

USE: Treatment of acute leukemia, esp pediatric lymphoblastic ▪ Treatment of Hodgkin's disease, lymphosarcoma, reticulum cell sarcoma, rhabdomyosarcoma, neuroblastoma, Wilms' tumor. **ACTION:** Antineoplastic activity due to microtubular protein binding, resulting in mitotic arrest during metaphase.

PHARMACOKINETICS: Limited studies indicate rapid distribution from blood into body tissue; drug metabolized in liver, exhibits high protein binding, long half-life; is excreted primarily via feces, c̄ some renal excretion.

CONTRAINDICATIONS: Demyelinating form of Charcot-Marie-Tooth disease. **CC:** For IV use only. Fatal if administered intrathecally.

DOSAGE

Pediatric	*IV*	$2mg/m^2$ at weekly intervals
Adult	*IV*	$1.4mg/m^2$ at weekly intervals

SIDE/ADVERSE EFFECTS: CNS: neuritic pain, sensory loss, paresthesia, slapping gait, loss of deep tendon reflexes, ***convulsions,*** footdrop, cranial nerve manifestations ▪ CV: hypertension ▪ EENT: photophobia, diplopia, transient cortical blindness ▪ GI: N/V, constipation, PO ulceration, cramps; paralytic ileus, esp in children ▪ HEM: anemia (rare), leukopenia ▪ INT: *alopecia* ▪ Other: syndrome attributed to inappropriate antidiuretic hormone secretion c̄ high degree of Na^+ excretion, jaw pain, bone pain, limb pain.

INTERACTIONS: Drug: Use of live vaccines best avoided during therapy ▪ Radiation therapy, bone marrow depressants produce additive bone marrow depression ▪ Use c̄ neurotoxic drugs produces additive neurotoxicity.

NURSING MANAGEMENT PRIORITIES

ADMINISTRATION: Assess pt for hx, recent course of radiation/antineoplastic agents; report to physician ▪ Assess hepatic function; ↓ dosage if impaired ▪ Avoid exposure to moisture/light in storage ▪ Reconstitute according to manufacturer's directions; may administer direct IV (over 1m)

▪ Avoid contact c̄ eyes during preparation ▪ Administer antiemetic before therapy ▪ Avoid IM injection during therapy ▪ Provide emotional support ▪ Rinse needle, syringe c̄ venous blood before withdrawal.

EVALUATION: Monitor VS (avoid rectal temperature) ▪ Monitor CBC throughout therapy; if WBC <4000, platelets <100,000/mm^3, do *not* administer ▪ Assess for infection, bleeding, anemia ▪ Monitor hepatic function ▪ Assess abdominal distention, bowel sounds; administer laxative as ordered for constipation ▪ Monitor IV site closely; avoid extravasation ▪ Assess hydration status (I&O, daily weight) ▪ Assess for mental depression, neurotoxicity (ataxia, ⬇ LOC, tremors).

EDUCATION: Store in tightly closed, light-resistant container ▪ ⬆ Fluid intake (8-10 glasses/d) ▪ Avoid exposure to infection ▪ Check c̄ physician before immunization (pt, family) ▪ Diet as tolerated; avoid spicy foods ▪ Maintain good oral hygiene; use soft-bristled toothbrush ▪ Notify physician of symptoms of bone marrow depression (fever, sore throat, bruising, bleeding, lethargy) ▪ Loss of hair may occur (reversible) ▪ Women: avoid breastfeeding ▪ Encourage ventilation of feelings ▪ Use contraception if sexually active.

NOTES:

vinorelbine tartrate • (vin-oh-rell-bean)

CATEGORY: *Antineoplastic:* semisynthetic vinca alkaloid — Rx; Preg Cat D

BRAND NAME	DOSAGE FORM
Navelbine (G-W)	Injection (IV): 10mg/ml

USE: Treatment of non–small cell lung cancer as a sole agent/in combination c̄ cisplatin. **ACTION:** Antineoplastic activity due to microtubular protein (tublin) binding, resulting in mitotic arrest during metaphase; drug also interferes c̄ cyclic adenosine monophosphate, glutathione metabolism, nucleic acid synthesis, cellular respiration.

PHARMACOKINETICS: Limited studies indicate rapid distribution from blood into body tissue; drug metabolized in liver, high protein binding (80%-92%), long half-life (up to 43.6h); excreted primarily via feces c̄ some renal excretion.

CONTRAINDICATIONS: Pretreatment granulocyte count <1000/mm². **CC:** Requires experienced physician for administration ▪ ⬆ Susceptibility to infection due to granulocytopenia ▪ Avoid extravasation by proper needle/catheter positioning.

DOSAGE

Adult	*IV*	30mg/m² over 6-10m once/wk. Dose for cisplatin combination therapy is 120mg/m² on day 1 & day 29, thereafter q6wks

SIDE/ADVERSE EFFECTS: CNS: paresthesia, hypesthesia ▪ CV: chest pain, ***rare MI***, chemical phlebitis at injection site ▪ GI: N/V/D, constipation ▪ HEM: anemia, ***granulocytopenia, leukopenia*** ▪ INT: *alopecia* ▪ Other: shortness of breath, fatigue, pain at injection site, jaw pain, hemorrhagic cystitis.

INTERACTIONS: Drug: Use c̄ cisplatin will produce additive granulocytopenia ▪ Use c̄ mitomycin can result in acute pulmonary rxs. **Lab:** ⬆ AST, bilirubin serum levels ▪ Transient ⬆ liver enzymes.

NURSING MANAGEMENT PRIORITIES

ADMINISTRATION: Check pt hx for recent course of radiation or antineoplastic agents; report to physician ▪ Assess hepatic function; ⬇ dosage if impaired ▪ Avoid exposure to moisture/light in storage ▪ Use gloves in preparation/handling; wash areas of contact thoroughly c̄ soap, water ■ Avoid contact c̄ eyes during preparation ■ Administer antiemetic before therapy ■ Avoid IM injections during therapy ■ Provide emotional support ■ Dilute according to manufacturer's directions; administer direct IV (over 6-10m); may store for 24h w/out loss of potency at room light & temperature; protect from light/freezing in storage.

EVALUATION: Monitor VS (avoid rectal temperature) ■ Monitor CBC throughout therapy; if WBC <4000, platelets <100,000/mm^3, do not administer ■ Assess for infection, bleeding, anemia ■ May produce ↑ serum uric acid level ■ Monitor hepatic function ■ Assess abdominal distention, bowel sounds; administer laxative as ordered for constipation ■ Monitor IV site closely; avoid extravasation ■ Assess hydration status (I&O, daily weight) ■ Assess for neurotoxicity, skin breakdown ■ Assess for mental depression.

EDUCATION: Store in tightly closed, light-resistant container ■ ↑ Fluid intake (8-10 glasses/d) ■ Avoid exposure to infection ■ Check c̄ physician before immunization (pt, family) ■ Diet as tolerated; avoid spicy foods ■ Maintain good oral hygiene; use soft-bristled toothbrush ■ Notify physician of symptoms of bone marrow depression (fever, sore throat, bruising, bleeding, lethargy) ■ Women: notify physician of possible pregnancy; avoid breastfeeding ■ Avoid exposure to direct sunlight, UV light (sun lamps); use sunscreen, protective clothing ■ Encourage ventilation of feelings ■ Use contraception if sexually active.

NOTES:

CATEGORY: *Coumarin anticoagulant* Rx; Preg Cat X

BRAND NAMES
Coumadin (Du Pont)

**Warfilone Sodium*

DOSAGE FORMS
Injection (IM/IV): 50mg/vial
Tablet: 1, 2, 2.5, 5, 7.5, 10mg
Tablet: 2, 2.5, 5, 7.5, 10mg

USE: Adjunct in coronary occlusion ▪ Treatment of thromboembolic complications associated c̄ atrial fibrillation, cardiac valve replacement ▪ Prophylaxis, treatment of venous thrombosis, pulmonary embolism. **ACTION:** Coumarin anticoagulants inhibit synthesis of prothrombin (factor II), proconvertin (factor VII), Christmas factor (factor IX), Stuart-Prower factor (factor X) in liver by interfering c̄ action of vitamin K.

CONTRAINDICATIONS: Hypersensitivity, subacute bacterial endocarditis, any bleeding/potential bleeding condition, pregnancy. **CC: Drug:** Use may enhance release of atheromatous plaque emboli, ⬆ risk of systemic cholesterol microembolization incl "purple toe syndrome," which indicates D/C of therapy ▪ Use c̄ caution in presence of known/suspected vitamin C deficiency, severe to moderate hypertension, hepatic/renal impairment, trauma. **Food:** Ingestion of green, leafy vegetables ⬇ therapeutic effects.

DOSAGE

Adult *PO*	PT determines maintenance dose, usually 2-10mg/d

SIDE/ADVERSE EFFECTS: GI/GU: ***hemorrhage*** ▪ HEM: ***agranulocytosis,*** leukopenia, anemia ▪ HEP: hepatitis, jaundice ▪ INT: dermatitis, urticaria, alopecia ▪ Other: fever.

INTERACTIONS: Drug: List of drug interactions extremely long; main interactions that ⬆ anticoagulant activity include enzyme ⬇ of biotransformation, displacement from inactive protein storage sites, ⬇ intestinal absorption of vitamin K, alteration of intestinal bacterial flora, alteration of platelet count/activity ▪ Main interaction that ⬇ anticoagulant activity is enzyme induction of biotransformation ▪ Drugs that ⬆ activity incl anabolic steroids, broad-spectrum antibiotics, clofibrate, dextrothyroxine, disulfiram, oxyphenbutazone, phenylbutazone, salicylates ▪ Drugs that ↓ activity incl barbiturates, cholestyramine, estrogens, glutethimide, PO contraceptives.

NURSING MANAGEMENT PRIORITIES

ADMINISTRATION: Assess for hx of coumarin anticoagulant hypersensitivity ▪ PO: administer as single daily dose c̄ food ▪ Avoid abrupt withdrawal ▪ Avoid exposure to moisture in storage ▪ Regulate dosage according to PT ▪ Have vitamin K available ▪ Elderly pts may require ↓ dosage.

EVALUATION: Monitor hepatic, renal status ▪ Monitor PT; maintain at 1.5-2.5 times control value ▪ Monitor serum for ↑ ALT, AST, LDH ▪ Observe pt for signs of hemorrhage, incl abdominal/lumbar pain; treat c̄ vitamin K/whole blood.

EDUCATION: Notify physician *immediately* of unusual bleeding/bruising, blood detected in urine/stool ▪ Take c̄ food ▪ Follow dosage exactly as prescribed by physician ▪ Use electric razor/depilatory for hair removal ▪ Check c̄ physician/pharmacist before taking OTC preparations ▪ Avoid aspirin-containing products ▪ Avoid engaging in contact sports, other potentially injurious activities ▪ Do *not* change dietary habits in relation to daily intake of fat, green leafy vegetables, fish, vitamin K, alcoholic beverages ▪ Keep laboratory appointments as scheduled for PT determination ▪ Women: avoid pregnancy, breastfeeding; report menstrual flow ▪ Carry identification (MedicAlert) if receiving anticoagulant therapy ▪ Notify physician/dentist of anticoagulant use before treatment ▪ May turn urine red/brown ▪ Avoid changing brand-name preparations.

NOTES:

zafirlukast/zileuton • (za-fear-lew-cast/zi-lew-ton)

CATEGORY: *Antiasthmatic:* leukotriene modifier Rx; Preg Cat B/C

BRAND NAMES	DOSAGE FORMS
zafirlukast	
Accolate (Zenica)	Tablet: 20mg
zileuton	
Zyflo (Abbott)	Tablet: 600mg

USE: Prophylaxis & treatment for adults/children >12y/o c̄ chronic asthma. **ACTION:** Antiasthmatic activity due to modification of physiologic activities of leukotriene agonists in pathogenesis of asthma. Leukotrienes produce bronchoconstriction, edema, inflammation, mucus secretions. Zafirlukast is a selective competitive antagonist of leukotrienic activity at leukotrienic receptor sites on respiratory smooth muscle resulting in antagonized muscular constriction. Zileuton is a specific inhibitor of the enzyme 5-lepoxygenase resulting in inhibition of leukotriene formation.

CONTRAINDICATIONS: Hypersensitivity, active liver disease or 43 times upper normal transaminase levels for zileuton. **CC:** Safety in children <12y/o, nursing mothers not established ▪ Not indicated for acute asthma attacks ▪ Use c̄ caution c̄ liver impairment & monitor ALT levels for toxicity ▪ Zafirlukast can ↑ incidence of infection in pts who are >55y/o.

DOSAGE: Adult/Children >12y/o *PO*

zafirlukast	20mg bid 1h ac or 2h pc
zileuton	600mg qid

SIDE/ADVERSE EFFECTS: CNS: headache, dizziness ▪ GI: N/V/D, abdominal pain, dyspepsia ▪ Other: ↑ ALT levels, myalgia, accidental injury.

INTERACTIONS: Drug: Use c̄ warfarin will ↑ plasma level, may require lower dosages of anticoagulant ▪ Theophylline use c̄ zafirlukast will ↓ its plasma levels & zileuton will ↑ theophylline plasma levels ▪ Terfenadine will ↓ zafirlukast plasma levels & aspirin will ↑ plasma levels ▪ Erythromycin will ↓ zafirlukast bioavailability ▪ zileuton will ↑ activity of propranolol.

NURSING MANAGEMENT PRIORITIES

ADMINISTRATION: Assess for hx of hypersensitivity ▪ Assess respiratory function, patency of nasal passages ▪ Avoid abrupt withdrawal ▪ Avoid exposure to heat/

light/moisture in storage ▪ zafirlukast: administer on empty stomach (1h ac or 2h pc) ▪ zileuton: administer c̄ food at hs.

EVALUATION: Monitor renal, hepatic function ▪ Assess respiratory status, adequate inhalation ▪ Monitor frequency of asthmatic attacks.

EDUCATION: Take as directed by physician; do *not* abruptly D/C drug ▪ Notify physician/dentist of use before treatment ▪ Notify physician *immediately* of wheezing, respiratory distress ▪ Do *not* use for acute asthma attacks (prophylaxis only) ▪ Notify physician if experiencing flu-like symptoms, jaundice, pruritus, right upper quadrant pain ▪ Full drug effects may require several days of therapy.

NOTES:

zalcitabine (dideoxycytidine) • (zal-sit-ah-bean)

CATEGORY: *Antiviral:* synthetic pyrimidine nucleoside analog — Rx; Preg Cat C

BRAND NAME
Hivid (Roche)

DOSAGE FORMS
Tablets: 0.375, 0.75mg

USE: Treatment of advanced HIV infections in pts c̄ disease progression c̄ or w/out intolerance to zidovudine ▪ In combination c̄ zidovudine in adult pts c̄ advanced HIV infection c̄ significant clinical or immunologic deterioration (CD4 cell count ≤300/mm³). **ACTION:** Antiviral activity due to inhibition of viral DNA synthesis.

PHARMACOKINETICS

PO absorption	Peak	Half-life	Excretion
80%	0.8-1.6h	1-3h	70% single dose in 24h via urine

CONTRAINDICATIONS: Hypersensitivity. **CC:** Use c̄ caution in pts c̄ preexisting neuropathy, renal impairment ▪ Use associated c̄ lactic acidosis in absence of hypoxemia, rare cases of hepatomegaly/fatal hepatic failure, pancreatitis ▪ Safety in children <13y/o not established.

DOSAGE

Adult *PO*	0.75mg q8h 0.75mg + 200mg zidovudine q8h

SIDE/ADVERSE EFFECTS: CNS: headache, seizures, Bell's palsy, confusion, loss of mental acuity, nervousness, peripheral sensorimotor neuropathy of distal extremities (numbness, burning dysesthesia) ▪ CV: hypertension, rhythm irregularities, rare cases of ***cardiomyopathy/CHF*** ▪ EENT: abnormal vision & taste, ear blockage, tinnitus, xerophthalmia ▪ GI: esophageal/oral ulcers, N/V/D, dyspepsia, glossitis, rectal bleeding, dry mouth, ***pancreatitis*** ▪ GU: ***acute renal failure, toxic neuropathy,*** hyperuricemia, calculus ▪ HEM: anemia, leukopenia, ***thrombocytopenia*** ▪ HEP: jaundice, hepatitis, ***hepatocellular damage*** ▪ INT: acne, alopecia, bulbous eruptions, follicular rash ▪ MS: arthralgia, myalgia, gout ▪ Other: fever, ⬇ weight, coughing, dyspnea, flulike symptoms.

INTERACTIONS: Drug: Use c̄ didanosine best avoided ▪ Use c̄ peripheral neurotoxic, nephrotoxic, pancreatoxic drugs can result in additive toxicity.

NURSING MANAGEMENT PRIORITIES

ADMINISTRATION: Assess for hx of hypersensitivity ▪ Administer 1h ac/2h pc ▪ Avoid exposure to light in storage.

EVALUATION: Monitor VS, esp temperature ▪ Monitor hepatic, renal status ▪ Monitor WBC counts (anemia, granulocytopenia); repeated blood transfusions may be necessary.

EDUCATION: Take as ordered by physician at equal intervals around clock to maintain blood levels; do *not* ↑ dose ▪ Do *not* share drug ▪ Women: avoid breastfeeding ▪ Used to control, *not* cure, HIV infections ▪ Notify physician of any change in health status ▪ Check c̄ physician/pharmacist before taking OTC preparations ▪ Avoid sexual contact/blood donation (risk of HIV transmission) ▪ Keep scheduled appointments c̄ physician/for blood work.

NOTES:

zidovudine (AZT) • (zye-doe-view-deen)

CATEGORY: *Antiviral*

Rx; Preg Cat C

BRAND NAME
Retrovir (G-W)

DOSAGE FORMS
Capsule: 100mg
IV infusion: 10mg/20ml
Syrup: 50mg/5ml

USE: Management (PO) of asymptomatic, symptomatic HIV infections in children >3mo/o & adults ▪ Management (IV) of selected adult symptomatic HIV infections & advanced ARC in pts c̄ confirmed *Pneumocystic carinii* pneumonia or lymphocyte (T_4 cells) count <200/mm³ ▪ Prophylaxis of maternal/fetal HIV transmission. **ACTION:** Antiviral activity due to inhibition of viral replication in selected retroviruses incl human immunodeficiency virus (HIV/HTLV III), etiologic agent of AIDS, ARC; drug is thymidine analog that inhibits HIV reverse transcriptase enzymes, required for DNA synthesis.

PHARMACOKINETICS

PO absorption	Peak	Half-life	Excretion
52%-75%	0.5-1.5h	0.78-1.93h	Via urine as metabolites (GAZT)

CONTRAINDICATIONS: Hypersensitivity rxs that are life threatening. **CC:** Full safety c̄ prolonged use not established ▪ Anemia can develop after 4-6wks of treatment, may require dosage adjustments.

DOSAGE: Must be individualized (adjusted to the degree of anemia &/or granulocytopenia present)

Pediatric *PO* (3mo-12y/o)	Recommended starting dose 180mg/m² q6h (720mg/m²/d). Do *not* exceed 200mg q6h
Adult *PO*	
Asymptomatic	100mg q4h while awake (500mg/d)
Symptomatic	Starting dose 200mg q4h (1200 mg/d). Dosage may be ⬇ to 100mg q4h (600mg/d) after 1mo
Maternal/Fetal	100mg 5 times/d until start of labor.
(>14wks pregnant)	During labor/delivery, 2mg/kg/IV over 1h, followed by 1mg/kg/h until clamping of umbilical cord. Infant dose after birth: 2mg/kg PO q6h starting w/in 12h of delivery for 6wks
IV	1-2mg infused over 1h q4h (6 times/d)

SIDE/ADVERSE EFFECTS: CNS: anxiety, dizziness, insomnia, loss of mental acuity/confusion, nervousness, somnolence, vertigo ▪ CV: ECG abnormalities, vasodilation, ***phlebitis (IV)*** ▪ GI: anorexia, dyspepsia, abdominal pain, N/V/D, bleeding from gums/rectum, oral ulcers, HEM: ***anemia, granulocytopenia*** ▪ EENT: pharyngitis, sinusitis, hoarseness, rhinitis, amblyopia, hearing loss, photophobia ▪ GU: dysuria, polyuria, urinary frequency/hesitancy ▪ INT: acne, pruritus, urticaria ▪ MS: arthralgia, muscle spasms/tremors ▪ Other: chills, chest pains, lip edema.

INTERACTIONS: Drug: Use c̄ acetaminophen can ↑ incidence of granulocytopenia ▪ Use c̄ nephrotoxic drugs, cytotoxic drugs, or bone marrow depressants can result in additive toxicity ▪ Use c̄ probenecid may ↓ zidovudine renal excretion.

NURSING MANAGEMENT PRIORITIES

ADMINISTRATION: Assess for hx of hypersensitivity ▪ Avoid administration of acetaminophen during therapy ▪ Avoid exposure to light in storage.

EVALUATION: Monitor VS, esp temperature ▪ Monitor hepatic, renal status ▪ Monitor WBC counts (anemia, granulocytopenia); repeated blood transfusions may be necessary.

EDUCATION: Take as ordered by physician at equal intervals around clock to maintain blood levels; do *not* ↑ dose ▪ Do *not* share drug ▪ Women: avoid breastfeeding ▪ Used to control, *not* cure, HIV infections ▪ Notify physician of any change in health status ▪ Avoid concurrent use of acetaminophen (↑ toxicity) ▪ Check c̄ physician/pharmacist before taking OTC preparations ▪ Avoid sexual contact/blood donation (risk of HIV transmission) ▪ Keep scheduled appointments c̄ physician/for blood work.

NOTES:

zolmitriptan • (zole-meh-trip-tan)

CATEGORY: *Antimigraine:* serotonin receptor agonist Rx; Preg Cat C

BRAND NAME	**DOSAGE FORMS**
Zomig (Zeneca)	Tablet: 2.5, 5mg

USE: Treatment of acute migraine c̄/w/out aura. **ACTION:** Migraine is associated c̄ selective cerebral vasodilation & release of sensory neuropeptides from the trigemovascular system that incl substance P, neurokinin A, other vasoactive peptides.

Antimigraine activity of zolmitriptan, a serotonin 5HT-1 receptor agonist, on selected cerebral blood vessels containing 5HT-1 receptors results in vasoconstriction & inhibition of sensory neuropeptide release from the trigemovascular system.

PHARMACOKINETICS

PO absorption	Peak serum	Half-life	Protein binding	Excretion
Good	2-3.5h	6h	25%	Via feces, urine primarily as metabolites

CONTRAINDICATIONS: Hypersensitivity, w/in 24h after administration of ergot-type medication, incl dihydroergotamine, ergotamine, methysergide, current &/or w/in 2wks of D/C MAO-I therapy, severe cardiovascular/peripheral syndrome, symptomatic Wolff-Parkinson-White syndrome, cardiac accessory pathway disease. **CC:** Use of 5HT-1 agonists requires a + diagnosis ▪ Use can produce significant cardiovascular events, incl MI, ventricular tachycardia/fibrillation, cardiac arrest, death ▪ Safety & efficacy not established in pediatric pts ▪ Use c̄ caution in pts c̄ moderate/severe liver impairment.

DOSAGE

Adult	*PO*	2.5mg or higher as a single dose & repeated if needed q2h to a maximum of 10mg in 24h

SIDE/ADVERSE EFFECTS: CNS: agitation, anxiety, sleep disorders, hallucination ▪ CV: ***abnormal EKG,*** hypertension, orthostatic hypotension, ***atrial/ventricular arrhythmias,*** ecchymosis, facial edema ▪ GI: gastroenteritis, ↑

appetite, excessive thirst, constipation, tongue edema ▪ GU: cystitis, hematuria, polyuria ▪ HEM: ***thrombocytopenia***, eosinophilia ▪ INT: pruritus, rash, urticaria ▪ RESP: bronchitis, bronchospasm, epistaxis ▪ Other: back pain, leg cramps, vision disturbances, tinnitus.

INTERACTIONS: Drug: Use c̄ cimetidine, PO contraceptives can ↑ zolmitriptan activity.

NURSING MANAGEMENT PRIORITIES

ADMINISTRATION: Assess for hx of hypersensitivity to serotonin 5HT-1 receptor agonists ▪ Assess CV, hepatic, renal function; use caution if impaired ▪ Assess severity of headache, associated symptoms ▪ Administer c̄ fluids at onset of attack ▪ Maintain quiet environment.

EVALUATION: Monitor neurologic, CV, hepatic, renal, status; notify physician if abnormal ▪ Monitor severity of headache & when relief is obtained ▪ Observe pt for signs of ↑ bleeding.

EDUCATION: Dizziness may occur; use caution in potentially hazardous activities ▪ Avoid foods containing tyramine (aged & fermented foods) ▪ Notify physician *immediately* of abnormal rxs (burning, numbness, tingling, bleeding) ▪ Check c̄ physician/pharmacist before taking any OTC preparations ▪ Women: avoid breastfeeding.

NOTES:

zolpidem tartrate • (zole-pih-dem)

CATEGORY: *Hypnotic*

Rx; Preg Cat C

BRAND NAME
Ambien (Searle)

DOSAGE FORMS
Tablet: 5, 10mg

USE: Short-term treatment of insomnia. **ACTION:** Hypnotic activity similar to that of benzodiazepines. Interacts c̄ omega receptor (benzodiazepine receptor) to produce hypnotic effect.

PHARMACOKINETICS

PO absorption	Half-life	Protein binding	Excretion
Rapid	2.5h	92.5h	Via urine primarily as metabolites

CONTRAINDICATIONS: Hypersensitivity. **CC:** Failure to treat insomnia after 7-10d of treatment requires medical reevaluation due to possible medical/psychiatric disorders.

DOSAGE

Adult *PO* — 10mg immediately before hs for 7-10d. Reevaluate if treatment is longer than 2-3wks. Elderly pts require 5-mg dose.

SIDE/ADVERSE EFFECTS: CNS: *headache, drowsiness,* dizziness, lethargy, drugged-type hangover, depression, abnormal dreams, amnesia, anxiety ▪ GI: N/V/D, dyspepsia, abdominal pain, constipation, anorexia, dry mouth ▪ INT: rash ▪ MS: myalgia, arthralgia ▪ RESP: URI, sinusitis, pharyngitis, flulike symptoms ▪ Other: chest & back pain, UTI, palpitations.

INTERACTIONS: Drug: Use c̄ CNS depressants will produce additive effects.

NURSING MANAGEMENT PRIORITIES

ADMINISTRATION: Assess for hx of benzodiazepine hypersensitivity ▪ Avoid exposure to heat/moisture/light in storage ▪ Avoid abrupt withdrawal ▪ Elderly pts may require ↓ dosage ▪ ↓ Environmental stimuli.

EVALUATION: Monitor renal, hepatic status ▪ Assess for symptoms of abrupt withdrawal (tremors, abdominal/muscle cramps, convulsions) c̄ prolonged use ▪ Check for signs of dependence (↑ drug request) ▪ Monitor activity status (safety precautions) ▪ Assess for tolerance to therapeutic dose ▪ Assess for paradoxic rxs (CNS stimulation), esp in elderly ▪ Check for depression, suicide precautions prn ▪ Assess pt sleep pattern.

EDUCATION: Drowsiness may occur; use caution in potentially hazardous activities ▪ Avoid use c̄ alcohol, other CNS depressants ▪ Indiscriminate use may lead to dependence ▪ Do *not* keep at bedside ▪ Take as directed by physician; do *not* ↑ dose ▪ Women: avoid breastfeeding ▪ Check c̄ physician/pharmacist before taking OTC preparations ▪ Practice relaxation exercises, ventilation of feelings ▪ Utilize sleep producers (reading, warm milk, soft music) ▪ Use sugarless gum/hard candy to diminish dry mouth.

NOTES:

DESCRIPTION: Large, varied group of drugs that can duplicate/mimic (sympathomimetic) effects of catecholamines, esp norepinephrine, at postganglionic adrenoreceptor in sympathetic nervous system; selected agents capable of central sympathomimetic activity ▪ Adrenoreceptors currently divided into α receptors, which produce stimulatory responses, & β receptors, which usually produce inhibitory responses, except in heart, which are stimulatory. Furthermore, α adrenoreceptors are subdivided into α_1, α_2 receptors, & β adrenoreceptors are subdivided into β_1 receptors (heart) & β_2 receptors (bronchi, GI tract, uterus) ▪ Predominant α-adrenergic agonist response is vasoconstriction, CNS stimulation. β-adrenergic agonist response results in relaxation of bronchial, GI, uterine smooth muscle (β_2 activity), cardiac stimulation (β_1 activity).

DRUGS: Predominant adrenergic activity listed ▪ α **Drugs**: amphetamine, amphetamine complex, benzphetamine *(Didrex)*, dextroamphetamine *(Dexedrine)*, diethylpropion *(Tenuate)*, mazindol *(Mazanor)*, methamphetamine *(Desoxyn)*, methoxamine *(Vasoxyl)*, naphazoline *(Privine)*, oxymetazoline *(Afrin)*, phendimetrazine *(Bontril)*, phentermine *(Fastin, Ionamin)*, phenylephrine *(Neo-Synephrine)*, phenylpropanolamine *(Acutrim, Control, Dexatrim)*, pseudoephedrine *(Sudafed)*, tetrahydrozoline *(Visine)*, xylometazoline *(Otrivin)* ▪ α_2 ***Drugs***: brimonidine tartrate *(Alphagan)* ▪ ***Central acting a_2 drugs:*** clonidine *(Catapress)*, guanabenz *(Wytensin)*, guanfacine *(Tenex)* ▪ α-β **Drugs**: dipivefrin *(Propine)*, ephedrine, epinephrine, ethylnorepinephrine *(Bronkephrine)*, mephentermine *(Wyamine)*, metaraminol *(Aramine)*, norepinephrine *(Levophed)* ▪ β **Drugs:** isoproterenol *(Isuprel)*, metaproterenol *(Alupent, Metaprel)*, ritodrine *(Yutopar)* ▪ β_1 **Drugs:** dobutamine *(Dobutrex)*, dopamine *(Intropin)* ▪ β_2 **Drugs:** albuterol *(Proventil, Ventolin)*, bitolterol *(Tornalate)*, salmeterol *(Serevent)*, terbutaline *(Brethine, Bricanyl)*.

THERAPEUTIC USE: Anorexiant: Several current references separate this group from adrenergic drugs, esp amphetamine-like drugs: amphetamine complex, amphetamine sulfate, benzphetamine hcl, dextroamphetamine sulfate, diethylpropion, fenfluramine hcl, mazindol, phendimetrazine tartrate, phenylpropanolamine hcl ▪ **Bronchodilator:** albuterol, albuterol sulfate, bitolterol mesylate, ephedrine & salts, epinephrine & salts, ethylnorepinephrine, isoetharine, isoproterenol hcl, isoproterenol sulfate, metaproterenol sulfate, salmeterol, terbutaline hcl ▪ **Glaucoma:** brimonidine tartrate ▪ **Hypertension:** clonidine, guanabenz, guanfacine ▪ **Nasal decongestant:** epinephrine hcl, ephedrine salts, naphazoline hcl, oxymetazoline hcl, phenylephrine hcl, phenylpropanolamine hcl, pseudoephedrine hcl, tetrahydrozoline hcl ▪ **Ophthalmic decongestant:** epinephrine hcl, naphazoline hcl, phenylephrine hcl, tetrahydrozoline hcl ▪ GLAUCOMA (open-angle): epinephrine hcl, dipivefrin ▪ MYDRIATIC: epinephrine hcl, hydroxyamphetamine HBr, phenylephrine hcl ▪ SHOCK (inotropic/vasopressor activity): dobutamine, dopamine hcl, ephedrine sulfate, epinephrine hcl, isoproterenol hcl, mephentermine sulfate, metaraminol bitartrate, methoxamine hcl, norepinephrine bitartrate, phenylephrine hcl ▪ *See* individual drug cards for further information.

MECHANISM OF ACTION: Sympathomimetics produce agonist effects by direct activity c̄ adrenoreceptor; by causing release of norepinephrine from storage vesicles in adrenergic neurons (indirect); combination of both mechanisms (mixed).

NURSING MANAGEMENT PRIORITIES

ASSESS: Hx of catecholamine hypersensitivity ▪ Adequate renal function ▪ ABGs, lung sounds ▪ CAUTION: diabetes ▪ **ndx: Therapeutic effects**: Ineffective airway clearance ▪ Ineffective breathing pattern ▪ ↓ Cardiac output ▪ **Adverse effects:** Risk for injury ▪ Sleep pattern disturbance ▪ Altered tissue perfusion ▪ Altered patterns of urinary elimination. **PLAN:** Check preparation, dosage calculations c̄ another nurse ▪ Maintain IV access site, cardiac monitoring, hydration ▪ **Special considerations:** G: caution, ↓ dosage (↑ sensitivity) ▪ P: caution, ↓ dosage (↑ sensitivity) ▪ OB: avoid breastfeeding ▪ **Dietary management**: Avoid caffeine ▪ **Lab test evaluation:** ABGs, FBS (diabetics). **IMPLEMENT**: Use infusion control device for regulation ▪ Monitor VS closely ▪ Monitor I&O, lung sounds ▪ **Patient education**: Maintain fluid intake ▪ Avoid exposure to allergens, URI ▪ Report abnormal rxs to drug therapy (irregular, rapid heartbeat; difficult breathing). **EVALUATE**: **Observe for therapeutic effects:** ↑ BP ▪ ↑ Heart rate ▪ ↑ Force of cardiac contraction ▪ ↑ Air exchange.

DESCRIPTION: Group of diverse chemicals that block effects of catecholamines & α adrenergics at α adrenoreceptors in sympathetic nervous system.

DRUGS: α **Blockers:** dihydroergotamine mesylate *(D.H.E. 45)*, ergoloid mesylates *(Gerimal, Hydergine)*, ergotamine tartrate *(Ergostat)*, methysergide maleate *(Sansert)*, phenoxybenzamine hcl *(Dibenzyline)*, phentolamine mesylate *(Regitine, *Rogitine HCl, *Rogitine Mesylate)*, tolazoline hcl *(Priscoline)* ▪ α_1 **Blockers:** doxazosin mesylate *(Cardura)*, prazosin *(Minipress)*, tamsulosin hcl *(Flomax)*, terazosin *(Hytrin)*.

THERAPEUTIC USE: Since introduction, these agents have been used for various conditions, esp hypertension, but poor clinical efficacy has ⬇ usefulness for vascular headaches, malignant hypertension ▪ α_1 Blockers are used to treat hypertension & benign prostatic hyperplasia (doxazosin, terazosin).

MECHANISM OF ACTION: α-Blocking agents exhibit varying degrees of competitive/noncompetitive α_1-adrenergic blocking activity; exhibit vasoconstrictor, oxytoxic, antiserotonin activity. α-Adrenergic blocking activity inhibits pressor effects of epinephrine on BP, opposes activity of norepinephrine. α_1 Blocker antihypertensive effect due to vasodilation.

CONTRAINDICATIONS: Hypersensitivity, MI, coronary artery disease, peripheral vascular disease, pregnancy. *See* individual drug cards; specific contraindications vary.

DOSAGE

Adult D.H.E.	Vascular headache: 1mg IM. May be repeated twice at 1-h intervals
doxazosin	Hypertension: ≤16mg/d divided
Benign prostatic hyperplasia	4-8mg/d PO
Hypertension	1-16mg/d PO
ergoloid	Symptomatic relief of senility: 1mg tid PO/sublingual
ergotamine	Vascular headache: 1-2mg PO. May be repeated twice at ½-h intervals
methysergide	Vascular headache: 4-8mg/d PO
phenoxybenzamine	Pheochromocytoma (hypertension): 10-40mg PO 2-3 times/d
phentolamine	Pheochromocytoma (surgery & dx): 5mg IM/IV prn during surgery

prazosin	Hypertension: ≤20mg divided
tamsulosin	Benign prostatic hyperplasia: 0.4mg once/d PO
terazosin	Benign prostatic hyperplasia: 10mg/d PO Hypertension: 1-5mg/d PO
Neonatal	
tolazoline	Neonatal pulmonary hypertension: 1-2mg/kg IV followed by infusion of 1-2mg/kg/h

CONTRAINDICATIONS: Hypersensitivity, MI, coronary artery disease, peripheral vascular disease, pregnancy. *See* individual drug cards; specific contraindications vary.

SIDE/ADVERSE EFFECTS: CV: postural hypotension ▪ EENT: nasal stuffiness ▪ GI: gastric upset ▪ GU: oliguria, hematuria ▪ Other: ergotism (for ergot derivatives), N/V/D, cramps, drowsiness, dizziness, headache, mental confusion.

DRUG INTERACTIONS: Disulfiramlike rx c̄ tolazoline, alcohol ▪ Phentolamine use in pediatric diabetics may ↑ antidiabetic effects ▪ Use of nonselective adrenergic agents c̄ phenoxybenzamine may produce hypotension, tachycardia.

NURSING MANAGEMENT PRIORITIES

ASSESS: Hx of hypersensitivity ▪ BP ▪ Peripheral circulation ▪ CAUTION**:** coronary artery disease ▪ **ndx: Therapeutic effects:** Risk for injury ▪ Altered tissue perfusion ▪ **Adverse effects:** Diarrhea ▪ Risk for fluid volume deficit ▪ Risk for injury ▪ Pain ▪ Altered tissue perfusion. **PLAN:** Prevent postural hypotension ▪ **Special considerations:** G: caution (↑ hypotensive effects) ▪ P: caution (immature systems) ▪ OB: caution if pregnant, breastfeeding ▪ **Dietary management:** Avoid use c̄ alcohol, high-Na^+ foods ▪ **Lab test evaluation**: Serum catecholamine, glucose. **IMPLEMENT:** Monitor BP ▪ Observe for hypotension ▪ Monitor peripheral circulation (skin color, temperature, pulses) ▪ Monitor CV, hepatic, renal status ▪ **Patient education:** Avoid sudden position changes (postural hypotension) ▪ Comply c̄ prescribed drug regimen ▪ Avoid smoking, use c̄ alcohol, constrictive clothing, extremely hot objects, OTC cough/cold/allergy preparations. **EVALUATE: Observe for therapeutic effects:** ↓ BP ▪ ↑ Peripheral circulation ▪ Relief of pain.

DESCRIPTION: Group of semisynthetic broad-spectrum, water-soluble, bactericidal antibiotics.

DRUGS: amikacin sulfate *(Amikin)*, gentamicin sulfate *(Garamycin, *Cidomycin)*, kanamycin sulfate *(Kantrex, *Anamid)*, neomycin sulfate *(Mycifradin, Myciguent, *Neocin)*, netilmicin sulfate *(Netromycin)*, paromomycin sulfate *(Humatin)*, streptomycin sulfate, tobramycin sulfate *(Nebcin, *Tobrex)*.

THERAPEUTIC USE: Treatment of infections caused (combined spectrums) by susceptible strains ▪ Specific gram-negative spectrum doses vary; selection of drug is based on causative organism ▪ Treatment of tularemia, plague, tuberculosis (streptomycin) ▪ In combined therapy for enterococcal endocarditis ▪ Alternate for penicillin-resistant *Staphylococcus* infections ▪ In combination c̄ carbenicillin for treating stubborn *Pseudomonas* infections.

MECHANISM OF ACTION: Bactericidal activity due to inhibition of ribosomal protein synthesis in susceptible organisms; neomycin limited to nonsystemic use because of high toxicity; paromomycin usually separated from group & classified c̄ amebicides.

PHARMACOKINETICS

	IM peak	Half-life	Protein binding	Excretion
amikacin	1h	2h	0%-11%	92% unchanged in urine in 8h
gentamicin	½-1h	2-2½h	0%-30%	70% unchanged in urine in 24h
kanamycin	1h	2-2½h	—	50% unchanged in urine in 4h
netilmicin	½-1h	2-2½h	0%-30%	80% unchanged in urine in 24h
streptomycin	1h	2-3h	35%	29%-89% unchanged in urine in 24h
tobramycin	½-1½	2h	—	84% unchanged in urine in 8h

CONTRAINDICATIONS: Hypersensitivity, hx of serious aminoglycoside toxicity.

DOSAGE: Usual adult IM/IV range. Dosage must be ↓ in pts c̄ impaired renal function.

amikacin	15mg/kg/d in 2-3 doses. Do *not* exceed 1.5g/d
gentamicin	3-5mg/kg/d in 3-4 doses
kanamycin	7.5-15mg/kg/d in 2-3 doses
netilmicin	3-6.5mg/kg/d in 2-3 doses
streptomycin	1-4g/d
tobramycin	3-5mg/kg/d in 3 doses

SIDE/ADVERSE EFFECTS: EENT: ***ototoxicity*** ▪ GI: N/V ▪ GU: ***nephrotoxicity***, casts, proteinuria, ↑ BUN, ↑ NPN, serum creatinine ▪ HEM: anemia ▪ Other: arthralgia, convulsions, fever, hypotension (rare).

DRUG INTERACTIONS: Avoid use c̄ neurotoxic/nephrotoxic drugs ▪ Dimenhydrinate can mask aminoglycoside toxicity ▪ Use c̄ succinylcholine, tubocurarine will ↑ their activity ▪ PO anticoagulant activity may ↑ .

NURSING MANAGEMENT PRIORITIES

ASSESS: Hx of hypersensitivity ▪ Baseline hearing status, renal function ▪ Peak, trough serum concentrations ▪ Pt weight for dose calculation ▪ CAUTION: renal failure ▪ **ndx: Therapeutic effects:** Risk for altered body temperature ▪ Risk for infection ▪ Impaired skin/tissue integrity ▪ **Adverse effects:** Diarrhea ▪ Risk for fluid volume deficit, injury ▪ Sensory/perceptual alteration (auditory) ▪ Risk for impaired skin integrity ▪ Altered patterns of urinary elimination. **PLAN:** Maintain hydration ▪ Administer at equal intervals around clock to maintain blood levels ▪ **Special considerations:** G: caution, ↓ dosage (renal dysfunction) ▪ P: caution, ↓ dosage (prolonged half-life) ▪ OB: not recommended if pregnant; avoid if breastfeeding ▪ **Dietary management:** Encourage alkaline ash foods (UTI) ▪ **Lab test evaluation:** Peak, trough serum concentrations; BUN, serum creatinine. **IMPLEMENT:** Obtain C&S; check results ▪ Observe for signs of superinfection (diarrhea, URI, coated tongue) ▪ Monitor for hearing dysfunction, nephrotoxicity, neuromuscular blockade, respiratory paralysis ▪ **Patient education:** Report hearing, balance difficulties to physician at once ▪ ↑ Fluid intake (10-12 glasses/d) ▪ Notify physician of symptoms of allergic rx (fever, difficult breathing, rash, burning/stinging in eyes). **EVALUATE: Observe for therapeutic effect:** Resolution of infection.

DESCRIPTION: Narcotics are natural opiate agonists, semisynthetic opiate agonists, or synthetic opiates (agonist opiates, agonist-antagonist opiates) ▪ Excellent analgesics; exhibit phenomenon of tolerance; have varying abuse/addiction potentials; most are schedule drugs.

DRUGS: Natural opiates: codeine phosphate (CII), codeine sulfate (CII), morphine sulfate (CII), opium preparations—deodorized tincture of opium (CII), opium (alkaloids), paregoric (CIII) ▪ **Semisynthetic opiates:** hydromorphone hcl (CII; *Dilaudid*), oxymorphone hcl (CII; *Numorphan*) ▪ **Synthetic opiates**—AGONIST: fentanyl citrate (CII; *Sublimaze*), levomethadyl acetate hcl (CII; *ORLAAM*), levorphanol tartrate (CII; *Levo-Dromoran*), meperidine hcl (CII; *Demerol*), methadone hcl (CII; *Dolophine*), oxycodone hcl (CII), sufentanil citrate (CII; *Sufenta*) ▪ AGONIST-ANTAGONIST: buprenorphine hcl (CV; *Buprenex*), butorphanol tartrate (*Stadol*), dezocine (*Dalgan*), nalbuphine hcl (*Nubain*), pentazocine (CIV; *Talwin*).

PHARMACOKINETICS: *See* individual drug cards.

THERAPEUTIC USE: Relief of severe pain ▪ Sedation/hypnosis when pain present ▪ Preanesthetic sedation; postop analgesia (obstetric); support of anesthesia ▪ Antitussive, antidiarrheal ▪ Maintenance of opiate addiction (levamethadyl, methadone).

MECHANISM OF ACTION: Analgesic activity probably due to interference c̄ pain impulses at subcortical level of brain. Narcotics significantly alter psychologic response to pain, suppress anxiety/apprehension by producing euphoria.

CONTRAINDICATIONS: Hypersensitivity.

DOSAGE: Adult

buprenorphine	*IM/IV*	0.3mg q6h
butorphanol	*IM*	2mg q3-4h
codeine	*PO*	15-60mg q4-6h
dezocine	*IV*	2-10mg q2-4h
fentanyl	*IM*	5-20mg q3-6h
hydromorphone	*PO*	2mg q4-6h
levomethadyl	*PO*	60-90mg or ↑ 3 times/wk
levorphanol	*PO/SC*	2-3mg q6-8h
meperidine	*PO/IM/SC*	50-150mg q3-4h
methadone	*IM/SC*	2.5-10mg q3-4h
	PO	≥40-120mg once/d
morphine	*SC*	10-15mg q4h
nalbuphine	*IM/IV/SC*	10-20mg

oxycodone	*PO*	5mg q6h
oxymorphone	*IM/SC*	1-1.5mg q6h
pantopon	*PO*	2-4mg q4-6h
pentazocine	*IM/IV/SC*	30mg q3-4h
sufentanil	*IV*	0.5-1μg/kg; 2-8μg/kg initially

SIDE/ADVERSE EFFECTS: CNS: *lightheadedness, dizziness, sedation, sweating,* euphoria, disorientation, transient hallucination, weakness ▪ CV: hypotension, palpitation; flushing of face, phlebitis after IV injection ▪ GI: dry mouth, constipation, anorexia, biliary tract spasm ▪ GU: urinary retention, ureteral spasm ▪ INT: pruritus, urticaria ▪ RESP: respiratory depression, apnea.

DRUG INTERACTIONS: Use c̄ alcohol, antihistamines, barbiturates, benzodiazepines, methotrimeprazine, phenothiazines, other CNS depressants can produce additive effects ▪ Use c̄ TCAs can produce respiratory depression ▪ Meperidine contraindicated c̄ MAO-I ▪ Methadone maintenance may produce withdrawal symptoms c̄ opiate agonist-antagonist drugs.

NURSING MANAGEMENT PRIORITIES

ASSESS: Hx of opioid hypersensitivity ▪ Respirations; do *not* administer if <12/m ▪ Pain characteristics ▪ Signs of dependence ▪ Signs of OD (coma, pinpoint pupils, respiratory depression); have naloxone hcl (*Narcan*) available ▪ Bowel function, abdominal distention ▪ Renal function, urinary retention ▪ CAUTION: recent CNS depressant administration; hepatic, renal, respiratory impairment; craniocerebral trauma ▪ **ndx: Therapeutic effects**: Pain ▪ **Adverse effects:** Risk for activity intolerance ▪ Ineffective breathing pattern ▪ Constipation ▪ Risk for injury ▪ Sensory/perceptual alterations (visual) ▪ Risk for impaired skin integrity ▪ Altered thought processes ▪ Altered tissue perfusion ▪ Altered patterns of urinary elimination. **PLAN:** Have emergency support measures available ▪ Administer *before* pain becomes severe ▪ Maintain safety precautions (raise bedrails, bed in low position, call bell) ▪ Maintain hydration ▪ Store under double lock/key; document use accurately ▪ **Special considerations:** G: caution, ↓ dosage (↑ sensitivity) ▪ P: caution (↑ sensitivity) ▪ OB: caution if pregnant, breastfeeding ▪ **Dietary management**: Avoid use c̄ alcohol; ↑ bulk-containing foods (constipation) ▪ **Lab test evaluation**: None specific. **IMPLEMENT:** Monitor VS, respirations, circulatory function ▪ Monitor activity status (safety precautions) ▪ Check for potentiation of CNS depressant effect ▪ **Patient education:** Comply c̄ prescribed drug regimen; indiscriminate use may lead to dependence ▪ Avoid use c̄ alcohol, other CNS depressants ▪ Use safety precautions c̄ ambulation, hazardous activity ▪ Avoid smoking after administration ▪ Avoid sudden position changes (postural hypotension) ▪ ↑ Fluids, dietary bulk. **EVALUATE: Observe for therapeutic effect:** ↓ Pain.

Analgesic-narcotic combinations are fixed dosage formulations of a narcotic & a nonnarcotic analgesic. Many preparations are available in a variety of narcotic/nonnarcotic dosage ratios. All preparations are Rx, have a controlled schedule assignment. Dosage of these preparations must be adjusted for the pt after initiation of treatment, depending on intensity of pain, pt narcotic tolerance. In addition, pain intensity may necessitate ↑ starting dose.

PRODUCT INFORMATION

Preparation	Dosage form	Manufacturer	Formula	Schedule	Usual starting dose
Aceta c̄ Codeine	Tablet	Century	Acetaminophen 300mg/Codeine 30mg	C-III	1 q4-6h
Acetaminophen c̄ Codeine	Tablet	Generic	Acetaminophen 300mg/Codeine 30mg	C-III	1 q4-6h
	Tablet	Generic	Acetaminophen 300mg/Codeine 60mg	C-III	1 q4-6h
Anexsia 5/500	Tablet	MAL	Acetaminophen 500mg/Hydrocodone 5mg	C-III	1-2 q4-6h
Anexsia 7.5/650	Tablet	MAL	Acetaminophen 650mg/Hydrocodone 7.5mg	C-III	1 q4-6h
Anexsia 10/666	Tablet	MAL	Acetaminophen 500mg/Hydrocodone 5mg	C-III	1 q4-6h
Aspirin c̄ Codeine #3	Tablet	Generic	Aspirin 325mg/Codeine 30mg	C-III	1 q4-6h
Aspirin c̄ Codeine #4	Tablet	Generic	Aspirin 325mg/Codeine 60mg	C-III	1 q4-6h
Bancap HC	Capsule	Forest	Acetaminophen 500mg/Hydrocodone 5mg	C-III	1-2 q4-6h
Capital c̄ Codeine	Suspension	Carnick	Acetaminophen 120mg/Codeine 12mg (15ml)	C-V	15ml q4h
Darvocet-N50	Tablet	Lilly	Acetaminophen 325mg/Propoxyphene 50mg	C-IV	1-2 q4h
Darvocet-N100	Tablet	Lilly	Acetaminophen 650mg/Propoxyphene 100mg	C-IV	1 q4h
Darvon Compound-65	Capsule	Lilly (puvule)	Aspirin 389mg/Caffeine 32.4mg/Propoxyphene 65mg	C-IV	1 q4-6h
Empirin c̄ Codeine #3	Tablet	G-W	Aspirin 325mg/Codeine 30mg	C-III	1 q4-6h

Preparation	Dosage form	Manufacturer	Formula	Schedule	Usual starting dose
Empirin c̄ Codeine #4	Tablet	G-W	Aspirin 325mg/Codeine 60mg	C-III	1 q4-6h
Fioricet c̄ Codeine	Capsule	Sandoz	Acetaminophen 325mg/Butalbital 50mg Caffeine 40mg/Codeine 30mg	C-III	1-2 q4-6h
Fiorinal c̄ Codeine	Capsule	Sandoz	Aspirin 325mg/Butalbital 50mg Caffeine 40mg/Codeine 30mg	C-III	1-2 q4-6h
Hydrocet	Capsule	Carnick	Acetaminophen 500mg/Hydrocodone 5mg	C-III	1q 4-6h
Lorcet-HD	Capsule	Forest	Acetaminophen 500mg/Hydrocodone 5mg	C-III	1 q4-6h
Lorcet Plus	Tablet	Forest	Acetaminophen 650mg/Hydrocodone 7.5mg	C-III	1 q4-6h
Lorcet 10/650	Tablet	Forest	Acetaminophen 650mg/Hydrocodone 10mg	C-III	1 q4-6h
Lortab	Elixir	UCB	Acetaminophen 500mg/Hydrocodone 7.5mg (15ml)	C-III	15ml q4-6h
Lortab 2.5/500	Tablet	UCB	Acetaminophen 500mg/Hydrocodone 2.5mg	C-III	1 q4-6h
Lortab 5/500	Tablet	UCB	Acetaminophen 500mg/Hydrocodone 5mg	C-III	1 q4-6h
Lortab 7.5/500	Tablet	UCB	Acetaminophen 500mg/Hydrocodone/7.5mg	C-III	1 q4-6h
Lortab 10/500	Tablet	UCB	Acetaminophen 500mg/Hydrocodone 10mg	C-III	1 q4-6h
Margesic #3	Tablet	Whitby	Acetaminophen 650mg/Codeine 30mg	C-III	1 q4-6h
Margesic H	Capsule	Marnel	Acetaminophen 500mg/Hydrocodone 5mg	C-III	1 q4-6h
Mepergan	Injection	W-A	Promethazine 25mg/Meperidine 50mg (1ml)	C-II	1-2ml q3-4h IM/IV
Mepergan Fortis	Capsule	W-A	Promethazine 25mg/Meperidine 50mg	C-II	1 q4-6h
Percocet	Tablet	Endo	Acetaminophen 325mg/Oxycodone 5mg	C-II	1 q6h
Percodan	Tablet	Endo	Aspirin 325mg/Oxycodone 4.88mg	C-II	1 q6h

Preparation	Dosage form	Manufacturer	Formula	Schedule	Usual starting dose
Percodan-Demi	Tablet	Endo	Aspirin 325mg/Oxycodone 2.44mg	C-II	1 q6h
Phenaphen c̄ Codeine #3	Capsule	Robins	Acetaminophen 325mg/Codeine 30mg	C-III	1 q4-6h
Phenaphen c̄ Codeine #4	Capsule	Robins	Acetaminophen 325mg/Codeine 60mg	C-III	1 q4-6h
Roxicet	Tablet	Roxane	Acetaminophen 325mg/Oxycodone 5mg	C-II	1 q6h
	PO solution		Acetaminophen 325mg/Oxydocone 5mg (5ml)	C-II	5ml q6h
Synalgos-DC	Capsule	W-A	Aspirin 356.4mg/Caffeine 30mg/ Dihydrocodeine 16mg	C-III	1-2 q4h
Tylenol c̄ Codeine #2	Tablet	McNeil	Acetaminophen 300mg/Codeine 15mg	C-III	1 q4-6h
Tylenol c̄ Codeine #3	Tablet	McNeil	Acetaminophen 300mg/Codeine 30mg	C-III	1 q4-6h
Tylenol c̄ Codeine #4	Tablet	McNeil	Acetaminophen 300mg/Codeine 60mg	C-III	1 q4-6h
Tylox	Capsule	McNeil	Acetaminophen 500mg/Oxycodone 5mg	C-II	1 q6h
Vicodin	Tablet	Knoll	Acetaminophen 500mg/Hydrocodone 5mg	C-III	1 q4-6h
Vicodin ES	Tablet	Knoll	Acetaminophen 750mg/Hydrocodone 7.5mg	C-III	1 q4-6h
Wygesic	Tablet	W-A	Acetaminophen 650mg/Propoxyphene 65mg	C-IV	1 q4-6h
Zydone	Capsule	Endo	Acetaminophen 500mg/Hydrocodone 5mg	C-III	1 q4-6h

DESCRIPTION: Large, chemically diverse group of drugs that produce main pharmacologic effects by inhibiting synthesis, release of prostaglandins. Chemically divided into salicylates, propionic acid derivatives, fenamates, indoles, oxicams, pyrazolines; several references classify these agents as prostaglandin inhibitors rather than NSAIAs ▪ Prostaglandins are naturally occurring fatty acid derivatives of prostanoic acid; possess potent physiologic activity; exhibit wide tissue distribution c̄ high concentrations in seminal fluid; are synthesized locally (by enzyme system prostaglandin synthetase), where they act as local tissue hormones; affect CV, GI, reproductive, respiratory smooth muscle; play role in blood platelet aggregation, inflammatory response, pain sensation, fever.

DRUGS: Acetic acid derivatives: bromfenac *(Duract)*, diclofenac sodium *(Voltaren)*, etodolac *(Lodine)*, sulindac *(Clinoril)* ▪ **Propionic acid derivatives:** fenoprofen calcium *(Nalfon)*, flurbiprofen *(Ansaid)*, ibuprofen *(Advil, Haltran, Nuprin, Motrin)*, ketoprofen *(Orudis)*, naproxen *(Anaprox, Naprosyn)*, oxaprozin *(Daypro)* ▪ **Fenamates:** meclofenamate sodium *(Meclomen)*, mefenamic acid *(Ponstel)* ▪ **Indoles:** etodolac *(Lodine)*, indomethacin *(Indocin)* ▪ **Oxicams:** piroxicam *(Feldene)* ▪ **Salicylates:** aspirin *(A.S.A., Ecotrin)*, choline magnesium trisalicylate *(Trilisate)*, choline salicylate *(Arthropan)*, diflunisal *(Dolobid)*, magnesium salicylate, salsalate *(Disalcid)*, sodium salicylate ▪ **Other:** celecoxib *(Celebrex)*, ketorolac tromethamine *(Toradol)*, nabumetone *(Relafen)*, tolmetin sodium *(Tolectin)*.

DOSAGE: Usual adult dose ranges *PO*

aspirin	325-6000mg/d
bromfenac	25-50mg q6-8h
celecoxib	100-200mg/d
choline salicylate	870-5220mg/d
diclofenac	100-200mg/d
diflunisal	250-2500mg/d
etodolac	200-1200mg/d
fenoprofen	300-3200mg/d
flurbiprofen	50-300mg/d
ibuprofen	200-3200mg/d
indomethacin	25-200mg/d
ketoprofen	25-300mg/d
ketorolac	10-60mg/d
magnesium salicylate	325-4800mg/d
meclofenamate	50-400mg/d
mefenamic acid	250-1250mg/d
nabumetone	500-2000mg/d
naproxen	250-1250mg/d

oxaprozin	600-1800mg/d
piroxicam	10-20mg/d
salsalate	500-3000mg/d
sodium salicylate	325-3900mg/d
sulindac	150-400mg/d
tolmetin sodium	200-2000mg/d

NURSING MANAGEMENT PRIORITIES

ASSESS: Hx of hypersensitivity ▪ Pain characteristics ▪ Bleeding, esp c̄ anticoagulant therapy ▪ CAUTION: GI bleeding/bleeding disorders; CV, hepatic, renal impairment ▪ **ndx: Therapeutic effects**: Impaired physical mobility ▪ Pain ▪ **Adverse effects:** Risk for activity intolerance ▪ Constipation ▪ Risk for fluid volume deficit ▪ Fluid volume excess ▪ Risk for injury ▪ Sensory/perceptual alterations (visual) ▪ Risk for impaired skin integrity ▪ Altered tissue perfusion ▪ Altered patterns of urinary elimination. **PLAN:** Observe for edema in extremities ▪ Evaluate vision, hearing ▪ Avoid use c̄ aspirin ▪ **Special considerations:** G: caution (↑ sensitivity; renal impairment) ▪ P: avoid use (Reye's syndrome) ▪ OB: avoid use if pregnant, breastfeeding ▪ **Dietary management**: Avoid use c̄ alcohol, GI-irritating foods ▪ **Lab test evaluation**: Blood glucose levels ↓ (diabetics). **IMPLEMENT:** Administer c̄ food to ↓ GI irritation; encourage upright position for 15-30m ▪ Monitor F/E status (I&O, daily weight, peripheral edema) ▪ Check for bleeding; D/C drug, notify physician ▪ **Patient education:** Comply c̄ prescribed drug regimen ▪ Notify physician *immediately* of bleeding, rash, flulike symptoms, swelling of feet/legs, GI distress, jaundice, ↓ urine output, visual disturbances ▪ Take c̄ food/milk ▪ Check c̄ physician/pharmacist before using OTC preparations ▪ Avoid use c̄ alcohol ▪ Use safety precautions c̄ hazardous activity (drowsiness, dizziness, visual disturbance). **EVALUATE: Observe for therapeutic effects:** ↓ Pain ▪ ↓ Inflammation.

DESCRIPTION: Chemical derivatives of salicylic acid that exhibit wide array of pharmacologic activity incl topical, systemic applications.

DRUGS: Systemic salicylates: aspirin *(A.S.A., Ecotrin),* systemic choline magnesium trisalicylate *(Trilisate),* choline salicylate *(Arthropan),* diflunisal *(Dolobid, *Trilisate),* magnesium salicylate *(Doan's pills, Magan),* olsalazine sodium *(Dipentum),* salsalate *(Disalcid, Mono-Gesic),* sodium salicylate *(*S-60),* sodium thiosalicylate ▪ **Topical salicylates:** salicylic acid *(*Keralyt Gel, *Salingel),* methyl salicylate, triethanolamine salicylate *(Aspercreme, Exocaine, *Royflex).*

THERAPEUTIC USE: Analgesic for mild-moderate pain ▪ Antipyretic ▪ Rheumatoid arthritis, osteoarthritis, other arthritic diseases ▪ Symptomatic treatment of rheumatic fever ▪ Prophylaxis (aspirin) of thrombotic diseases, esp coronary artery disease ▪ Remission of ulcerative colitis in pts intolerant to sulfasalazine (olsalazine sodium) ▪ Topical salicylates are used as rubefacients (heat producing on skin) except for salicylic acid (antifungal & keratolytic).

MECHANISM OF ACTION: Analgesic/antiinflammatory effect may be due to effect on prostaglandin synthesis. Antipyresis due to effect on thermoregulatory areas in hypothalamus, resulting in dilation of peripheral blood vessels, marked sweating. Antithrombotic effect due to inhibition

PHARMACOKINETICS

	Absorption						
	PO	Rectal	Peak	Duration	Half-life	Protein binding	Excretion
aspirin	80%-100%	70%-100%	15m-2h	4-6h	15-30m	90%	98% in urine as metabolites
diflunisal	98%-100%	—	2-3h	8-12h	8-12h	99%	90% in urine as metabolites
olsalazine	2.4%	—	1h	NA	0.9h	99%	>90% urine, feces as metabolites

of platelet aggregation (limited to aspirin). Salicylates may interfere c̄ synthesis of hepatic coagulation factors.

CONTRAINDICATIONS: Hypersensitivity, active ulcers, magnesium salicylate c̄ advanced renal impairment.

DOSAGE: Adult *PO*

aspirin	325-650mg 4-6 times/d
choline salicylate	870mg 5-8 times/d
diflunisal	250-500mg q8-12h
magnesium salicylate	325-650mg 3-4 times/d
olsalazine sodium	500mg bid
salsalate	500mg 4-6 times/d
sodium salicylate	325-600mg q4h

SIDE/ADVERSE EFFECTS: CNS: tinnitus (use in febrile pediatric pts c̄ selected virus infections may induce ***Reye's syndrome***) ▪ GI: epigastric distress, nausea, ***bleeding, ulcers*** ▪ HEM: hypothrombinemia ▪ HEP: ↑ AST, ALT.

DRUG INTERACTIONS: Use c̄ other ulcerogenic drugs best avoided ▪ Salicylates ↑ effects of PO anticoagulants, antidiabetics ▪ Use c̄ alcohol ↑ GI bleeding ▪ Salicylates ↓ PO absorption, uricosuric effects of indomethacin, other NSAIAs ▪ Use c̄ antacids ↓ salicylate PO absorption.

NURSING MANAGEMENT PRIORITIES

ASSESS: Hx of hypersensitivity ▪ GI irritation ▪ Bleeding ▪ Toxicity (CNS disturbances, tinnitus, hyperventilation) ▪ Pain characteristics ▪ CAUTION**:** active ulcers, renal impairment ▪ **ndx: Therapeutic effects:** Risk for altered body temperature ▪ Impaired physical mobility ▪ Pain ▪ Altered tissue perfusion ▪ **Adverse effects:** Risk for injury ▪ Pain ▪ Sensory/perceptual alterations (auditory) ▪ Altered tissue perfusion. **PLAN:** Avoid concurrent administration c̄ large amounts of antacids ▪ **Special considerations:** G: caution (↑ sensitivity; renal impairment) ▪ P: avoid use (Reye's syndrome) ▪ OB: avoid use if pregnant, breastfeeding ▪ **Dietary management:** Avoid use c̄ GI-irritating foods ▪ **Lab test evaluation:** ↓ Blood glucose levels (diabetics). **IMPLEMENT:** Administer c̄ food to ↓ GI irritation ▪ Check for bleeding; D/C drug, notify physician ▪ Monitor VS, esp temperature ▪ **Patient education:** Comply c̄ prescribed drug regimen ▪ Take c̄ food/milk ▪ Notify physician immediately of bleeding, rash, hearing disturbances ▪ Check c̄ physician/pharmacist before taking OTC preparations. **EVALUATE: Observe for therapeutic effects:** ↓ Fever ▪ ↓ Pain ▪ ↓ Inflammation ▪ ↓ Clot formation.

Drug	Type	Brand name	Use	Dose range	Legal status
acetaminophen	p-aminophenol	Anacin-3, Datril, Tempra, Tylenol	Analgesic, antipyretic	325-4000mg/d PO	OTC
alfentanil hcl	Synthetic narcotic	Alfenta	Opioid analgesic adjunct during anesthesia	8-245µg/kg IV	Rx, C-II, C
aspirin	Salicylate NSAIA	Bufferin, Ecotrin	Analgesic, antiinflammatory, antipyretic, anti rheumatic, antithrombotic	325-6000mg/d PO	OTC
bromfenac Na	NSAIA	Duract	Short-term analgesic	25-150mg/d PO	Rx, C
buprenorphine hcl	Synthetic agonist-antagonist narcotic	Buprenex	Opioid analgesic	0.3mg IM/IV	Rx, C-V, C
butorphanol tartrate	Synthetic agonist-antagonist narcotic	Stadol	Opioid analgesic	2mg q3-4h IM 1mg q3-4h IV	Rx, C
choline/magnesium salicylate	Combination salicylate NSAIA	Trilisate	Antiinflammatory	1500-3000mg/d PO	Rx, C
choline salicylate	Salicylate NSAIA	Arthropan	Antiinflammatory; antipyretic	870mg/d 5-8 times/d	OTC
clonidine hcl	Central analgesic	Duracolon	In combination c̄ opiates for severe pain in cancer pts	30µg/hr by continuous epidural infusion	Rx, C

Drug	Type	Brand name	Use	Dose range	Legal status
codeine phosphate/ sulfate	Natural opium alkaloid narcotic	None	Opioid analgesic, antitussive	15-60mg q4-6h PO	Rx, C-II, C
dezocine	Synthetic agonist-antagonist narcotic	Dalgan	Opioid analgesic	5-20mg q3-6h IM 2.5-10mg q2-4h IV	Rx, C
diclofenac K/NA▲	NSAIA	Cataflam, Voltaren	Analgesic, antiinflammatory; postop ocular analgesic▲	100-200mg/d PO 1gtt qid starting 24h after surgery	Rx, C
diflunisal	Salicylate derivative NSAIA	Dolobid	Analgesic, antiinflammatory	250-2500mg/d PO	Rx, C
etodolac	NSAIA	Lodine	Analgesic, antiinflammatory	200-1200mg/d PO	Rx, C
fenoprofen Ca	NSAIA	Nalfon	Analgesic, antiinflammatory	200-3200mg/d PO	Rx
fentanyl citrate	Synthetic narcotic	Duragesic (transdermal), Fentanyl Oracet (transmucosal), Sublimaze (IM/IV)	Opioid analgesic	IM/IV: Variable $\bar{c}$ procedure Transdermal: 25-100µg/h Transmucosal: 5-10µg/kg	Rx, C-II, C
flurbiprofen/Na▲	NSAIA	Ansaid, Ocufen▲	Analgesic, antiinflammatory, mioisis inhibitor during ocular surgery▲	50-300mg/d PO 1gtt q½h starting 2h before surgery	Rx, B

Drug	Type	Brand name	Use	Dose range	Legal status
hydrocodone bitartrate	Synthetic narcotic	None—component for analgesic, antitussive combination formulation	Antitussive, opioid analgesic	5-10mg q4-6h PO	Rx, C-II/III, C
hydromorphone hcl	Semisynthetic narcotic	Dilaudid	Opioid analgesic	2mg q4-6h PO 1-2mg q4-6h IM/SC	Rx, C-II, C
ibuprofen	NSAIA	Advil▲, Motrin, MotrinB▲, Nuprin▲	Analgesic, antiinflammatory, antipyretic	200-3200mg/d PO	Rx, OTC▲
indomethacin/Na trihydrate▲	NSAIA	Indocin	Antiinflammatory, infant PD closure▲ (<48h old)	25-200mg/d PO 0.1-0.2mg/kg, doses 2 & 3 0.1mg/kg IV	Rx
ketoprofen	NSAIA	Agron▲, Orudis, Oruvail	Analgesic, antiinflammatory	25-300mg/d PO	Rx, OTC▲
ketorolac tromethamine	NSAIA	Acular▲, Toradol	Short-term analgesic seasonal allergic conjunctivitis▲	10-60mg/d PO 1 gtt/qid▲	Rx, C
levomethadyl acetate hcl	Synthetic narcotic	ORLAAM	Maintenance of opiate addiction	60-90mg 3 times/wk PO	Rx, C-II
levophanol tartrate	Synthetic narcotic	Levo-Dromoran	Opioid analgesic, preanesthetic sedation	2-3mg q6-8h PO 1-2mg q6-8h IM/SC	Rx, C-II, C

Note: Side/adverse effects: common in *italic;* serious in ***boldface italic.*** *Available in Canada only.

Drug	Type	Brand name	Use	Dose range	Legal status
magnesium salicylate	Salicylate NSAIA	Doan's pills, Magan	Analgesic, antiinflammatory	325-650mg 3-4 times/d PO	OTC
meclofenamate Na	NSAIA	None	Analgesic, antiinflammatory	50-400mg/d PO	Rx
mefenamic acid	NSAIA	Ponstel	Analgesic	250-1250mg/d PO	Rx, C
meperidine hcl	Synthetic narcotic	Demerol	Opioid analgesis, preop sedation, support of anesthesia	50-150mg q3-4h PO/SC/IM	Rx, C-II, C
methadone hcl	Synthetic narcotic	Dolophine	Opioid analgesic, maintenance of opiate addiction▲	2.5-10mg q3-4h IM/SC ≥40-120mg once/d▲	Rx, C-II, C
methotrimeprazine hcl	Phenothiazine	Levoprome	Analgesic, preop sedation	2-20mg preop IM 10-20mg q4-6h IM	Rx
morphine sulfate	Natural opium, alkaloid narcotic	None	Opioid analgesic, preop/postop sedation/analgesic	10-30mg PO 5-20mg q4h IM/SC 2.5-15mg IV 10-20mg q4h rectally	Rx, C-II, C
nabumetone	NSAIA	Relafen	Antiinflammatory	500-2000mg/d PO	Rx, C
nalbuphine hcl	Synthetic agonist-antagonist narcotic	Nubain	Opioid analgesic, preop sedation	10-20mg q3-6h IM/IV/SC	Rx, C
naproxen/Na▲	NSAIA	Aleve▲, Anaprox▲, Naprelan, Naprosyn	Analgesic, antiinflammatory	250-1250mg/d	Rx, OTC▲, B

Drug	Type	Brand name	Use	Dose range	Legal status
opium tincture, camphorated (paregoric)	Natural 0.43% extract tincture of opium	None	Diarrhea	5-10ml (2-4mg of morphine) 1-4 times/d PO	Rx, C-III
opium tincture, deodorized (laudanum)	Natural 10% extract tincture of opium	None	Diarrhea	0.6ml (6mg of morphine) 1-4 times/d PO	Rx, C
oxaprozin	NSAIA	Daypro	Analgesic, antiinflammatory	600-1800mg/d PO	Rx, C
oxycodone	Synthetic narcotic	Roxicodone	Opioid analgesic	5mg q6h PO	Rx, C-II
oxymorphone hcl	Semisynthetic narcotic	Numorphan	Opioid analgesic, preop sedation, anxiety c̄ dyspnea associated c̄ acute left ventricular failure & pulmonary edema	1-1.5mg q6h IM/SC 5mg suppository q4-6h	Rx, C-II
pentazocine lactate	Synthetic agonist-antagonist narcotic	Talwin	Opioid analgesic, preop sedation	30mg q3-4h IM/IV/SC	Rx, C-IV, C
piroxicam	NSAIA	Feldene	Antiinflammatory	10-20mg/d PO	Rx
propoxyphene hcl/napsylate▲	Opioidlike synthetic analgesic (related to methadone)	Darvon, Darvon-N▲	Analgesic	65mg q4h PO 100mg q4h PO▲	Rx, C-IV

Note: Side/adverse effects: common in *italic;* serious in ***boldface italic.*** ▲Available in Canada only.

Drug	Type	Brand name	Use	Dose range	Legal status
remifentanil hcl	Rapid/short-acting synthetic narcotic	Ultiva	Opioid analgesic for induction/maintenance of general anesthesia & as an analgesic component for monitored anesthesia care	0.025-1µg/kg/m	Rx, C
salsalate	Salicylate NSAIA	Disalcid, Mono-Gesic, Salflex	Antiinflammatory	500-mg 4-6 times/d PO	Rx, C
sodium salicylate	Salicylate NSAIA	None	Analgesic	325-650mg q4h PO	OTC
sodium thiosalicylate	Salicylate NSAIA	Rexolate	Analgesic, antiinflammatory gout	50-100mg/d PO 100-150mg/d PO for rheumatic fever 100mg q3-4h for gout	Rx
sulindac	NSAIA	Clinoral	Antiinflammatory	150-400mg/d PO	Rx
sufentanil citrate	Synthetic narcotic	Sufenta	Opioid analgesic supplement for maintenance of balanced general anesthesia, general anesthesia	Variable $\bar{c}$ procedure (1-30µg/kg IV)	Rx, C-II, C
tolmetin Na	NSAIA	Tolectin/DS	Antiinflammatory	200-2000mg/d PO	Rx, C
tramadol hcl	Central analgesic	Ultram	Analgesic	50-400mg/d PO	Rx, C

DESCRIPTION: Group of antihypertensive drugs that inhibit ACE, resulting in a hypotensive effect.

DRUGS: Rx; Preg Cat C/D benazepril hcl *(Lotensin)*, captopril *(Capoten)*, enalapril maleate *(Vasotec)*, enalaprilat *(Vasotec I.V.)*, fosinopril sodium *(Monopril)*, lisinopril *(Prinivil, Zestril)*, moexipril *(Univasc)*, quinapril hcl *(Accupril)*, ramipril *(Altace)*, trandolapril *(Mavik)*.

THERAPEUTIC USE: Treatment of hypertension as sole agent/in combination c̄ other antihypertensives. (Preg Cat C for 1st trimester, Preg Cat D for 2nd & 3rd trimesters) ▪ Adjunct for CHF (lisinopril, trandolapril) ▪ Treatment of heart failure (captopril, enalapril, lisinopril, quinapril) ▪ Treatment of left ventricular dysfunction (captopril, enalapril, lisinopril, trandolapril) ▪ Treatment of diabetic neuropathy (captopril) ▪ Treatment of acute MI w/in 24h (lisinopril).

MECHANISM OF ACTION: Antihypertensive activity appears related to suppression of renin-angiotensin aldosterone system by competitive inhibition of ACE, which produces angiotensin II from angiotensin I, resulting in a ↓ of peripheral arterial resistance, ↓ in aldosterone secretion.

PHARMACOKINETICS

	PO absorption	Peak	Half-life	Protein binding	Excretion
benazepril	37%	0.5-1h	10-11h	96.7%	Via urine as metabolites
captopril	75%	1h	1-1.5h	25%-30%	95% via urine
enalapril	60%	1h	1.5h	NA	95% via urine in 24h
fosinopril	35%	3h	2-3h	95%	50% via urine, 50% via feces in 24h
lisinopril	25%	7h	6-7h	NA	98%-100% via urine in 24h
moexipril	13%	1.5h	2-9h	50%	40% via urine, 52% via feces
quinapril	60%	1h	2-3h	97%	96% via urine as metabolites
ramipril	50%-60%	1h	1h	73%	60% via urine, 40% via feces in 24h
trandolapril	NA	1h	6h	80%	66% via urine, 33% via feces

CONTRAINDICATIONS: Hypersensitivity. D/C during pregnancy as soon as possible. **CC:** Use of ACE-I during 2nd & 3rd trimesters is associated c̄ fetal harm.

DOSAGE: Adult *PO*

benazepril	20-40mg/d
captopril	50-100mg/d
enalapril	10-40mg/d
fosinopril	10mg/d
lisinopril	20-40mg/d
moexipril	7.5-30mg/d
quinapril	10-80mg/d
ramipril	2.5-20mg/d
trandolapril	2-8mg/d

SIDE/ADVERSE EFFECTS: CNS: headache, dizziness, mood changes ▪ CV: hypotension, tachycardia, chest pain, palpitation, ***MI*** (rare), ***Raynaud's syndrome*** ▪ GI: V/D, pain, dyspepsia, gastroenteritis ▪ HEM: ***agranulocytosis***, anemia, *thrombocytosis*, neutropenia ▪ INT: rash, pruritus ▪ Other: loss of taste, proteinuria, hyperkalemia.

DRUG INTERACTIONS: Use c̄ aspirin, indomethacin, other NSAIAs may antagonize therapeutic response ▪ Use K^+-sparing diuretics c̄ caution due to hyperkalemia ▪ Concurrent use c̄ lithium can ↑ its toxicity.

NURSING MANAGEMENT PRIORITIES

ASSESS: Hx of hypersensitivity ▪ BP ▪ Adequate renal function ▪ CAUTION: CV, hepatic, renal impairment ▪ **ndx: Therapeutic effects**: ↓ Cardiac output ▪ Altered tissue perfusion ▪ **Adverse effects:** Risk for activity intolerance ▪ ↓ Cardiac output ▪ Fatigue ▪ Risk for injury ▪ Sensory/perceptual alterations ▪ Risk for impaired skin integrity. **PLAN**: Observe for edema in extremities ▪ Prevent postural hypotension ▪ **Special considerations:** G: caution, ↓ dosage (renal impairment) ▪ P: not recommended ▪ OB: avoid use if pregnant, breastfeeding ▪ **Dietary management**: Avoid high-Na^+/high-K^+ foods, alcohol; calorie restrictions ▪ **Lab test evaluation**: Electrolytes. **IMPLEMENT:** Monitor BP; observe for hypotension ▪ Monitor I&O, daily weight ▪ Monitor CV, hepatic, renal status ▪ **Patient education:** Avoid sudden position changes (postural hypotension) ▪ Comply c̄ prescribed drug regimen ▪ Avoid smoking, use c̄ alcohol, constrictive clothing, extremely hot objects, OTC cough/cold/allergy preparations ▪ Follow low-Na^+ diet ▪ Have BP checked regularly ▪ Keep appointments c̄ physician ▪ Carry medical identification (Medic-Alert). **EVALUATE: Observe for therapeutic effect:** ↓ BP.

DESCRIPTION: Large group of OTC preparations available in assorted dosage preparations c̄ single/multiple antacid formulations; recent mass media advertisements stress Ca^{++}-containing formulas for osteoporosis, low-Na^{+}/Na^{+}-free preparations. Many preparations contain simethicone, which ↓ gas, bloating.

THERAPEUTIC USE: Treatment of hyperacidity. Effects on BM, Na^{+} content vary c̄ formulation. Na^{+} >0.2mEq must be stated & >5mEq in total daily dose is contraindicated c̄ restricted salt diet.

MECHANISM OF ACTION: Chemical neutralization rx. Must be able to ↑ gastric pH to ≥3.5 w/in 10m.

SIDE/ADVERSE EFFECTS: GI: diarrhea c̄ Mg preparations, esp Milk of Magnesia; constipation c̄ Al-, Ca-containing products ▪ MET: alkalosis (systemic products).

DRUG INTERACTIONS: Concurrent administration c̄ any drug *not* recommended because of poor PO absorption ▪ Contraindicated c̄ tetracycline therapy.

NURSING MANAGEMENT PRIORITIES

ASSESS: GI, renal status ▪ Characteristics of discomfort ▪ CHF, hypertension, fluid retention (avoid Na^{+}-containing preparations) ▪ Renal impairment (avoid Mg^{++}-containing preparations) ▪ CAUTION: abdominal pain ▪ **ndx: Therapeutic effects**: Pain ▪ **Adverse effects:** Constipation ▪ Diarrhea. **PLAN:** Avoid concurrent administration c̄ any drug; poor PO absorption results ▪ **Special considerations:** G: caution (↓ GI motility; renal impairment) ▪ P: caution <6y/o (vague symptoms) ▪ OB: no reported precautions ▪ **Dietary management**: Avoid GI-irritating foods ▪ **Lab test evaluation**: Serum electrolytes (long-term). **IMPLEMENT:** Shake PO suspensions well before pouring; follow c̄ H_2O to ensure reaching stomach ▪ Avoid concurrent drug administration, esp tetracycline, enteric-coated preparations ▪ Administer 1-3h pc & at hs ▪ **Patient education:** Comply c̄ prescribed dosage regimen ▪ Comply c̄ dietary restrictions ▪ Notify physician if GI distress persists or worsens (black, tarry stools; coffee-ground emesis). **EVALUATE: Observe for therapeutic effect:** ↓ GI distress.

DOSAGE/PRODUCT INFORMATION: Effervescent powder/tablet, suspension formulations have greater efficacy than capsule, powder, tablet formulations.

KEY:

$Al(OH)_3$	Aluminum hydroxide	$2MgO3SiO_2$	Magnesium trisilicate
$CaCO_3$	Calcium carbonate	$Mg(OH)_2$	Magnesium hydroxide
$KHCO_3$	Potassium bicarbonate	NaCl	Sodium chloride
MgO	Magnesium oxide	$NaHCO_3$	Sodium bicarbonate

PRODUCT INFORMATION

Brand name	Dosage form	Formula (per 5ml/tab)	Sodium content (per 5ml/tab)	Dose
Alka-Seltzer	Eff tab	Citric acid 312mg/$NaHCO_3$ 958mg/ $KHCO_3$, 312mg	311mg (13.5mEq)	1-2 tab c̄ H_2O q4h
AlternaGEL	Susp	$Al(OH)_3$, 600mg	0.109mEq	5-10ml prn between meals, at hs. Do *not* exceed 120ml/d
Aludrox	Susp	$Al(OH)_3$, 307mg; $Mg(OH)_2$, 103mg	0.10mEq	10ml q4h. Do *not* exceed 60ml/d
Amphojel	Susp	$Al(OH)_3$, 320mg	0.10mEq	10ml 5-6 times/d between meals, at hs. Do *not* exceed 60ml/d
	Tab	$Al(OH)_3$, 300mg or 600mg	0.08mEq or 0.13mEq	0.6g 5-6 times/d between meals, at hs. Do *not* exceed 3.6g/d
Citrocarbonate	Eff pwd	Citric acid, 1.19g; $NaHCO_3$, 2.34g; NaCl, 79mg; sodium citrate, 254mg/3.9g of pwd	30.46mEq	4-8g in H_2O pc. Do *not* exceed 20g/d
Di-Gel	Susp	$Al(OH)_3$, 200mg; $Mg(OH)_2$, 200mg; simethicone, 20mg	0.22mEq	10ml or 2 tab q2h or after or between meals at the hour. Do *not* exceed 100ml or 24/d
	Tab	$Ca(CO_3)$, 200mg; $Mg(OH)_2$, 128mg; simethicone, 20mg		

Brand name	Dosage form	Formula (per 5ml/tab)	Sodium content (per 5ml/tab)	Dose
Gaviscon	Susp	$Al(OH)_3$, 200mg; $Mg(CO)_3$, 358mg	1.7mEq	15 30ml qid. Do *not* exceed 120ml/d
	Tab	$Al(OH)_3$, 80mg; $2MgO3SiO_2$, 20mg	0.8mEq	2-4 qid. Do *not* exceed 16/d
Gaviscon Extra Strength	Susp	$Al(OH)_3$, 508mg; $MgCO_3$, 475mg	0.9mEq	10-20ml qid. Do *not* exceed 80ml/d
	Tab	$Al(OH)_3$, 160mg; $MgCO_3$, 105mg	1.3mEq	2-4 qid. Do *not* exceed 16/d
Gaviscon-2	Tab	$Al(OH)_3$, 160mg; $2Mg3SiO_2$, 40mg	1.6mEq	1-2 qid. Do *not* exceed 8/d
Gelusil	Susp/Tab	$Al(OH)_3$, 200mg; $Mg(OH)_2$, 200mg simethicone, 25mg	0.03mEq	10ml or 2 tab 1h pc, at hs. Do *not* exceed 60ml or 12 tabs/d
Maalox Heart-burn Relief	Susp	$Al(OH)_3$, 140mg; $MgCO_3$, 175mg	—	10-20ml pc, at hs. Do *not* exceed 80ml/d
Maalox Plus	Tab	$Al(OH)_3$, 250mg; $Mg(OH)_2$, 250mg simethicone, 25mg	0.03mEq	1-4pc, hs. Do *not* exceed 16/d
Maalox Extra Strength	Susp	$Al(OH)_3$, 500mg; $Mg(OH)_2$, 450mg; simethicone, 40m	0.05mEq	10-20ml pc, at hs. Do *not* exceed 60ml/d
	Tab	$Al(OH)_3$, 350mg; $Mg(OH)_2$, 350mg; simethicone, 30mg	0.03mEq	1-3pc, at hs. Do *not* exceed 12/d
Milk of Magnesia	Susp	$Mg(OH)_2$,400mg	0.005mEq	5-15ml $\bar{c}$ H_2O up to 4 times/d. Do *not* exceed 60ml/d
Mylanta	Gelcaps	$CaCO_3$, 311mg; $MgCO_3$, 232mg	0.1087mEq	2-4 prn. Do *not* exceed 24/d
	Susp/Tab	$Al(OH)_3$, 200mg; $Mg(OH)_2$, 200mg simethicone, 20mg	0.03/0.33mEq	10-20ml or 2-4 tab qid. Do *not* exceed 24 doses/d

Brand name	Dosage form	Formula (per 5ml/tab)	Sodium content (per 5ml/tab)	Dose
Mylanta Double Strength	Susp/Tab	$Al(OH)_3$, 400mg; $Mg(HO)_2$, 400mg simethicone, 40mg	0.05mEq	10-20ml or 2-4 tab qid. Do *not* exceed 12 doses/d
Mylanta Gas	Tab	Simethicone 40, 80, 125mg		40-125mg qid. Do *not* exceed 480mg/d
Mylicon	gtt	Simethicone, 40mg/0.6ml		<2y/o: 0.3ml qid pc, at hs
Riopan	Susp/Tab	Magaldrate, 540/480mg	0.013/0.004mEq	5-10ml or 1-2 tab qid. Do *not* exceed 90ml or 20/d
Riopan Plus	Susp/Tab	Magaldrate, 540/480mg; simethicone, 20mg	0.013/0.004mEq	5-10ml or 1-2 tab qid. Do *not* exceed 60ml or 25/d
Riopan Plus 2	Susp/Tab	Magaldrate, 1080mg; simethicone, 20mg	0.013/0.021mEq	5-10ml or 1-2 tab qid. Do *not* exceed 60ml or 25/d
Rolaids Calcium Rich	Tab	$CaCO_3$, 550mg	0.017mEq	1-2 prn. Do *not* exceed 14/d
Titralac	Tab	$CaCO_3$, 420mg; glycine, 180mg	0.01mEq	1-2 tabs pc. Do *not* exceed 19/d
Tums	Tab	$CaCO_3$, 500mg	0.087mEq	1-2 prn. Do *not* exceed 16/d
Tums E-X	Tab	$CaCO_3$, 750mg	0.087mEq	1-2 prn. Do *not* exceed 10/d
Tums Plus	Tab	$CaCO_3$, 500mg; simethicone, 20mg	0.087mEq	1-2 prn. Do *not* exceed 16/d
Wingel	Susp/Tab	$Al(OH)_3$, 180mg; $Mg(OH)_2$, 160mg	0.1mEq	5-10ml or 2 tab qid. Do *not* exceed 40ml or 8/d

DESCRIPTION: A small group of drugs used in treatment of helminth (parasitic worm) infections. Helminth infections are indigenous to every country. Incidence of worm infections is much higher in underdeveloped countries than in countries c̄ adequate sewage treatment facilities. In the United States helminth infections are usually limited to selective causative organisms c̄ enterobiasis being the most common worm infection. Helminth parasites belong to two animal phyla: (1) Platyhelminthes (flat worms), which are subdivided into Cestodes (segmented) & Trematodes (nonsegmented) and (2) Nemathelminthes or Nematodes (round worms). Selected helminth infections include *Cestodes* (flat segmented worms): *Diphyllobothrium latum* (fish), *Echinococcus granulosus* (dog), *Taenia saginata* (beef), *Taenia solium* (pork), *Nematodes* (round worms): *Ancylostoma duodenale* (Old World hookworm), *Ascaris lumbricoides, Enterobiasis vermicularis* (oxyuriasis, pinworms, seat worms), *Necator americanus* (New World hookworms), *Trichinella spiralis* (trichinosis), *Trichuris trichiura* (whipworms).

DRUGS: albendazole, mebendazole, pyrantel pamoate, thiabendazole.

THERAPEUTIC USE: Ascaris: mebendazole, pyrantel ▪ Hookworm: mebendazole ▪ Pinworm: mebendazole, pyrantel ▪ Tapeworm: albendazole (larval pork neurocysticercosis ▪ Trichinosis: thiabendazole (invasive phase) ▪ Whipworm: mebendazole.

MECHANISM OF ACTION: albendazole: inhibition of tubulin polymerization resulting in ↓ of microtubules ▪ mebendazole: inhibition of glucose uptake ▪ pyrantel: depolarizing neuromuscular blocking activity ▪ thiabendazole: enzyme inhibition (fumarate reductose).

NURSING MANAGEMENT PRIORITIES

ASSESS: Hx of hypersensitivity ▪ Hepatic, renal function ▪ Signs of toxicity (CNS, neurotoxicity) ▪ **ndx: Therapeutic effects:** Risk for infection ▪ **Adverse effects:** Risk for injury ▪ Diarrhea ▪ Impaired tissue integrity ▪ Risk for peripheral neurovascular dysfunction ▪ Sensory/perceptual alterations. **PLAN:** Take c̄ food to ↓ GI irriation ▪ Maintain hydration ▪ Strict handwashing ▪ Seizure precautions ▪ **Special considerations:** G: caution, ↓ dosage (neurotoxicity) ▪ P: caution (↑ sensitivity) ▪ OB: caution if pregnant, breastfeeding ▪ **Dietary management:** None specific ▪ **Lab test evaluation:** Culture for ova & parasites. **IMPLEMENT:** Monitor VS ▪ **Patient education:** ▪ Safety precautions c̄ hazardous activity ▪ All family members must be treated ▪ Disinfect bathroom facilities. **EVALUATE: Observe for therapeutic effect:** Resolution of helminth infection.

Drug name	Dosage form	Dosage	Contraindications	Adverse effects	Legal status
albendazole *(Albenza)*	Tab: 200mg	*C/A:* Hydatid disease <60kg-15mg/kg/d divided bid >60kg-400mg. Each for 28d. For 3 cycles c̄ 14d rest period between cycles *C/A:* Neurocysticerosis <60kg-15mg/kg/d divided bid & >60kg 400mg bid for 8-30d	Hypersensitivity	Hydatid: N/V, headache, abdominal pain; Neurocysticerosis: N/V, headache	Rx-C
mebendazole *(Vermox)*	Chewable tab: 100mg	*C/A:* Pinworms—100mg/d for 3d Ascaris Hookworm } 100mg bid for 3d Whipworm }	Hypersensitivity	Diarrhea, abdominal pain	Rx-C
pyrantel *(Antiminth)*	PO Susp: 250mg/5ml	*C/A:* Ascaris/pinworm 11mg/kg as a single dose. Do *not* exceed 1g	Hypersensitivity, hepatic disease	N/V/D, anorexia, headache	Rx-NA
thiabendazole *(Mintezol)*	PO Susp: 500mg/5ml Chewable tab: 500mg	*C/A:* Trichinosis 25mg/kg bid for 2-4d	Hypersensitivity	N/V/D, anorexia, dizziness, headache	Rx-C

DESCRIPTION: Antiarrhythmics (antidysrhythmics) are used to treat various cardiac arrhythmias.

DRUGS: Classified by pharmacologic/therapeutic drug categories, effect produced on action potential of cardiac electrophysiology ▪ **Pharmacologic/therapeutic**: β BLOCKERS: acebutolol *(Sectral)*, esmolol *(Brevibloc)*, propranolol hcl *(Inderal)*, sotalol hcl *(Betapace)* ▪ CALCIUM BLOCKERS: diltiazem hcl *(Cardizem)*, verapamil hcl *(Calan, Isoptin)* ▪ CARDIAC GLYCOSIDES: digoxin *(Lanoxin)*, digitoxin *(Crystodigin)* ▪ LOCAL ANESTHETICS/DERIVATIVES: flecainide acetate *(Tambocor)*, lidocaine hcl, mexiletine hcl *(Mexitil)*, procainamide hcl *(Pronestyl)*, propafenone hcl *(Rythmol)*, tocainide hcl *(Tonocard)* ▪ QUINIDINE SALTS: quinidine gluconate *(Quinaglute)*, quinidine polygalacturonate *(Cardioquin)*, quinidine sulfate *(Quinidex Extentabs)* ▪ MISCELLANEOUS: amiodarone hcl *(Cordarone)*, bretylium tosylate *(Bretylol)*, disopyramide *(Norpace)*, moricizine hcl *(Ethmozine)* ▪ **Miscellaneous:** ibutilide fumarate *(Convert)* ▪ **Action potential:** Phase 0, rapid depolarization of ventricular cardiac tissue *(QRS complex of ECG)*; phases 1, 2, 3, repolarization; phase 4, resting ▪ CLASS I DRUGS: *(membrane stabilizing)* depress phase 0: I—moricizine hcl *(Ethmozine)*; IA—quinidine salts, disopyramide, procainamide; IB—lidocaine, mexiletine, tocainide; IC—flecainide, propafenone ▪ CLASS II DRUGS: β-adrenergic blockers, depress phase 4 depolarization: acebutolol, esmolol, propranolol hcl ▪ CLASS III DRUGS: prolong repolarization in phase 3: amiodarone hcl, bretylium tosylate, ibutilide fumarate ▪ CLASS IV DRUGS: calcium blockers, depress phase 4 depolarization, prolong repolarization of phases 1, 2: cardiac glycosides, diltiazem, verapamil hcl.

DOSAGE: Usual adult range

acebutolol	*PO*	600-1200mg/d divided
amiodarone	*PO*	800-1600mg/d divided
bretylium	*IV*	5-10mg/kg
digitoxin	*PO*	0.05-0.3mg/d
digoxin	*PO*	0.125-0.5mg/d
diltiazem	*PO*	180-240mg/d divided
	IV	0.25mg/kg over 2m
disopyramide	*PO*	400-800mg/d divided
esmolol	*IV*	500μg/kg/m, then 50-100μg/kg/4m
flecainide	*PO*	100-600mg/d divided
ibutilide	*IV*	<60kg: 0.01mg/kg over 10m >60kg: 1mg over 10m
lidocaine	*IV*	50-100mg c̄ 1-4mg/m maintenance
mexiletine	*PO*	200mg q8h
moricizine	*PO*	600-900mg/d divided

procainamide	*PO*	0.5-1g q4-6h (atrial) 50mg/kg divided q3h, then adjusted (ventricular)
propafenone	*PO*	450-900mg/d divided
propranolol	*PO*	10-30mg 3-4 times/d. 180-240 mg/d divided (MI prevention)
quinidine gluconate	*PO*	324-648mg q8-12h
quinidine polygalacturonate	*PO*	275mg 3-4 times/d
quinidine sulfate	*PO*	0.2-0.3g 3-4 times/d (premature atrial/ventricular contractions)
sotalol	*PO*	160-320mg/d divided
tocainide	*PO*	1200-1800mg in 3 doses
verapamil	*PO*	320-480mg/d divided

NURSING MANAGEMENT PRIORITIES

ASSESS: Hx of hypersensitivity ▪ Apical pulse, BP, ECG ▪ Lung sounds ▪ Therapeutic blood level ▪ CAUTION: heart failure ▪ **ndx: Therapeutic effects:** ⬇ Cardiac output ▪ Altered tissue perfusion ▪ **Adverse effects:** Risk for activity intolerance ▪ ⬇ Cardiac output ▪ Constipation ▪ Diarrhea ▪ Risk for fluid volume deficit ▪ Altered thought processes ▪ Impaired tissue integrity (PO mucous membrane) ▪ Altered patterns of urinary elimination. **PLAN:** Institute cardiac monitoring (IV, initial PO) ▪ Administer at equal intervals around clock to maintain blood levels ▪ **Special considerations:** G: caution, ⬇ dosage (⬇ metabolism; chronic illness) ▪ P: caution (immature systems) ▪ OB: caution if pregnant; breast- feeding not recommended ▪ **Dietary management:** Avoid use c̄ caffeine, alcohol, Na^+-containing foods ▪ **Lab test evaluation:** Therapeutic blood levels. **IMPLEMENT:** Assess apical pulse for 1m ▪ Monitor F/E status (I&O, daily weight, peripheral edema) ▪ **Patient education:** Procedure for checking radial pulse ▪ Comply c̄ prescribed dosage regimen ▪ Report abnormal rxs to physician (difficult breathing; rapid, irregular heart rate) ▪ Check c̄ physician/pharmacist before taking OTC preparations ▪ Keep appointments c̄ physician ▪ Carry identification (Medic-Alert). **EVALUATE: Observe for therapeutic effects:** ⬇ Cardiac arrhythmias ▪ Normal heart rate, rhythm.

DESCRIPTION: Large, diverse group of natural, semisynthetic & synthetic drugs that block effects of acetylcholine at postganglionic parasympathetic muscarinic receptors; also known as antimuscarinics, parasympatholytics. Natural drugs obtained from deadly nightshade plants, including *Atropa belladonna, Hyoscyamus* (henbane).

DRUGS: Natural: atropine sulfate, belladonna extract/tincture *(*Belladenal, *Belladenal Spacetabs)*, hyoscyamine sulfate *(Anaspaz, Cystospaz, Cystospaz-M, Levsin)*, *hyoscine hydrobromide, scopolamine *(Transderm-Scop)*, scopolamine hydrobromide *(Triptone)* ▪ **Semisynthetic:** homatropine hydrobromide *(*Isopto Homatropine)* ▪ **Synthetic:** anisotropine methylbromide, clidinium bromide *(Librax, Menrium, Quarzan)*, dicyclomine hcl *(Bentyl, Byclomine)*, glycopyrrolate (*Robinul*), ipratropium bromide *(Atrovent)*, mepenzolate bromide *(Cantil)*, methantheline bromide *(Banthine)*, oxyphencyclimine hcl *(Daricon)*, propantheline bromide *(Pro-Banthine)*, tolterodine tartrate (Detrol), tridihexethyl chloride *(Pathilon)*.

THERAPEUTIC USE: Treat/manage/cause bradycardia, bronchial asthma (cholinergic mediated), cardiospasm, colitis, dilation of pupils, dysmenorrhea relief, enuresis control, GI spasm; inhibition of bronchial/gastric secretions, salivation, sweating; paralysis of accommodation, pylorospasm; secretion due to coryza, hay fever, rhinitis; spastic/rigid states due to CNS injury; ureteral colic, urinary frequency reduction.

MECHANISM OF ACTION: Anticholinergic activity due to competition c̄ acetylcholine for receptors at postganglionic fiber of parasympathetic nervous system, resulting in biliary dilation, bronchial dilation, cycloplegia, ↓ gastric secretion, ↓ GI motility, ↓ salivation, ↓ sweating, drying of mucous membranes, ↑ IOP, mydriasis, tachycardia, urinary retention.

CONTRAINDICATIONS: Adhesions, advanced hepatic/renal impairment, asthma, hiatal hernia associated c̄ reflux esophagitis, hypersensitivity, intestinal atony, myasthenia gravis, narrow-angle glaucoma, obstructive diseases of GI/urinary tract, severe ulcerative colitis.

DOSAGE: Usual adult *PO*

anisotropine	50mg tid
atropine	0.1-0.5mg q4-6h
belladonna extract	15mg 3-4 times/d
belladonna tincture	0.3-1ml 3-4 times/d
clidinium	2.5-5mg 3-4 times/d

dicyclomine	40mg qid
glycopyrrolate	1-2mg tid
homatropine	5-10mg tid
hyoscyamine	0.15-0.3mg qid
ipratropium	2 inhalation qid
mepenzolate	25-50mg qid
methantheline	50-100mg q6h
methscopolamine	2.5-3mg qid
oxyphencyclimine	5-10mg bid
propantheline	15mg tid
scopolamine	0.4-0.8mg 3-4 times/d
tolterodine tartrate	2mg bid
tridihexethyl chloride	25-50mg 3-4 times/d

SIDE/ADVERSE EFFECTS: CNS: mental confusion ▪ CV: tachycardia ▪ EENT: blurred vision, cycloplegia, mydriasis ↓ ocular tension, photophobia ▪ GU: urinary retention ▪ GI: N/V, constipation ▪ Other: suppression of lactation/ body secretions, rash.

DRUG INTERACTIONS: Use c̄ antihistamines, phenothiazines, TCAs produces ↑ anticholinergic effects ▪ MAO-I ↑ activity by ↓ anticholinergic biotransformation ▪ Use c̄ other drugs ↑ their GI absorption.

NURSING MANAGEMENT PRIORITIES

ASSESS: Hx of hypersensitivity ▪ VS, esp heart rate, BP ▪ Urinary retention ▪ Bowel sounds, GI status ▪ CAUTION: hepatic/renal impairment, cardiopulmonary disease, GI/urinary tract obstruction ▪ **ndx: Therapeutic effects:** ↓ Cardiac output ▪ Diarrhea ▪ Fluid volume deficit ▪ Impaired physical mobility. **Adverse effects:** ↓ Cardiac output ▪ Sensory/perceptual alterations (visual) ▪ Altered thought processes ▪ Impaired tissue integrity (PO mucous membrane) ▪ Urinary retention. **PLAN:** Check all dosages carefully ▪ **Special considerations:** G: caution, ↓ dosage (↑ sensitivity) ▪ P: not recommended ▪ OB: caution if pregnant; avoid breastfeeding ▪ **Dietary management:** ↑ Bulk-containing foods (constipation) ▪ **Lab test evaluation:** None specific. **IMPLEMENT:** Monitor VS, esp heart rate ▪ Observe for exaggerated anticholinergic effects ▪ Monitor I&O, GI function ▪ **Patient education:** Expect anticholinergic side effects (dry mouth, photophobia, constipation) ▪ Blurred vision may occur ▪ Protect eyes in sunlight ▪ Use sugarless gum/hard candy to diminish dry mouth ▪ Frequent oral hygiene is required ▪ Avoid OTC cough/cold/ allergy preparations. **EVALUATE: Observe for therapeutic effect:** ↓ Parasympathetic activity.

DESCRIPTION: Anticonvulsants (antiepileptics) comprise several chemically distinct groups of drugs that selectively depress the CNS to prevent epileptic seizures w/out impairing consciousness. Epilepsy is not a specific disease, but an assortment of convulsive symptoms precipitated by abnormal focus of neuronal discharges that originate in the brain, esp motor cortex ▪ Disease categorized by specific EEG patterns & clinical nature of seizures. Therapy must always be individualized to specific seizure patterns because no anticonvulsant drug is equally effective in treating various forms of epilepsy ▪ It is generally accepted that anticonvulsant drugs prevent seizures by acting on nonneuronal cells & therefore have some indirect effect on seizure center (eg, vascular blood supply) ▪ Acting to prevent hyperactive neuron discharge located in the epileptic seizure focus ▪ Acting to prevent seizure spread to normal neurons located near seizure focus.

DRUGS: Barbiturates: phenobarbital (*Luminal*), primidone *(Mysoline)* ▪ **Benzodiazepines:** clonazepam *(Klonopin)*, clorazepate dipotassium *(Tranxene)*, diazepam *(Valium)* ▪ **Hydantoins:** ethotoin *(Peganone)*, fosphenytoin *(Cerebyx)*, mephenytoin *(Mesantoin)*, phenytoin *(Dilantin)* ▪ **Oxazolidinediones:** trimethadione *(Tridione)* ▪ **Succinimides:** ethosuximide *(Zarontin)*, methsuximide *(Celontin)*, phensuximide *(Milontin)* ▪ **Miscellaneous:** acetazolamide *(Diamox)*, carbamazepine *(Tegretol)*, divalproex sodium *(Depakote)*, felbamate *(Felbatol)*, gabapentin *(Neurontin)*, lamotrigine *(Lamictal)*, magnesium sulfate, phenacemide *(Phenurone)*, tiagabine hcl *(Gabatril)*, topiramate *(Topamax)*, valproic acid *(Depakene)*.

THERAPEUTIC USE: Absence seizures: acetazolamide, clonazepam, clorazepate, felbamate, gabapentin, lamotrigine, oxazolidinediones, succinimides (esp ethosuximide), tiagabine, topiramate, valproic acid ▪ **Generalized tonic-clonic/focal seizures:** barbiturates (esp phenobarbital), carbamazepine, hydantoins (esp phenytoin) ▪ **Psychomotor:** carbamazepine, hydantoin, phenacemide, primidone ▪ **Status epilepticus:** diazepam, phenytoin ▪ **Miscellaneous:** (seizures associated c̄ preeclampsia, eclampsia, cerebral edema, glomerulonephritis): magnesium sulfate.

DOSAGE: Usual adult *PO* range[†]

divalproex sodium	15-60mg/kg/d
ethotoin	2-3g/d in 4-6 divided doses
felbamate	1200-3600mg/d divided

[†]Consult category cards or individual drug card for other doses.

fosphentoin	*IM/IV*	10-20mg PE/kg then 4-6mg PE/kg/d for status epilepticus
gabapentin		900-1800mg/d divided
lamotrigine		300-500mg/d divided w/out valproic acid. 100-150mg/d divided c̄ valproic acid
magnesium sulfate	*IM*	1-5g prn
mephenytoin		0.2-0.6g/d
mephobarbital		400-600mg/d
methsuximide		0.3-1.2g/d
phenacemide		1.5-5g/d
phensuximide		1-3g/d
primidone		250-500mg 3-4 times/d
tiagabine		4-56mg/d divided
topiramate		50-400mg/d divided
trimethadione		300-600mg 3-4 times/d

NURSING MANAGEMENT PRIORITIES

ASSESS: Hx of hypersensitivity ▪ Neurologic status ▪ Seizure activity characteristics ▪ Therapeutic blood levels ▪ CAUTION: hepatic, hemopoietic, renal impairment ▪ **ndx: Therapeutic effects:** Risk for injury ▪ Sensory/perceptual alterations ▪ **Adverse effects:** Risk for injury ▪ Sensory/perceptual alterations (visual) ▪ Risk for impaired skin integrity ▪ Altered thought processes ▪ Impaired tissue integrity. **PLAN:** Institute seizure precautions ▪ Maintain safety precautions ▪ Administer at equal intervals around clock to maintain blood levels ▪ **Special considerations:** G: caution, ↓ dosage (↓ metabolism) ▪ P: caution (check dosage forms carefully) ▪ OB: caution if pregnant; avoid breast-feeding ▪ **Dietary management:** Avoid use c̄ alcohol ▪ **Lab test evaluation:** Therapeutic blood levels. **IMPLEMENT:** Monitor VS ▪ PO: administer c̄ food to ↓ GI irritation ▪ Avoid mixing parenteral dosage forms c̄ other IV preparations ▪ Avoid abrupt withdrawal ▪ Monitor neurologic status, incl seizure characteristics ▪ **Patient education:** Comply c̄ prescribed therapy; take at equal intervals, do *not* omit doses ▪ Avoid use c̄ alcohol ▪ Take safety precautions c̄ hazardous activity ▪ Frequent oral hygiene is required (phenytoin) ▪ Keep scheduled appointments c̄ physician/ for blood work ▪ Carry medical identification (MedicAlert). **EVALUATE: Observe for therapeutic effects:** ↓/Absent seizure activity.

DESCRIPTION: A small group of drugs/preparations available in a variety of Rx, OTC dosage forms. They are divided by their antidiarrheal activity into (1) agents that ↓ intestinal motility, (2) insoluble adsorbing PO agents, (3) bacterial cultures.

DRUGS: Decrease intestinal motility: Rx: difenoxin/atropine (Motofen-C-IV, Preg Cat C), diphenoxylate/atropine (Lomotil, C-V, Preg Cat C [*see* card #112), loperamide (Rx▲/OTC, Preg Cat B) Imodium▲, Imodium AD, Kaopectate II, Maalox Antidiarrheal, Pepto Diarrhea Control (*see* card #186) ▪ **Adsorbing oral agents (OTC):** Attapulgite: a hydrated magnesium aluminum silicate (Kaopectate) ▪ kaolin: a hydrated aluminum silicate ▪ pectin: a carbohydrate obtained from the inner portion of citrus fruit rinds & from apple pomace (kaolin/pectin preparation—generic) ▪ **Bacterial cultures:** Contain *Lactobacillus acidophilus*, an acid-producing bacteria (Bacid).

PHARMACOKINETICS: Attapulgite: not applicable ▪ difenoxin: extensive & rapid PO absorption c̄ peak serum levels w/in 40-60m ▪ kaolin: not applicable ▪ pectin: not applicable.

MECHANISM OF ACTION: Decreased intestinal motility: difenoxin & diphenoxylate are synthetic analogs of the narcotic, meperidine. Antidiarrheal affect is due to slowing of intestinal motility. Atropine is added in subtherapeutic doses to discourage substance misuse. In addition, a lower drug schedule classification is possible because of the presence of atropine ▪ **Adsorbing insoluable PO agents:** These agents adsorb & remove bacteria & toxic substances c̄ defecation ▪ **Bacterial cultures:** *L. acidophilus* is an acid-producing bacillus bacteria that helps reestablish the normal flora of the colon that was altered by use of antibiotics.

CONTRAINDICATIONS/SIDE EFFECTS: Attapulgite: essentially none c̄ occasional constipation ▪ difenoxin/atropine: hypersensitivity c̄ diarrhea associated c̄ pseudomembranous colitis or toxigenic/enterotoxins from bacteria (*Escherichia coli, Salmonella, Shigella*) that are capable of penetrating intestinal mucosa. Most significant side/adverse effects are toxic megacolon, paralytic ileus. In addition, use in children <2y/o not recommended ▪ kaolin/pectin: essentially none c̄ occasional constipation ▪ *L. acidophilus:* hypersensitivity to lactose (milk). No significant adverse effects; use in children <3y/o or use for >2d c̄ elevated fever not recommended.

DOSAGE

Drug / Form / Age	Route	Dosage
Attapulgite		
Chewable tablets	*PO*	
Pediatric		3-6y/o: 1 tab after each BM 6-12y/o: 2 tab after each BM
Adult		4 tab after each BM
Concentrate		
Pediatric		3-6y/o: 7.5ml after each BM 6-12y/o: 15ml after each BM
Adult		30ml after each BM
Maximum strength tablets (c̄ pectin)		
Pediatric		6-12y/o: 1 tab after each BM
Adult		2 tab after each BM
Difenoxin/atropine		
Tablets	*PO*	
>12y/o-Adults		Start c̄ 2 tab (2mg difenoxin), then 1 tab q3h prn
L. acidophilus	*PO*	Dosage varies c̄ strength of preparation. Check OTC label for specific dosage

NURSING MANAGEMENT PRIORITIES

ASSESS: GI status ▪ Characteristics of stools ▪ Fluid/electrolyte status ▪ CAUTION: abdominal pain ▪ **ndx: Therapeutic effects:** Diarrhea ▪ Fluid volume deficit ▪ Risk for impaired skin integrity ▪ Pain ▪ **Adverse effects:** Constipation ▪ Risk for infection. **PLAN:** Do *not* administer w/in 48h of suspected food poisoning ▪ Evaluate frequency, consistency of stools ▪ Assess bowel sounds ▪ **Special considerations:** G: caution (↓ GI motility, ↑ sensitivity) ▪ P: caution (immature systems, ↑ sensitivity) ▪ OB: caution (fetal sensitivity to narcotic preparations) ▪ **Dietary management:** Avoid GI-irritating foods ▪ **Lab test evaluation:** Serum electrolytes (initial). **IMPLEMENT:** Avoid concurrent tetracycline administration ▪ Encourage adequate fluid intake ▪ **Patient education:** Comply c̄ prescribed dosage regimen ▪ Maintain adequate fluid intake ▪ Notify physician if diarrhea, GI distress persists or worsens. **EVALUATE: Observe for therapeutics:** Resolution of diarrhea ▪ Regular BMs.

DESCRIPTION: Chemically diverse group of drugs that competitively antagonize (block) physiologic effects of histamine, an endogenous agonist at histamine receptor sites. These agents can antagonize most effects of histamine & are subdivided according to type of histamine receptor they block. Histamine receptors are currently divided into peripheral H_1 & parietal H_2 receptors.

H_1 blockers (H_1 receptor antagonists) are original & largest group of antihistamines. Term *antihistamine* usually associated c̄ H_1 blockers.

DRUGS: Classical antihistamines. H_1 antihistamines can be classified according to their chemical derivation, duration of activity, anticholinergic activity, potential ability to cross blood-brain barrier to produce sedation ▪ **Alkylamines:** short acting (4-6h) c̄ moderate anticholinergic & low sedation activity. brompheniramine maleate *(Dimetane)*, chlorpheniramine maleate *(Chlor-Trimeton, *Chlorophen, *Novapheniram)*, dexchlorpheniramine maleate *(Polaramine)* ▪ **Ethanolamines:** moderate acting (6-8h) c̄ high anticholinergic & sedation activity. clemastine fumarate *(Tavist)*, diphenhydramine hcl *(Benadryl, *Allerdyl, *Insomnal)*, doxylamine succinate *(Unisom)* ▪ **Ethylenediamines:** short acting (4-6h) c̄ low anticholinergic & high sedation activity. tripelennamine hcl *(PBZ)* ▪ **Phenothiazines:** moderate to long acting (6-24h) c̄ high anticholinergic & sedation activity. methdilazine hcl *(Tacaryl, *Dilosyn)*, promethazine hcl *(Phenergan, *Histanil)* (*see* drug card) ▪ **Piperazines:** high anticholinergic & low to moderate sedation activity. buclizine hcl *(Bucladin-S)* (short acting), cyclizine hcl *(Marezine)* (short acting), meclizine hcl *(Antivert, Bonine)* (short acting) ▪ **Miscellaneous:** astemizole *(Hismanal)*, azatadine maleate *(Optimine)*, cetirizine hcl *(Zyrtec)*, cyproheptadine hcl *(Periactin, *Vimicon)*, dimenhydrinate *(Dramamine)*, fexofenadine hcl *(Allegra)*, loratadine *(Claritin)*.

THERAPEUTIC USE: Allergic conditions: all medications listed (piperazines are usually omitted for allergic conditions). However, current prescribing trends for allergic conditions indicate preference for nonsedating &/or long-acting H_1 blockers that include astemizole, cetrizine, fexofenadine, or loratadine ▪ **Motion sickness:** buclizine, cyclizine, dimenhydrinate, diphenhydramine, meclizine, promethazine ▪ **Parkinsonism:** diphenhydramine ▪ **Sleep:** diphenhydramine, doxylamine ▪ **Vertigo:** buclizine, dimenhydrinate, meclizine.

MECHANISM OF ACTION: H_1 antihistaminic activity caused by competitive inhibition of histamine at H_1-histamine receptors on peripheral cells. They do not inhibit synthesis or release of histamine. All antihistamines employed for allergic conditions have approximately same clinical efficacy & differ primarily in dosing schedules & sedative activity. Antihistamines c̄ ↑ anticholinergic activity are employed for treatment/prevention of motion sickness, vertigo, Parkinson's disease.

CONTRAINDICATIONS: Hypersensitivity, neonates, nursing mothers, lower respiratory tract symptoms (c̄ asthma). **CC:** Use c̄ extreme caution c̄ narrow-angle glaucoma, pyloroduodenal obstruction, stenosing peptic ulcer, prostatic hypertrophy, bladder neck obstruction.

DOSAGE: Adult *PO*

azatadine	1-2mg bid
brompheniramine	4-8mg 3-4 times/d
buclizine	50mg q4-6h
chlorpheniramine	4mg q4-6h
clemastine	1.35-2.68mg 1-3 times/d
cyclizine	50mg q4-6h
cyproheptadine	4mg 3-4 times/d
dexchlorpheniramine	2mg 3-4 times/d
dimenhydrinate	50-100mg 3-4 times/d
diphenhydramine	20-50mg 3-4 times/d
doxylamine	25mg at hs
meclizine	25-50mg once/d
methdilazine	8mg 2-4 times/d
promethazine	12.5-25mg tid
tripelennamine	25-50mg q4-6h

SIDE/ADVERSE EFFECTS: CNS: drowsiness, dizziness, euphoria, paresthesias ▪ CV: hypotension, palpitations, extrasystole, tachycardia ▪ EENT: blurred vision, nasal stuffiness ▪ GI: N/V, anorexia ▪ HEM: *agranulocytosis, hemolytic anemia, thrombocytopenia* ▪ RESP: wheezing, thickening of bronchial secretions ▪ Other: anticholinergic effects.

DRUG INTERACTIONS: Use c̄ anticholinergics or CNS depressants produces additive sedation effects ▪ MAO-I can ↑ anticholinergic effects of antihistamines.

NURSING MANAGEMENT PRIORITIES

ASSESS: Hx of hypersensitivity ▪ Allergy symptoms ▪ Lung sounds ▪ CAUTION: GI, cardiac, hepatic impairment; pregnancy, lactation ▪ **ndx: Therapeutic effects:** Ineffective airway clearance ▪ Anxiety ▪ Ineffective breathing pattern ▪ Risk for fluid volume deficit ▪ Risk for injury ▪ Impaired skin integrity ▪ **Adverse effects:** Risk for activity intolerance ▪ Sensory/perceptual alterations (visual) ▪ Risk for impaired skin integrity ▪ Impaired tissue integrity (PO mucous membrane) ▪ Altered patterns of urinary elimination. **PLAN:** Maintain hydration ▪ **Special considerations:** G: caution, ↓ dosage (↑ sensitivity; chronic illness) ▪ P: caution, ↓ dosage (paradoxic rx) ▪ OB: caution if pregnant; avoid breastfeeding ▪ **Dietary management:** Avoid use c̄ alcohol ▪ **Lab test evaluation:** CBC (c̄ prolonged therapy). **IMPLEMENT:** Administer PO forms c̄ meals ▪ Monitor VS, esp BP ▪ Monitor activity status ▪ Monitor children for paradoxic rxs (CNS stimulation) ▪ **Patient education:** Drowsiness, dizziness may occcur ▪ Avoid potentially hazardous activity ▪ Take PO forms c̄ meals ▪ ↑ Fluid intake ▪ Avoid CNS depressants, incl alcohol ▪ Use sugarless gum/hard candy to diminish dry mouth. **EVALUATE: Observe for therapeutic effects:** ↓ Cold/allergy symptoms.

---

astemizole: 2nd-generation H_1 blocker (nonsedating) Rx; Preg Cat C

BRAND NAME	**DOSAGE FORM**
Hismanal (Janssen)	Tablet: 10mg

USE: Symptomatic treatment of seasonal allergic rhinitis & chronic idiopathic urticaria. Drug exhibits low to no anticholinergic activity, does not readily cross blood-brain barrier.

PHARMACOKINETICS: Good PO absorption ac c̄ a duration up to 24h, protein binding is 96%, a half-life of 1-2d for unchanged drug, excretion via feces primarily as metabolites.

CONTRAINDICATIONS: Hypersensitivity, erythromycin, ketoconazole, itraconazole, quinine. **CC:** Exceeding recommended doses can result in Q-T prolongation/ventricular arrhythmias ▪ Food ↓ PO absorption by 60% ▪ Use c̄ azithromycin, clarithromycin, fluconazole, metronidazole, meconazole not recommended ▪ Use c̄ quinine tonic waters is best avoided ▪ Safety in children <12y/o not established.

DOSAGE: *PO*

Adult/Children >12y/o 10mg ac once/d

---

cetirizine hcl: Long-acting H_1 blocker Rx; Preg Cat B

BRAND NAME	**DOSAGE FORMS**
Zyrtec (Pfizer)	Tablet: 5, 10mg

USE: Symptomatic treatment of seasonal/perennial rhinitis, chronic idiopathic urticaria. Drug is an active metabolite of hydroxyzine.

PHARMACOKINETICS: Good PO absorption ac c̄ a duration up to 24h, protein binding is 93%, half-life is 8.3±1.8h, excretion is primarily via urine.

CONTRAINDICATIONS: Hypersensitivity. **CC:** Use c̄ caution c̄ hepatic or renal impairment ▪ Use in nursing mothers not recommended ▪ Safety in children <12y/o not established.

DOSAGE: *PO*

Adult/Children >12y/o — 5 or 10mg once/d

---

fexofenadine hcl: 2nd-generation H_1 blocker (nonsedating) — Rx; Preg Cat C

BRAND NAME	DOSAGE FORM
Allegra (H-M-R)	Capsule: 60mg

USE: Symptomatic treatment of seasonal allergic rhinitis.

PHARMACOKINETICS: Good PO absorption c̄ a duration of 10-12h.

CONTRAINDICATIONS: Hypersensitivity. **CC:** Use in nursing mothers requires caution ▪ Safety in children <12y/o not established ▪ Use c̄ caution c̄ renal impairment.

DOSAGE: *PO*

Adult/Children >12y/o — 60mg bid & 60mg once/d for renal impairment

---

loratadine: Long-acting H_1 blocker tricyclic antihistamine — Rx; Preg Cat B

BRAND NAMES	DOSAGE FORMS
Claritin (Schering)	Syrup: 5mg/5ml RediTab/tablet: 10mg
Claritin-D (Schering)	5mg loratidine/100mg pseudoephrine/tab

USE: Symptomatic treatment of nasal, nasal seasonal allergic rhinitis, chronic idiopathic urticaria ▪ Claritin-D when nasal decongestion is desired.

PHARMACOKINETICS: Rapid PO absorption ac c̄ an onset of 1-3h; peak 8-12h; duration 24; protein binding is 97%; half-life is 8.4h; excretion via urine, feces primarily as metabolites.

CONTRAINDICATIONS: Hypersensitivity. Claritin-D: severe hypertension or coronary artery disease, MAO-I use, urinary retention. **CC:** Lower doses are required c̄ caution c̄ diabetes, hypertension, hyperthyroidism, ischemic heart disease, prostatic hypertrophy.

DOSAGE: *PO*

Adult/Children >12y/o — 10mg once/d on empty stomach. Pts c̄ liver/renal dysfunction, 10mg qod. Claritin-D: 1 q12h ac

DRUGS: cimetidine/hcl▲ *(Tagamet, Tagamet injection,▲ Tagamet HB, *Peptol)*; famotidine *(Pepcid, Pepcid AC)*; nizatidine *(Axid, Axid AR)*; ranitidine *(Zantac, Zantac 75 AR)*.

MECHANISM OF ACTION: H_2 blockers are chemical analogs of histamine & cimetidine is the prototype drug. H_2 antihistaminic activity due to competitive inhibition of histamine on gastric parietal cells resulting in ↓ gastric acid daytime & nocturnal secretions. These agents lack anticholinergic activity & do not affect H_1 histamine receptors.

CONTRAINDICATIONS: Hypersensitivity. **CC:** Clinical response to therapy does not preclude possible GI malignancies ▪ Use c̄ caution in nursing mothers ▪ Safety in children not established.

SIDE/ADVERSE EFFECTS: These drugs are well tolerated & most rxs occur at low percentages or are rare. CNS: anxiety, dizziness, depression, somnolence, headache, mental confusion ▪ CV: arrhythmias, palpitations ▪ END: gynecomastia ▪ GI: anorexia, N/V/D, dry mouth, constipation, ***pancreatitis*** ▪ GU: urinary retention, ***interstitial nephritis*** ▪ HEM: neutropenia, ***thrombocytopenia*** ▪ INT: rash, reversible alopecia, pruritus ▪ Other: hepatitis, arthralgia, bronchospasm.

DRUG INTERACTIONS: Antacids can ↓/propantheline can ↑ PO absorption of H_2 blockers ▪ Smoking can ↓ therapeutic effects of H_2 blockers ▪ *cimetidine* & *ranitidine* can ↑ activity of coumarin anticoagulants, phenytoin, propranolol, theophylline ▪ *nizatidine* can ↑ salicylate levels in pts c̄ ↑ salicylate doses.

NURSING MANAGEMENT PRIORITIES

ASSESS: Hx of hypersensitivity ▪ GI symptoms ▪ Bowel sounds ▪ CAUTION: GI, cardiac, hepatic impairment; pregnancy, lactation; abdominal pain ▪ **ndx: Therapeutic effects:** Pain ▪ Impaired tissue integrity (GI) ▪ **Adverse effects:** Sensory/perceptual alterations ▪ Diarrhea ▪ Risk for impaired skin integrity ▪ Activity intolerance ▪ Impaired tissue integrity ▪ Altered thought processes. **PLAN:** Monitor GI status ▪ Maintain hydration ▪ **Special considerations:** G: caution (↑ sensitivity) ▪ P: not recommended ▪ OB: caution if pregnant; avoid breastfeeding ▪ **Dietary management:** Avoid GI-irritating foods ▪ Avoid use c̄ alcohol ▪ **Lab test evaluation:** CBC (c̄ prolonged therapy). **IMPLEMENT:** Administer PO forms c̄ meals ▪ Monitor VS, esp BP ▪ Monitor activity status ▪ Institute safety precautions ▪

Administer antacids 1h before or 1h after (if ordered) ▪ **Patient education:** Drowsiness, dizziness may occur ▪ Avoid potentially hazardous activity ▪ Take PO forms c̄ meals ▪ ↑ Fluid intake ▪ Avoid CNS depressants, incl alcohol ▪ Avoid anxiety-producing situations ▪ Avoid GI-irritating foods, OTC preparations (pepper, caffeine, aspirin). **EVALUATE: Observe for therapeutic effects:** Relief of pain associated c̄ gastric/duodenal ulcers.

---

cimetidine/cimetidine hcl▲: Rx/OTC†; Preg Cat B
H_2 receptor antagonist

BRAND NAMES	DOSAGE FORMS
Tagamet (SKB)	Injection▲: 300mg/2ml, 300mg/50ml
	Liquids▲: 300mg/5ml
Tagamet HB† (SKB)	Tablet: 100mg

USE: Short-term treatment of gastric/duodenal ulcers ▪ Duodenal ulcer prophylaxis ▪ Treatment of pathologic hypersecretory conditions (Zollinger-Ellison syndrome, systemic mastocytosis, multiple endocrine adenomas) ▪ Treatment of gastroesophageal reflux disease (GERD) ▪ Prevention of upper GI bleeding in critically ill pts.

PHARMACOKINETICS: Rapid PO absorption, peak 45-90m, protein binding 15%-20%, half-life is 2h, excretion via urine primarily as metabolites.

CC: Rapid IV bolus injection has resulted in rare cases of arrhythmias & hypotension.

DOSAGE

Adult	*PO*	
Ulcers		800mg at hs is preferred dose or 300mg qid c̄ meals/at hs or 400mg bid. Usual maintenance dose is 400mg at hs
Pathologic hypersecretion		300mg qid c meals/at hs. Do *not* exceed 2400mg/d
GERD		800mg bid or 400mg qid for 12wks
Tagamet HB		200mg q12h
Adult parenteral	*IM/IV*	300mg q6-8h or more prn. Do *not* exceed 2400mg/d
	Intermittent IV infusion	300mg q6-8h infused over 15-20m. Do *not* exceed 2400mg/d
	Continuous IV infusion	Usual dose 37.5mg/h. If required, a 150-mg IV loading dose may precede start of infusion
GI bleeding	*IV*	Continuous infusion of 50mg/h

famotidine: H_2 receptor antagonist — Rx/OTC†; Preg Cat B

BRAND NAMES	DOSAGE FORMS
Pepcid (Merck)	IV injection: 0.4mg/ml; 10mg/ml Tablet: 20, 40mg
Pepcid† (Merck)	Chewable tablet: 10mg

USE: Short-term treatment of gastric/duodenal ulcers ▪ Duodenal ulcer prophylaxis ▪ Short-term treatment of gastroesophageal reflux disease (GERD) ▪ Treatment of pathologic hypersecretory conditions ▪ Relief of acid indigestion (OTC).

PHARMACOKINETICS: Moderate PO absorption, peak 1-3h, protein binding 15%-20%, half-life 2.5-3.5h, excretion is 30% PO dose/65%-70% IV dose as unchanged drug via urine.

CC: Severe renal insufficiency may require lower doses.

DOSAGE

Adult	*PO*	
Ulcers		40mg/d or 20mg bid. Usual maintenance dose is 20mg/d at hs
GERD		20mg bid for up to 6wks
Pathologic hypersecretions		20-160mg q6h
	IV	20mg q12h
Pepcid AC		10mg bid

---

nizatidine: H_2 receptor antagonist — Rx/OTC†; Preg Cat B

BRAND NAMES	DOSAGE FORMS
Axid (Lilly)	Capsule: 150, 300mg
Axid AR† (Whitehall)	Tablet: 75mg

USE: Short-term treatment of gastric/duodenal ulcers ▪ Duodenal ulcer prophylaxis ▪ Treatment of GERD ▪ Relief of acid indigestion (OTC).

PHARMACOKINETICS: Very high PO absorption, peak 1-3h, protein binding 35%, half-life 1-2h, 90% excretion via urine in 12h.

CC: Severe renal insufficiency may require lower doses.

Note: Side/adverse effects: common in *italic;* serious in ***boldface italic.*** *Available in Canada only.

DOSAGE

Adult	*PO*	
Ulcers		300mg/d or 150mg bid. Maintenance dose is 150mg/d at hs
GERD		150mg bid
Axid AR		75mg 1-2 times/d ac

---

ranitidine hcl: H_2 receptor antagonist — Rx/OTC[†]; Preg Cat B

BRAND NAMES	DOSAGE FORMS
Zantac (G-W)	Capsule (GEL dose): 150, 300mg Granules (EFFER dose): 150mg/packet Syrup: 75mg/5ml Tablet: 75, 150, 300mg
Zantac-75 AR[†] (G-W)	Tablet: 75mg

USE: Short-term treatment of gastric/duodenal ulcers ▪ Gastric/duodenal ulcer prophylaxis ▪ Treatment of GERD ▪ Treatment of pathologic hypersecretory conditions (Zollinger-Ellison syndrome, systemic mastocytosis) ▪ Relief of acid indigestion (OTC).

PHARMACOKINETICS: Rapid PO absorption in moderate amounts (50% bioavailability), peak 2-3h, protein binding 10%-20%, 30% excreted unchanged via urine in 24h.

CC: Lower doses may be required c̄ hepatic & renal impairment ▪ Use c̄ caution in pts c̄ acute porphyria due to rare episodes of acute attacks ▪ Effervescent granules contain phenylalanine.

DOSAGE

Adult	*PO*	150mg bid for all indications *except* for erosive esophagitis. 150mg qid c̄ a maintenance dose of 150mg bid. Maintenance dose for ulcers is 150mg/d at hs
	IM/IV	50mg q6-8h
	Infusion	6.25mg/h
Zantac-75		75mg 1-2 times/d

DESCRIPTION: Drugs used in treatment of essential (1°), malignant (2°) hypertension; antihypertensives are large category of therapeutic drugs that exhibit various hypotensive pharmacologic mechanisms.

DRUGS: Adrenergic activity: Hypotensive effects due to agonist, antagonist receptor activity ▪ α **blockers:** Hypotensive effect due to antagonism of peripheral α_1-α_2 receptors: phenoxybenzamine *(Dibenzyline),* phentolamine *(Regitine)* ▪ α_1 **blockers:** Hypotensive effect due to antagonism of peripheral α_1 receptors: doxazosin mesylate *(Cardura),* prazosin *(Minipress),* terazosin *(Hytrin)* ▪ α_2 **agonists:** Hypotensive effect due to central α_2 agonist activity: clonidine hcl *(Catapres),* guanabenz acetate (*Wytensin*), guanfacine hcl *(Tenex)* ▪ α-β **blockers:** Hypotensive effect due to antagonism of α_1, β_1, β_2 receptors: carvedilol *(Coreg),* labetalol hcl *(Normodyne)* ▪ β **blockers:** Exact antihypertensive mechanisms not determined ▪ β_1-β_2 **blockers:** carteolol *(Cartrol),* nadolol *(Corgard),* penbutolol *(Levatol),* pindolol *(Visken),* propranolol *(Inderal),* timolol maleate *(Blocadren)* ▪ β_1 **blockers:** acebutolol *(Sectral),* atenolol *(Tenormin),* betaxolol hcl *(Kerlone),* bisoprolol *(Zebeta),* metoprolol *(Lopressor)* ▪ **Alteration of catecholamine synthesis:** Hypotensive mechanism that ↓ catecholamine synthesis (metyrosine) or produces synthesis of α-methyl norepinephrine (methyldopa), which stimulates central inhibitory α-adrenergic receptors: methyldopa *(Aldomet),* metyrosine *(Demser)* ▪ **Norepinephrine depletors:** Hypotensive effect probably due to slow depletion of norepinephrine in adrenergic fibers, esp in vascular smooth muscle: guanadrel *(Hylorel),* guanethidine monosulfate *(Ismelin),* reserpine ▪ **Angiotensin inhibition (ACE-I):** Inhibition of ACE blocks conversion of angiotensin I to angiotensin II, resulting in hypotensive effect: benazepril *(Lotensin),* captopril *(Capoten),* enalapril maleate *(Vasotec),* fosinopril *(Monopril),* lisinopril *(Prinivil, Zestril),* moexipril hcl *(Univasc),* quinapril hcl *(Accupril),* ramipril *(Altace),* trandolapril *(Mavik)* ▪ **Angiotensin II blocker:** Hypotensive effect due to antagonism of angiotension II receptors: *candesartan* cilexetil *(Atacand),* irbesartan *(Avapro),* losartan potassium *(Cozaar),* valsartan *(Diovan)* ▪ **Calcium blockers:** amlodipine *(Norvasc),* diltiazem *(Cardizem*—only SR dosage forms), felodipine *(Plendil),* isradipine *(DynaCirc),* nicardipine *(Cardene),* nifedipine *(Procardia*—only SR dosage forms), nisoldipine *(Sular),* verapamil *(Calan, Isoptin, Verelan*—only SR dosage forms) ▪ **Direct vasodilators:** diazoxide *(Hyperstat IV),* hydralazine hcl *(Apresoline),* minoxidil *(Loniten),* prazosin hcl *(Minipress),* sodium nitroprusside *(Nitropress)* ▪ **Diuretics:** bendroflumethiazide *(Naturetin),* chlorothiazide *(Diuril),* chlorthalidone *(Hygroton, Thalitone),* furosemide *(Lasix),* hydrochlorothiazide *(Esidrix, Hydro-DIURIL),* hydroflumethiazide *(Diucardin, Saluron),* indapamide *(Lozol),* methyclothiazide *(Aquatensen, Enduron),* metolazone *(Zaroxolyn),* polythiazide *(Renese),* quinethazone *(Hydromox),* spironolactone *(Aldactone),* trichlormethiazide *(Metahydrin, Naqua)* ▪ **Ganglionic blockers:** Produce hypotensive effect by blocking autonomic ganglia transmission; primarily used in treatment of malignant hypertension (mecamylamine hcl *[Inversine]*) ▪ **Miscellaneous:** nitroglycerin IV *(Nitro-Bid, Nitrol IV, Nitrostat IV, Tridil).*

DOSAGE: Adult *PO*†

carvedilol	12.5-50mg/d
guanadrel	20-75mg/d
mecamylamine	2.5-25mg/d
metyrosine	1-4g/d
reserpine	0.1-0.25mg/d
terazosin	1-5mg/d
torsemide	5-10mg/d
trandolapril	2-8mg/d

†Consult category cards or individual drug card for other dosages.

NURSING MANAGEMENT PRIORITIES

ASSESS: Hx of hypersensitivity ▪ BP ▪ Adequate renal function ▪ CAUTION: CV, hepatic, renal impairment ▪ **ndx: Therapeutic effects:** ↓ Cardiac output ▪ Altered tissue perfusion ▪ **Adverse effects:** Risk for activity intolerance ▪ ↓ Cardiac output ▪ Fatigue ▪ Risk for injury ▪ Sensory/perceptual alterations ▪ Sexual dysfunction ▪ Risk for impaired skin integrity. **PLAN:** Observe extremities for edema ▪ Prevent postural hypotension ▪ **Special considerations:** G: caution (↑ hypotensive effects; chronic illness) ▪ P: caution (immature systems) ▪ OB: caution if pregnant, breastfeeding ▪ **Dietary management:** Avoid high-Na^+ foods, use c̄ alcohol; calorie restrictions ▪ **Lab test evaluation:** Electrolytes. **IMPLEMENT:** Monitor BP; observe for hypotension ▪ Monitor I&O, daily weight ▪ Monitor CV, hepatic, renal status ▪ **Patient education:** Avoid sudden position changes (postural hypotension) ▪ Comply c̄ prescribed drug regimen ▪ Avoid smoking, alcohol, constrictive clothing, extremely hot objects, OTC cough/cold/allergy preparations ▪ Follow low-Na^+ diet ▪ Have BP checked regularly ▪ Keep appointments c̄ physician ▪ Carry identification (MedicAlert). **EVALUATE: Observe for therapeutic effect:** ↓ **BP.**

The antihypertensive combinations are fixed dosage formulations of a diuretic (usually a thiazide) & a 2nd antihypertensive drug. Many preparations are available in a variety of diuretic/antihypertensive dosage ratios. All preparations are Rx, & the dosage must be adjusted to the pt after initiation of treatment.

PRODUCT INFORMATION

Preparation	Dosage form	Manufacturer	Formula	Preg Cat	Usual starting dose
Aldoclor 150; 250	Tablet	Merck	Methyldopa 250mg/Chlorothiazide 150/250mg	B	1 2-3 times/d
Aldoril-15; 25	Tablet	Merck	Methyldopa 250mg/Hydrochlorothiazide 15/25mg	C	1 2-3 times/d
Aldoril D30; 50	Tablet	Merck	Methyldopa 250mg/Hydrochlorothiazide 30/50mg	C	1 2-3 times/d
Apresazide 25/25; 50/50	Capsule	Novartis	Hydralazine 25/50mg/Hydrochlorothiazide 25/50mg	C	1 bid
Apresazide 100/50	Capsule	Novartis	Hydralazine 100mg/Hydrochlorothiazide 50mg	C	1 bid
Capozide 25/15; 25/25	Tablet	Squibb	Captopril 25mg/Hydrochlorothiazide 15/25mg	C/D	1/d
Capozide 50/15; 50/25	Tablet	Squibb	Captopril 50mg/Hydrochlorothiazide 15/25mg	C/D	1/d
Combipres 0.1; 0.2; 0.3	Tablet	B-I	Clonidine HCl 0.1/0.2/0.3mg/Chlorthalidone 15mg	C	1 bid
Corzide 40/5; 80/5	Tablet	Bristol	Nadolol 40/80mg/Bendroflumethiazide 5mg	C	1 bid
Diupres 250; 500	Tablet	Merck	Reserpine 0.125mg/Chlorothiazide 250/500mg	C	1 1-2 times/d
Enduronyl, Forte	Tablet	Abbott	Deserpidine 0.25/0.5mg/Methyclothiazide 5mg	NA	½-2/d
Esimil	Tablet	Novartis	Guanethidine 10mg/Hydrochlorothiazide 25mg	B	1/d
Hydropres 25; 50	Tablet	Merck	Reserpine 0.125mg/Hydrochlorothiazide 25/50mg	C	1/d
Inderide 40/25; 80/50	Tablet	W-A	Propranolol HCl 40/80mg/Hydrochlorothiazide 25/50mg	C	1 1-2 times/d
Inderide LA 80/50; 120/50	Capsule	W-A	Propranolol HCl 80/120mg/Hydrochlorothiazide 50mg	C	1/d
Lopressor HCT 50/25 100/25	Tablet	Novartis	Metoprolol HCl 50/100mg/Hydrochlorothiazide 25mg	C	1-2/d

Preparation	Dosage form	Manu-facturer	Formula	Preg Cat	Usual starting dose
Lopressor HCT 100/50	Tablet	Novartis	Metoprolol HCl 100mg/Hydrochlorothiazide 50mg	C	1/d
Minizide 1; 2; 3	Capsule	Pfizer	Prazosin HCl 1/2/3mg/Polythiazide 0.5mg	C	1 2-3 times/d
Prinzide 12.5; 25	Tablet	Merck	Lisinopril 20mg/Hydrochlorothiazide 12.5/25mg	C/D	1-2/d
Rauzide	Tablet	Squibb	Rauwolfia Serpentina 50mg/Bendroflumethiazide 4mg	C	1/d
Tenoretic 50; 100	Tablet	ICI	Atenolol 50/100mg/Chlorthalidone 25mg	C	1/d
Timolide 10/25	Tablet	Merck	Timolol Maleate 10mg/Hydrochlorothiazide 25mg	C	1 bid
Vaseretic	Tablet	Merck	Enalapril Maleate 25mg/Hydrochlorothiazide 25mg	C/D	1/d
Zestoretic 20/12.5; 20/25	Tablet	Stuart	Lisinopril 20mg/Hydrochlorothiazide 12.5/25mg	C/D	1/d

NURSING MANAGEMENT PRIORITIES

ASSESS: Hx of hypersensitivity ▪ BP ▪ Adequate renal function ▪ CAUTION: CV, hepatic, renal impairment ▪ **ndx: Therapeutic effects:** ↓ Cardiac output ▪ Altered tissue perfusion ▪ **Adverse effects:** Risk for activity intolerance ▪ ↓ Cardiac output ▪ Fatigue ▪ Risk for injury ▪ Sensory/perceptual alterations ▪ Sexual dysfunction ▪ Risk for impaired skin integrity. **PLAN:** Observe extremities for edema ▪ Prevent postural hypotension ▪ **Special considerations:** G: caution (↑ hypotensive effects; chronic illness) ▪ P: caution (immature systems) ▪ OB: caution if pregnant, breastfeeding ▪ **Dietary management:** Avoid high-Na^+ foods, alcohol; calorie restrictions ▪ **Lab test evaluation:** Electrolytes. **IMPLEMENT:** Monitor BP; observe for hypotension ▪ Monitor I&O, daily weight ▪ Monitor CV, hepatic, renal status ▪ **Patient education:** Avoid sudden position changes (postural hypotension) ▪ Comply c̄ prescribed drug regimen ▪ Avoid smoking, alcohol, constrictive clothing, extremely hot objects, OTC cough/cold/allergy preparations ▪ Follow low-Na^+ diet ▪ Have BP checked regularly ▪ Keep appointments c̄ physician ▪ Carry identification (MedicAlert). **EVALUATE: Observe for therapeutic effect:** ↓ BP.

DESCRIPTION: Large group of highly reactive cytotoxic cycle phase nonspecific agents that have polyfunctional alkylating properties; main alkylating effect on DNA, resulting in disruption of DNA replication; many alkylating agents also interfere c̄ RNA transcription.

DRUGS: busulfan *(Myleran)*, carboplatin *(Paraplatin)*, carmustine *(BiCNU)*, chlorambucil *(Leukeran)*, cisplatin *(Platinol)*, cyclophosphamide *(Cytoxan, Neosar, *Procytox)*, dacarbazine *(*DTIC, DTIC-Dome)*, ifosfamide *(Ifex)*, lomustine *(*CCNU, CeeNU)*, mechlorethamine *(Mustargen)*, melphalan *(Alkeran)*, streptozocin *(Zanosar)*, thiotepa *(Thioplex)*.

THERAPEUTIC USE: Treatment of various neoplasms as sole agent/in combination. Combination antineoplastic chemotherapy is usually preferred because it produces greater results, ↑ remissions in many types of carcinomas.

MECHANISM OF ACTION: These agents add alkyl groups (alkylation) to DNA in exchange for hydrogen ions; resulting alkylation interferes c̄ DNA replication, RNA transcription, which is usually cytoxic, most lethal type of alkylation produces crosslinking of DNA strands. Alkylating agents not specific in cytoxic effects, & interact c̄ rapidly dividing normal body cells; therefore they are highly toxic agents c̄ array of significant adverse effects, esp bone marrow & immune suppression.

CONTRAINDICATIONS: Hypersensitivity, pts who exhibit unacceptable toxic effect from previous chemotherapy/radiation.

SIDE/ADVERSE EFFECTS: GI: N/D, oral ulcers, hemorrhagic colitis ▪ GU: cystitis, hemorrhagic cystitis, fibrosis, amenorrhea ▪ HEM: ***bone marrow depression*** resulting in anemia, leukopenia, neutropenia, pancytopenia, ***thrombocytopenia*** ▪ HEP: ***hepatotoxicity*** ▪ INT: alopecia, pigmentation ▪ Other: ***2° malignancies, pulmonary fibrosis.***

DRUG INTERACTIONS: Vaccinations c̄ live vaccines contraindicated during therapy ▪ Use c̄ steroids produces addictive immunosuppressant activity ▪ Radiation therapy, other myelosuppressive drugs produce additive bone marrow depression.

Note: Side/adverse effects: common in *italic;* serious in ***boldface italic.***

*Available in Canada only.

NURSING MANAGEMENT PRIORITIES

ASSESS: Hx of previous radiation, antineoplastic therapy ▪ Infection, bleeding, anemia ▪ CAUTION: bone marrow depression, acute infection, sexually active females ▪ **ndx: Therapeutic effects:** Impaired tissue integrity ▪ **Adverse effects:** Risk for activity intolerance ▪ Diarrhea ▪ Fatigue ▪ Risk for fluid volume deficit ▪ Risk for infection ▪ Altered nutrition: less than body requirements ▪ Impaired tissue integrity (PO mucous membrane). **PLAN:** Maintain optimum hydration ▪ Administer antiemetic as ordered ▪ Display hopeful approach ▪ Encourage ventilation of feelings ▪ **Special considerations:** G: caution, ↓ dosage (↑ sensitivity) ▪ P: caution (immature systems) ▪ OB: avoid use if pregnant, breastfeeding ▪ **Dietary management:** Avoid spicy foods, institute methods to stimulate appetite ▪ **Lab test evaluation:** CBC, platelets, serum uric acid. **IMPLEMENT:** Force fluids ▪ Observe for infection, bleeding, anemia ▪ Monitor hepatic, renal function ▪ IV: check site closely, avoid extravasation ▪ Observe for gout symptoms (↑ serum uric acid) ▪ Monitor I&O, daily weight ▪ Provide emotional support ▪ **Patient education:** Comply c̄ prescribed dosage regimen ▪ ↑ Fluid intake (10-12 glasses/d) ▪ Avoid exposure to infection ▪ Diet as tolerated; avoid spicy foods ▪ Maintain good oral hygiene; use soft-bristled toothbrush ▪ Notify physician of symptoms of bone marrow depression (fever, sore throat, bruising, bleeding, lethargy) ▪ Side effects are reversible ▪ Take measures to conserve energy ▪ Use contraceptives if sexually active ▪ Check c̄ physician before immunization ▪ Keep scheduled appointments c̄ physician/for blood work. **EVALUATE: Observe for therapeutic effects:** ↓ Proliferation of malignant cells ▪ Regression of tumor.

DESCRIPTION: Small, diverse group of cytotoxic drugs that are chemical analogs of folic acid, nucleic acid purines, or pyrimidines; produce antineoplastic effects by interfering c̄ various cellular metabolic pathways.

DRUGS: Folic acid antagonists: Inhibit metabolism of folic acid by blocking enzyme dihydrofolate reductase: methotrexate (amethopterin mtx), (*Folex PFS*, Rheumatrex dose pack) ▪ **Purine antagonists:** Antineoplastic activity due to inhibition of purine pathways, ultimately resulting in DNA, RNA synthesis inhibition: cladribine *(Leustatin)*, fludarabine phosphate (*Fludara*), mercaptopurine *(Purinethol)*, thioguanine ▪ **Pyrimidine antagonists:** Inhibit DNA, RNA synthesis by interfering c̄ pyrimidine metabolic pathways: cytarabine *(Cytosar-U)*, floxuridine *(FUDR)*, fluorouracil (5FU) *(Adrucil)*, gemcitabine hcl *(Gemzar)*.

NURSING MANAGEMENT PRIORITIES

ASSESS: Hx of previous radiation, antineoplastic therapy ▪ Infection, bleeding, anemia ▪ CAUTION: bone marrow depression, acute infection, sexually active females ▪ **ndx: Therapeutic effects:** Impaired tissue integrity ▪ **Adverse effects:** Risk for activity intolerance ▪ Diarrhea ▪ Fatigue ▪ Risk for fluid volume deficit ▪ Risk for infection ▪ Altered nutrition: less than body requirements ▪ Impaired tissue integrity (PO mucous membrane). **PLAN:** Maintain optimum hydration ▪ Administer antiemetic as ordered ▪ Display hopeful approach ▪ Encourage ventilation of feelings ▪ **Special considerations:** G: caution, ↓ dosage (↑ sensitivity) ▪ P: caution (immature systems) ▪ OB: avoid use if pregnant, breastfeeding ▪ **Dietary management:** Avoid spicy foods, institute methods to stimulate appetite ▪ **Lab test evaluation:** CBC, platelets, serum uric acid. **IMPLEMENT:** Force fluids ▪ Observe for infection, bleeding, anemia ▪ Monitor hepatic, renal function ▪ IV: check site closely, avoid extravasation ▪ Observe for gout symptoms (↑ serum uric acid) ▪ Monitor I&O, daily weight ▪ Provide emotional support ▪ **Patient education:** Comply c̄ prescribed dosage regimen ▪ ↑ Fluid intake (10-12 glasses/d) ▪ Avoid exposure to infection ▪ Diet as tolerated; avoid spicy foods ▪ Maintain good oral hygiene; use soft-bristled toothbrush ▪ Notify physician of symptoms of bone marrow depression (fever, sore throat, bruising, bleeding, lethargy) ▪ Side effects are reversible ▪ Take measures to conserve energy ▪ Use contraceptives if sexually active ▪ Check c̄ physician before immunization ▪ Keep scheduled appointments c̄ physician/for blood work. **EVALUATE: Observe for therapeutic effects:** ↓ Proliferation of malignant cells ▪ Regression of tumor.

DESCRIPTION: Symptoms of Parkinson's disease primarily due to imbalance between central dopaminergic & cholinergic mechanisms; pathophysiology of disorder due to tissue degeneration w/in basal ganglia of brain, resulting in low concentrations of dopamine, esp in corpus striatum, substantia nigra; cholinergic transmission becomes hyperactive, intensifying symptoms ▪ Dopamine has inhibitory effect in nigrostriatal system, acetylcholine produces excitatory effects; drug therapy must either restore dopamine levels or antagonize hyperactive cholinergic activity. Until recently, classic treatment for disorder incl anticholinergic drugs that could penetrate blood-brain barrier to ↓ cholinergic activity. Most effective treatment currently available is dopamine replacement therapy c̄ levodopa (biologic precursor of dopamine); levodopa enters brain after administration, is converted into dopamine by enzyme dopa decarboxylase. Dopamine cannot be used because it does not penetrate blood-brain barrier. Centrally acting direct/indirect dopaminergics also used ▪ Activity of levodopa can be augmented by concurrent use of carbidopa (dopa decarboxylase enzyme inhibitor that cannot enter brain), which inhibits peripheral dopa decarboxylase activity, & therefore more levodopa available to cross blood-brain barrier.

DRUGS: Anticholinergic drugs: benztropine mesylate *(Cogentin)*, biperiden hcl *(Akineton)*, procyclidine hcl (*Kemadrin*), trihexyphenidyl hcl *(Artane)* ▪ **Antihistamines** (c̄ anticholinergic activity): diphenhydramine hcl *(Benadryl)*, ethopropazine hcl *(Parsidol)* ▪ **Dopaminergic agents:** REPLACEMENT: carbidopa *(Lodosyn)*, levodopa *(Dopar, Larodopa)*, levodopa-carbidopa *(Sinemet 10/100, 25/100, 25/250, 50/200)* ▪ DIRECT ACTING: (on dopamine receptors); bromocriptine mesylate *(Parlodel)*, pergolide mesylate *(Permax)*, pramipexole *(Mirapex)*, ropinirole *(Requip)* ▪ INDIRECT ACTING: (may block dopamine reuptake/cause its release/inhibit enzyme breakdown of levodopa): amantadine hcl *(Symmetrel)*, selegiline *(Eldepryl)*, tolcapone *(Tasmar)*.

DOSAGE: Usual adult *PO*

amantadine	100-400mg/d divided
benztropine	1-2mg/d c̄ range of 0.5-6mg/d
biperiden	2mg 3-4 times/d
bromocriptine	Maximum of 100mg/d divided
carbidopa	Maximum of 200mg/d in combination c̄ levodopa
diphenhydramine	25-50mg 3-4 times/d
ethopropazine	100-600mg/d divided

pergolide	Maximum of 5mg/d in combination c̄ levodopa-carbidopa
pramipexole	0.375-4.5mg/d divided
procyclidine	2.5-5mg tid
ropinirole	0.75-3mg/d or higher if required
selegiline	5mg bid in combination c̄ levodopa-carbidopa
tolcapone	100 or 200mg tid
trihexyphenidyl	6-10mg/d divided

NURSING MANAGEMENT PRIORITIES

ASSESS: Hx of hypersensitivity ▪ BP ▪ Parkinson & extrapyramidal symptoms ▪ GI, renal status ▪ CAUTION: cardiac dysfunction, prostatic hypertrophy ▪ **ndx: Therapeutic effects**: Risk for aspiration ▪ Risk for injury ▪ Impaired physical mobility ▪ Self-care deficit ▪ Impaired swallowing ▪ **Adverse effects:** Risk for activity intolerance ▪ Risk for fluid volume deficit ▪ Impaired physical mobility ▪ Sensory/perceptual alterations ▪ Risk for impaired skin integrity ▪ Altered thought processes ▪ Altered tissue perfusion. **PLAN:** Avoid abrupt withdrawal ▪ Assess for therapeutic dose tolerance ▪ Prevent postural hypotension ▪ **Special considerations:** G: caution, ↓ dosage (↓ tolerance, ↑ CNS sensitivity, ↑ fractures) ▪ P: not recommended ▪ OB: avoid use if pregnant, breastfeeding ▪ **Dietary management:** Avoid use c̄ alcohol ▪ **Lab test evaluation:** CBC, H&H, serum creatinine. **IMPLEMENT:** Administer c̄ food to ↓ GI irritation ▪ Monitor VS, esp BP ▪ Monitor activity status (safety precautions) ▪ Observe for visual problems ▪ Monitor bowel function, I&O, IOP ▪ Observe for exaggerated anticholinergic effects ▪ Assess for muscle weakness ▪ Monitor GI, GU, CV status ▪ **Patient education:** Comply c̄ prescribed drug therapy ▪ Full drug effects may take several mos of therapy ▪ Avoid use c̄ alcohol ▪ Use sugarless gum/hard candy to diminish dry mouth ▪ Frequent oral hygiene necessary ▪ Protect eyes in sunlight ▪ Use safety precautions c̄ ambulation, hazardous activity ▪ Avoid sudden position changes (postural hypotension) ▪ Avoid extremes in exercise, climate ▪ Check c̄ physician/pharmacist before taking OTC preparations. **EVALUATE: Observe for therapeutic effect:** ↑ Neuromuscular function.

DESCRIPTION: Group of antibiotics & synthetic anti-infective agents classified into first-line (1°), second-line (2°) drugs according to their antimycobacterial activity, efficacy, & potential adverse & toxic effects.

DRUGS: **First line:** ethambutol *(Myambutol)*, isoniazid *(Laniazid, Nydrazid)*, pyrazinamide, rifabutin *(Mycobutin)*, rifampin *(Rifadin, Rimactane)*, rifapentine *(Priftin)*, streptomycin ▪ **Second line:** aminosalicylate sodium *(PAS)*, capreomycin *(Capastat)*, cycloserine *(Seromycin)*, ethionamide *(Trecator-SC)*, kanamycin *(Kantrex)* ▪ **Combinations:** isoniazid/rifampin *(Rifamate,* 150mg/300mg; *Rimactane/INH,* 300mg/300mg).

THERAPEUTIC USE: Treatment of tuberculosis or prophylaxis. The effectiveness of antimycobacterial therapy is de-

PHARMACOKINETICS

	PO absorption	Peak	Half-life	Excretion
aminosalicylate	Well	3-4h	1h	77% metabolites via urine in 24h
capreomycin	IM	1-2h	4-6h	57% unchanged via urine in 24h
cycloserine	70%-90%	3-4h	10h	60%-70% unchanged via urine in 24h
ethambutol	75%-80%	2-4h	3.3h	50% unchanged via urine in 24h
ethionamide	80%	3h	3h	95% unchanged via urine in 24h
isoniazid	Well	1-2h	1-4h	50%-70% unchanged via urine in 24h
kanamycin	IM	1h	2-2.5h	50% unchanged via urine in 24h
pyrazinamide	Well	2h	9-10h	70% unchanged via urine in 24h
rifabutin	53%	2-4h	16-69h	>50% metabolites via urine in 24h
rifampin	Well	2-4h	3h	60% unchanged via urine in 24h
rifapentine	70%	5-6h	1-4h	70% metabolites via feces
streptomycin	IM	1h	2-3h	29%-89% unchanged via urine in 24h

pendent on type of infection, adequate dosing, sufficient treatment period(s), & effective drug combinations when required (usually resistant strains & retreatment). Effective combinations include isoniazid/rifampin; isoniazid/ethambutol; isoniazid/ethambutol/streptomycin; isonazid/ethambutol/rifampin/pyrazinamide ▪ HIV-infected pts are at risk for infection, incl *Mycobacterium avium-intracellulare* complex ▪ Treatment during pregnancy is not w/out risk; ethambutol, isoniazid, rifampin are good choices.

MECHANISM OF ACTION

aminosalicylate sodium	Tuberculostatic—inhibits folic acid synthesis
capreomycin	Tuberculostatic—unknown mechanism
cycloserine	Tuberculocidal/static†—inhibits cell wall synthesis
ethambutol	Tuberculostatic—inhibits RNA synthesis
ethionamide	Tuberculocidal/static†—inhibits peptide synthesis
isoniazid	Tuberculocidal/static†—inhibits transaminase activity
kanamycin	Tuberculocidal—inhibits protein synthesis, cell wall synthesis
pyrazinamide	Tuberculocidal/static†—unknown mechanism, may be due to conversion of active metabolite pyrazinoic acid by tuberculosis bacteria
rifabutin	Tuberculostatic—unknown mechanism
rifampin	Tuberculocidal/static†—inhibits DNA dependent RNA polymerase activity
rifapentine	Tuberculocidal—inhibits DNA-dependent RNA polymerase activity
streptomycin	Tuberculocidal—inhibits protein synthesis

NURSING MANAGEMENT PRIORITIES

ASSESS: Hx of hypersensitivity (incl ethionamide, pyrazinamide, niacin) ▪ Hepatic function (↓ dose if impaired) ▪ Visual disturbances (ocular toxicity) ▪ CAUTION: hepatic impairment ▪ **ndx: Therapeutic effects**: Ineffective airway clearance ▪ Risk for altered body temperature ▪ Ineffective feeding ▪ **Dietary management:** Avoid alcohol, tyramine-containing (aged, fermented) foods; vitamin B_6 supplements (neurotoxicity) ▪ **Lab test evaluation:** Serum uric acid, AST, ALT; use Clinistix/Diastix for urine glucose. **IMPLEMENT:** Obtain C&S; check results ▪ Monitor VS, esp temperature, BP ▪ Monitor hepatic, renal status ▪ **Patient education:** Comply c̄ prescribed drug regimen ▪ Avoid sudden position changes ▪ Keep appointments for eye

†Depends on concentration of drug at site of injection & susceptibililty of tubercular bacilli.

DOSAGE/ADVERSE EFFECTS

Drug	Usual adult dose	Adverse effects
aminosalicylate	10-12g/d	GI disturbances, hepatotoxicity
capreomycin	15mg/kg/d IM	Ototoxicity, nephrotoxicity
cycloserine	500mg-1g/d	Psychotic behavior, seizures
ethambutol	15mg/kg as single dose	Optic toxicity
ethionamide	750mg-1g/d	GI disturbances, hepatotoxicity
isoniazid		Hepatitis; peripheral neuropathy
prophylaxis	300mg once/d	
active tuberculosis	5-10mg/kg once/d	
kanamycin	0.5-1g/d IM	Hepatotoxicity, ototoxicity, nephrotoxicity
pyrazinamide	15-30mg/kg once/d	Hepatotoxicity, hyperuricemia
rifabutin	300mg once/d	GI disturbances, hepatotoxicity
rifampin	600mg once/d	Hematologic, hepatotoxicity
rifapentine	600mg twice/wk c̄ an internal of ≥3d between doses for 2mo	GI disturbance, hematologic, nephrotoxicity
streptomycin	1g IM once/d	Hepatotoxicity, ototoxicity, nephrotoxicity

exams/c̄ physician ▪ Notify physician *immediately* of visual problems, tingling/numbness of hands/feet, jaundice, lethargy, dark urine ▪ Safety precautions c̄ ↑ activity ▪ Full drug effects may require several wks of therapy.

EVALUATE: Observe for therapeutic effect: Resolution of tubercular infection.

Note: Side/adverse effects: common in *italic;* serious in ***boldface italic.***

*Available in Canada only.

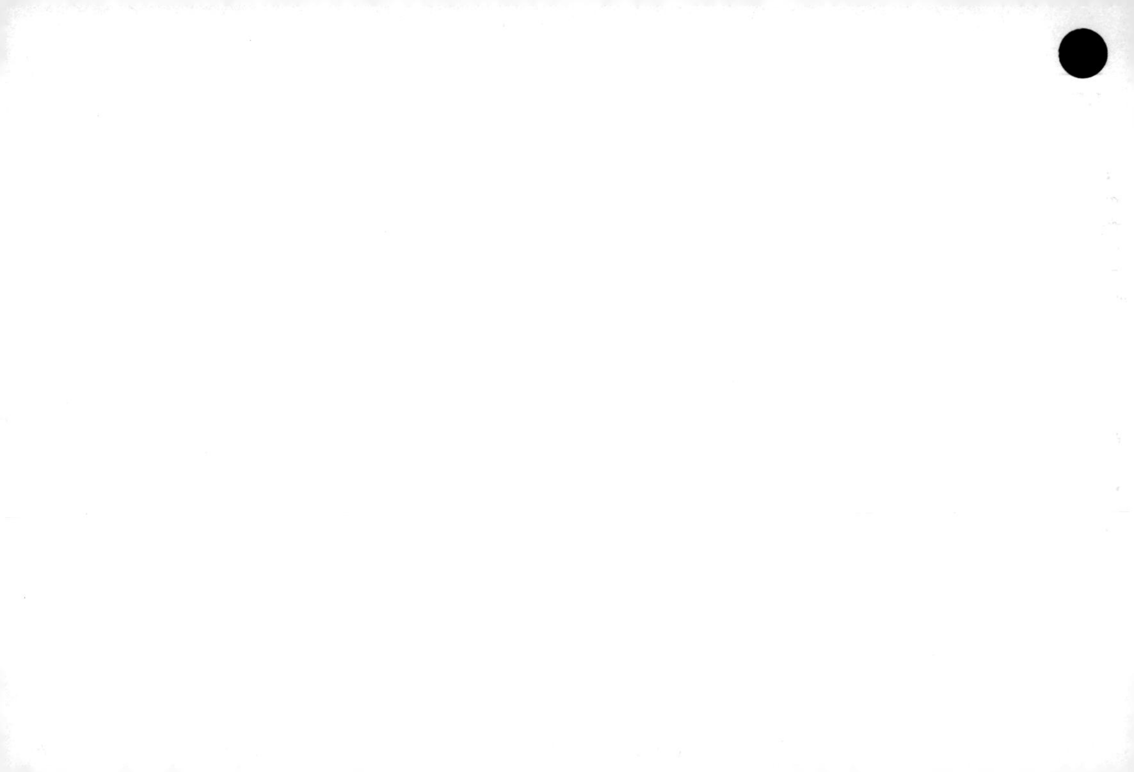

DESCRIPTION: A large group of drugs c̄ limited antiviral spectrums that are broadly divided into two chemical groups: (1) synthetic nucleoside analogs and, the largest group, (2) nonnucleoside agents.

A nucleoside is composed of a purine nitrogen base (either adenine or guanine) or a pyrimidine nitrogen base (either cytosine or thymine) combined c̄ a pentose (5-carbon) sugar.

In addition, these agents can also be classified by their main mechanism(s) of antiviral activity that include (1) alteration/inhibition of viral DNA synthesis, (2) inhibition of viral protease enzyme, (3) inhibition of viral (HIV) reverse transcript enzyme in retrovirals. Ultimately, all antiviral agents either alter or inhibit viral RNA, DNA, or protein synthesis, resulting in inhibition or faulty viral replication.

DRUGS: acyclovir *(Zovirax),* amantadine *(Symmetrel),* cidofovir *(Vistide),* delavirdine mesylate *(Rescriptor),* didanosine *(Videx),* famciclovir *(Famvir),* foscarnet *(Foscavir),* ganciclovir *(Cytovene),* idoxuridine *(Herplex),* indinavir sulfate *(Crixivan),* lamivudine *(Epivir),* nelfinavir mesylate *(Viracept),* nevirapine *(Viramune),* penciclovir *(Denavir),* ribavirin *(Virazole),* rimantadine hcl *(Flumadine),* ritonavir *(Norvir),* saquinavir mesylate *(Invirase),* stavudine *(Zerit),* trifluridine *(Viroptic),* valacyclovir *(Valtrex),* vidarabine *(Vira-A),* zalcitabine *(Hivid),* zidovudine *(Retrovir).* **Other:** imiquimod *(Aldara).*

THERAPEUTIC USE: *acyclovir:* initial & recurrent cutaneous mucosal HSV-1, HSV-2 infection, herpes zoster (shingles); *amantadine:* prevention/treatment of influenza A; *cidovudine:* cytomegalovirus (CMV), retinitis in AIDS pts; *delavirdine:* HIV infection in combination c̄ appropriate antiretroviral agents; *didanosine:* alternative for advanced HIV infection; *famciclovir:* herpes zoster, recurrent genital herpes; *foscarnet:* CMV, retinitis in AIDS pts; *ganciclovir:* CMV disease in AIDS pts; *idoxuridine:* HSV keratitis; *indinavir:* HIV infection; *lamivudine:* HIV infection in combination c̄ AZT; *nelfinavir:* HIV infection; *nevirapine:* HIV infection in combination c̄ nucleoside analog; *penciclovir:* recurrent cold sores (herpes labialis); *ribavirin:* severe respiratory syncytial virus infection; *rimantadine:* used for prevention/treatment of influenza-A; *ritonavir:* HIV infection in combination c̄ nucleoside analog; *saquinavir:* advanced HIV infection, prevention of CMV in transplant pts; *stavudine:* advanced HIV infection; *trifluridine:* HSV-1 & HSV-2 keratoconjunctivitis, recurrent epithelial keratitis; *valacyclovir:* herpes zoster; *vidarabine:* HSV-1 & HSV-2 keratoconjunctivitis, recurrent epithelial keratitis; *zalcitabine:* in combination c̄ *zidovudine* for advanced HIV infection; *zidovudine:* asymptomatic, symptomatic HIV infection & prophylaxis of maternal/fetal HIV transmission.

MECHANISM OF ACTION: (1) **Alteration/inhibition of DNA synthesis:** interferes c̄ viral DNA synthesis, resulting in inhibition of viral replication: acyclovir (purine nucleoside), cidofovir (purine nucleoside), famciclovir (purine nucleoside), foscarnet (nonnucleoside), ganciclovir (purine nucleoside), idoxuridine (pyrimidine nucleoside), penciclovir (purine nucleoside), ribavirin (purine nucleoside), trifluridine (purine nucleoside), valacyclovir (purine nucleoside), vidarabine (purine nucleoside); (2) **inhibition of viral protease enzyme:** interferes c̄ viral protein synthesis, resulting in formation of immature noninfectious viral particles: indinavir (nonnucleoside), nelfinavir (nonnucleoside), ritonavir (nonnucleoside), saquinavir (nonnucleoside); (3) **inhibition of reverse transcript enzyme (antiretroviral agents):** inhibits HIV reverse transcript enzymes required for DNA synthesis: delavirdine (nonnucleoside), didanosine (purine nucleoside), lamivudine (pyrimidine nucleoside), nevirapine (nonnucleoside), stavudine (pyrimidine nucleoside), zalcitabine (pyrimidine nucleoside), zidovudine (pyrimidine nucleoside); (4) **other:** nonnucleosides that appear to prevent viral uncoating, resulting in inhibition of early viral replication: amantadine, rimantadine.

NURSING MANAGEMENT PRIORITIES

ASSESS: Hx of hypersensitivity ▪ Hepatic, renal function ▪ Signs of toxicity (CNS, neurotoxicity) ▪ Therapeutic drug level ▪ CAUTION: hepatic, renal impairment ▪ **ndx: Therapeutic effects**: Risk for infection ▪ Impaired skin integrity ▪ **Adverse effects:** Risk for activity intolerance ▪ ↓ Cardiac output ▪ Risk for injury ▪ Sensory/perceptual alterations ▪ Risk for impaired skin integrity ▪ Altered thought processes ▪ Impaired tissue integrity. **PLAN**: Administer at equal intervals around clock to maintain blood levels ▪ Maintain hydration. **Special considerations:** G: caution (renal impairment) ▪ P: avoid use if <3mos (↑ sensitivity) ▪ OB: avoid use if pregnant, breastfeeding. **Dietary management**: None specific. **Lab test evaluation**: BUN, serum creatinine (IV); therapeutic drug levels. **IMPLEMENT:** Monitor VS ▪ Monitor F/E, hepatic, renal status ▪ Topical: use gloves to prevent herpes transmission ▪ **Patient education:** Comply c̄ prescribed drug regimen ▪ Safety precautions c̄ hazardous activity ▪ ↑ Fluid intake (8-10 glasses/d) ▪ Procedure for topical/ophthalmic preparations ▪ Use condoms if sexually active ▪ Information on herpes (symptoms, hygiene, transmission). **EVALUATE: Observe for therapeutic effects:** Prevention/resolution of viral infection.

DOSAGE/ADVERSE EFFECTS†

Drug	Usual adult dose	Adverse effects
amantadine	100mg bid or 200mg once/d	Dizziness, GI disturbances
cidofovir	5mg/kg IV over 1h once/wk for 2wks. Maintenance dose is 5mg/kg IV over 1h once q2wks	GI disturbances, headache, hematologic, nephrotoxicity
delavirdine	400mg tid	GI disturbances, fatigue, headache
famciclovir	500mg q8h for 7d	GI disturbances, fatigue, headache
ganciclovir	Induction dose 5mg/kg IV at a constant rate q12h for 14-21d. Maintenance dose is 5mg/kg IV over 1h/d or 6mg/kg/d for 5d qwk; PO dose is 1g tid c̄ food or 500mg 6 times/d q3h c̄ food	GI disturbances, fever, hematologic
idoxuridine	1gtt qh to infected eye during day, q2h at night	Edema, inflammation, corneal clouding
imiquimod	Usual dose: apply cream to genital/perianal warts 3 times/wk	Headache, local skin rxs
indinavir	800mg q8h	Asthenia, GI disturbances, headache
lamivudine	150mg bid	GI disturbances, headache, nasal symptoms
nelfinavir	750mg tid in combination c̄ nucleoside	GI disturbances, hematologic
nevirapine	200mg/d for 14d then 200mg bid in combination c̄ antiretroviral agents	GI disturbances, headache, hepatotoxicity
penciclovir	Apply cream to cold sores q2h while aware for 4d	Local disturbances

*Available in Canada only
†Consult category cards or individual drug cards for remaining dosages/adverse effects.

Note: Side/adverse effects: common in *italic;* serious in ***boldface italic.***

DOSAGE/ADVERSE EFFECTS†

Drug	Usual adult dose	Adverse effects
ribavirin	Aerosol treatment c̄ SPAG-2 for 12-18h/d c̄ drug concentration of 20mg/ml in drug reservoir of unit. Average concentration for 12-h period is 190μg/L of air	Cardiovascular, pulmonary
rimantadine	100mg bid	GI disturbances, insomnia, nervousness
ritonavir	600mg bid c̄ food	Asthenia, GI & neurological disturbances
saquinavir	200mg tid w/in 2h after full meal in combination c̄ AZT	Asthenia, GI disturbances
trifluridine	1gtt q2h to affected eye	Burning, epithelial keratopathy
valacyclovir	1g tid for 7d	GI disturbances, headache
vidarabine	Ocular: ½ inch of ointment in lower conjunctival sac 5 times/d at 3 h intervals	Lacrimation, uveitis

DESCRIPTION: Group of CNS depressant drugs that are chemical derivatives of barbituric acid; exhibit similar pharmacologic activity; classified according to onset, duration of activity.

DRUGS: Ultrashort: methohexital sodium *(Brevital Sodium),* thiamylal sodium, thiopental sodium *(Pentothal)* ▪ **Short:** pentobarbital *(Nembutal, *NovaRecal, *Pentagen),* pentobarbital sodium *(Nembutal Sodium),* secobarbital *(Seconal),* secobarbital sodium *(Seconal Sodium)* ▪ **Intermediate:** amobarbital *(Amytal, *Isabec),* amobarbital sodium *(Amytal Sodium),* aprobarbital *(Alurate),* butabarbital sodium *(Butisol Sodium)* ▪ **Long:** mephobarbital *(Mebaral),* phenobarbital *(Luminal),* phenobarbital sodium *(Luminal Sodium).*

THERAPEUTIC USE: Ultrashort: anesthesia induction, surgical procedures, convulsive states, narcoanalysis, narcosynthesis ▪ **Short:** sedation, hypnotic, acute convulsive states ▪ **Intermediate**: sedation, hypnotic, acute convulsive states ▪ **Long:** sedation, hypnotic, convulsive prophylaxis.

MECHANISM OF ACTION: Barbiturates act primarily on brainstem reticular formation to produce dose-related sedative, hypnotic effects. In high doses barbiturates can produce surgical anesthesia (ultrashort) ▪ Capable of raising convulsive threshold; selective barbiturates used for epileptic seizure prophylaxis ▪ Barbiturates are scheduled drugs because of potential for misuse/addiction.

CONTRAINDICATIONS: Hypersensitivity, severe liver/respiratory impairment, porphyria, addiction.

DOSAGE: *PO* (daily ranges)

	Convulsive	Hypnotic	Sedation
amobarbital	—	65-200mg	50-400mg
aprobarbital	—	40-160mg	120mg
butabarbital	—	50-100mg	45-120mg
mephobarbital	400-600mg	—	90-400mg
pentobarbital	—	100mg	40-160mg
phenobarbital	100-300mg	100-320mg	30-120mg
secobarbital	—	100-200mg	40-120mg

Note: Side/adverse effects: common in *italic;* serious in ***boldface italic.***

*Available in Canada only.

SIDE/ADVERSE EFFECTS: CNS: *drowsiness, lethargy, hangover,* headache, dizziness, paradoxic restlessness/excitement ▪ GI: N/V ▪ INT: morbilliform rash, ***Stevens-Johnson syndrome***, urticaria ▪ Other: asthma, ***angioneurotic edema.***

DRUG INTERACTIONS: Use c̄ alcohol, antihistamines, benzodiazepines, methotrimeprazine, narcotics, tranquilizers produces ↑ depressant effects ▪ Barbiturates are enzyme inducers; can ↓ effects of PO anticoagulants, other drugs ▪ MAO-I ↑ barbiturate activity ▪ Barbiturates ↓ PO absorption of griseofulvin.

NURSING MANAGEMENT PRIORITIES

ASSESS: Hx of hypersensitivity ▪ Recent CNS depressant administration (hold drug) ▪ Respiratory status; do *not* administer if <12/m ▪ Therapeutic blood levels ▪ Signs of dependence ▪ Actual swallowing of PO forms ▪ CAUTION: hepatic, renal, respiratory impairment ▪ **ndx: Therapeutic effects**: Anxiety ▪ Ineffective individual coping ▪ Sleep pattern disturbance ▪ **Adverse effects:** Risk for activity intolerance ▪ Ineffective breathing pattern ▪ Constipation ▪ Diarrhea ▪ Risk for fluid volume deficit ▪ Risk for injury ▪ Impaired physical mobility ▪ Risk for impaired skin integrity ▪ Altered thought processes. **PLAN:** Have emergency support measures available ▪ Avoid abrupt withdrawal ▪ Assess for tolerance of therapeutic dose ▪ Maintain safety precautions (raise bedrails, bed in low position, call bell) ▪ **Special considerations:** G: caution (paradoxic rxs) ▪ P: caution (paradoxic rxs), premies (↑ CNS sensitivity) ▪ OB: avoid use if pregnant, breastfeeding ▪ **Dietary management**: Avoid use c̄ alcohol ▪ **Lab test evaluation**: PT (anticoagulants), therapeutic blood levels. **IMPLEMENT:** Monitor VS, esp c̄ parenteral doses ▪ Check for signs of dependence ▪ Monitor occurrence/characteristics of seizure activity ▪ Monitor activity status (safety precautions) ▪ Assess for paradoxic rxs (CNS stimulation) esp in elderly ▪ Check for depression; suicide precautions prn ▪ **Patient education:** Comply c̄ prescribed drug regimen; indiscriminate use may lead to dependence ▪ Store properly (do *not* keep at bedside) ▪ Avoid use c̄ alcohol/other CNS depressants ▪ Use safety precautions c̄ ambulation, hazardous activity ▪ Avoid smoking after administration ▪ Use relaxation techniques, sleep producers (reading, warm milk, soft music). **EVALUATE: Observe for therapeutic effects:** ↓ Anxiety ▪ ↓ Insomnia ▪ ↓ Convulsive episodes ▪ ↑ Induction of anesthesia (ultrashort).

DESCRIPTION: Large group of anxiolytic agents that are chemical congeners of original prototype drug chlordiazepoxide.

DRUGS: alprazolam *(Xanax),* chlordiazepoxide *(Libritabs),* chlordiazepoxide hcl *(*Apo-Chlorax, Librium, *Medilium, *Novopoxide, *Solium),* clonazepam *(Klonopin, *Rivotril),* clorazepate dipotassium *(Tranxene),* diazepam *(Valium),* estazolam *(ProSom),* flurazepam hcl *(Dalmane, *Novoflupam),* lorazepam *(Ativan),* oxazepam *(*Ox-Pam, Serax, *Zapex),* prazepam, quazepam *(Doral),* temazepam *(Restoril),* triazolam *(Halcion).*

THERAPEUTIC USE: Alcoholism: chlordiazepoxide, clorazepate, diazepam, oxazepam ▪ **Anxiety**: alprazolam, chlordiazepoxide, clorazepate dipotassium, diazepam, lorazepam, oxazepam, prazepam ▪ **Convulsive states:** clonazepam, clorazepate, diazepam ▪ **Hypnotic:** estazolam, flurazepam, temazepam, triazolam ▪ **Muscle spasms:** diazepam.

MECHANISM OF ACTION: Benzodiazepines appear to potentiate the inhibitory effects of gamma aminobutyric acid in central mediated neurotransmission. Anxiolytic activity appears related to depression of CNS at brainstem formation, limbic systems. Benzodiazepines also depress polysynaptic reflex arcs in spinal cord, which may result in mild skeletal relaxation. They exhibit sedative, appetite-stimulating, weak analgesic, varying degrees of anticonvulsant activity.

CONTRAINDICATIONS: Hypersensitivity, narrow-angle glaucoma.

DOSAGE: Adult *PO*

alprazolam	0.25-0.5mg tid
chlordiazepoxide	5-25mg 3-4 times/d
clonazepam	Up to 20mg/d divided
clorazepate dipotassium	15-60mg/d divided
diazepam	2-10mg 3-4 times/d
estazolam	1-2mg at hs
flurazepam	15-30mg at hs
lorazepam	2-6mg/d divided
oxazepam	10-30mg 3-4 times/d
prazepam	20-60mg/d divided
quazepam	7.5-15mg at hs
temazepam	15-30mg at hs
triazolam	0.25-0.5mg at hs

SIDE/ADVERSE EFFECTS: CNS: *drowsiness, fatigue, ataxia,* headache ▪ GI: N/V ▪ GU: urinary retention ▪ HEM: neutropenia (rare) ▪ INT: rash, urticaria, pruritus ▪ PSYCH: paradoxic anxiety, depression, hallucinations, hyperexcited states.

OVERDOSE TREATMENT: Administer competitive antagonist flumazenil (*Mazicon*). Initial dose of 0.2mg IV over 15s. Subsequent doses if required must be individualized; be prepared for possible seizures.

DRUG INTERACTIONS: Use c̄ other CNS depressants produces additive effects ▪ Use c̄ MAO-I, disulfiram can produce serious toxic effects due to ↓ metabolism of benzodiazepines ▪ Smoking can ↓ effects of benzodiazepines.

NURSING MANAGEMENT PRIORITIES

ASSESS: Hx of hypersensitivity ▪ Recent CNS depressant administration (hold drug) ▪ Respiratory status ▪ Signs of dependence ▪ Pt sleep patterns ▪ CAUTION: hepatic, renal, respiratory impairment ▪ **ndx: Therapeutic effects**: Anxiety ▪ Ineffective individual coping ▪ Impaired physical mobility ▪ Sleep pattern disturbance ▪ **Adverse effects:** Risk for activity intolerance ▪ Ineffective breathing pattern ▪ Constipation ▪ Diarrhea ▪ Risk for fluid volume deficit ▪ Risk for injury ▪ Impaired physical mobility ▪ Risk for impaired skin integrity ▪ Altered thought processes. **PLAN:** Have emergency support measures available ▪ Avoid abrupt withdrawal ▪ Assess for tolerance to therapeutic dose ▪ Maintain safety precautions (raise bedrails, bed in low position, call bell) ▪ **Special considerations:** G: caution, ↓ dosage (↑ CNS sensitivity) ▪ P: caution, ↓ dosage (↑ sensitivity) ▪ OB: not recommended if pregnant, breastfeeding ▪ **Dietary management**: Avoid alcohol ▪ **Lab test evaluation**: CBC (long-term), serum creatinine. **IMPLEMENT:** Monitor VS, esp c̄ parenteral doses ▪ Check for signs of dependence ▪ Monitor occurrence/characteristics of seizure activity ▪ Monitor activity status (safety precautions) ▪ Assess for paradoxic rxs (CNS stimulation), esp in elderly ▪ Check for depression; suicide precautions prn ▪ **Patient education:** Comply c̄ prescribed drug regimen; indiscriminate use may lead to dependence ▪ Store properly (do *not* keep at bedside) ▪ Avoid use c̄ alcohol, other CNS depressants ▪ Use safety precautions c̄ ambulation, hazardous activity ▪ Avoid smoking after administration ▪ Use relaxation techniques, sleep producers (reading, warm milk, soft music). **EVALUATE: Observe for therapeutic effects:** ↓ Anxiety ▪ ↓ Insomnia.

DESCRIPTION: Nonselective (β_1, β_2) & selective (β_1) agents that block normal agonist response at β-adrenergic receptors in sympathetic nervous system; carvedilol, labetalol also exhibit α blockage.

DRUGS: Nonselective blockers: carteolol *(Cartrol)*, carvedilol *(Coreg)*, labetalol *(Normodyne, Trandate)*, nadolol *(Corgard)*, penbutolol *(Levatol)*, pindolol *(Visken)*, propranolol *(Inderal)*, sotalol *(Betapace)*, timolol *(Blocadren)* ▪ **Selective blockers:** acebutolol *(Sectral)*, atenolol *(Tenormin)*, betaxolol hcl *(Kerlone)*, bisoprolol *(Zebeta)*, esmolol hcl *(Brevibloc)*, metoprolol *(Lopressor)* ▪ **Topical:** betaxolol *(Betoptic 0.25, 0.5%)*, levobunolol *(Betagan 0.5%)*, metipranolol *(OptiPranolol 0.3%)*, timolol *(Timoptic 0.25, 0.5%)*.

THERAPEUTIC USE: Antianginal: nadolol, propranolol ▪ **Antiarrhythmic:** acebutolol, esmolol, propranolol, sotalol ▪ **Antihypertensive:** acebutolol, atenolol, betaxolol, bisoprolol, carteolol, labetalol, metoprolol, nadolol, penbutolol, pindolol, propranolol, timolol ▪ **MI**: metoprolol, propranolol, timolol ▪ **Migraine:** propranolol ▪ Topical treatment of glaucoma (usual dose 1gtt 1-2 times/d) ▪ **Congestive heart failure:** carvedilol.

MECHANISM OF ACTION: β blockers competitively prevent access of catecholamine neurotransmitters at β receptors in sympathetic nervous system. Nonselective agents block both β_1-, β_2-adrenergic receptors, whereas selective agents only block β_1 receptors, primarily located in cardiac tissue; selective β_1 blockers also inhibit β_2 receptors in high doses. β_2 receptors mainly located in bronchial, vascular smooth muscle ▪ β_1-adrenoreceptor blockage produces ↓ heart rate, ↓ cardiac output, ↓ conduction velocity at SA & AV nodes, myocardial automaticity, contractility; ↓ myocardial O_2 consumption, ↑ cardiac volume, quinidinelike membrane-stabilizing effect.

CONTRAINDICATIONS: Hypersensitivity, bronchial asthma (nonselective blockers), heart block, cardiac failure, cardiogenic shock.

DOSAGE†

betaxolol	10-20mg/d
bisoprolol	2.5-20mg/d
carteolol	2.5-10mg/d
carvedilol	12.5-50mg/d
esmolol	50-200mg/d
labetalol	200-800mg/d

*Available in Canada only
†Consult individual drug cards for remaining dosages.

metoprolol	100-450mg/d
nadolol	80-320mg/d
penbutolol	20-40mg/d
pindolol	10-60mg/d
sotalol	160-320mg/d
timolol	20-60mg/d

SIDE/ADVERSE EFFECTS: CNS: dizziness, mental depression, fatigue, hallucinations ▪ CV: bradycardia, CHF, hypotension, peripheral vascular insufficiency, exacerbation of AV block ▪ EENT: visual disturbances; dry mouth, eyes ▪ GI: N/V/D, cramps, constipation, ischemic colitis ▪ GU: impotence ▪ HEM: ***agranulocytosis,*** thrombocytopenic purpura ▪ INT: rash, pruritus, alopecia ▪ MS: joint pain ▪ RESP: bronchospasm.

DRUG INTERACTIONS: Use c̄ reserpine, other catecholamine-depleting drugs can result in serious adrenergic blockage ▪ Nonselective β adrenergics antagonize therapeutic effects.

NURSING MANAGEMENT PRIORITIES

ASSESS: Hx of hypersensitivity ▪ BP, apical pulse, respiratory distress ▪ CAUTION: hepatic, respiratory impairment, diabetics ▪ **ndx: Therapeutic effects**: ↓ Cardiac output ▪ Pain ▪ Altered tissue perfusion ▪ **Adverse effects:** Risk for activity intolerance ▪ Ineffective breathing pattern ▪ ↓ Cardiac output ▪ Diarrhea ▪ Fatigue ▪ Risk for fluid volume deficit ▪ Self-esteem disturbance ▪ Sensory/perceptual alterations ▪ Sexual dysfunction ▪ Altered thought processes ▪ Altered tissue perfusion. **PLAN:** Prevent postural hypotension ▪ Institute cardiac monitoring (IV) ▪ **Special considerations:** G: caution, ↓ dosage (↓ metabolism, ↑ sensitivity) ▪ P: not recommended ▪ OB:caution if pregnant, breastfeeding ▪ **Dietary management**: Avoid high-Na^+ foods, use c̄ alcohol; do *not* abstain from food for >12h (diabetics) ▪ **Lab test evaluation**: FBS (diabetics). **IMPLEMENT:** Assess apical pulse: if <60/m hold drug ▪ Monitor BP; observe for hypotension ▪ Monitor I&O, daily weight ▪ Monitor blood glucose in diabetics (hypoglycemia) ▪ **Patient education:** Avoid sudden position changes (postural hypotension) ▪ Comply c̄ prescribed drug regimen ▪ Avoid smoking, use c̄ alcohol, constrictive clothing, extremely hot objects, OTC cough/cold/allergy preparations ▪ Follow low-Na^+ diet ▪ Check for leg/foot swelling ▪ Check c̄ physician/pharmacist before taking OTC preparations ▪ Have BP checked regularly ▪ Keep appointments c̄ physician ▪ Carry identification (MedicAlert). **EVALUATE: Observe for therapeutic effects:** ↓ BP ▪ Normal sinus rhythm.

DESCRIPTION: Obtained from dried leaves of *Digitalis lanata* (Grecian foxglove), which yields digoxin; *D. purpurea* (purple foxglove) yields powdered digitalis leaf, digitoxin. Synthetic amrinone lactate & milrinone often listed c̄ dig drugs.

DRUGS: amrinone lactate *(Inocor)*, digitoxin *(Crystodigin)*, digoxin *(Lanoxicaps, Lanoxin, *Novodigoxin)*, milrinone *(Primacor)*.

THERAPEUTIC USE: Glycosides have same clinical efficacy, PO route preferred, digitoxin indicated in pts c̄ renal impairment ▪ Treatment of CHF ▪ Treatment of supraventricular arrhythmias incl atrial flutter/fibrillation, sinus tachycardia due to CHF ▪ Use in cardiogenic shock controversial.

MECHANISM OF ACTION: Produces dramatic changes in cardiac contractility (inotropic), electrophysiologic activity; + inotropic effect due to membrane electrolyte transport system (Na^+-K^+ pump) changes; Ca^{++}-dependent cardiac contractile mechanism altered because more intracellular Ca^{++} ions available to cardiac myofibrils. Digitalization in CHF produces + inotropic effect w/out corresponding ↑ O_2 consumption, ↑ stroke volume, ↓ coronary circulation ▪ ↓ Heart rate, conductivity in atrioventricular node, bundle of His ▪ ↓ Diastolic heart size, venous BP, vein engorgement ▪ Prolonged atrial, ventricular refractory periods ▪ Diuresis c̄ ↓ edema, palliation of exertional/paroxysmal nocturnal dyspnea, cough, cyanosis.

THERAPEUTIC USE: Glycosides have same clinical efficacy, PO route preferred, digitoxin indicated in pts c̄ renal impairment ▪ Treatment of CHF ▪ Treatment of supraventricular arrhythmias incl atrial flutter/fibrillation, sinus tachycardia due to CHF ▪ Use in cardiogenic shock controversial.

CONTRAINDICATIONS: Hypersensitivity, ventricular tachycardia, toxic effects.

DOSAGE: Adult: Usual dig; usual maintenance

amrinone	*IV*	0.75mg/kg (direct); 5-10µg/kg/m
digitoxin	*PO/IV*	1.2mg/24h; 0.15mg/d
digoxin	*PO/IV*	1-1.5mg/24h; 0.125-0.5mg/d
milrinone	*IV*	50µg/kg over 10m then 0.375-0.75 µg/kg/m

SIDE/ADVERSE EFFECTS: CNS: apathy, fatigue, headache, psychosis ▪ CV: bradycardia, arrhythmias ▪ GI: *N/V*, anorexia, diarrhea ▪ EENT: blurred/yellow vision ▪ Other: estrogenlike effects (long-term use).

DRUG INTERACTIONS: Acetazolamide, amphotericin B, chlorthalidone, ethacrynic acid, furosemide, laxatives, thiazides ↑ dig toxicity by inducing hypokalemia ▪ Parenteral Ca administration can produce serious arrhythmias ▪ Barbiturates, hydantoins, phenylbutazone may ↓ dig activity by enzyme induction ▪ Ion-exchange resins inhibit PO dig absorption ▪ Quinidine ↑ dig, digitoxin levels.

NURSING MANAGEMENT PRIORITIES

ASSESS: Hx of hypersensitivity ▪ Apical pulse ▪ Lung sounds ▪ Renal function ▪ Therapeutic blood levels ▪ CAUTION: renal impairment, ventricular arrhythmias ▪ **ndx: Therapeutic effects:** ↓ Cardiac output ▪ Altered tissue perfusion ▪ **Adverse effects:** Risk for activity intolerance ▪ ↓ Cardiac output ▪ Risk for fluid volume deficit ▪ Altered nutrition: less than body requirements ▪ Sensory/perceptual alterations (visual) ▪ Altered tissue perfusion. **PLAN:** Institute cardiac monitoring (IV) ▪ Identify exact dig preparation, dosage form ▪ **Special considerations:** G: caution (hepatic, renal impairment) ▪ P: caution, may require ↑ dosage to achieve effect ▪ OB: caution if pregnant, breastfeeding ▪ **Dietary management:** ↑ K^+, ↓ Na^+ ▪ **Lab test evaluation:** Electrolytes (K^+, Ca^{++}, Mg^{++}) therapeutic blood levels. **IMPLEMENT:** Assess apical pulse for 1m (hold dose if <60) ▪ Monitor VS, esp heart rate, BP ▪ Monitor F/E status (I&O, daily weight, peripheral edema) ▪ Check for toxicity before administering each dose (N/V, bradycardia, arrhythmias) ▪ **Patient education:** Procedure for checking radial pulse ▪ Comply c̄ prescribed drug regimen ▪ Report signs of toxicity to physician (loss of appetite, N/D, visual problems, irregular heartbeat) ▪ Follow low-Na^+, high-K^+ diet ▪ Check for leg/foot swelling ▪ Keep appointments c̄ physician **EVALUATE: Observe for therapeutic effects:** ↑ Cardiac output ▪ ↑ Urinary output ▪ ↓ Dyspnea.

OVERDOSE MANAGEMENT: Toxic dose 3/5 (60%) of therapeutic dose ▪ Principal symptoms: visual, conduction disturbances (arrhythmias) ▪ Treatment: adult—KCl 3-6g divided; pediatric—1-1.5mEq/kg divided ▪ Digoxin immune Fab (ovine) indicated in life-threatening OD; administered by IV infusion over 30m; bolus IV dose recommended in imminent cardiac arrest. Dosage variable; follow manufacturer's recommendation.

DESCRIPTION: Large diverse group of β-lactam antibiotics that are semisynthetic, H_2O soluble, broad spectrum, bactericidal against array of microbes; chemically related to penicillins ▪ Divided into 1st-, 2nd-, 3rd-generation cephalosporins on basis of bacterial spectrum of drugs, not chronologic development ▪ Cefoxitin, cefotetan (cephamycin antibiotics) usually classified c̄ cephalosporins.

DRUGS: First generation: Active against gram-positive bacteria, selected gram-negative organisms: cefadroxil *(Duricef, Ultracef)*, cefazolin sodium *(Ancef, Kefzol)*, cephalexin *(Keflex)*, cephalothin *(Keflin)*, cephapirin *(Cefadyl)*, cephradine *(Anspor, Velosef)* ▪ **Second generation:** Similar spectrum of organisms susceptible to 1st-generation drugs but more active against greater variety of gram-negative organisms: cefaclor *(Ceclor)*, cefamandole nafate *(Mandol)*, cefmetazole *(Zefazone)*, cefmetazole sodium *(Zefazone)*, cefonicid sodium *(Monocid)*, cefoxitin sodium *(Mefoxin)*, cefpodoxime proxetil *(Vantin)*, cefprozil *(Cefzil)*, cefuroxime sodium *(Kefurox, Zinacef)* ▪ **Third generation:** Less active against gram-positive organisms, expanded spectrum against gram-negative bacteria: cefdinir *(Omnicef)*, cefepime hcl *(Maxipime)*, cefixime *(Suprax)*, cefoperazone sodium *(Cefobid)*, cefotaxime sodium *(Claforan)*, cefotetan disodium *(Cefotan)*, ceftazidime *(Fortaz, Tazicef, Tazidime)*, ceftibuten *(Cedax)*, ceftizoxime *(Cefizox)*, ceftriaxone sodium *(Rocephin)*.

MECHANISM OF ACTION: Bactericidal activity due to inhibition of mucopeptide cell wall synthesis in susceptible organisms.

CAUTION: Coagulation irregularities can occur c̄ cefamandole, cefoperazone, moxalactam; observe for signs of hemorrhage ▪ Overgrowth of nonsusceptible organisms, pseudomembranous colitis can occur c̄ broad-spectrum antibiotics.

NURSING MANAGEMENT PRIORITIES

ASSESS: Hx of hypersensitivity (incl penicillin) ▪ VS, hepatic, renal function ▪ CAUTION: hepatic, renal impairment ▪ **ndx: Therapeutic effects**: Risk for altered body temperature ▪ Risk for infection ▪ **Adverse effects:** Diarrhea ▪ Risk for fluid volume deficit ▪ Risk for injury ▪ Risk for impaired skin integrity. **PLAN:** Administer at equal intervals around clock to maintain blood levels ▪ Maintain hydration ▪ **Special considerations:** G: caution, ↓ dosage (renal impairment, ↑ superinfection, coagulopathy) ▪ P: caution, ↓ dosage (prolonged half-life) ▪ OB: caution if pregnant, breastfeeding ▪ **Dietary management**: Avoid use c̄ alcohol ▪ **Lab test evaluation**: CBC; use Clinistix/Diastix for urine glucose. **IMPLEMENT:** Obtain C&S; check results ▪ Observe for signs of superinfection (diarrhea, URI, coated tongue) ▪ Administer on empty stomach ▪ **Patient education:** Comply c̄ prescribed drug regimen ▪ ↑ Fluid intake (8-10 glasses/d) ▪ Take on empty stomach ▪ Diarrhea may occur ▪ Notify physician of symptoms of allergic rx (fever, difficult breathing, rash). **EVALUATE: Observe for therapeutic effect:** Resolution of infection.

DESCRIPTION: Two exogenous biosynthetic agents produced by microbial DNA recombinant technology that influence proliferation differentiation (leukopoiesis) & activity of selected leukocytes. Both biosynthetic factors are almost identical to the two natural endogenous hemopoietic factors: (1) granulocyte colony stimulating factor (G-CSF), which is produced by endothelial cells, fibroblasts, & monocytes & (2) granulocyte-macrophage colony stimulating factor (GM-CSF), which is produced by endothelial cells, fibroblasts, macrophages, & T-cells.

DRUGS: Rx; Preg Cat C. filgrastim *(Neupogen)* is a G-CSF produced by DNA-modified *Escherichia coli* bacteria sargramostim *(Leukine),* a GM-CSF produced by DNA-modified *Saccharomyces cerevisiae.*

THERAPEUTIC USE: filgrastim: ↓ infections (febrile neutropenia) in pts receiving myelosuppressive antineoplastics for nonmyeloid malignancies ▪ In pts c̄ nonmyeloid malignancies undergoing myeloablative chemotherapy followed by bone marrow transplants ▪ Severe chronic neutropenia, peripheral blood progenitor cell (PBPC) collection. sargramostim: bone marrow transplantation delay/failure ▪ PBPC collection ▪ ↓ Infection ↑ neutrophil recovery following induction therapy for acute myelogenous leukemia ▪ Myeloid recovery following allogenic or autologous bone marrow transplantation in Hodgkin's/non-Hodgkin's lymphoma, acute lymphoblastic leukemia.

MECHANISM OF ACTION: Both natural & biosynthetic colony stimulating factors are glycoproteins that bind to leukocyte progenitor cells & induce proliferation, differentiation, & activity of leukocytes. Filgrastim (G-CSF) primarily influences neutrophils, whereas sargramostim (GM-CSF) affects granulocytes & macrophages.

CONTRAINDICATIONS: G-CSF/GM-CSF hypersensitivity, excessive leukemic myeloid blast cells ≥10% in blood or bone marrow.

DOSAGE

filgrastim

Myelosuppressive chemotherapy	*IV/SC*	5μg/kg/d as single bolus or short or continuous infusion given no earlier than 24h after treatment (not in the 24h before treatment) for up to 2wks
BMT	*IV/SC*	10μg/kg/d as 4h or 24h IV infusion or as continuous SC infusion

PBPC collection	*SC*	10μg/d 4 or more d before first collection and during collection period
Severe neutropenia		
Congenital	*SC*	6μg/kg bid qd
Idiopathic	*SC*	5μg once/d qd
sargramostim		
AML neutrophil recovery	*IV*	250μg/m²/d starting on day 11 or 4d following completion of therapy
BMT delay/ failure	*IV*	250μg/m²/d in 2-h infusion for 14d. May be repeated in 7d. A third course of 500μg/m²/d for 14d may be required
Myeloid recovery	*IV*	250μg/m²/d in 2-h infusion for 21d starting 2-4h after allogenic/autologous transplant infusion
PBPC collection	*IV/SC*	250μg/m²/d & continued during collection period

SIDE/ADVERSE EFFECTS: CV: edema ▪ GI: anorexia, N/V/D, hemorrhage, stomatitis ▪ INT: alopecia, rash ▪ RESP: cough, dyspnea, sore throat ▪ Other: fever, ***blood dyscrasias***, headache, medullary bone pain.

DRUG INTERACTIONS: Use c̄ corticosteroids, lithium can produce ↑ myeloprolific effects.

NURSING MANAGEMENT PRIORITIES

ASSESS: Hx of hypersensitivity to *E. coli*-derived proteins ▪ CBC, platelet counts ▪ Renal, hepatic function ▪ CAUTION: myeloid malignancies; cardiac conditions; renal, hepatic dysfunction ▪ **ndx: Therapeutic effects**: Impaired tissue integrity ▪ Risk for infection ▪ **Adverse effects:** Risk for activity intolerance ▪ Risk for altered temperature ▪ Fatigue ▪ Fluid volume excess ▪ Pain (bone). **PLAN:** Observe for edema in extremities ▪ Maintain hydration ▪ **Special considerations:** G: caution (renal impairment) ▪ P: caution (immature systems) ▪ OB: caution if pregnant; breastfeeding ▪ **Dietary management**: Adequate protein intake; well-balanced diet ▪ **Lab test evaluation**: CBC, platelets, neutrophil count. **IMPLEMENT:** Monitor VS, esp temperature ▪ Monitor F/E, hepatic, renal status ▪ Avoid administration 24h before, after cytotoxic chemotherapy, radiation ▪ Do not dilute c̄ saline (precipitation) ▪ **Patient education:** Comply c̄ prescribed drug regimen ▪ Safety precautions c̄ hazardous activity ▪ Procedure for self-administration ▪ Procedure for proper disposal of drug, used syringes, needles ▪ Notify physician of abnormal rxs (rash, wheezing, hypotension, tachycardia). **EVALUATE: Observe for therapeutic effects:** ↑ Neutrophil production ▪ Prevention/resolution of infection.

DESCRIPTION: The adrenal gland is regulated by the pituitary gland & is divided into cortex & medulla ▪ Cortex produces glucocorticoids (glucosteroids) & mineralocorticoids (mineralosteroids) ▪ Glucosteroids regulate metabolism of carbohydrates, lipids, proteins, to lesser extent minerals; potent inhibitors of inflammatory process, immune response; other significant effects incl ↓ number of circulating eosinophils, lymphocytes ▪ Glucosteroids are not curative agents but are used for potent antiinflammatory, immune suppressive activity in various pathophysiologic conditions. Prolonged administration of natural/synthetic steroids produces fluid & salt retention, suppression of hypothalamus, pituitary, adrenal glands. Synthetic glucosteroids are preferred because of lower salt & fluid retention properties ▪ Mineralosteroids regulate electrolyte metabolism, H_2O balance; used in maintenance treatment of Addison's disease in conjunction c̄ glucosteroids ▪ In addition to corticosteroids is small group of adrenal inhibitors consisting of aminoglutethimide, trilostane; used in treatment of Cushing's syndrome.

DRUGS: Glucosteroids: beclomethasone dipropionate *(Beclovent, Vanceril),* betamethasone *(Celestone),* cortisone acetate *(Cortone Acetate),* dexamethasone *(Decadron),* dexamethasone acetate *(Decadron-LA),* dexamethasone sodium phosphate *(Decadron Phosphate),* fludrocortisone acetate *(Florinef),* hydrocortisone *(Cortef),* hydrocortisone acetate *(Hydrocortone Acetate),* hydrocortisone cypionate *(Cortef Suspension),* hydrocortisone sodium phosphate *(Hydrocortisone Sodium Phosphate),* hydrocortisone sodium succinate *(Solu-Cortef),* methylprednisolone *(Medrol),* methylprednisolone acetate *(Depo-Medrol),* methylprednisolone sodium succinate *(A-Methapred, Solu-Medrol),* prednisolone *(Delta-Cortef),* prednisolone acetate *(Key-Pred),* prednisolone sodium phosphate *(Hydeltrasol),* prednisolone tebutate *(Hydeltra-T.B.A.),* prednisone *(Deltasone, Meticorten, Orasone),* triamcinolone *(Aristocort, Kenacort),* triamcinolone acetonide *(Kenalog-10),* triamcinolone diacetate *(Aristocort Syrup, Kenacort Diacetate Syrup),* triamcinolone hexacetonide *(Aristospan)* ▪ **Mineralosteroids:** fludrocortisone acetate *(Florinef Acetate)* ▪ **Adrenal inhibitors:** aminoglutethimide, trilostane *(Modrastane).*

NURSING MANAGEMENT PRIORITIES

ASSESS: Hx of hypersensitivity ▪ Adrenal insufficiency (lethargy, N/V, hypotension, confusion) ▪ CAUTION: infection, long-term therapy ▪ **ndx: Therapeutic effects**: Activity intolerance ▪ Ineffective airway clearance ▪ Risk for injury ▪ Impaired physical mobility ▪ Pain ▪ Impaired tissue integrity ■ **Adverse effects:** Fluid volume excess ■ Risk for infection ■ Impaired physical mobility ■ Altered nutrition: less than body requirement ■ Self-esteem disturbance ■ Sensory/perceptual alterations (visual) ■ Risk for impaired skin integrity ■ Impaired tissue perfusion. **PLAN:** Maintain hydration ■ Administer in AM ■ **Special considerations:** G: caution (↓ metabolism, chronic illness) ■ P: caution (↓ bone growth) ■ OB: caution if pregnant; avoid breastfeeding ■ **Dietary management**: ↑ K^+, protein; ↓ Na^+ ■ Avoid black licorice ■ **Lab test evaluation**: Electrolytes; blood/urine glucose (diabetics). **IMPLEMENT:** Monitor VS, esp BP ■ Monitor F/E status (I&O, daily weight, peripheral edema) ■ PO: administer c̄ food to ↓ GI irritation ■ Avoid abrupt withdrawal ■ **Patient education:** Comply c̄ prescribed drug regimen; take c̄ food/milk in AM ■ Check c̄ physician before vaccinations ■ Avoid exposure to infection ■ Notify physician of black/tarry stools, slow wound healing, blurred vision, bruising/bleeding, emotional changes ■ Keep scheduled appointments c̄ physician ■ Body image changes may occur c̄ prolonged use (reversible) ■ Carry identification (MedicAlert). **EVALUATE: Observe for therapeutic effects:** ↓ Inflammation ■ ↓ Immune response.

DESCRIPTION: A large, chemically/clinically similar group of antiinflammatory drugs that are synthetic derivatives of the natural glucosteroid hydrocortisone. Most of the synthetic derivatives are halogenated (addition of a chlorine or fluorinated atom) to enhance their antiinflammatory activity. They are subdivided clinically into groups according to their antiinflammatory response (potency), which is determined by their effectiveness in treating psoriasis or by vasoconstrictor measurements. Therapeutic efficacy for steroids in the same subgroup is approximately the same. Corticosteroids have a pregnancy category of C.

DRUG FORMULATIONS: Topical corticosteroids are usually applied to the skin by use of aerosols, creams, lotions, ointments, solutions. **Aerosol (A):** Formulations that spray the medication (usually a gas under pressure or hand-type pump spray) onto the skin as a foam, liquid, powder. **Cream (C):** Semisolid preparations of medication that is usually formulated c̄ water-soluble bases (for easy removal by washing) & intended to be rubbed onto the skin. **Lotions (L):** Liquid (usually aqueous) suspension of insoluble medication that is applied to the skin by rubbing the mixture onto the skin. **Ointment (O):** Semisolid preparation of medication that is formulated c̄ petroleum base (petrolatum) that liquefies by body temperature after being rubbed onto the skin. **Solutions (S):** A homogenous mixture of dissolved (solute) medication in a suitable solvent such as alcohol, H_2O that is applied to the skin.

DRUGS: Potency subdivision of topical steroids are (1) Group I: super potent, (2) Group II: potent, (3) Group III: moderately potent, (4) Group IV: low potency. Some reference standards use a sixth and seventh subdivision in describing the potency of topical corticosteroids (see accompanying product information chart for details).

THERAPEUTIC USE: Treatment of inflammatory, pruritic dermatoses ▪ In combination c̄ antibiotics or antifungals for treating cutaneous infection caused by susceptible bacteria or candidiasis.

MECHANISM OF ACTION: Application of corticosteroid to skin produces a significant antiinflammatory & antipruritic effect via several biologic pathways that incl (1) inhibiting synthesis & release of destructive endogenous agonists responsible for inflammation that incl histamine, kinins, prostaglandins; (2) reducing leukocyte adhesion to capillaries & stabilizing their lyosomal membranes;

(3) retarding migration of macrophages to areas of inflammation by vasoconstriction, ⬇ capillary wall permeability, subsequent edema reduction.

CONTRAINDICATIONS: Hypersensitivity. **CC:** Extended use can result in development of tolerance.

SIDE/ADVERSE EFFECTS: Local: burning, irritation, dryness, possible systemic absorption, which can produce corticosteroid systemic effects.

NURSING MANAGEMENT PRIORITIES

ASSESS: Hx of hypersensitivity ▪ Affected area; if open, weeping area do *not* apply ▪ CAUTION: Infection, long-term therapy ▪ **ndx: Therapeutic effects:** Risk for injury ▪ Pain ▪ Impaired tissue integrity ▪ **Adverse effects:** Risk for infection ▪ Risk for injury ▪ Risk for impaired skin integrity. **PLAN:** Monitor site of application for local rxs (burning, itching, erythema) ▪ Avoid contact c̄ eyes ▪ Continue treatment for several days after improvement is noted ▪ **Special considerations;** G: none specific ▪ P: apply sparingly (thin epidermis ▪ OB: none specific ▪ **Dietary management:** none specific ▪ **Lab test evaluation:** none specific. **IMPLEMENT:** Cleanse area before application ▪ Apply as directed by physician to affected area; use gloves & nonocclusive dressings (if needed) ▪ Monitor VS ▪ **Patient education:** Comply c̄ prescribed drug regimen ▪ Avoid exposure to infection ▪ Notify physician of slow wound healing ▪ Notify physician *immediately* of fever; D/C drug. **EVALUATE: Observe for therapeutic effects:** ⬇ Inflammation ▪ ⬇ Itching.

Drug	Brand names	Type	Potency	Dosage forms	Legal status
alclometasone dipropionate	Alcovate (G-W)	Halogenated	GP IV	Cream, ointment 0.05%	Rx
amcinonide	Cyclocort (Lederle)	Halogenated	GP II	Cream, lotion, ointment 0.1%	Rx
betamethasone dipropionate	Diprolene (Schering), Diprosone (Schering), Maxivate (Westwood)	Halogenated	GP I or II (GP I c̄ special formulation)	Cream, lotion, ointment 0.05% Aerosol 0.1% Cream, lotion, ointment 0.05%	Rx
betamethasone valerate	Valisone (Schering)	Halogenated	GP II	Cream 0.01%; cream, lotion, ointment 0.1%	Rx
clobetasol propionate	Temovate (G-W)	Halogenated	GP I	Cream, lotion, ointment 0.05%	Rx
clocortolone pivalate	Cloderm (Hermal)	Halogenated	GP III	Cream 0.1%	Rx
desonide	DesOwen (Owen/Gladerma)	Nonhalogenated	GP IV	Cream, lotion, ointment 0.05%	Rx
	Tridesilon (Bayer)			Cream, ointment 0.05%	Rx
desoximetasone	Topicort (H-M-R)	Halogenated	GP III	Cream 0.25, 0.05%; gel 0.05%; ointment 0.25%	
dexamethasone	Decaspray (Merck)	Halogenated	GP IV	Spray 0.01%, 0.04%	Rx

Note: Side/adverse effects: common in *italic;* serious in ***boldface italic.***

*Available in Canada only.

Drug	Brand names	Type	Potency	Dosage forms	Legal status
dexamethasone sodium phosphate	Decadron Phosphate (Merck)	Halogenated	GP IV	Cream 0.1%	Rx
diflorasone diacetate	Florone (Dermik) Maxiflor (Allergan)	Halogenated	GP I	Cream, ointment 0.05%	Rx
fluocinolone acetonide	Fluonid (Allergan) Synalar (Roche)	Halogenated	GP IV	Solution 0.01% Cream 0.01%, 0.025%, 0.2%; ointment 0.025%	Rx
fluocinonide	Lidex (Roche)	Halogenated	GP II	Cream, gel, ointment, solution, 0.05%	Rx
flurandrenolide	Cordan (Oclassen)	Halogenated	GP III	Cream 0.025, 0.05% Tape 4µg/cm^2 Lotion 0.05%; ointment 0.025, 0.05%	Rx
fluticasone propionate	Cultivate (Glaxo)	Halogenated	GP III	Cream 0.05%; ointment 0.005%	Rx
halcinonide	Halog (Westwood)	Halogenated	GP II	Cream 0.025, 0.1%; ointment, solution 0.1%	Rx
halobetasol	Ultravate (Westwood)	Halogenated	GP I	Cream, ointment 0.05%	Rx
mometasone furoate	Elocon (Schering)	Halogenated	GP III	Cream, lotion, ointment 0.1%	Rx
prednicarbate	Dermatop (H-M-R)	Nonhalogenated	GP IV	Cream 0.1%	Rx
triamcinolone acetate	Aristocort (Fujisawa) Kenalog (Westwood)	Halogenated	GP III	Aerosol, cream, lotion, ointment, solution—variable strengths	Rx

DESCRIPTION: Small group of drugs that promote diuresis, electrolyte excretion; bumetanide, furosemide are sulfonamidelike; ethacrynic acid is not.

DRUGS: bumetanide *(Bumex)*, ethacrynate sodium *(Edecrin Sodium)*, ethacrynic acid *(Edecrin)*, furosemide *(*Furoside, Lasix, *Neo-Renal, *Uritol)*, torsemide *(Demadex)*.

PHARMACOKINETICS: *See* individual drug cards.

THERAPEUTIC USE: Treatment of edema due to CHF, renal, hepatic dysfunction ▪ Treatment of hypertension (furosemide, torsemide) ▪ Short-term management of ascites due to malignancy, idiopathic edema, lymphedema, pediatric congenital heart disease, nephrotic syndrome (ethacrynate sodium, ethacrynic acid).

MECHANISM OF ACTION: Promote excretion of H_2O, Na^+, Cl^-, other electrolytes (esp K^+) by inhibiting tubular reabsorption, esp in medullary, cortical portions of ascending limb of loop of Henle ▪ Antihypertensive activity due to ↓ peripheral vascular resistance.

CONTRAINDICATIONS: Hypersensitivity, anuria, severe electrolyte imbalance, hepatic coma, watery diarrhea during treatment, nursing mothers (ethacrynic acid or ethacrynate sodium).

DOSAGE: Adult

bumetanide	*PO*	0.5-2mg/d to maximum 10mg
ethacrynate sodium	*IV*	50mg or 0.5-1mg/kg
ethacrynic acid	*PO*	50-300mg/d
furosemide	*PO*	20-80mg/d to maximum 600mg for refractory cases
torsemide	*PO/IV*	5-20mg once/d

SIDE/ADVERSE EFFECTS: CNS: dizziness, headache, encephalopathy in preexisting liver disease (bumetanide only) ▪ CV: hypotension ▪ EENT: blurred vision, hearing loss, tinnitus ▪ GI: N/V, abdominal pain, watery diarrhea, bleeding (ethacrynic acid only) ▪ HEM: anemia, ***thrombocytopenia, aplastic anemia*** (rare; furosemide only), neutropenia, Henoch-Schönlein purpura (ethacrynic acid only) ▪ INT: rash, urticaria, ***exfoliative dermatitis, erythema multiforme*** (furosemide only) ▪ MS: muscle cramps, arthritic pain (bumetanide only).

Note: Side/adverse effects: common in *italic;* serious in ***boldface italic.***

*Available in Canada only.

DRUG INTERACTIONS: Use c̄ neurotoxic drugs incl aminoglycosides, capreomycin, chloroquine, vancomycin can result in significant toxicity ▪ Induced hypokalemia, ↑ dig toxicity ▪ Avoid use c̄ nephrotoxic drugs, lithium, probenecid, indomethacin ▪ Antihypertensives may require dosage adjustments ▪ Use c̄ corticosteroids can produce severe hypokalemia.

NURSING MANAGEMENT PRIORITIES

ASSESS: Hx of hypersensitivity (incl sulfonamides) ▪ Adequate renal function ▪ Serum K^+ (normal level: 3.5-5mEq/L) ▪ Hydration status ▪ CAUTION: ascites, renal failure, gout, diabetes ▪ **ndx: Therapeutic effects**: Fluid volume excess ▪ Altered tissue perfusion ▪ **Adverse effects:** Risk for activity intolerance ▪ Ineffective breathing pattern ▪ ↓ Cardiac output ▪ Diarrhea ▪ Risk for fluid volume deficit ▪ Sensory/perceptual alterations (auditory, visual) ▪ Risk for impaired skin integrity ▪ Altered patterns of urinary elimination. **PLAN:** Maintain hydration ▪ **Special considerations:** G: caution, ↓ dosage (↑ sensitivity) ▪ P: caution (↑ electrolyte imbalance) ▪ OB: caution if pregnant; breastfeeding not recommended ▪ **Dietary management**: ↑ K^+, ↓ Na^+ ▪ **Lab test evaluation**: Electrolytes, FBS, BUN, serum uric acid. **IMPLEMENT:** Administer on awakening ▪ Monitor BP, K^+, I&O, daily weight, edema, lung sounds, skin turgor/mucous membranes ▪ Observe for changes in hearing & visual acuity ▪ **Patient education:** Expect ↑ urine output; have bathroom facilities close ▪ Eat foods high in K^+; avoid black licorice, high-Na^+ foods ▪ Take on arising qd ▪ Watch for signs of hypokalemia (muscle cramps, lethargy, anorexia), hyponatremia (thirst, dry mouth, drowsiness). **EVALUATE: Observe for therapeutic effects:** ↑ Urine output ▪ ↓ Edema ▪ ↓ BP.

DESCRIPTION: Large group of diuretic-antihypertensive agents that are sulfonamidelike chemical derivatives of benzothiadiazine.

DRUGS: ▪ **Thiazide diuretics:** bendroflumethiazide *(Naturetin),* benzthiazide *(Exna),* chlorothiazide *(Diuril),* hydrochlorothiazide *(*Diuchlor H, Esidrix, HydroDIURIL, *Nefrol, *Neo-Codema, Oretic, *Urozide),* hydroflumethiazide *(Diucardin, Saluron),* methyclothiazide *(Aquatensen, Enduron),* polythiazide *(Renese),* trichlormethiazide *(Metahydrin, Naqua)* ▪ **Thiazidelike diuretics:** chlorthalidone *(Hygroton, Thalitone, *Uridon),* indapamide *(*Lozide, Lozol),* metolazone *(Zaroxolyn),* quinethazone *(*Aquamox, Hydromox).*

PHARMACOKINETICS: *See* individual drug cards.

THERAPEUTIC USE: Treatment of hypertension as sole agent/in combination c̄ other antihypertensives ▪ Treatment of edema due to renal dysfunction ▪ Adjunct in treating edema due to CHF, hepatic cirrhosis, corticosteroid/estrogen therapy.

MECHANISM OF ACTION: Thiazides promote excretion of H_2O, Na^+, Cl^- by inhibiting reabsorption of Na^+, primarily in ascending loop of Henle & in early distal tubule of nephron; enhance excretion of K^+, bicarbonate, other ions w/out significantly altering pH of urine; lower peripheral vascular resistance, resulting in significant antihypertensive activity; exhibit similar clinical efficacy.

CONTRAINDICATIONS: Hypersensitivity due to any thiazide, other sulfonamide-derivative drug; anuria.

DOSAGE: Usual adult range *PO*

bendroflumethiazide	2.5-15mg/d
benzthiazide	50-200mg/d
chlorothiazide	0.5-2g/d
chlorthalidone	50-100mg/d; 100mg qod
hydrochlorothiazide	50-200mg/d
hydroflumethiazide	50-200mg/d
indapamide	2.5-5mg/d
methyclothiazide	2.5-10mg/d
metolazone	2.5-10mg/d
polythiazide	2-4mg/d
quinethazone	50-100mg/d
trichlormethiazide	2-4mg/d

SIDE/ADVERSE EFFECTS: CNS: *dizziness,* vertigo, paresthesia, headache ▪ EENT: blurred vision, xanthopsia ▪

GI: anorexia, N/V/D, jaundice ▪ HEM: ***agranulocytosis, aplastic anemia,*** leukopenia, ***thrombocytopenia*** ▪ INT: purpura, urticaria, photosensitivity ▪ MET: hypokalemia, glycosuria, hyperglycemia, hyperuricemia, hypochloremic alkalosis ▪ MS: *fatigue, leg cramps* ▪ RESP: respiratory distress ▪ Other: necrotizing angiitis.

DRUG INTERACTIONS: ↑ Dig toxicity due to hypokalemia ▪ Use c̄ corticosteroids ↑ hypokalemia ▪ Antidiabetic agents may require dose adjustments ▪ Use c̄ diazoxide can produce significant diabetogenic effects.

NURSING MANAGEMENT PRIORITIES

ASSESS: Hx of hypersensitivity (incl sulfonamides) ▪ Adequate renal function ▪ Serum K^+ (normal level: 3.5-5mEq/L) ▪ Hydration status ▪ CAUTION: ascites, renal failure, gout, diabetes ▪ **ndx: Therapeutic effects**: Fluid volume excess ▪ Altered tissue perfusion ▪ **Adverse effects:** Risk for activity intolerance ▪ Ineffective breathing pattern ▪ ↓ Cardiac output ▪ Diarrhea ▪ Risk for fluid volume deficit ▪ Sensory/perceptual alterations (visual) ▪ Risk for impaired skin integrity ▪ Altered patterns of urinary elimination. **PLAN:** Maintain hydration ▪ **Special considerations:** G: caution, ↓ dosage (↑ sensitivity) ▪ P: caution (↑ electrolyte imbalance) ▪ OB: caution if pregnant; breastfeeding not recommended ▪ **Dietary management**: ↑ K^+, ↓ Na^+ ▪ **Lab test evaluation**: Electrolytes, FBS, BUN, serum uric acid. **IMPLEMENT:** Administer on awakening ▪ Monitor BP, K^+, I&O, daily weight, edema, lung sounds, skin turgor/mucous membranes ▪ Observe for changes in hearing & visual acuity ▪ **Patient education:** Expect ↑ urine output; have bathroom facilities ▪ Eat foods high in K^+; avoid black licorice, high-Na^+ foods ▪ Take on arising qd ▪ Watch for signs of hypokalemia (muscle cramps, lethargy, anorexia), hyponatremia (thirst, dry mouth, drowsiness). **EVALUATE: Observe for therapeutic effects:** ↑ Urine output ▪ ↓ Edema ▪ ↓ BP.

DESCRIPTION: A group of synthetic broad-spectrum bactericidal antiinfective agents that are chemically divided into fluorinated & nonfluorinated quinolones. The fluoroquinolones are newer & contain a fluorine atom (fluorinated), which results in a greatly expanded bacterial spectrum & greater potency.

DRUGS: Fluoroquinolones: ciprofloxacin *(Cipro),* enoxacin *(Penetrex),* grepafloxacin hcl *(Raxar),* levofloxacin *(Levaquin),* lomefloxacin *(Maxaquin),* norfloxacin *(Noroxin),* ofloxacin *(Floxin),* sparfloxacin *(Zagam)* ▪ **Quinolones:** cinoxacin *(Cinobac),* nalidixic acid *(NegGram).*

THERAPEUTIC USE: Fluoroquinolones are primarily employed for treatment of gram-negative & selected gram-positive infections of bone, joint, lower respiratory tract, skin & skin structure, & urinary tract ▪ Treatment of infectious diarrhea, prostatitis, sinusitis, & STDs ▪ Prevention of postop infections from transurethral surgical procedures ▪ **Quinolones** have a narrow gram-negative bacterial spectrum & are limited to UTI.

MECHANISM OF ACTION: Bactericidal activity caused by interference c̄ DNA gyrase enzyme (DNA topoisomerase), which is required for DNA synthesis in sus-

PHARMACOKINETICS

Drug	PO absorption	Peak serum	Half-life	Protein binding	Excretion
ciprofloxacin	Good	1-2h	4h	20%-40%	50% via urine as unchanged drug
cinoxacin	High	2h	1-1.5h	NA	60% via urine as unchanged drug
enoxacin	Excellent	1-3h	3-6h	40%	40% via urine as unchanged drug
levofloxacin	Excellent	1-2h	6-8h	24%-38%	87% via urine as unchanged drug
lomefloxacin	Excellent	1.5h	8h	10%	65% via urine as unchanged drug
nalidixic acid	Excellent	1-2h	6h	90%	85% via urine as unchanged drug
norfloxacin	Moderate	1-2h	3-4h	10%-15%	26%-32% via urine as unchanged drug
ofloxacin	Excellent	1-2h	9h	32%	65%-80% via urine as unchanged drug
sparfloxacin	Good	3-6h	20h	45%	50% via urine & feces primarily as metabolites

ceptible organisms, esp gram-negative bacteria. In addition, fluoroquinolones are active against selected chlamydia, mycoplasmal, & mycobacterial infections.

Antimicrobial spectra of fluoroquinolones are similar & ciprofloxacin (prototype drug), norfloxacin, & ofloxacin have largest spectrum of activity. Cross-resistance exists between fluoroquinolones & is usually absent c̄ other antimicrobial agents, esp c̄ antibiotics.

CONTRAINDICATIONS: Hypersensitivity to drug or other quinolones or fluoroquinolones. **CC:** Use can result in overgrowth of nonsusceptible organism & pseudomembranous colitis.

SIDE/ADVERSE EFFECTS (COMMON): CNS: headache, restlessness, dizziness, drowsiness, ***convulsive seizures,*** insomnia ▪ GI: N/V/D, abdominal distress, dyspepsia, flatulence, ***pseudomembranous colitis*** ▪ Other: rash, photosensitivity, visual disturbance, mycotic infection.

DRUG INTERACTIONS: Al, Fe, Mg products, sucralfate may ↓ PO absorption ▪ Use c̄ theophylline may ↑ theophylline toxicity ▪ Probenecid will ↓ renal excretion ▪ Use c̄ PO anticoagulants requires caution because of possible alteration of interstitial flora ▪ Use c̄ caffeine will ↑ its effects. **Food:** Food can delay/↓ PO absorption.

NURSING MANAGEMENT PRIORITIES

ASSESS: Hx of hypersensitivity ▪ Hepatic, renal function ▪ CAUTION: hepatic, renal impairment ▪ **ndx: Therapeutic effects:** risk for altered body temperature ▪ Risk for infection ▪ **Adverse effects:** diarrhea ▪ Risk for fluid volume deficit ▪ Risk for injury ▪ Risk for impaired skin integrity ▪ Risk for sensory/perceptual impairment. **PLAN:** Administer at equal intervals around the clock to maintain blood levels ▪ Maintain hydration ▪ **Special considerations:** G: caution, ↓ dosage (renal impairment, ↑ superinfection) ▪ P: caution (↑ sensitivity) ▪ OB: caution if pregnant, breastfeeding ▪ **Dietary management:** none specific ▪ **Lab test evaluation:** CBC, blood glucose (diabetics). **IMPLEMENT:** Obtain C&S, check results ▪ Observe for signs of superinfection (diarrhea, URI, coated tongue) ▪ Administer on empty stomach ▪ Assess for tremors, seizures; notify physician ▪ **Patient education:** Comply c̄ prescribed drug regimen ▪ ↑ Fluid intake (8-10 glasses/d) ▪ Take on empty stomach ▪ CNS alterations may occur ▪ Diarrhea may occur ▪ Notify physician of symptoms of allergic rx (fever, difficult breathing, rash) &/or visual disturbances. **EVALUATE: Observe for therapeutic effect:** Resolution of infection.

cinoxacin: Quinolone Rx; Preg Cat B

BRAND NAME	DOSAGE FORMS
Cinobac (Oclassen)	Capsule: 250, 500mg

USE: Treatment of UTI caused by susceptible strains of *Enterobacter* spp, *Escherichia coli, Klebsiella* spp, *Proteus* spp.

CC: Use c̄ caution in pts c̄ renal impairment ▪ Avoid alkalinization of urine during treatment ▪ Avoid exposure to sunlight ▪ Safety in nursing mothers, children <12y/o not established.

DOSAGE

Adult	*PO*	1g/d in 2-4 divided doses for 7-14d

---

ciprofloxacin: Fluoroquinolone Rx; Preg Cat C

BRAND NAME	DOSAGE FORMS
Cipro (Bayer)	IV injection: 200, 400mg/vial Tablet: 100, 250, 500, 750mg

USE: Treatment of bone, joint infection, infectious diarrhea, lower respiratory, skin, & urinary tract infection caused by susceptible strains of *Campylobacter jejuni, Morganella morganii, Citrobacter* spp, *Enterobacter cloacae, Escherichia coli, Haemophilus influenzae, Klebsiella pneumoniae, Proteus* spp, *Providencia* spp, *Pseudomonas aeruginosa, Serratia marcescens, Shigella* spp, *Staphylococcus* spp, *Streptococcus* spp ▪ Treatment of gonorrhea, typhoid fever.

CC: Safety during pregnancy, in nursing mothers, children <18y/o not established ▪ Not indicated for syphilis treatment ▪ Avoid alkalinization of urine during treatment ▪ D/C use c̄ inflammation, pain in or rupture of a tendon ▪ IV administration must extend over a 1-h period ▪ Use may cause crystalluria ▪ Use c̄ glyburide can cause rare episodes of severe hypoglycemia.

DOSAGE: For normal renal function. Treatment should continue for at lease 2d after pt is asymptomatic.

Adult *PO*

Bone/joint	500mg q12h & 750mg q12h for more complicated infections for 4-6wks
Gonorrhea	250mg as single dose. Many clinicians use 500mg as single dose
Infectious diarrhea	500mg q12h for 5-7d

Lower respiratory/ skin	500mg q12h & 750mg q12h for more complicated infections for 7-14d
Typhoid fever	500mg q12h for 10d
UTI	
Acute	100mg q12h for 3d
Mild/moderate	250mg q12h for 7-14d
Complicated	500mg q12h for 7-14d
IV	200mg q12h for renal infections 400mg q12h for bone, joint, lower respiratory, skin, & more complicated renal infections

SIDE/ADVERSE EFFECTS: CV: angina, atrial flutter, ***MI***, palpitations, hypertension, ***cerebral thrombosis, cardiopulmonary arrest, ventricular ectopy*** ▪ GI: ***intestinal perforation*** ▪ GU: vaginitis, ***interstitial nephritis, nephritis, renal failure,*** urethral bleeding, voiding irregularities ▪ HEM: eosinophilia, leukopenia ▪ HEP: ↑ ALT, AST, alkaline phosphatase, BUN ▪ INT: erythema nodosum, edema of face, lips, neck, hyperpigmentation, ***Stevens-Johnson syndrome, toxic epidermal necrolysis.***

---

enoxacin: Fluoroquinolone Rx; Preg Cat C

BRAND NAME	**DOSAGE FORMS**
Penetrex (RPR)	Tablet 200, 400mg

USE: Treatment of STDs & UTIs caused by susceptible strains of *Enterobacter cloacae, Escherichia coli, Klebsiella pneumoniae, Neisseria gonorrhoeae, Proteus mirabilis, Pseudomonas aeruginosa, Staphylococcus epidermidis, S. saprophyticus.*

CONTRAINDICATIONS: Tendinitis or tendon rupture associated c̄ quinolone group of agents. **CC:** Safety during pregnancy, in nursing mothers, children <18y/o not established ▪ Not indicated for syphilis treatment ▪ D/C use c̄ inflammation, pain in or rupture of a tendon ▪ Use c̄ bismuth subsalicylate should be avoided.

DOSAGE

Adult *PO*

Uncomplicated gonorrhea (STD)	400mg as single dose
Uncomplicated UTI	200mg q12h for 7d
Complicated UTI	400mg q12h for 14d

SIDE/ADVERSE EFFECTS: CV: palpitations, tachycardia, vasodilation ▪ GU: ***renal failure*** ▪ INT: ***erythema multiforme, Stevens-Johnson syndrome, toxic epidermal necrolysis*** ▪ RESP: cough, dyspnea, epistaxis ▪ Other: asthenia, arthralgia, myalgia, purpura.

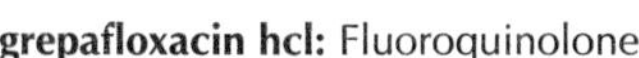

grepafloxacin hcl: Fluoroquinolone Rx; Preg Cat C

BRAND NAME	DOSAGE FORM
Raxar (GW)	Tablet: 200mg

USE: Treatment of acute exacerbation of chronic bronchitis, community-acquired pneumonia, uncomplicated gonorrhea, nongonococcal cervicitis & urethritis caused by susceptible strains of *Chlamydia trachomatis, Haemophilus influenzae, Moraxella catarrhalis, Mycoplasma pneumoniae, Neisseria gonorrhoeae, Streptococcus pneumoniae.*

CONTRAINDICATIONS: Hepatic failure, known QT cardiac prolongation interval. **CC:** Use c̄ medication that can produce an ↑ in QT interval or torsades de pointes requires extensive & appropriate cardiac monitoring. If this is not feasible, drug is contraindicated.

DOSAGE

Adult *PO*

Bronchitis	400 or 600mg once/d for 10d
Pneumonia	600mg once/d for 10d
Gonorrhea	400mg as single dose
Nongonococcal	400mg once/d for 7d

levofloxacin: Fluoroquinolone Rx; Preg Cat C

BRAND NAME	DOSAGE FORMS
Levaquin (McNeil)	IV injection: 500-mg vial, 250mg/50ml D_5, 500mg/100ml D_5 Tablet: 250, 500mg

USE: Treatment of acute exacerbation of chronic bronchitis, acute maxillary sinusitis, community-acquired pneumonia, acute pyelonephritis, UTIs & skin/skin structure infections caused by susceptible strains of *Chlamydia pneumoniae, Enterobacter cloacae, Enterococcus faecalis, Escherichia coli, Haemophilus influenzae, H. parainfluenzae, Klebsiella pneumoniae, Legionella pneumophilia, Moraxella catarrhalis, Mycoplasma pneumoniae, Proteus mirabilis, Pseudomonas aeruginosa, Staphylococcus aureus, Streptococcus pneumoniae, S. pyogenes.*

CC: Safety in pregnant women, nursing mothers, children <18y/o not established ▪ D/C use c̄ inflammation, pain in or rupture of a tendon ▪ Use c̄ caution c̄ renal impairment.

DOSAGE: For normal renal function

Adult *PO*

Bronchitis	500mg/d for 7d

Pneumonia	500mg/d for 7-14d
Pyelonephritis	250mg/d for 10d
Sinusitis	500mg/d for 10-14d
Skin	500mg/d for 10d
UTIs	250mg/d for 10d

SIDE/ADVERSE EFFECTS: CV: edema hypertension, ***cardiac failure*** ▪ EENT: pharyngitis, rhinitis, tinnitus, taste changes, visual disturbances ▪ INT: rash, pruritus, urticaria ▪ Other: abdominal/back/chest pain, leukocytosis.

---

lomefloxacin: Fluoroquinolone Rx; Preg Cat C

BRAND NAME	DOSAGE FORM
Maxaquin (Searle)	Tablet: 400mg

USE: Treatment of lower respiratory infection caused by susceptible strains of *Haemophilus influenzae, Moraxella catarrhalis* ▪ Treatment of UTIs caused by susceptible strains of *Citrobacter diversum, Enterobacter cloacae, Escherichia coli, H. influenzae, Klebsiella pneumoniae, M. catarrhalis, Proteus mirabilis, Pseudomonas aeruginosa, Staphylococcus saprophyticus* ▪ Prophylaxis of postop infections from transurethral surgical procedures.

CC: Safety during pregnancy, in nursing mothers, children <18y/o not established ▪ Use in treating pseudomonas bacteremia not established ▪ Drug produces highest rate of fluoroquinolone photosensitivity rxs.

DOSAGE

Adult *PO*

Respiratory infection	400mg/d for 10d
UTIs	400mg/d for 10d & 400mg qd for complicated infections
Postop prophylaxis	400mg q2-6h when prophylaxis for transurethral procedure is appropriate

SIDE/ADVERSE EFFECTS: CV: ***angina, arrhythmia, cardiac failure, cardiomyopathy, pulmonary embolism,*** edema, phlebitis ▪ GI: anorexia, bleeding, taste changes ▪ GU: dysuria, leukorrhea, intermenstrual bleeding ▪ HEM: ↑ fibrinolysis, ***thrombocytopenia,*** thrombocytopenia purpura ▪ Other: bronchospasm, back pain, ↓ heat tolerance, flulike symptoms.

nalidixic acid: Quinolone Rx; Preg Cat C

BRAND NAME	DOSAGE FORMS
NegGram (S-W)	PO suspension: 250mg/5ml Caplet: 250, 500mg; 1g

USE: Treatment of UTIs caused by susceptible strains of *Enterobacter* spp, *Escherichia coli, Klebsiella* spp, *Proteus* spp, & other sensitive gram-negative organisms.

CONTRAINDICATIONS: Hx of convulsive disorders. **CC:** Use c̄ caution c̄ epilepsy, severe cerebral arteriosclerosis, hepatic or renal dysfunction ▪ Safety in infants <3m/o not established ▪ Use in pregnancy or nursing mothers, children <18y/o only when potential benefits are > potential risks.

DOSAGE: *PO*

Children ≤12y/o	25mg/lb/d in 4 equally divided doses. Extended treatment dose may be ↓ to 15mg/lb/d
Adult	1g qid for 1-2wks. Extended treatment dose may be ↓ to 2g/d

SIDE/ADVERSE EFFECTS: CNS: drowsiness, dizziness, headache, convulsions ▪ INT: pruritus, rash, urticaria, photosensitivity ▪ Other: visual disturbances, overbrightness of light.

---

norfloxacin: Fluoroquinolone Rx; Preg Cat C

BRAND NAMES	DOSAGE FORMS
Chibroxin Sterile (Merck)	Ophthalmic solution: 0.3%
Noroxin (Merck)	Tablet: 400mg

USE: Treatment of UTI infections caused by susceptible strains of *Citrobacter freundii, Enterobacter* spp, *Enterococcus faecalis, Escherichia coli, Klebsiella pneumoniae, Proteus* spp, *Pseudomonas aeruginosa, Serratia marcescens, Staphylococcus* spp, *Streptococcus agalactiae* ▪ Treatment of gonorrhea & *E. coli* prostatitis ▪ Ophthalmic solution: treatment of conjunctivitis caused by selected gram-positive & gram-negative organisms.

CONTRAINDICATIONS: Tendinitis or tendon rupture associated c̄ quinolone group of agents. **CC:** Not effective against syphilis ▪ Safety in pregnant women, nursing mothers, children <18y/o not established ▪ Ophthalmic solution not for ocular injection.

DOSAGE: For normal renal function

Adult *PO*	400mg bid 1h ac or 2h pc for 7-10d & up to 21d for complicated infections. Gonorrhea dose is 800mg as a single dose. Prostatitis dose 400mg bid for 28d
Ophthalmic solution	1-2gtt qid for up to 7d for adults, children ≥1y/o

SIDE/ADVERSE EFFECTS: HEM: eosinophilia, neutropenia, ↓ in hematocrit ▪ HEP: ↑ in ALT, AST, alkaline phosphatase, BUN ▪ Other: ***Stevens-Johnson syndrome,*** visual disturbances.

---

ofloxacin: Fluoroquinolone Rx; Preg Cat C

BRAND NAMES	**DOSAGE FORMS**
Floxin (McNeil)	Tablet: 200, 300, 400mg
	IV injection: 200, 400mg/container
Ocuflox (Allergan)	Ophthalmic solution: 0.3%

USE: Treatment of lower respiratory, skin, urinary tract infections caused by susceptible strains of *Citrobacter diverus, Enterobacter aerogenes, Escherichia coli, Haemophilus influenzae, Klebsiella pneumoniae, Proteus mirabilis, Pseudomonas aeruginosa, Staphylococcus aureus, Streptococcus pneumoniae, S. pyogenes* ▪ Treatment of STDs: gonorrhea, nongonococcal & cervicitis caused by chlamydia trachomatis ▪ Treatment of *E. coli* prostatitis ▪ Ophthalmic solution: treatment of selected gram-positive, gram-negative organisms & trachoma.

CC: Not indicated for syphilis ▪ Safety during pregnancy, in nursing mothers & children <18y/o not established ▪ Use c̄ caution c̄ hepatic or renal impairment ▪ Keep pt well hydrated ▪ Ophthalmic solution: not for ocular injection & use in infants <1y/o not recommended.

DOSAGE: For normal renal function

Adult *PO*	LRI/skin: 400mg q12h for 10d; UTIs: 200-300mg q12h for 10d; gonorrhea: 400mg as single dose, 300mg q12h for 7d for complicated infections; chlamydial STDs: 300mg q12h for 7-10d; prostatitis: 300mg q12h for 6wks
IV	200-400mg q12h by infusion
Ophthalmic solution	Conjunctivitis: 1-2gtt q2-4h for 2d then 1-2gtt qid; corneal ulcers: 1-2gtt q30m while awake & at 4 & 6h dur-

ing sleep time for 2d for corneal ulcers, then 1-2gtt/h while awake for 5-7d & completed c̄ 1-2gtt qid for 1-2d.

SIDE/ADVERSE EFFECTS: CV: edema, hypertension, palpitation ▪ GU: vaginitis, dysmenorrhea, dysuria, glycosuria, proteinuria, hematuria ▪ HEM: leukocytosis, lymphocytopenia ▪ HEP: ↑ serum glutamate pyruvate transaminase ▪ Other: diaphoresis, vasculitis.

---

sparfloxacin: Fluoroquinolone Rx; Preg Cat C

BRAND NAME	DOSAGE FORM
Zagam (RPR)	Tablet: 200mg

USE: Treatment of acute exacerbation of chronic bronchitis & community acquired pneumonia caused by susceptible strains of *Chlamydia pneumoniae, Enterobacter cloacae, Haemophilus influenzae/parainfluenzae, Klebsiella pneumoniae, Moraxella catarrhalis, Mycoplasma pneumoniae, Staphylococcus aureus, Streptococcus pneumoniae.*

CC: Safety in pregnant women, nursing mothers, children <18y/o not established ▪ Use c̄ disopyramide or amiodarone can produce torsade de pointes ▪ Avoide medication that prolongs QT cardiac interval: astemizole, cisapride, erythromycin, pentamidine, terfenadine ▪ D/C use c̄ inflammation, pain in or rupture of tendon ▪ Use c̄ caution in pts who are predisposed to seizures ▪ Use can result in a false − culture for tuberculosis.

DOSAGE: For normal renal function

Adult *PO*	400-mg loading dose on day 1 followed by 200mg/d for 10d

SIDE/ADVERSE EFFECTS: CV: arrhythmias, hypertension, palpitations, QT interval prolonged, vasodilation ▪ EENT: visual disturbances, photophobia, tinnitus ▪ GU: dysuria, dysmenorrhea, vulvovaginal disorders ▪ Other: breast pain, asthma, epistaxis, exfoliative dermatitis, herpes simplex infections.

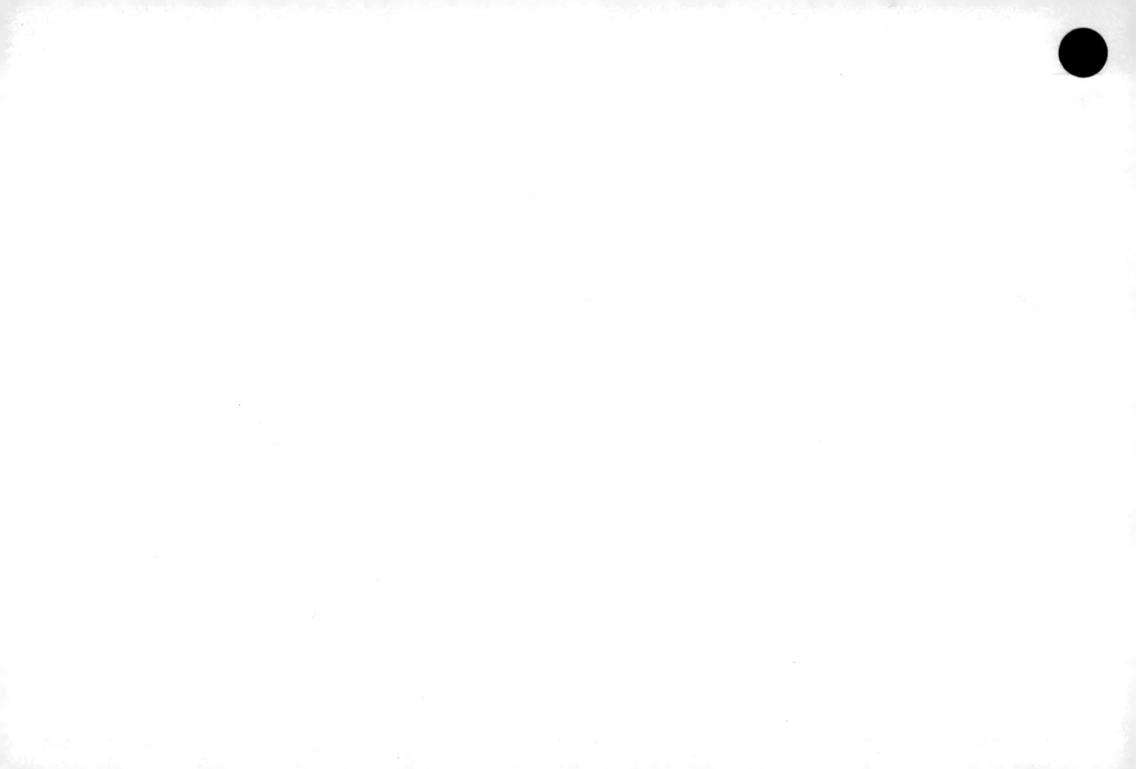

DESCRIPTION: Hydroxy methylglutaryl-coenzyme A (HMG-Co A) reductase inhibitors are antilipemic (lipid altering) drugs that are chemically, pharmacologically related. The prototype drug (lovastatin) is obtained from *Aspergillus* fermentation.

DRUGS

Drug	Brand name	Dosage forms
atorvastatin calcium	Lipitor (P-D)	Tablet: 10, 20, 40mg
cerivistatin	Baycol (Bayer)	Tablet: 0.2, 0.3mg
fluvastatin	Lescol (Sandoz)	Capsule: 20, 40mg
lovastatin	Mevacor (Merck)	Tablet: 10, 20, 40mg
pravastatin sodium	Pravachol (Squibb)	Tablet: 10, 20mg
simvastatin	Zocor (Merck)	Tablet: 5, 10, 15, 20mg

THERAPEUTIC USE: Adjunct to diet in management of type IIa, IIb primary hypercholesterolemia ▪ ⬇ Progress rate of coronary atherosclerosis (lovastatin) ▪ ⬇ Coronary heart disease mortality (pravastatin, simvastatin) ▪ ⬇ Risk of recurrent MI (pravastatin).

MECHANISM OF ACTION: The HMG-Co A reductase inhibitors are potent & reversible inhibitors of the enzyme HMG-Co A reductase. This enzyme (HMG-Co A reductase) converts the substrate HMG-Co A into mevalonate, a required precursor in synthesis of cholesterol. Also, it appears that these agents also inhibit the hepatic synthesis of very low density lipoproteins (VLDL), a required precursor for LDLs. The overall result of HMG-Co A reductase inhibitors is a marked ⬇ in hypercholesterolemia & hyper-

PHARMACOKINETICS

Drug	PO absorption	Peak	Protein binding	Excretion
atorvastatin	12%	NA	98%	98% via urine
cerivistatin	60%	2.5h	99%	24% via urine, 70% via feces
fluvastatin	98%	1h	98%	5% via urine, 90% via feces
lovastatin	30%	2-4h	95%	10% via urine, 83% via feces
pravastatin	34%	1-1.5h	50%	20% via urine, 70% via feces
simvastatin	85%	1.3-2.4h	95%	13% via urine, 60% via feces

lipidemia. Maximum response of treatment usually requires 4-6wks.

Lovastatin & simvastatin are inactive lactone-derivative drugs that are converted (hydrolyzed) in the body to activate HMG-Co A reductase inhibitors, & approximately 5% PO dose is available for enzyme inhibition.

CONTRAINDICATIONS: Hypersensitivity, pregnancy/lactation, active liver dysfunction/elevated serum transaminase of unknown cause.

DOSAGE: Adult *PO*

atorvastatin	10-80mg once/d
cerivistatin	0.3mg once/d in PM
fluvastatin	Initial dose of 20mg/d at hs. Usual daily range 20-40mg as a single dose
lovastatin	Initial dose 20mg/d c̄ PM meal. Usual daily range 20-80mg
pravastatin	Initial dose 10-20mg/d at hs. Usual daily range 10-40mg at hs
simvastatin	Initial dose 5-10mg c̄ PM meal. Usual range 5-40mg

SIDE/ADVERSE EFFECTS: Simvastatin produces the least amount (primarily CNS & GI effects), whereas fluvastatin produces the greatest array of adverse effects. CNS: headache, dizziness, insomnia (fluv, lov) ▪ CV: chest pain (lov, prav) ▪ GI: N/V/D, cramps/pain, constipation, flatulence, dyspepsia ▪ INT: rash, pruritus, alopecia (lov) ▪ MS: arthralgia (lov), cramps/pain (fluv, lov, prav) ▪ RESP: URI (lov, sim), common cold (prav), cough/rhinitis/influenza (fluv, prav), bronchitis/pharyngitis/sinusitis (flav) ▪ Other: blurred vision (lov), fatigue (fluv, prav), urinary abnormality (fluv).

DRUG INTERACTIONS: Use c̄ erythromycin, gemfibrozil, niacin can invoke rare cases of rhabdomyolysis ▪ Use c̄ PO anticoagulants requires PT monitoring.

NURSING MANAGEMENT PRIORITIES

ASSESS: Hx of hypersensitivity ▪ Adequate hepatic function ▪ CAUTION: hepatic impairment, alcoholism ▪ **ndx: Therapeutic effects**: Altered tissue perfusion ▪ Altered nutrition: more than body requirements ▪ **Adverse effects:** Constipation ▪ Diarrhea ▪ Risk for injury ▪ Pain (abdominal, musculoskeletal) ▪ Sensory/perceptual alterations ▪ Risk for impaired skin integrity. **PLAN:** Administer c̄ meals ▪ Observe extremities for edema ▪ Assess for visual disturbances c̄ prolonged use ▪ **Special considerations:** G: caution (↑ sensitivity) ▪ P: not recommended ▪ OB: avoid if pregnant, breastfeeding ▪ **Dietary management**: Avoid high-Na^+, high-cholesterol foods, alcohol ▪ **Lab test evaluation**: Serum cholesterol levels. **IMPLEMENT:** Monitor I&O, daily weight

▪ Monitor hepatic status (liver function tests) ▪ **Patient education:** Notify physician of muscle pain/tenderness, esp c̄ fever/weakness ▪ Comply c̄ prescribed drug regimen ▪ Avoid alcohol ▪ Follow low-cholesterol, low-Na^+ diet; maintain optimum body weight ▪ Keep appointments c̄ physician/for blood work. **EVALUATE: Observe for therapeutic effect:** ↓ Blood cholesterol levels.

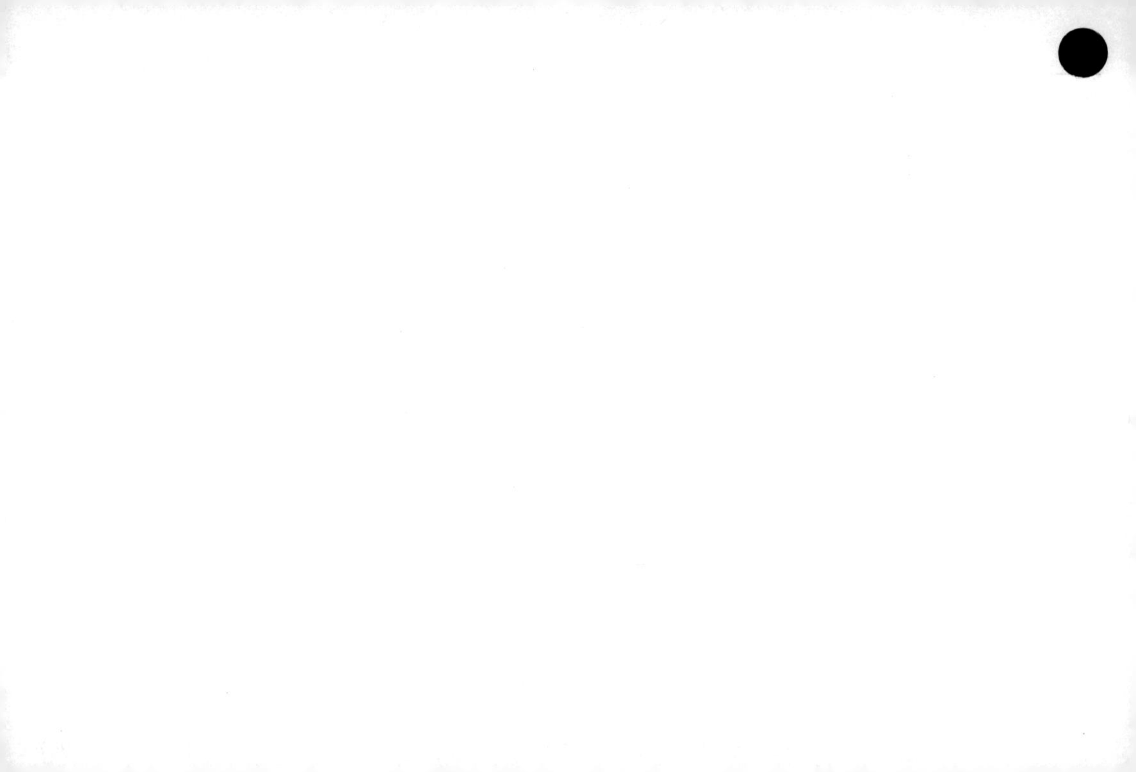

DESCRIPTION: Small protein endocrine hormone secreted by pancreatic β cells; required for proper metabolism of glucose. Deficiency of endogenous insulin results in diabetes mellitus, a serious metabolic disease. Insulin treatment of diabetes can utilize exogenous insulin obtained from (1) beef or pork pancreas extraction, (2) recombinant DNA strains of bacteria *(Escherichia coli)* & yeast, which produce human insulin & human insulin analog, (3) human insulin obtained semisynthetically from pork insulin ▪ Exogenous insulin is presently modified according to onset, peak, duration of activity into rapid-, intermediate-, long-acting insulin preparations. This manipulation of insulin activity is required to help-satisfy various metabolic demands for insulin in pts c̄ diabetes. Further individual modification possible by mixing compatible insulin preparations before administration.

Insulin preparations composed of insulin extracted from animal pancreas contain trace amounts of proinsulin, a protein prohormone that can cause allergic rxs in a very small percentage of diabetics ▪ FDA regulations state that all insulin preparations must not exceed 25ppm proinsulin. Insulin products labeled "purified" must not exceed 10ppm proinsulin; all other preparations, no more that 20ppm proinsulin ▪ Insulin products usually contain 40U/ml or 10U/ml.

PREPARATIONS: Rapid acting: *Insulin injection (regular):* *Humulin R* (human); *Iletin I* (beef-pork); *Iletin II* (purified

PHARMACOKINETICS

	Onset	Peak	Duration
Rapid			
Insulin injection	0.5h	2-3h	5-7h
Insulin lispro	<0.5h	0.5-1.5h	<8h
Intermediate acting			
Insulin zinc suspension (lente)	2.5h	7-15h	Up to 24h
Isophane insulin suspension (NPH)	1-2h	4-12h	Up to 24h
Long acting			
Extended insulin zinc suspension (ultralente)	4-8h	10-30h	Up to 36h

pork); *Insulin Regular* (purified pork); *Novolin R* (human); *Velosulin BR* (human) ▪ ***Insulin lispro:*** (human analog); Humalog ▪ **Intermediate acting: *Insulin suspension, isophane (NPH):*** *Humulin N* (human); *Iletin I, NPH* (beef-pork); *Iletin II, NPH* (purified pork); *Insulin, NPH-N* (purified pork); *Novolin N* (human) ▪ ***Insulin zinc suspension (lente):*** *Humulin L* (human); *Iletin I, Lente* (beef-pork); *Iletin II, Lente* (purified pork); *Insulin, Lente* (purified pork); *Novolin L* (human) ▪ **Long acting: *Insulin suspension, extended (ultralente):*** *Humulin U* (human) ▪ ***Other:*** *Humulin 50/50* (human) (50% regular insulin, 50% isophane insulin); *Humulin 70/30* (human); *Novolin 70/30* (70% isophane insulin, 30% regular insulin).

THERAPEUTIC USE: Management of diabetic coma (regular insulin), diabetes mellitus (all insulins). Human insulin is more advantageous in pts c̄ hypersensitivity rxs to animal-derived insulins, lipoatrophy at injection sites, insulin resistance ▪ Pts requiring temporary insulin therapy, during pregnancy.

MECHANISM OF ACTION: Insulin required for transport of monosaccharides, amino acids, through cell membrane of insulin-sensitive cells, incl skeletal muscle, cardiac muscle, mammary glands, anterior pituitary, aorta, lens of eye ▪ Pork insulin differs from human insulin in one amino acid (alanine [P] for threonine [H]) of 51 amino acids in insulin molecule; therefore they are extremely similar. Beef insulin differs in three amino acids, is less similar to human insulin.

CONTRAINDICATIONS: Hypersensitivity. **CC:** Close supervision required when changing insulin preparation due to possible differences in purity, strength, origin of insulin.

DOSAGE: Must be individualized.

SIDE/ADVERSE EFFECTS: *Hypoglycemia* due to OD, insulin resistance, localized urticarial lesions (usually disappear), atrophy of subcutaneous fat, hypersensitivity rxs include ***anaphylactic shock,*** angioneurotic edema, urticaria.

DRUG INTERACTIONS: Use c̄ chlorthalidone, corticosteroids, diazoxide, epinephrine, ethacrynic acid, furosemide, glucagon, phenytoin, thiazides, thyroid hormones will antagonize hypoglycemic effects of insulin ▪ Use c̄ alcohol, anabolic steroids, guanethidine, MAO-I, propranolol, salicylates will intensify hypoglycemic effects of insulin.

NURSING MANAGEMENT PRIORITIES
ASSESS: Hx of hypersensitivity ▪ Hypoglycemic/hyperglycemic rxs ▪ Hepatic, renal function ▪ CAUTION: hypoglycemia, CV, hepatic, renal impairment ▪ **ndx: Therapeutic effects**: Risk for altered nutrition: less than body requirements ▪ **Adverse effects:** Risk for infection ▪ Risk for injury ▪ Risk for impaired skin integrity. **PLAN:** Obtain proper equipment (appropriate insulin syringe c̄ 25-gauge needle) ▪ Check solution for discoloration/precipitation; do *not* use ▪ Check calculation/preparation (strength/type) c̄ another nurse ▪ Administer single AM dose before breakfast ▪ Assess pt need to change dosage in relation to exercise, stress, appetite ▪ **Special considerations:** None (individualized dosage) ▪ **Dietary management**: Avoid use c̄ alcohol; ADA diet (↓ carbohydrate, ↓ fat); calorie restrictions ▪ **Lab test evaluation**: FBS, urine glucose/ketones. **IMPLEMENT:** Monitor FBS; blood/urine glucose/ketones ac & at hs or as ordered ▪ Administer single AM dose before breakfast ▪ IV: administer *regular* insulin only ▪ Monitor for hypoglycemic/hyperglycemic rxs ▪ **Patient education:** Comply c̄ prescribed drug regimen ▪ Follow special diet (↓ carbohydrate, ↓ fat) ▪ Proper storage (refrigerate), preparation (roll between palms; do *not* shake) ▪ Procedure for subcutaneous administration (rotate sites) ▪ Mixing insulins: draw clear (regular) into syringe before cloudy (NPH suspension) ▪ Signs of hypoglycemia/hyperglycemia ▪ Procedure for blood/urine, glucose/ketone testing ▪ Keep medical appointments/for blood work ▪ Avoid use c̄ alcohol ▪ Carry identification (MedicAlert) ▪ Procedure for hypoglycemia rx (always carry sugar source) ▪ Long-term therapy; used to control, *not* cure, diabetes ▪ Avoid changing brand-name preparations/equipment ▪ Report infection. **EVALUATE: Observe for therapeutic effects:** ↓ Blood sugar ▪ ↓ Hyperglycemic manifestations.

DESCRIPTION: A group of endogenous body proteins &/or glycoproteins produced in response to selective infections, esp RNA-containing viruses & other inducer antigens. They exhibit complex, variable immunologic activity & are produced primarily by fibroblasts, leukocytes (usually identified as lymphokines or cytokines), infected body cells. When first discovered in late 1950s, interferon was believed to be a single entity that could be used for treating viral infections due to its antiviral activity.

However, this expectation was not realized because interferons are highly species specific. That is, interferons had to be of human origin to be effective. Accordingly, the supply of human interferons was extremely limited because exogenous animal sources would be ineffective. In addition, early experiments c̄ interferons produced limited success.

Since then, ongoing research has been able to identify three different types of interferons (alfa, beta, gamma) based on antigenic, biologic activity c̄ many subtypes in each group & produce adequate amounts of human interferons from genetically modified *Escherichia coli* bacteria (recombinant DNA technology). Also, interferons are obtained from pooled human leukocytes that have been stimulated (challenged) c̄ various natural, synthetic inducers (antigens).

DRUGS: Rx; Preg Cat C ▪ **Interferons Alfa:** Interferon alfa-2a recombinant *(Roferon-A),* interferon alfa-2b recombinant *(Intron A),* interferon alfa-n3 leukocyte origin *(Alferon N),* interferon alfacon-1 *(Infergen)* ▪ **Interferons Beta:** Interferon beta-1a *(Avonex),* Interferon beta-1b recombinant *(Betaseron)* ▪ **Interferons Gamma:** Interferon gamma-1b recombinant *(Actimmune)* ▪ **Combination Product:** Rebetron (Interferon alfa-2b SC injection c̄ ribavirin capsules 200mg).

MECHANISM OF ACTION: Interferons possess a broad antiviral spectrum & selected antineoplastic activity. These effects are not direct but result from a series of complex modulating mechanisms. Also, they can modulate the immune system response & are useful for treating selected immune disorders. Accordingly, interferons are described as biologic response modifiers ▪ **Antiviral effect:** Interferons have no effect in host cells that are already infected. They protect uninfected cells by stimulating cells to produce antiviral proteins (enzymes) that prevent subsequent viral replication if infected. It has also been suggested that interferons may inhibit viral penetration into uninfected cells ▪ **Antineoplastic effect:** Produced by several mechanisms that are not fully understood. Antineoplastic effect involves inhibition of cell division, inhibition of oncogene expression, augmentation of macrophages, monocytes, natural killer cell activity ▪ **Immune effect:** Interferons can restore, augment, modulate the immune response. This effect is involved c̄ cancer therapy, is useful for treating autoimmune diseases.

CONTRAINDICATIONS: Hypersensitivity.

THERAPEUTIC USE/DOSAGE

Interferon alfa-2a *IM/SC*	
Chronic myelogenous leukemia	9 million IU/d (Philadelphia chromosome positive). Pt tolerance can be ↑ by giving 3 million IU/d & ↑ by 3 million IU q3d to reach 9 million IU/d dose
Hairy cell leukemia	3 million IU/d for 16-24wks. Maintenance dose 3 million IU 3 times/wk
Kaposi's sarcoma (AIDS related)	36 million IU/d for 10-12wks. Maintenance dose 36 million IU 3 times/wk
Interferon alfa-2b *IM/SC*	
Chronic hepatitis B	≥18y/o: 30-35 million IU/wk as 5 million IU/d or 10 million IU 3 times/wk for 16wks
Chronic hepatitis C	≥18y/o: 3 million IU 3 times/wk for up to 6mo
Hairy cell leukemia	≥18y/o: 2 million IU/m² 3 times/wk
Kaposi's sarcoma (AIDS related)	≥18y/o: 30 million IU/m² 3 times/wk
Condylomata acuminata (Genital/perianal warts)	≥18y/o: 1 million IU into each wart (lesion) 3 times/wk PM
Malignant melanoma	20 million IU/m² IV for 5 consecutive d/wk for 4wks. Maintenance dose 10 million IV/m² SC 3 times/ wk for 48wks
Interferon alfa-n3	
Condylomata acuminata	≥18y/o: 250,000 IU/wart twice/ wk for up to 8wks. Do *not* exceed 2.5 million IU/treatment session
Interferon alfacon-1	
Hepatitis C	≥18y/o: 9μg SC tid for 24wks
Interferon beta-1a	
Multiple sclerosis	30μg once a wk IM
Interferon beta-1b	
Multiple sclerosis	0.25mg (8 million IU) subcutaneously qod
Interferon gamma-1b	
Reducing frequency/ severity of infections associated c̄ chronic granulomatous disease	Body surface >0.5m²: 50μg/m² SC 3 times/wk Body surface ≤0.5m²: 1.5μg/kg 3 times/wk

Rebetron	
Relapsed chronic hepatits C (following alfa interferon treatment)	Interferon alfa-2b (Intron): 3 million IU 3 times/wk for 6mo
	Ribavirin (Rebetol): ≤75kg, 400mg in AM & 600mg in PM; ≥75kg, 600mg in AM & PM for 6mo

SIDE/ADVERSE EFFECTS: CNS: depression, dizziness, headache ▪ GI: N/V/D, anorexia, abdominal pain ▪ INT: rash, alopecia, sweating, dryness, photosensitivity (beta-1b) ▪ GYN: menstrual disorders (beta-1b) ▪ RESP: coughing, flulike syndrome, sinusitis (beta-1b) ▪ Other: fever, chills, weight loss, myalagia, arthralgia, fatigue.

DRUG INTERACTIONS: Alfa-2a, -2b use c̄ aminophylline will ⬇ its metabolism due to inhibition of cytochrome P-450 enzyme system ▪ Gamma-1b use c̄ myelosuppressive agents can produce additive effects.

NURSING MANAGEMENT PRIORITIES

ASSESS: Hx of hypersensitivity ▪ Hepatic, renal function ▪ Signs of toxicity (CNS, neurotoxicity) ▪ **ndx: Therapeutic effects**: Risk for infection ▪ Impaired skin integrity ▪ **Adverse effects:** Risk for altered body temperature ▪ Risk for injury ▪ Altered nutrition: less than body requirements ▪ Pain (headache) ▪ Impaired physical mobility ▪ Sensory/perceptual alterations (visual) ▪ Altered thought processes ▪ Impaired tissue integrity. **PLAN:** Maintain hydration ▪ UV radiation precautions ▪ **Special considerations:** G: caution (renal impairment) ▪ P: caution (⬆ sensitivity) ▪ OB: caution if pregnant, breastfeeding ▪ **Dietary management**: None specific ▪ **Lab test evaluation**: WBC count, BUN, serum creatinine. **IMPLEMENT:** Monitor VS ▪ Monitor F/E, hepatic, renal status ▪ Seizure precautions in pts c̄ hx of convulsive disorders ▪ **Patient education:** Comply c̄ prescribed drug regimen ▪ Safety precautions c̄ hazardous activity ▪ Procedure for self-administration ▪ Procedure for proper disposal of drug, used syringes, needles ▪ Avoid direct sunlight/UV light (photosensitivity) ▪ Notify physician of abnormal rxs (flulike symptoms: fever, headache, chills). **EVALUATE: Observe for therapeutic effects:** Prevention/resolution of infection.

DESCRIPTION: Diverse group of drugs that promote defecation (BM) c̄ varied mechanisms of action are available primarily as OTC preparations. Laxatives produce a BM c̄ a soft, formed stool. Laxatives that produce a rapid, forceful BM c̄ a loose stool are called *cathartics* (pergatives). This term is obsolete because the intensity of the BM is primarily a dose-related, cause-and-effect relationship.

DRUGS: Bowel evacuant: Polyethylene glycol electrolyte solution (Rx: *Colovage, CoLyte, GoLYTELY, OCL)* ▪ **Bulk-forming:** methylcellulose *(Citrucel),* polycarbophil *(Fiberall, FiberCon, Mitrolan),* psyllium *(Metamucil, Modane Bulk, Perdiem Fiber, Syllact)* ▪ **Fecal softener:** docusate calcium *(Pro-Cal-Sof),* docusate potassium *(Kasof),* docusate sodium *(Colace, Dialose)* ▪ **Lubricant:** mineral oil, mineral oil emulsion *(Agoral Plain, Kondremul Plain)* ▪ **Saline:** magnesium citrate, magnesium hydroxide *(Milk of Magnesia)* ▪ **Stimulant:** bisacodyl *(Dulcolax),* cascara sagrada, castor oil, phenolphthalein *(Alophen, Ex-Lax, Modane)* senna/sennosides *(Fletcher's Castoria, Senokot)* ▪ **Miscellaneous:** glycerin suppositories, lactulose (Rx: *Cephulac, Chronulac).*

MECHANISM OF ACTION/THERAPEUTIC USE: Bowel evacuant: Hyperosmotic activity produces H_2O retention, resulting in diarrhea & a complete cleansing of intestines before GI diagnostic procedures ▪ **Bulk-forming:** Absorbs H_2O, resulting in an ↑ in stool mass, which stimulates evacuation. Used for treating constipation, irritable bowel syndrome, diverticulosis ▪ **Fecal softeners:** Lowers the surface tension of intestinal fluids, resulting in H_2O & lipid passage into fecal mass. Used for constipation to soften fecal impacts, to facilitate easy defecation c̄ painful anorectal conditions ▪ **Lubricant:** Retards intestinal H_2O reabsorption, which softens, expands stool; same use as fecal softeners. **Saline:** Hyperosmotic activity produces H_2O retention, resulting in an H_2O stool. Used for treating constipation & c̄ anthelmintics for removal of drug & parasite. Also used before diagnostic or intestinal surgical procedures ▪ **Stimulant:** Directly stimulates peristaltic activity of the intestinal tract, ↑ fluid level that results in defecation. Used for general constipation ▪ **Miscellaneous:** Glycerin suppositories promote defecation in 15-30m via hyperosmotic activity, irritation to rectum. Lactulose is a disaccharide that is metabolized by the intestinal flora into hyperosmotic metabolites (acids) that promote H_2O retention & defecation. Used for constipation (*Chronulac*), for management of portal-systemic encephalopathy (*Cephulac*).

CONTRAINDICATIONS: Acute surgical abdomen, undiagnosed pain, appendicitis, fecal impaction, obstruction of intestinal tract.

DOSAGE: Usual *PO* dose

bisacodyl	Adult/Children >12y/o: 5-15mg single daily dose Children >3y/o: 5-10mg single daily dose
cascara sagrada	Adult: 325mg at hs
castor oil	Adult: 15-60ml Children: 5-15ml
docusate Ca	Adult/Children ≥12y/o: 100-240mg/d
docusate K	Adult: 50-240mg/d
docusate Na	Adult/Children ≥12y/o: 50-360mg/d Children 2-11y/o: 50-150mg/d Children <2y/o: 25mg/d
glycerin suppositories (rectal), one each for adult, children, or pediatric size	
lactulose	Adult: laxative 15-60ml/d Encephalopathy: 30-45ml 3-4 times/d
magnesium citrate	Adult: 200ml as single dose Children: 100ml as single dose
magnesium hydroxide	Adult/Children ≥12y/o: 30-60ml/d Children 6-11y/o: 15-30ml/d Children 2-5y/o: 5-15ml/d
methylcellulose	Adult/Children ≥12y/o: ≤6g/d divided
phenolphthalein	Adult/Children ≥12y/o: 30-270mg at hs Children 6-11y/o: 30-60mg at hs Children 2-5y/o: 15-30mg at hs
polyethylene glycol electrolyte solution	Adult: 4L in 240-ml doses q10m
psyllium	Adult/Children ≥12y/o: ≤30g/d divided Children 6-11y/o: ≤15g/d divided
senna	Adult: 0.5-2g
sennosides	Adult: 12-50mg

NURSING MANAGEMENT PRIORITIES

ASSESS: Hx of hypersensitivity ▪ Health, nutritional status ▪ Bowel sounds, GI status ▪ Duration of constipation ▪ Medication hx contributing to constipation ▪ CAUTION: abdominal pain ▪ **ndx: Therapeutic effects:** Risk for activity intolerance ▪ Constipation ▪ Pain ▪ Impaired physical mobility ▪ **Adverse effects:** Diarrhea ▪ Fatigue ▪ Risk for fluid volume deficit ▪ Risk for impaired skin integrity ▪ Impaired tissue integrity. **PLAN:** Administer on empty stomach at hs unless otherwise directed ▪ Administer at appropriate times for diagnostic study preparation ▪ Provide appropriate toileting facilities ▪ Establish regular defecation schedule ▪ **Special considerations:** G: caution (↑ illness-related restrictions) ▪ P: caution (immature systems) ▪ OB: caution if pregnant, avoid breastfeeding ▪ **Dietary management:** ↑ Fluids, bulk-containing foods, prunes ▪ **Lab test evaluation:** None specific. **IMPLEMENT:** Monitor for dehydration, electrolyte imbalance ▪ Encourage ↑ fluid intake, ↑ activity ▪ Monitor bowel function ▪ **Patient education:** Avoid chronic use ▪ ↑ Exercise ▪ Promote regular bowel habits ▪ Notify physician of abdominal pain ▪ Keep well hydrated ▪ Follow high-fiber diet ▪ ↑ Activity/mobility. **EVALUATE: Observe for therapeutic effects:** Relief of constipation ▪ Regular BMs.

DESCRIPTION: Small group of drugs that inhibit activity of MAO enzyme system.

DRUGS: phenelzine *(Nardil)*, tranylcypromine *(Parnate)*.

PHARMACOKINETICS: Not available.

THERAPEUTIC USE: Treatment of reactive depression not responsive to other drugs ▪ Treatment of panic disorder syndromes (phenelzine).

MECHANISM OF ACTION: Antidepressant activity appears related to inhibition of MAO enzyme system, resulting in ↑ levels of epinephrine, norepinephrine, serotonin at adrenergic neuron storage sites ▪ pargyline has hypotensive activity by an unknown mechanism.

CONTRAINDICATIONS: Hypersensitivity; cerebrovascular defects, cardiovascular disorders, pheochromocytoma; in combination c̄ benzodiazepines, adrenergics, tyramine-rich foods, narcotics, hypotensive agents; severe liver & renal impairment; geriatric pts.

DOSAGE: Adult

phenelzine	Initial dose 45-90mg/d, maintenance dose 15mg/d or qod
tranylcypromine	30mg/d divided to a maximum of 60mg/d

SIDE/ADVERSE EFFECTS: CNS: restlessness, insomnia, drowsiness, dizziness, headache ▪ CV: tachycardia, edema, palpitations, postural hypotension ▪ EENT: blurred vision ▪ GI: anorexia, dry mouth, N/D, abdominal cramps ▪ GU: impotence ▪ HEP: ↑ Serum AST, ALT, bilirubin; hepatitis ▪ INT: skin rash.

DRUG INTERACTIONS: Serious/fatal results can occur c̄ adrenergics, benzodiazepines, narcotics, TCAs.

NURSING MANAGEMENT PRIORITIES

ASSESS: Hx of hypersensitivity ▪ BP ▪ Signs of hypertensive crisis (tachycardia, stiff neck, chest pain) ▪ CAUTION: hepatic, renal impairment ▪ **ndx: Therapeutic effects:** Ineffective individual coping ▪ Self-esteem disturbance ▪ Risk for self-directed violence ▪ **Adverse effects:** Risk for activity intolerance ▪ ↓ Cardiac output ▪ Diarrhea ▪ Fluid volume excess ▪ Risk for injury ▪ Pain ▪ Sensory/perceptual alterations ▪ Sexual dysfunction ▪ Risk for impaired skin integrity. **PLAN:** Prevent postural hypotension ▪ Avoid abrupt withdrawal ▪ Institute suicide precautions ▪ Ensure drug ingestion ▪ **Special considerations:** G: not recommended ▪ P: not recommended ▪ OB: caution if pregnant, breastfeeding ▪ **Dietary management:** Avoid use c̄ alcohol, caffeine, tyramine-containing foods ▪ **Lab test evaluation:** CBC. **IMPLEMENT:** Monitor BP ▪ Suicide precaution prn ▪ Monitor hepatic, renal status ▪ **Patient education:** Comply c̄ prescribed drug regimen ▪ Avoid sudden position changes (postural hypotension) ▪ Use safety precautions c̄ hazardous activity ▪ Full drug effects may require several wks of therapy ▪ Use sugarless gum/hard candy to diminish dry mouth ▪ Check c̄ physician before taking OTC preparations ▪ Avoid use c̄ alcohol, caffeine, tyramine-containing foods ▪ Symptoms of hypertensive crisis ▪ Carry identification (MedicAlert). **EVALUATE: Observe for therapeutic effects:** ↓ Depression ▪ Mood elevation.

DESCRIPTION: Group of skeletal (striated) muscle relaxants subdivided into surgical neuromuscular blocking agents, central-, direct-acting muscle relaxants.

The surgical blocking agents are subdivided into depolarizing agents, large group of nondepolarizing agents.

DRUGS: Depolarizing neuromuscular blocking agents: succinylcholine chloride *(Anectine, Quelicin, Sucostrin)* ▪ **Nondepolarizing neuromuscular blocking agents:** atracurium besylate *(Tracrium)*, cisatracurium besylate *(Nimbex)*, doxacurium chloride *(Nuromax)*, gallamine triethiodide *(Flaxedil)*, metocurine iodide *(Metubine)*, mivacurium chloride *(Mivacron)*, pancuronium bromide *(Pavulon)*, pipecuronium *(Arduan)*, rocuronium bromide *(Zemuron)*, tubocurarine chloride, vecuronium bromide *(Norcuron)* ▪ **Central-acting relaxants:** baclofen *(Lioresal)*, carisoprodol *(Soma)*, chlorphenesin chloride carbamate *(Maolate)*, chlorzoxazone *(Paraflex, Parafon Forte DSC)*, cyclobenzaprine hcl *(Flexeril)*, metaxalone *(Skelaxin)*, methocarbamol *(Robaxin)*, orphenadrine citrate *(Norflex)*, tizanidine hcl *(Zanaflex)* ▪ **Direct-acting relaxants:** dantrolene sodium *(Dantrium)*.

THERAPEUTIC USES: Neuromuscular blocking agents: Adjunct to anesthesia to enhance skeletal muscle relaxation. ↓ Of muscle contractions of drugs or electrically induced convulsions. To facilitate endotracheal intubation, management of mechanical respiration. Agents are potent, must be administered by qualified surgical personnel ▪ **Central-acting agent:** Adjunct for relief of discomfort associated c̄ acute, painful musculoskeletal conditions. Treatment of spasticity resulting from multiple sclerosis esp for flexor spasms (baclofen) ▪ **Direct-acting agent:** Treatment of spasticity resulting from upper motor neuron disorders associated c̄ cerebral palsy, multiple sclerosis, spinal cord injury, stroke.

MECHANISMS OF ACTION: Depolarizing agents: Causes skeletal muscle paralysis by combining c̄ cholinergic receptors on motor end-plate neuromuscular junction to produce depolarization, which is followed by initial transient muscular contraction often visible as fasciculation. Neuromuscular transmission becomes inhibited & remains so as long as there is adequate concentration of drug at receptor site.

Onset of activity is about 1m after single effective IV dose. Muscular relaxation persists for about 2m, returns to normal in 8-10m ▪ **Nondepolarizing agents:** Causes skeletal muscle paralysis by combining c̄ cholinergic receptors on neuromuscular junction. Therefore normal agonist effect of acetylcholine is prevented. Repeated doses may be accompanied by cumulative effect. Acetylcholinesterase drugs can antagonize effect of these agents. Various depolarizing agents differ in potency, onset, duration of activity ▪ **Central-acting agents:** Skeletal muscle relaxant effect due to activity in CNS, esp spinal cord. Exact mechanism of activity not determined. Agents are primarily CNS depressants c̄ sedative properties. Muscle relaxation not direct, minimal.

Baclofen activity appears related to inhibition of monosynaptic, polysynaptic reflexes in spinal cord.

DOSAGE: Usual adult range

baclofen	*PO*	40-80mg/d divided
carisoprodol	*PO*	350mg tid & at hs
chlorphenesin	*PO*	400mg qid
chlorzoxazone	*PO*	250mg 3-4 times/d
cyclobenzaprine	*PO*	10mg tid
dantrolene	*PO*	25-400mg/d divided
	IV	1-10mg/kg
metaxalone	*PO*	800mg 3-4 times/d
methocarbamol	*PO*	4g/d divided
	IV	1-3g/d
orphenadrine	*PO*	100mg bid
	IM/IV	60mg q12h
tizanidine	*PO*	8mg q6-8h

NURSING MANAGEMENT PRIORITIES

ASSESS: Hx of hypersensitivity ▪ Recent CNS depressant administration (hold drug) ▪ Neurologic, respiratory status ▪ CAUTION: hepatic, renal impairment ▪ **ndx: Therapeutic effects:** Impaired physical mobility ▪ Pain ▪ **Adverse effects:** Risk for activity intolerance ▪ Constipation ▪ Diarrhea ▪ Risk for injury ▪ Impaired physical mobility ▪ Risk for impaired skin integrity ▪ Sensory/perceptual alterations ▪ Sleep pattern disturbance ▪ Altered thought processes. **PLAN:** Assess for tolerance to therapeutic dose ▪ Maintain safety precautions ▪ **Special considerations:** G: caution, ↓ dosage (↑ CNS sensitivity) ▪ P: caution, ↓ dosage (↑ sensitivity) ▪ OB: not recommended if pregnant, breastfeeding ▪ **Dietary management:** Avoid use c̄ alcohol ▪ **Lab test evaluation:** CBC, hepatic function tests (long-term). **IMPLEMENT:** Monitor VS ▪ Check for signs of dependence ▪ Monitor activity status (safety precautions) ▪ Monitor neurologic, respiratory status ▪ **Patient education:** Comply c̄ prescribed drug regimen; indiscriminate use may lead to dependence ▪ Store properly (do *not* keep at bedside) ▪ Avoid use c̄ alcohol, other CNS depressants ▪ Use safety precautions c̄ ambulation, hazardous activity ▪ Avoid smoking after administration ▪ Use relaxation techniques. **EVALUATE: Observe for therapeutic effects:** Relief of spasms ▪ ↑ Musculoskeletal function.

DESCRIPTION: An array of estrogen-progestin combination products ("pill") or progestin preparations ("mini-pill") ▪ Combinations may be low-, intermediate-, or high-dose ratio preparations and most contain estradiol/norethindrone.

FORMULATIONS: Estrogen-progestin combination products: ***Monophasic:*** Fixed estrogen-progestin dosage ratio for qd of cycle in 21-d or 28-d dosage formulations: *Brevicon, Demulen, Loestrin, Lo/Ovral, Modicon, Nelova, Nordette, Norinyl, Ortho-Cept, Ortho-Novum, Ovcon, Ovral* ▪ ***Biphasic:*** Fixed estrogen dose c̄ low progestin dose 1st 10d, higher progestin dose rest of cycle in 21-d or 28-d dosage formulations: *Nelova 10/11, Ortho-Novum 10/11-21, Ortho-Novum 10/11-28* ▪ ***Triphasic:*** Three different estrogen/progestin dose ratios, administered sequentially during cycle in 21-d or 28-d dosage formulations: *Ortho-Novum 7/7/7, Tri-Levlen, Tri-Norinyl, Triphasil* ▪ ***Progestin products:*** norethindrone *(Micronor, Nor-Q.D.),* norgestrel *(Ovrette).*

PHARMACOKINETICS: Good absorption patterns, wide tissue distribution, high protein binding, variable half-lives; excretion via feces/urine primarily as conjugated metabolites.

THERAPEUTIC USE: Prevention of pregnancy ▪ Treatment of endometriosis, hypermenorrhea; to produce cyclic withdrawal bleeding (high-dose combination formulations).

MECHANISM OF ACTION: Prevent ovulation by inhibiting release of gonadotropins & by ↑ uterine mucous viscosity, which ↓ sperm movement, fertilization, possibility of zygote implantation.

CONTRAINDICATIONS: Known/suspected pregnancy; present/past thrombophlebotic disorders; known/suspected breast cancer, estrogen neoplasia; undiagnosed abnormal genital bleeding; cerebrovascular coronary artery disease; benign/malignant liver tumors associated c̄ estrogen-containing products.

DOSAGE: Monophasic combinations: Dosage starts on 5th day of cycle or on 1st Sunday after menstruation starts; 1 tablet/d from day 5 to day 24/25 of cycle ▪ **Biphasic combinations:** Dosage starts on 1st day of cycle if Sunday or on 1st Sunday after menstruation starts; 1 tablet/d (in correct sequence) for 21/28 days, depending on product ▪ **Triphasic combinations:** Dosage starts on 1st day of cycle if Sunday or on 1st Sunday after menstruation starts; 1 tablet/d (in correct sequence) for 21d.

SIDE/ADVERSE EFFECTS: CNS: migraine, mental depression ▪ CV: ***cerebral hemorrhage/thrombosis, coronary thrombosis, arterial thromboembolism, mesenteric thrombosis, pulmonary embolism,*** Raynaud disease, ***thrombosis,*** optic neuritis, corneal curvature changes ▪ GI: N/V, bloating, colitis, cramps ▪ GU: breakthrough bleeding, spotting, amenorrhea, dysmenorrhea, vaginal candidiasis, cervical erosion, ↑ size of uterine leiomyomas ▪ HEP: liver tumors, cholestatic jaundice ▪ INT: rash, melasma ▪ Other: congenital anomalies; breast enlargement, tenderness, secretions; weight changes; ↓ tolerance to carbohydrate; prolactin-secreting pituitary tumors.

DRUG INTERACTIONS: Use c̄ nicotine (smoking) ↑ risk of MI, stroke, hypertension, thromboembolism, visual disturbances, liver tumor, gallbladder disease, teratogenic fetal effects ▪ Drugs that ↓ effectiveness of PO contraceptives incl ampicillin, analgesics, antihistamines, barbiturates, chloramphenicol, griseofulvin, isoniazid, migraine preparations, neomycin, nitrofurantoin, penicillin V, phenytoin, primidone, rifampin, sulfonamides, tetracyclines, tranquilizers ▪ PO contraceptives can ↓ therapeutic effects of anticonvulsants, β blockers, guanethidine, hypnotics, hypoglycemic agents, PO anticoagulants, theophylline, tranquilizers, TCAs, vitamins.

NURSING MANAGEMENT PRIORITIES

ASSESS: Hx of estrogen/progestin hypersensitivity ▪ Pregnancy; do *not* administer, notify physician ▪ CAUTION: thrombophlebotic disorders, coronary artery disease, hepatic impairment ▪ **ndx: Therapeutic effects**: Sexual dysfunction ▪ **Adverse effects:** Risk for fluid volume deficit ▪ Fluid volume excess ▪ Pain ▪ Risk for impaired skin integrity ▪ Impaired tissue perfusion. **PLAN:** Administer *exactly* as scheduled ▪ **Special considerations:** G: caution (chronic illness) ▪ P: avoid use (immature systems) ▪ OB: caution if pregnant, breastfeeding ▪ **Dietary management**: Avoid caffeine, high-Na^+ foods ▪ **Lab test evaluation**: FBS; hepatic, thyroid function tests. **IMPLEMENT:** Administer c̄ food/milk to ↓ GI irritation ▪ Monitor for thromboembolic phenomena; notify physician ▪ **Patient education:** Use alternative method of birth control during 1st mo after starting & for 3mo after D/C birth control pills ▪ Take *exactly* as scheduled c̄ food/milk ▪ Notify physician *immediately* of unusual bleeding, severe headache, difficult breathing, changes in vision/coordination, chest/leg pain ▪ Avoid smoking ▪ Keep appointments c̄ physician ▪ Describe administration of specific product, review package insert c̄ pt ▪ Instruct pt on procedure for missed dose: 1st day, take as soon as remembered; if not until 2nd day, take 2; continue regular dose schedule; use 2nd method of birth control until end of cycle; notify physician; 3rd day D/C drug, use another method of birth control; notify physician *immediately*. **EVALUATE: Observe for therapeutic effect:** Prevention of pregnancy.

DESCRIPTION: PO hypoglycemics comprise one biguanide derivative, several first-, second-generation sulfonylurea derivatives, & one oligosaccharide derivative.

DRUGS: Biguanides: metformin *(Glucophage)* ▪ **Meglitinides:** repaglinide *(Prandin)* ▪ **Oligosaccharides:** acarbose *(Precose),* miglitol *(Glyset)* ▪ **Sulfonylureas:** ***First-generation sulfonylureas:*** acetohexamide *(Dymelor),* chlorpropamide *(Diabinese, *Novopropamide),* tolazamide *(Tolinase),* tolbutamide *(Orinase)* ▪ ***Second-generation sulfonylureas:*** glimepiride *(Amaryl),* glipizide *(Glucotrol),* glyburide *(DiaBeta, Glynase PresTab, Micronase).*

THERAPEUTIC USE: Management of type 2 (noninsulin-dependent) diabetes that cannot be controlled by diet alone.

MECHANISM OF ACTION: Biguanides: Antidiabetic activity appears related to ↓ in gluconeogenesis ▪ **Oligosaccharides:** Local inhibition of ingested carbohydrate digestion w/in GI tract. Acarbose has extremely poor absorption, is excreted primarily in feces; miglitol varies $\bar{c}$

PHARMACOKINETICS

	PO absorption	Peak	Duration	Half-life	Excretion
acetohexamide	Rapid	3h	12-24h	1.3h	80% via urine in 24h
chlorpropamide	Rapid	2-4h	Up to 24h	36h	80%-90% via urine in 96h
glipizide	Rapid	1-3h	Up to 24h	2-4h	90% as metabolites in urine
glyburide	Rapid	2-4h	Up to 24h	10h	50% via urine, 50% via bile
metformin	Good	NA	6-17.6h	6.2h	90% unchanged via urine
miglitol	Good	2-3h	4-8h	2h	95% unchanged via urine
repaglinide	Complete	1h	4-8h	2h	90% as metabolites via feces
tolazamide	Slow	2-6h	10h	7h	85% via urine
tolbutamide	Rapid	3-5h	6-12h	4-7h	75% via urine

*Available in Canada only.

dose ▪ **Meglitinides/sulfonylureas:** Antidiabetic activity due to stimulation of insulin release from functioning β cells of pancreas; second-generation sulfonylureas have not demonstrated clear advantage over first-generation drugs.

CONTRAINDICATIONS: Hypersensitivity; diabetic ketoacidosis c̄, w/out coma.

DOSAGE: Usual adult *PO* range†

acarbose	75-300mg/d
miglitol	50mg tid

†Consult individual drug cards for other doses.

SIDE/ADVERSE EFFECTS: GI: *nausea, epigastric fullness,* heartburn ▪ HEM: ***aplastic anemia, agranulocytosis,*** leukopenia, ***hemolytic anemia,*** pancytopenia, ***thrombocytopenia*** ▪ INT: erythremia, morbilliform/maculopapular eruptions, photosensitivity ▪ MET: hypoglycemia.

DRUG INTERACTIONS: Use c̄ alcohol, MAO-I, phenylbutazones, β blockers can significantly ↑ hypoglycemic effects ▪ Use c̄ anabolic steroids, chloramphenicol, guanethidine, PO anticoagulants, probenecid, salicylates, sulfinpyrazone, sulfonamides ↑ hypoglycemic effects ▪ Use c̄ adrenergics, corticosteroids, phenytoin, thiazides, thyroid preparations ↓ hypoglycemic effects.

NURSING MANAGEMENT PRIORITIES

ASSESS: Hx of hypersensitivity ▪ Hypoglycemic/hyperglycemic rxs ▪ Hepatic, renal function ▪ CAUTION: hypoglycemia, CV, hepatic, renal impairment ▪ **ndx: Therapeutic effects:** Risk for altered nutrition: less than body requirements ▪ **Adverse effects:** Risk for infection ▪ Risk for injury ▪ Risk for impaired skin integrity. **PLAN:** Administer as single AM dose c̄ breakfast, divided doses c̄ meals ▪ Assess pt need to change dosage in relation to exercise, stress, appetite ▪ **Special considerations:** G: caution, ↓ dosage (↑ sensitivity) ▪ P: not recommended (use insulin) ▪ OB: caution if pregnant (use insulin) ▪ **Dietary management:** Avoid alcohol; American Diabetes Association diet (↓ carbohydrate, ↓ fat); calorie restrictions ▪ **Lab test evaluation:** FBS, urine glucose/ketones. **IMPLEMENT:** Monitor FBS; blood/urine glucose/ketones ac & at hs or as ordered ▪ Administer single AM dose c̄ breakfast, divided doses c̄ meals ▪ Monitor for hypoclycemic/hyperglycemic rxs ▪ **Patient education:** Comply c̄ prescribed drug regimen ▪ Follow special diet (↓ carbohydrate, ↓ fat) ▪ Proper storage ▪ Signs of hypoclycemia/hyperglycemia ▪ Procedure for blood/urine, glucose/ketone testing ▪ Keep scheduled appointments ▪ Avoid use c̄ alcohol ▪ Procedure for hypoglycemia rx (always carry sugar source) ▪ Carry identification (Medic-Alert) ▪ Report infection. **EVALUATE: Observe for therapeutic effect:** ↓ Hyperglycemic manifestations.

DESCRIPTION: Amino: Bactericidal, acid-stable, penicillinase-labile, penicillin derivatives ▪ **Penicillinase resistant:** Bactericidal, acid-stable (except methicillin) penicillinase-stable penicillin derivatives.

DRUGS: Amino: amoxicillin *(Amoxil, *Apo-Amoxi, Biomox, *Novomoxin, Trimox),* ampicillin *(*Ampicin, *Ampilean, *Apo-Ampi, *Novoampicillin, Omnipen, *Penbriten, Principen),* bacampicillin hcl *(*Penglobe, Spectrobid)* ▪ **Penicillinase resistant:** cloxacillin sodium *(*Apo-Cloxi, *Bactopen, Cloxapen, *Novocloxin, *Orbenin),* dicloxacillin sodium *(Dycill, Dynapen, Pathocil),* methicillin sodium *(Staphcillin),* nafcillin sodium *(Nallpen, Unipen),* oxacillin sodium *(Bactocill).*

THERAPEUTIC USE: Amino: Spectrum similar to penicillin G/V but more effective against wider variety of gram-negative bacteria. Use should be limited to organisms that are not sensitive to penicillin G/V. Bacampicillin changed to ampicillin in body. Treatment of infections caused by susceptible strains of *Escherichia coli, Haemophilus influenzae, Neisseria meningitidis, Proteus mirabilis, Salmonella* spp, *Shigella* spp, *Neisseria gonorrhoeae* ▪ Treatment of subacute bacterial endocarditis, enterococcal infections ▪ Ampicillin drug of choice for treating typhoid fever *(Salmonella typhi)* resistant to chloramphenicol ▪ **Penicillinase resistant:** methicillin exhibits greatest activity, oxacillin, the lowest ▪ Indicated in treatment of infections due to penicillinase-producing staphylococci ▪ Resistance to any penicillinase-stable penicillin should be interpreted as resistance to all ▪ Cross-resistance c̄ cephalosporins occurs frequently.

MECHANISM OF ACTION: Bactericidal activity due to inhibition of mucopeptide cell wall synthesis in susceptible organisms.

CONTRAINDICATIONS: Hypersensitivity to any penicillin.

DOSAGE: Adult

amoxicillin, ampicillin	*PO*	250-500mg qid
bacampicillin	*PO*	400-800mg bid
cloxacillin	*PO*	250-500mg or more q6h
dicloxacillin	*PO*	125-500mg or more q6h
methicillin	*IM*	1g q4-6h
	IV	1g q6h
nafcillin	*PO*	250mg-1g q4-6h
	IM	500mg q4-6h
	IV	500mg-1g q4-6h

oxacillin	*PO*	250-500mg or more q4-6h
	IM/IV	250mg-1g or more q4-6h

SIDE/ADVERSE EFFECTS: CNS: neuropathy usually associated c̄ high parenteral doses ▪ CV: edema ▪ GI: PO incl *N/V/D, epigastric distress*, black hairy tongue, flatulence, smell/taste disturbances ▪ GU: ***interstitial nephritis*** (rare) usually associated c̄ methicillin ▪ HEM: anemia, eosinophilia, leukopenia, neutropenia, ***thrombocytopenia*** ▪ HEP: ↑ Serum levels of AST, ALT, LDH ▪ INT: maculopapular rashes (most frequent), ***erythema multiforme, exfoliative dermatitis*** (infrequent), rash, pruritus, urticaria ▪ MS: arthralgia ▪ Other: *local irritation at injection site*, fever, ***anaphylaxis***, laryngeal edema.

DRUG INTERACTIONS: Do *not* use PO dosage forms c̄ antacids, antidiarrheal suspensions, ion-exchange resins ▪ Use c̄ bacteriostatic antibiotics can result in antibiotic antagonism ▪ Avoid concurrent use of bacampicillin, disulfiram ▪ PO anticoagulant therapy may require dose adjustments esp c̄ amino penicillins.

NURSING MANAGEMENT PRIORITIES

ASSESS: Hx of hypersensitivity (incl cephalosporins) ▪ Hepatic, renal function ▪ CAUTION: hepatic, renal impairment ▪ **ndx: Therapeutic effects:** Risk for altered body temperature ▪ High risk for infection ▪ **Adverse effects:** Diarrhea ▪ Risk for fluid volume deficit ▪ Risk for injury ▪ Risk for impaired skin integrity. **PLAN:** Administer at equal intervals around clock to maintain blood levels ▪ Maintain hydration ▪ **Special considerations:** G: caution, ↓ dosage (renal impairment, ↑ superinfection) ▪ P: caution (↑ sensitivity) ▪ OB: caution if pregnant, breastfeeding ▪ **Dietary management:** None specific ▪ **Lab test evaluation:** CBC. **IMPLEMENT:** Obtain C&S, check results ▪ Observe for signs of superinfection (diarrhea, URI, coated tongue) ▪ Administer on empty stomach ▪ **Patient education:** Comply c̄ prescribed drug therapy ▪ ↑ Fluid intake (8-10 glasses/d) ▪ Take on empty stomach ▪ Diarrhea may occur ▪ Notify physician of symptoms of allergic rx (fever, difficult breathing, rash). **EVALUATE: Observe for therapeutic effect:** Resolution of infection.

DESCRIPTION: Group of semisynthetic penicillins that exhibit ↑ spectrum against gram-negative organisms that is vastly superior to penicillin G/V, greater than the amino penicillins.

DRUGS: carbenicillin indanyl sodium *(Geocillin)*, mezlocillin *(Mezlin)*, piperacillin *(Pipracil)*, ticarcillin *(Ticar)*.

PHARMACOKINETICS: *See* individual drug cards.

THERAPEUTIC USE: Individual gram-negative spectrum varies. The combined spectrum incl *Acinetobacter* spp, *Bacteroides* spp, *Enterobacter* spp, *Escherichia coli, Haemophilus influenzae, Klebsiella* spp, *Neisseria* spp, *Peptococcus* spp, *Peptostreptococcus* spp, *Proteus* spp, *Pseudomonas aeruginosa, Providencia rettgeri, Serratia* spp, *Streptococcus faecalis, S. pneumoniae* ▪ Treatment of bacterial septicemia; bone/joint, gynecologic, intraabdominal, respiratory, skin infections, UTIs caused by susceptible microorganisms ▪ Initial treatment of mixed infections before identification of causative organism ▪ In combination c̄ aminoglycoside for treatment of stubborn gram-negative infections, esp *Pseudomonas.*

MECHANISM OF ACTION: Bactericidal activity due to inhibition of mucopeptide cell wall synthesis in susceptible organisms.

CONTRAINDICATIONS: Hypersensitivity to any penicillin.

DOSAGE: All extended-spectrum penicillins but carbenicillin indanyl sodium administered parenterally.

carbenicillin indanyl sodium	382mg PO qid
mezlocillin	100-300mg/kg/d divided
piperacillin	125-300mg/kg/d divided
ticarcillin	150-300mg/kg/d divided

SIDE/ADVERSE EFFECTS: GI: N/V/D, flatulence, smell/taste disturbances ▪ HEM: anemia, eosinophilia, leukopenia, neutropenia, ***thrombocytopenia*** ▪ HEP: ↑ Serum AST, ALT, LDH ▪ INT: rash, pruritus, urticaria ▪ MS: arthralgia, neuromuscular hyperirritability ▪ Other: *discomfort at site of injection, esp c̄ continuous administration;* ***anaphylaxis.***

DRUG INTERACTIONS: Use of bacteriostatic antibiotics c̄ any penicillin can lead to antibiotic antagonism ▪ PO anticoagulant therapy may require dose adjustment.

NURSING MANAGEMENT PRIORITIES

ASSESS: Hx of hypersensitivity (incl cephalosporins) ▪ Hepatic, renal function ▪ CAUTION: hepatic, renal impairment ▪ **ndx: Therapeutic effects:** Risk for altered body temperature ▪ Risk for infection ▪ **Adverse effects:** Diarrhea ▪ Risk for fluid volume deficit ▪ Risk for injury ▪ Risk for impaired skin integrity. **PLAN:** Administer at equal intervals around clock to maintain blood levels ▪ Maintain hydration ▪ **Special considerations:** G: caution, ↓ dosage (renal impairment, ↑ superinfection) ▪ P: caution (↑ sensitivity) ▪ OB: caution if pregnant, breastfeeding ▪ **Dietary management:** None specific ▪ **Lab test evaluation:** CBC. **IMPLEMENT:** Obtain C&S; check results ▪ Observe for signs of superinfection (diarrhea, URI, coated tongue) ▪ Administer on empty stomach ▪ **Patient education:** Comply c̄ prescribed drug therapy ▪ ↑ Fluid intake (8-10 glasses/d) ▪ Take on empty stomach ▪ Diarrhea may occur ▪ Notify physician of symptoms of allergic rx (fever, difficult breathing, rash). **EVALUATE: Observe for therapeutic effect:** Resolution of infection.

DESCRIPTION: Large group of antipsychotic (neuroleptic) agents that are chemical derivatives of phenothiazine ring. Several phenothiazinelike antipsychotic agents are chemically different but clinically similar.

DRUGS: acetophenazine maleate *(Tindal),* chlorpromazine *(*Chlor-Promanyl, *Largactil, *Novochlorpromazine, Thorazine suppositories),* chlorpromazine hcl *(Thorazine),* fluphenazine decanoate *(*Moditen, Prolixin Decanoate),* fluphenazine enanthate *(Prolixin Enanthate),* fluphenazine hcl *(Permitil, Prolixin),* mesoridazine besylate *(Serentil),* perphenazine *(*Apo-Perphenazine, Trilafon),* prochlorperazine *(Compazine suppositories, *Stemetil),* prochlorperazine edisylate *(Compazine injection, syrup; *Stemetil),* prochlorperazine maleate *(Compazine),* promazine hcl *(*Promanyl, Sparine),* thioridazine *(*Apo-Thioridazine, Mellaril-S, *Novoridazine, *PMS Thioridazine),* trifluoperazine hcl *(Stelazine),* triflupromazine hcl *(Vesprin)* ▪ Other antipsychotics: haloperidol *(Haldol),* haloperidol lactate *(Haldol concentrate, IM),* loxapine hcl *(*Loxapac, Loxitane C concentrate, IM),* loxapine succinate *(Loxitane),* molindone hcl *(Moban),* olanzapine *(Zyprexa),* quetiapine fumarate *(Seroquel),* thiothixene *(Navane),* thiothixene hcl *(Navane concentrate, IM).*

PHARMACOKINETICS: *See* individual drug cards.

THERAPEUTIC USE: Treatment of psychotic states ▪ Antiemetics (eg, chlorpromazine) ▪ Treatment of intractable hiccups, intermittent porphyria (chlorpromazine).

MECHANISM OF ACTION: Antipsychotic activity appears associated $\bar{c}$ ⬇ neural transmissions in central dopamine-dependent pathways. These agents block postsynaptic dopamine receptors in limbic system, basal ganglia, resulting in tranquilizing effect in psychotic pts ▪ Various phenothiazines, other antipsychotic agents do not differ significantly in antipsychotic efficacy but exhibit significant differences in adverse effects, potency ▪ Agents also possess anti–α adrenergic, anticholinergic activity; varying degrees of antiemetic activity; antihistamine, antiserotonin, sedative, ganglionic blocking activity.

CONTRAINDICATIONS: Hypersensitivity, comatose states, bone marrow depression, presence of large amounts of CNS depressants.

DOSAGE: Adult *PO.* Usual antipsychotic range

acetophenazine	40-600mg/d
chlorpromazine	30-1000mg/d
fluphenazine	0.5-20mg/d
haloperidol	2-100mg/d
loxapine	20-100mg/d
mesoridazine	100-400mg/d
molindone	20-225mg/d
olanzapine	50-400mg/d
perphenazine	6-100mg/d
prochlorperazine	15-150mg/d
promazine	40-1200mg/d
quetiapine	5-20mg once/d
thioridazine	200-800mg/d
thiothixene	6-30mg/d
trifluoperazine	5-40mg/d
triflupromazine	30-150mg/d

SIDE/ADVERSE EFFECTS: CNS: drowsiness, extrapyramidal rxs, tardive dyskinesia ▪ CV: postural hypotension, tachycardia, ECG changes in Q&T waves ▪ EENT: blurred vision, corneal/lenticular changes, epithelial keratopathy, ***pigmentary retinopathy,*** nasal congestion ▪ END: lactation/moderate breast enlargement in women ▪ HEM: ***agranulocytosis,*** eosinophilia, leukopenia, ***hemolytic anemia,*** thrombocytopenic purpura ▪ HEP: cholestatic jaundice ▪ INT: urticaria, photosensitivity, ***exfoliative dermatitis,*** skin pigmentation (rare) ▪ PSYCH: adverse behavioral changes incl catatoniclike states ▪ Other: fever, hyperpyrexia, ***neuroleptic malignant syndrome,*** hypothermia.

DRUG INTERACTIONS: Aluminum-magnesium antacid preparations ↓ absorption ▪ Use c̄ narcotics, barbiturates, other CNS depressants ↑ CNS depression ▪ Guanethidine, other related antihypertensive effects antagonized.

NURSING MANAGEMENT PRIORITIES

ASSESS: Hx of hypersensitivity ▪ BP ▪ Extrapyramidal rxs (spasm, trembling, shuffling gait) ▪ CAUTION: hepatic disease, seizure disorder, myasthenia gravis, Parkinson's disease ▪ **ndx: Therapeutic effects:** Defensive coping ▪ Ineffective individual coping ▪ Altered thought processes ▪ **Adverse effects:** Risk for activity intolerance ▪ Risk for altered body temperature ▪ ↓ Cardiac output ▪ Hypothermia ▪ Risk for injury ▪ Impaired physical mobility ▪ Sensory/perceptual alterations (visual) ▪ Risk for impaired skin integrity. **PLAN:** Prevent postural hypotension ▪ Avoid skin contact c̄ liquid forms (contact dermatitis) ▪ Position vomiting pt to avoid aspiration ▪ Avoid abrupt withdrawal ▪ Maintain hydration ▪ **Special considerations:** G: caution, ↓ dosage (↑ sensitivity) ▪ P: caution, avoid use if <6mos ▪ OB: caution if pregnant; avoid breastfeeding ▪ **Dietary**

management: Avoid use c̄ alcohol ▪ ↑ Bulk-containing foods (constipation) ▪ **Lab test evaluation:** CBC. **IMPLEMENT:** Assess VS, esp BP ▪ Monitor hepatic, ophthalmic, renal status ▪ Monitor fluid retention (I&O, daily weight), constipation ▪ Assess for extrapyramidal rx ▪ Seizure precautions in pts c̄ hx of convulsive disorders ▪ Assess for neuroleptic malignant syndrome (fever, convulsions, muscle rigidity, sweating); D/C drug, notify physician ▪ Long-term therapy: assess for jaundice, agranulocytosis ▪ **Patient education:** Avoid sudden position changes (postural hypotension) ▪ Use safety precautions c̄ hazardous activity ▪ Comply c̄ prescribed drug regimen ▪ Avoid use c̄ alcohol, other CNS depressants ▪ Use sugarless gum/hard candy to diminish dry mouth ▪ Constipation may occur; ↑ fluids, bulk-containing foods ▪ May turn urine pink/red/brown ▪ Full drug effects may take several wks ▪ Avoid temperature extremes ▪ Avoid direct sunlight/UV light (photosensitivity) ▪ Notify physician of fever, sore throat, bruising/bleeding, tics/spasms, trembling, shuffling gait. **EVALUATE: Observe for therapeutic effect:** ↓ Psychotic manifestations.

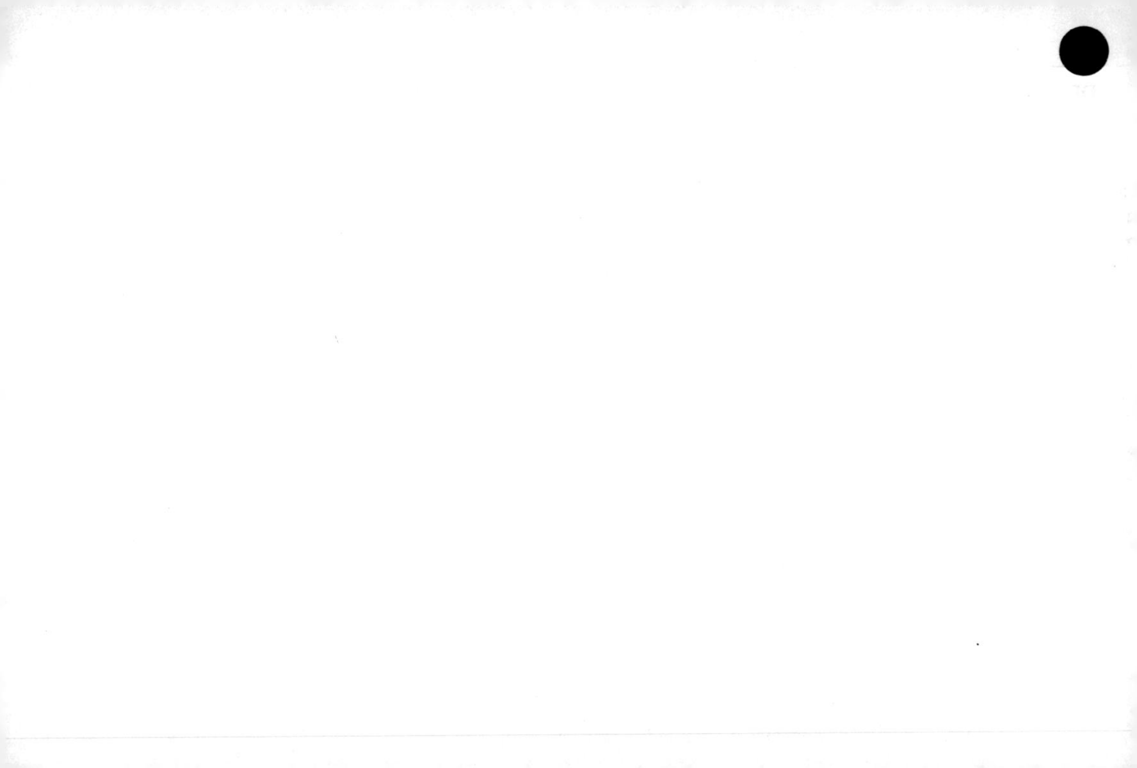

DESCRIPTION: Bacteriostatic sulfonamide derivatives of *p*-aminobenzene sulfonamide (sulfanilamide).

DRUGS: sulfacytine, sulfadiazine, sulfamethizole *(Thiosulfil Forte)*, sulfamethoxazole *(*Apo-Sulfamethoxazole, Gantanol)*, sulfapyridine, sulfasalazine *(Azulfidine)*, sulfisoxazole *(*Apo-Sulfisoxazole, Gantrisin, *Novosoxazole)*, trisulfapyrimidines.

PHARMACOKINETICS: *See* individual drug cards.

THERAPEUTIC USE: Antibacterial: SYSTEMIC: sulfacytine, sulfadiazine, sulfamethizole, sulfamethoxazole, sulfisoxazole, trisulfapyrimidines ▪ GI TRACT: sulfasalazine (ulcerative colitis) ▪ **Dermatitis herpetiformis:** sulfapyridine ▪ **Nocardiosis:** sulfadiazine, sulfamethoxazole, sulfisoxazole, trisulfapyrimidines.

MECHANISM OF ACTION: Bacteriostatic activity due to inhibition of folic acid synthesis in susceptible microorganisms.

CONTRAINDICATIONS: Hypersensitivity, pregnancy at term, nursing mothers, infant <2mo (except in treatment of congenital toxoplasmosis), urinary acidifiers.

DOSAGE: Adult *PO*

sulfacytine	500mg loading dose followed by 250mg qid
sulfadiazine	2-4g loading dose followed by 1g q4-6h
sulfamethizole	0.5-1g 3-4 times/d
sulfamethoxazole	2g loading dose followed by 1g 2-3 times/d
sulfapyridine	500mg qid until improvement. ⬇ Dose by 500mg q3d until symptom-free maintenance achieved
sulfasalazine	3-4g/d divided. Maintenance dose 2g
sulfisoxazole	2-4g loading dose followed by 4-8g/d in 4-6 doses
trisulfapyrimidines	2-4g loading dose followed by 2-4g/d in 3-6 doses

SIDE/ADVERSE EFFECTS: CNS: headache, peripheral neuritis, depression, ataxia, ***convulsions*** ▪ GI: N/V/D, anorexia, abdominal pain, ***pancreatitis***, stomatitis ▪ GU: ***crystalluria, toxic nephrosis*** ▪ HEM: ***agranulocytosis, aplastic anemia, hemolytic anemia, thrombocytopenia***, purpura, methemoglobinemia, hypoprothrombinemia, leukopenia ▪ INT: maculopapular/bullous eruptions, ***Stevens-Johnson syndrome, epidermal necrolysis, exfoliative dermatitis***, urticaria, photosensitivity ▪ MS: arthralgia ▪ Other: serum sickness, allergic myocarditis, periorbital edema.

DRUG INTERACTIONS: Avoid *p*-aminobenzoic preparations during therapy ▪ Use c̄ PO anticoagulant may require dosage adjustment due to ↓ vitamin K synthesis in gut ▪ Sulfonamides can enhance activity of PO hypoglycemics, methotrexate.

NURSING MANAGEMENT PRIORITIES

ASSESS: Hx of hypersensitivity (incl furosemide, thiazide diuretics) ▪ Hepatic, renal function ▪ CAUTION: hepatic, renal impairment ▪ **ndx: Therapeutic effects**: Risk for altered body temperature ▪ Risk for infection ▪ **Adverse effects:** Diarrhea ▪ Risk for fluid volume deficit ▪ Risk for injury ▪ Risk for impaired skin integrity ▪ Altered patterns of urinary elimination. **PLAN:** Administer at equal intervals around clock to maintain blood levels ▪ Maintain hydration ▪ **Special considerations:** G: caution (hepatic, renal impairment) ▪ P: caution; avoid use if <2mos ▪ OB: caution if pregnant, breastfeeding ▪ **Dietary management**: Avoid urinary acidifiers (crystalluria) ▪ **Lab test evaluation**: CBC, UA. **IMPLEMENT:** Obtain C&S; check results ▪ Observe for signs of superinfection (diarrhea, URI, coated tongue) ▪ Administer on an empty stomach ▪ **Patient education:** Comply c̄ prescribed drug regimen ▪ ↑ Fluid intake (8-10 glasses/d) ▪ Take on empty stomach ▪ Diarrhea may occur ▪ Avoid exposure to UV light ▪ Notify physician of fever, sore throat, difficult breathing, rash, bruising/bleeding. **EVALUATE: Observe for therapeutic effect:** Resolution of infection.

DESCRIPTION: Broad-spectrum bacteriostatic antibiotics obtained semisynthetically or from natural *Streptomyces* spp fermentation.

DRUGS: demeclocycline hcl *(Declomycin)*, doxycycline hyclate *(Vibramycin)*, minocycline hcl *(Minocin)*, oxytetracycline hcl *(Terramycin)*, tetracycline hcl *(*Achromycin, Achromycin V, *Apo-tetra, *Medicycline, *Neo-Tetrine, *Novetetra, Sumycin, *Tetracyn)*.

THERAPEUTIC USE: Drug(s) of choice for *Chlamydia*: lymphogranuloma venereum; psittacosis; nonspecific endocervical, rectal, urethral infections ▪ *Mycoplasma: Mycoplasma* pneumonia ▪ *Rickettsia*: Q fever, rickettsialpox, Rocky Mountain spotted fever, scrub typhus, typhus ▪ Drug(s) of choice for acne control, balantidiasis, brucellosis, chancroid, cholera, granuloma inguinale, shigellosis, spirochetal relapsing fever ▪ Alternative in penicillin allergy (esp for gonorrhea, syphilis), infections in which bacteriologic testing indicates good pathogen susceptibility.

MECHANISM OF ACTION: Bacteriostatic effect due to inhibition of ribosomal protein synthesis in susceptible microorganisms.

CONTRAINDICATIONS: Hypersensitivity to any tetracycline; pregnancy, nursing mothers, neonates, children <8y/o.

PHARMACOKINETICS

	PO absorption					
	No food	Food	Half-life	Protein binding	MIC	Excretion
demeclocycline	60%-80%	10%-30%	10-16h	35%-85%	4μg/ml	Renal, feces
doxycycline	90%-100%	70%-80%	14-24h	30%-90%	4μg/ml	Renal, feces
minocycline	90%-100%	70%-80%	11-26h	55%-80%	4μg/ml	Renal, feces
oxytetracycline	60%-80%	10%-30%	6-10h	20%-40%	4μg/ml	Renal, feces
tetracycline	60%-80%	10%-30%	6-12h	20%-65%	4μg/ml	Renal, feces

DOSAGE: Adult *PO*†

demeclocycline	150mg qid
doxycycline, minocycline	50-100mg bid
oxytetracycline, tetracycline	250mg qid

†Consult individual drug cards for other doses.

SIDE/ADVERSE EFFECTS: GI: *gastric upset, diarrhea,* bleeding, enterocolitis ▪ GU: dose-related ↑ BUN ▪ HEM: ***hemolytic anemia, thrombocytopenia*** ▪ INT: *Monilia overgrowth,* maculopapular rash, ***exacerbation of SLE,*** photosensitivity ▪ MS: reversible bulging fontanel in neonates, fetal skeletal retardation, tooth discoloration (<8y/o).

DRUG INTERACTIONS: Antacids, antidiarrheals, dairy products ↓ PO absorption ▪ Use c̄ methoxyflurane may produce nephrotoxicity ▪ PO anticoagulant activity may ↑ due to ↓ intestinal vitamin K synthesis ▪ Tetracyclines antagonize effects of bactericidal antibiotics.

NURSING MANAGEMENT PRIORITIES

ASSESS: Hx of hypersensitivity ▪ Hepatic, renal function ▪ CAUTION**:** hepatic, renal impairment ▪ **ndx: Therapeutic effects**: Risk for altered body temperature ▪ Risk for infection ▪ **Adverse effects:** Diarrhea ▪ Risk for fluid volume deficit ▪ Risk for injury ▪ Risk for impaired skin integrity.

PLAN: Administer at equal intervals around clock to maintain blood levels ▪ Maintain hydration ▪ **Special considerations:** G: caution (renal impairment) ▪ P: avoid use if <8y/o (permanent tooth discoloration; ↓ bone growth) ▪ OB: avoid use if pregnant, breastfeeding ▪ **Dietary management**: Avoid taking c̄ dairy products, antacids, antidiarrheals ▪ **Lab test evaluation:** CBC. **IMPLEMENT:** Obtain C&S; check results ▪ Observe for signs of superinfection (diarrhea, URI, coated tongue) ▪ Administer on empty stomach ▪ Check for ↑ PO anticoagulant activity ▪ Monitor for phlebitis c̄ IV use ▪ **Patient education:** Comply c̄ prescribed drug regimen ▪ Take on empty stomach ▪ Diarrhea may occur ▪ Avoid exposure to UV light ▪ Avoid use c̄ dairy products, antacids. **EVALUATE: Observe for therapeutic effect:** Resolution of infection.

DESCRIPTION: Natural, synthetic thyroid agents.

DRUGS: Natural preparations: Thyroid: obtained from fresh desiccated domesticated animal thyroid glands; active thyroid hormones levothyroxine (T_4), liothyronine (T_3), l-triiodothyroxine present in natural states, ratio ▪ **Synthetically produced preparations:** levothyroxine sodium (T_4; *Levothroid, Synthroid*), liothyronine sodium (T_3; *Cytomel*), liotrix *(Thyrolar):* combination of synthetic microcrystalline T_4 sodium, T_3 sodium in various specific amounts, as indicated by the label of the preparation.

THERAPEUTIC USE: Treatment of hypothyroidism ▪ Suppression of pituitary TSH in prevention/treatment of various types of goiters (T_3) ▪ Diagnostic T_3 suppression test for hyperthyroidism (T_3).

MECHANISM OF ACTION: Thyroid hormones regulate general body metabolism by controlling cellular oxidative process; influence growth; tissue differentiation, maturation.

CONTRAINDICATIONS: Thyrotoxicosis, uncorrected adrenocortical deficiency, acute MI.

DOSAGE: Must be individualized to approximate deficient thyroid activity; normal protein-bound iodine values 4-8μg/dl; values <4μg suggest hypothyroidism, need for supplemental thyroid therapy.

Adult *PO* maintenance dose

levothyroxine	50-200μg/d
liothyronine	25-100μg/d
liotrix	Based on thyroid equivalent (30 180mg thyroid)
thyroid	65-200mg/d

SIDE/ADVERSE EFFECTS: CNS: headache, insomnia, nervousness, tremors ▪ CV: angina, ***cardiac arrhythmias,*** palpitations, tachycardia ▪ GI: diarrhea ▪ Other: intolerance to heat; sweating, weight loss.

DRUG INTERACTIONS: Use c̄ epinephrine in coronary disease may induce coronary insufficiency ▪ Use c̄ PO anticoagulants ↑ their activity, requires lower anticoagulant doses ▪ Use c̄ cholestyramine ↓ PO absorption of thyroid preparations ▪ Use in diabetic pts may require ↑ dosage of hypoglycemic agents.

NURSING MANAGEMENT PRIORITIES

ASSESS: Hx of hypersensitivity ▪ Heart rate ▪ Signs of toxicity (nervous, chest pain, rapid/irregular heartbeat) ▪ CAUTION: CV impairment ▪ **ndx: Therapeutic effects**: Altered nutrition: less than body requirements ▪ **Adverse effects:** Risk for anxiety ▪ ↓ Cardiac output ▪ Diarrhea ▪ Fatigue ▪ Pain ▪ Altered thought processes ▪ Altered tissue perfusion. **PLAN:** Administer daily dose before breakfast ▪ **Special considerations:** G: caution, ↓ dosage (↓ metabolism) ▪ P: temporary alopecia may occur ▪ OB: caution if pregnant, breastfeeding ▪ **Dietary management:** Avoid use c̄ high-iodine foods (soybean, cabbage, shellfish) ▪ **Lab test evaluation:** Thyroid function tests (T_3, T_4, TSH); blood glucose (diabetics). **IMPLEMENT:** Monitor VS, esp heart rate ▪ Observe for signs of OD (chest pain, fever, nervousness, rapid heartbeat) ▪ Monitor thyroid function tests; evaluate pt use of iodine-containing substances before exam ▪ Diabetics: closely monitor blood glucose level (hyperglycemia) ▪ **Patient education:** Comply c̄ prescribed drug regimen ▪ Procedure for checking radial pulse; take pulse on arising qd, notify physician if irregular, D/C drug ▪ Notify physician/dentist of use before treatment ▪ Avoid use c̄ high-iodine foods ▪ Keep scheduled appointments for lab work/ c̄ physician ▪ Do *not* change brand-name preparations ▪ Avoid use c̄ alcohol ▪ Notify physician *immediately* of difficult breathing, chest pain, rapid/irregular heartbeat; D/C drug ▪ Check c̄ physician/pharmacist before taking OTC preparations. **EVALUATE: Observe for therapeutic effects:** ↑ Metabolic rate ▪ ↓ Manifestations of hypothyroidism.

DESCRIPTION: Topical fungal infections primarily caused by *Candida* spp (candidiasis, moniliasis), dermatophytes, *Malassezia furfur* (tinea versicolor).

Candidiasis is caused by *Candida albicans* (& other spp), a yeastlike opportunistic fungus. Organism is present in flora of mouth & in vaginal, intestinal tracts. Two significant factors that commonly predispose an individual to *Candida* infections are broad-spectrum antibiotic therapy that produces overgrowth of nonsusceptible organisms in the natural body flora & immunodeficiency disorders. Topical candidiasis can be oral (thrush) (esp in infants), vaginal, cutaneous, & nail infectious.

Dermatophytes are a group of three closely related genera (*Epidermophyton* spp, *Microsporum* spp, *Trichophyton* spp) that use keratin for growth. They produce superficial mycotic (fungal) infections of keratinized tissue: hair, skin, nails. Infections due to dermatophytes are collectively called tinea or ringworm infections. The body location identifies the tinea infection: tinea pedis (foot), t. cruris (groin), t. corporis (body), t. capitis (scalp). Tinea infections are spread by direct contact c̄ infected persons & animals or from indirect environmental contamination (locker floors, showers, etc.).

T. versicolor is a mild superficial infection of the skin. The lesions are usually located on the chest, back, & shoulders. Exposure to sunlight highlights the infected areas of the skin. *Malassezia* is usually part of the normal flora of the skin & appears to affect only selected individuals.

PRODUCT INFORMATION

Drug	Brand name	Dosage forms	Use	Legal status
amphotericin B	Fungizone	Cream, lotion, ointment 3%	Candidiasis	Rx
butenafine hcl	Mentax	Cream 1%	Dermatophytes	Rx
ciclopirox olamine	Loprox	Cream, lotion 1%	Candidiasis, dermotophytes, tinea versicolor	Rx

Drug	Brand name	Dosage forms	Use	Legal status
clioquinol	Vioform	Cream, ointment 3%	Dermatophytes	OTC
clotrimazole	Gyne-Lotrimin	Cream 1%, vaginal tabs 100, 500mg	Candidiasis	Rx
	Lotrimin	Cream 1%, lotion 1%, solution 1%	Candidiasis, tinea versicolor	Rx
	Lotrimin AF	Cream 1%, lotion 1%, solution 1%	Dermatophytes	OTC
	Mycelex	Cream 1%, solution 1%	Dermatophytes	OTC
	Mycelex	Troches 10mg	Oropharyngeal candidiasis	Rx
	Mycelex-7	Vaginal cream 1%, vaginal tabs 100mg	Candidiasis	OTC
	Mycelex-G	Vaginal tabs 500mg	Candidiasis	Rx
econazole nitrate	Spectazole	Cream 1%	Candidiasis dermatophytes	Rx
haloprogin	Halotex	Cream 1%, solution 1%	Dermatophytes, tinea versicolor	Rx
ketoconazole	Nizoral	Cream 2%, shampoo 2%	Candidiasis, dermatophytes, tinea versicolor	Rx
miconazole nitrate	Micatin	Cream 2%, powder 2%, spray 2%	Dermatophytes	OTC
	Monistat-Derm	Cream 2%	Candidiasis, dermatophytes, tinea versicolor	Rx
naftifine hcl	Naftin	Cream 1%, gel 1%	Dermatophytes	Rx
natamycin	Natacyn	Ophthalmic suspension 5%	Ocular fungal infections	Rx

Drug	Brand name	Dosage forms	Use	Legal status
nystatin	Nilstat/Mycostatin	Creams, ointment, powder 100,000mg	Candidiasis	Rx
oxiconazole nitrate	Oxistat	Cream 1%, lotion 1%	Dermatophytes, tinea versicolor	Rx
sodium thiosulfate	None	25% solution	Tinea versicolor	OTC
sulconazole	Exelderm	Cream 1%, solution 1%	Dermatophytes	Rx
terbinafine hcl	Lamisil	Cream 1%	Dermatophytes	Rx
terconazole	Terazol 3	Vaginal cream 0.8%, vaginal suppository 80mg	Candidiasis	Rx
	Terazol 7	Vaginal cream 0.4%	Candidiasis	Rx
tioconazole	Vagistat-1	Vaginal ointment 6.5%	Candidiasis	Rx
tolnaftate	NP-27	Cream 1%, solution 1%	Dermatophytes	OTC
	Tinactin	Cream 1%, solution 1%		
	Ting	Cream 1%		

NURSING MANAGEMENT PRIORITIES
ASSESS: Hx of hypersensitivity ▪ CAUTION: diabetics, impaired circulation ▪ **ndx: Therapeutic effects**: Risk for infection ▪ **Adverse effects:** Risk for injury ▪ Risk for impaired skin integrity. **PLAN:** Maintain hydration ▪ Maintain intact skin ▪ **Special considerations:** G: none specific ▪ P: caution (↑ sensitivity) ▪ OB: none specific ▪ **Dietary management:** None specific ▪ **Lab test evaluation:** CBC, C&S. **IMPLEMENT:** Obtain C&S, check results ▪ Cleanse, dry area well before application ▪ **Patient education:** Comply c̄ prescribed drug regimen; complete full course of treatment ▪ Apply after cleansing/drying affected area ▪ Avoid application near eyes, mucous membranes ▪ Notify physician of symptoms of allergic rx (burning, rash, itching). **EVALUATE: Observe for therapeutic effect:** Resolution of infection.

DESCRIPTION: Local anesthetics are a relatively small group of drugs that can be classified according to chemical structure or their method of application. They can be administered by injection or applied topically to produce local anesthesia. When local anesthetics are injected, the anesthetized area is distal to the point of injection. Topical local anesthetics produce anesthesia at their site of application.

DRUGS: benzocaine *(Dermoplast, Lanacaine, Solarcaine),* butamben picrate *(Butesin Picrate),* cocaine hcl (generic), dibucaine *(Nupercainal),* dyclonine hcl *(Dyclone),* lidocaine hcl *(Xylocaine),* pramoxine hcl *(Tronothane Hcl),* proparacaine hcl *(Alcaine, Ophthaine, Ophthetic),* tetracaine *(Pontocaine).*

THERAPEUTIC USES: To relieve discomfort/pain of mucous membranes, skin. In addition, they are used to produce anesthesia for various diagnostic, surgical procedures on mucous membrane structures.

MECHANISM OF ACTION: Local anesthetics reversibly block the generation & conduction of nerve impulses by inhibiting the opening of the slow sodium channels in the axon of the nerve cell, resulting in a loss of sensation & motor activity w/out producing a loss of consciousness.

NURSING MANAGEMENT PRIORITIES
ASSESS: Hx of hypersensitivity **ndx: Therapeutic effects:** Pain ▪ **Adverse Effects:** Risk for impaired skin integrity ▪ Risk for injury ▪ Sensory/perceptual alterations. **PLAN:** Safety precautions to prevent injury to anesthetized body parts ▪ Monitor for local rxs ▪ **Special considerations:** G: caution (↑ sensitivity) P: caution (↑ sensitivity) OB: none specific ▪ **Dietary management:** None specific ▪ **Lab test evaluation:** None specific. **IMPLEMENT:** Protect pt from injury ▪ **Patient education:** Assure pt that feeling will return ▪ **EVALUATE: Observe for therapeutic effects:** Relief of local pain ▪ Production of local anesthesia.

Drug	Brand name	Dosage form	Application	Usual dose	Legal status
benzocaine	Dermoplast	Lotion 8%,	Skin	Apply 2-3 times/d	OTC
	Lanacaine	Aerosol 20%, lotion	Skin		
		Cream 6%, Spray 6%	Skin		
	Solarcaine	Spray 20%	Skin		
butamben picrate	Butesin picrate	Ointment 1%	Skin	Apply 2-3 times/d	OTC
cocaine hcl	None	Topical soln 4, 10% Topical visous soln 4, 10%	Mucous membranes	Maximum single dose of 1mg/kg	Rx-CII
dibucaine	Nupercainal	Cream 0.5%	Skin	Apply 2-3 times/d	OTC
		Ointment 1%	Skin		
dyclonine hcl	Dyclone	Solution 0.5, 1%	Mucous membranes	Variable procedure & area to be anesthetized	Rx
	Sucrets Maximum Strength	Lozenge 3mg	Mucous membranes	1g q2-3h prn	OTC
lidocaine hcl	Xylocaine	Ointment 2.5%	Skin	Apply 2-3 times/d	OTC
		Ointment 5%	Skin	Apply 2-3 times/d	Rx
		Oral spray 10%	Mucous membranes	Physician determined	Rx
pramoxine hcl	Tronothane Hcl	Cream 10%	Skin	Apply 2-3 times/d	OTC
proparcaine hcl	Alcaine Ophthaine	Solution 0.5%	Ophthalmic	Variable c̄ ophthalmic procedure	Rx
tetracaine hcl	Ophthetic				
	Pontocaine	Cream 0.5%	Skin	Apply 2-3 times/d	OTC
		Ointment 1%	Skin		
		Solution 0.5%	Ophthalmic	1-2gtt	Rx

Topical local anesthetics

DESCRIPTION: Immunizing biologicals that produce acquired active artificial immunity against selected viral & bacterial diseases ▪ Toxoids are antigenic preparations of G^+ bacterial exotoxins that are detoxified c̄ formaldehyde &/or heat. Highly antigenic, cannot revert back to a toxic form. Stimulate specific antitoxin antibodies that neutralize tissue, destroying bacterial exotoxins. Immunity is effective & long lasting. Available preparations incl Diphtheria, Tetanus, & a combination c̄ Pertussis vaccine (DTwP) ▪ *Vaccines* induce the immune system to produce immunity (humoral or cell-mediated) against specific microorganisms. Vaccine-induced immunity varies c̄ the specific vaccine utilized & ranges from poor to excellent. Classic vaccines contain the actual pathogen (except smallpox, cowpox), which is either living, attenuated (weakened), or inactivated (killed). The attenuating &/or killing agent is usually formaldehyde or heat. Attenuation is also accomplished by the repeated passage through some animal or tissue. Live vaccines produce greater & longer lasting immunity than inactivated vaccines.

Newer vaccines utilize some extract or synthetic extract (genetic engineering) of the pathogen rather than the actual microbe. Because the microbe is not present in the vaccine, they are really viral, or bacterial, antigenic preparations. Hepatitis B & influenza vaccine contain either the natural or synthetic viral surface antigens of the virus. In addition, influenza vaccine may contain the whole virus or the split virus particle. Meningitis (meningococcal), *Haemophilus*, & pneumococcal vaccines contain selected bacterial capsular polysaccharides that are extracted from the respective microbes.

PREPARATIONS: Toxoids: Diphtheria toxoid adsorbed, diphtheria & tetanus toxoid adsorbed, tetanus toxoid fluid, tetanus toxoid adsorbed, diphtheria & tetanus toxoids & pertussis vaccine—DTwP, diphtheria & tetanus toxoids & acellular pertussis vaccine (DTaP) & *Haemophillus influenzae* type B conjugate vaccine (DTwP-HIB) ▪ **Vaccines:** *Bacterial:* Bacille Calmette-Guérin (BCG) vaccine, cholera vaccine, *Haemophilus b* conjugate vaccine, meningitis vaccine, plague vaccine, pneumococcal vaccine polyvalent ▪ *Viral:* hepatitis A vaccine inactivated, hepatitis b vaccine, influenza vaccine, measles vaccine live, measles & rubella vaccine live, measles, mumps, & rubella vaccine live, mumps vaccine live, polio virus vaccine inactivated-Salk, polio virus vaccine live-Sabin, rabies vaccine, rubella vaccine live, rubella & mumps vaccine live, varicella vaccine live, yellow fever vaccine. In addition, the Centers for Disease Control and Prevention provides an assortment of rare vaccines, incl smallpox.

THERAPEUTIC USE: Production of active artificial immunity to infectious diseases.

CONTRAINDICATIONS: Hypersensitivity, tuberculin-positive individuals (BCG), immune deficiencies or immunosuppressive therapy (esp for live vaccines), acute febrile infections, pt age &/or pregnancy for selected vaccines.

PEDIATRIC IMMUNIZATION SCHEDULES

diphtheria toxoid	*IM*	2, 4, 6, 18mo; 4-6yr
haemophillus B vaccine	*IM*	2, 4, 6, 12-15mo
hepatitis B vaccine	*IM*	Birth, 1-2, 6mo
measles vaccine	*SC*	≥12mo; 4-6 or 11-12yr
MMR	*IM*	≥15mo; 4-6yr, 11-12yr
mumps vaccine	*SC*	≥12mo; 4-6 or 11-12yr
oral polio vaccine		2, 4, 6, 18mo; 4-6yr
pertussis vaccine	*IM*	2, 4, 6, 18mo; 4-6yr
rotavirus	SC	2, 4, 6mo
rubella vaccine	*SC*	≥12mo; 4-6 or 11-12yr
tetanus toxoid	*IM*	2, 4, 6, 18mo; 4-6yr
varicella vaccine	*SC*	Given once from 1-12 y/o

DRUG INTERACTIONS: Use c̄ immunosuppressive drugs will antagonize effects (immunity), may induce serious infections c̄ live or attenuated vaccines.

NURSING MANAGEMENT PRIORITIES

ASSESS: Hx of hypersensitivity to any component of the vaccine ▪ Injection site for redness, edema, pain ▪ CAUTION: immunocompromised pts ▪ **ndx: Therapeutic effects**: Risk for infection ▪ **Adverse effects:** Risk for injury ▪ Risk for impaired skin integrity ▪ Impaired tissue integrity. **PLAN:** Have epinephrine (1:1000), oxygen, support equipment available for anaphylaxis ▪ Document immunization for pt; notify when repeat vaccine/booster is needed ▪ **Special considerations:** G: caution (chronic illness) ▪ P: caution (immature systems) ▪ OB: avoid use if pregnant, breastfeeding ▪ **Dietary management: None specific** ▪ **Lab test evaluation:** None specific. **IMPLEMENT:** Parenteral: administer IM via deltoid muscle or SC as directed; do *not* administer IV; rotate sites ▪ Trivalent PO poliovaccine: may be mixed c̄ H_2O, milk, syrup or placed on bread, sugar cube ▪ Monitor for hypersensitivity rxs (difficult breathing, chest pain, pruritus) ▪ Assess for discomfort following injection; provide comfort measures prn ▪ **Patient education:** Notify physician/nurse of chest pain, difficult breathing, any unusual rx to immunization ▪ Comfort measures postimmunization (analgesics, moist heat to injection site). **EVALUATE: Observe for therapeutic effect:** Prevention of specific disease.

DESCRIPTION: Large group of antidepressants chemically similar to phenothiazines.

DRUGS: amitriptyline hcl *(*Apo-Amitriptylline, Elavil, Endep, Enovil, *Levate, *Meravil, *Novotriptyn),* amoxapine *(Asendin),* clomipramine hcl *(Anafranil),* clozapine *(Clozaril),* desipramine hcl *(Norpramin, Pertofrane),* doxepin hcl *(Sinequan),* imipramine hcl *(*Apo-Imipramine, *Impril, Janimine, *Novopramine, Tofranil),* imipramine pamoate *(Tofranil-PM),* maprotiline hcl *(Ludiomil),*† mirtazapine *(Remeron),* nortriptyline hcl *(Aventyl),* protriptyline hcl *(Vivactil, *Triptil),* trimipramine maleate *(Surmontil).*

PHARMACOKINETICS: *See* individual drug cards.

THERAPEUTIC USE: Treatment of endogenous depression ▪ Imipramine: adjunct for treating enuresis (children >6y/o).

MECHANISM OF ACTION: Antidepressant activity appears related to inhibition of norepinephrine reuptake in central adrenergic neurons after its release. They affect serotonin, possess strong anticholinergic activity, produce varying degrees of sedation.

CONTRAINDICATIONS: Hypersensitivity, MAO-I therapy, MI (acute recovery period) ▪ Doxepin: glaucoma, urinary retention.

DOSAGE: Adult *PO*

amitriptyline	75-150mg/d
amoxapine	150-300mg/d
clomipramine	25-250mg/d
desipramine	100-200mg/d
doxepin	75-100mg/d
imipramine hcl	75-200mg/d
imipramine pamoate	75-200mg/d
maprotiline†	75-225mg/d
mirtazapine	15-30mg/d at hs
nortriptyline	25-100mg/d
protriptyline	15-60mg/d
trimipramine	75-200mg/d

SIDE/ADVERSE EFFECTS: CNS: drowsiness, dizziness, headache, incoordination, tremors, extrapyramidal symptoms, paresthesia (extremities), insomnia ▪ CV: ***arrhythmias,*** MI, stroke, ***heart block,*** postural hypotension ▪ EENT: tinnitus ▪ END: gynecomastia, testicular swelling, galactorrhea, breast enlargement (women) ▪ GI: anorexia,

*Available in Canada only.
†Tetracyclic antidepressant.

N/V/D, stomatitis, cramps, black hairy tongue, dry mouth, constipation ▪ GU: urinary hesitancy ▪ HEM: ***agranulocytosis,*** eosinophilia, ***thrombocytopenia*** ▪ HEP: cholestatic jaundice ▪ INT: skin rash, photosensitivity, alopecia ▪ PSYCH: disorientation, delusions, hallucinations, exacerbation of psychosis, confusion ▪ Other: parotid swelling.

DRUG INTERACTIONS: Significant depressant effects c̄ alcohol ▪ Anticholinergics, chlorpromazine produce ↑ atropinelike effects; paralytic ileus could occur ▪ Significant ↑ activity c̄ epinephrine, levarterenol, other adrenergic agents ▪ Significant antagonism of effects of reserpine, clonidine, guanethidine-type antihypertensives.

NURSING MANAGEMENT PRIORITIES

ASSESS: Hx of hypersensitivity ▪ BP ▪ CAUTION: hepatic, renal impairment ▪ **ndx: Therapeutic effects**: Ineffective individual coping ▪ Self-esteem disturbance ▪ Risk for violence: self-directed ▪ **Adverse effects:** Risk for activity intolerance ▪ ↓ Cardiac output ▪ Diarrhea ▪ Risk for fluid volume deficit ▪ Risk for injury ▪ Impaired physical mobility ▪ Sensory/perceptual alterations ▪ Sexual dysfunction ▪ Risk for impaired skin integrity. **PLAN:** Prevent postural hypotension ▪ Heavy smokers may require ↑ dosage ▪ Avoid abrupt withdrawal ▪ Institute suicide precautions ▪ Ensure drug ingestion ▪ **Special considerations:** G: caution (↑ sensitivity) ▪ P: not recommended ▪ OB: avoid use if pregnant, breastfeeding ▪ **Dietary management:** Avoid use c̄ alcohol ▪ **Lab test evaluation:** CBC. **IMPLEMENT:** Monitor BP ▪ Suicide precautions prn ▪ Monitor hepatic, renal status ▪ **Patient education:** Comply c̄ prescribed drug regimen ▪ Avoid sudden position changes (postural hypotension) ▪ Use safety precautions c̄ hazardous activity ▪ Full drug effects may take several wks ▪ Use sugarless gum/hard candy to diminish dry mouth ▪ Check c̄ physician before taking OTC preparations ▪ Avoid use c̄ alcohol ▪ Carry identification (MedicAlert). **EVALUATE: Observe for therapeutic effects:** ↓ Depression ▪ Mood elevation.

Management procedures usually involve (1) removal of drug from GI tract or ↓ delayed GI absorption, (2) ↑ in rate of drug/active metabolite(s) excretion, (3) ↑ in threshold of drug required to produce toxic effects (specific physiologic or pharmacologic antidotes), (4) providing general & symptomatic treatment.

REMOVAL OF DRUG FROM GI TRACT: Emesis: Use of ipecac syrup or gagging. Not recommended for convulsant agents (or during convulsions), corrosive chemicals, narcotics, petroleum distillates. **Gastric lavage:** Can be effective for several hours after ingestion. Not recommended for convulsant agents (or during convulsions), corrosive chemicals, petroleum distillates.

DECREASED/DELAYED GI ABSORPTION: Physical antagonism: Use of activated charcoal (adsorbent), which adsorbs toxic agent & physically interferes c̄ absorption. **Chemical antagonism:** Use of 2% tannic acid solution to form insoluble complexes, esp c̄ alkaloid drugs. **Delayed gastric emptying:** Milk or starch water will ↓ gastric emptying time.

INCREASE RATE OF DRUG/ACTIVE METABOLITE(S) EXCRETION: Antibody inactivation: Use of digoxin immune fab, which combines c̄ free digoxin/digitoxin to form a complex that is then excreted in urine. **Catharsis:** Cathartics can remove unabsorbed toxic substances from intestine. Use is controversial, not recommended for pts c̄ electrolyte imbalances or corrosive substances. **Chelating agents:** Use of chelating agents, which combine (chelate) c̄ a variety of metallic ions (heavy metal poisoning). Metal complex formed is slowly excreted over time in urine. Not recommended for use in pts c̄ severe renal disease, anuria. Calcium disodium edetate: Used to ↓ serum, deposit levels of lead (plumbism). Limited value in treating gold, cadmium, chromium, copper, nickel poisoning. Deferoxamine mesylate: Used to treat iron (ferrous & ferris) poisoning. Dimercaprol (BAL): Used to treat arsenic, gold, mercury poisoning. Also can be used c̄ calcium disodium edetate in treating severe pediatric plumbism. Use is restricted in hepatic insufficiency. Disodium edetate (EDTA): Used in emergency treatment of hypercalcemia & arrhythmias induced by digitalis OD. Penicillamine: Used for removal of copper in hepatolenticular degeneration (Wilson's disease). Also used in treating cystinuria, rheumatoid arthritis. Not recommended for use in penicillin-allergic pts. Succimers: Used for pediatric plumbism (>45μg/dl). Other: Trientine hcl for Wilson's disease in pts intolerant to penicillamine.

Dialysis: Used for removing selected drugs esp by hemodialysis. **Diuresis:** Renal excretion is dependent on glomerular filtration, active tubular secretion, tubular reabsorption. Rate of drug excretion in urine can be significantly ↑ by modifying conditions of kidneys to favor diuresis or forced diuresis. Alteration of urinary pH: Adjusting pH to favor ionization of toxic substances. Ionized chemicals exhibit lower tubular reabsorption & therefore ↑ their rate of execution. Excretion of weak acidic toxic chemicals will ↑ when urine is alkalinized. Weak basic toxic chemicals ↑ when urine is acidified. Osmotic diuretics: Effective in forcing excretion of certain drugs because of ↓ H_2O reabsorption in proximal tubules. Combining osmotic diuretics (mannitol, urea) c̄ urinary pH adjustments can ↑ renal clearance of many substances, esp barbiturate, salicylate intoxication. Not recommended for use c̄ CHF, renal disease.

RAISING TOXIC THRESHOLDS: Toxic rxs are dose related, require a minimum threshold (concentration) of toxic substance to produce toxic effects. Accordingly, toxic rxs can be minimized by ↑ toxic threshold. ↑ Of toxic thresholds can implore either physiologic or pharmacologic antagonism. ↑ Toxic threshold does not ↓ concentration of toxic substance in the body. **Physiologic antagonism:** Use of an antidote that has an opposite effect on the physiologic system being affected by toxic substances or augments a 2nd physiologic system that opposes, antagonizes the system being affected. However, antagonistic physiologic mechanisms have limited value. **Pharmacologic (competitive) antagonism:** Occurs when antidote, toxic substance compete for the same receptor site (competitive inhibitions). The following are selected examples:

Antidote	Drug/chemical
atropine sulfate	Anticholinesterase insecticide Cholinergic drugs
flumazenil	Benzodiazepines
fomepizole	Antifreeze
nalmefene hcl	Narcotics
naloxone hcl	Narcotics Propoxyphene
naltrexone	Narcotics
pilocarpine	Atropine

Drug dosage (posology) determinations are usually calculated on the basis of (1) patient age (least reliable method), (2) patient weight (more reliable method), (3) patient body surface area (most reliable method). However, it is best to remember that no dosage calculation method can incorporate all of the physiologic and pathologic conditions associated with patients. This is especially true for neonates, infants, & pediatric patients due to the uniqueness for these special groups. Accordingly, any rule and the resulting dose is just a guide and may require adjustments to suit a particular patient's clinical situation.

The dosage recommended for a patient is usually provided by the pharmaceutical manufacturer(s). For example, tetracycline, 250mg qid, is a typical medication order regardless of patient size. The required dose for a 90-lb woman is not the same as the required dose for a 210-lb man. Pharmaceutical manufacturers are currently expanding their dosing schedules to include such variables as patient body size, age, special patient physiologic parameters (eg, hepatic/renal function) & dosage based on square meter size.

PEDIATRIC AGE DOSING RULES

These rules are the most numerous and, as mentioned previously, the least reliable.

AUGSBURGER'S RULE

$$\text{Dose} = \frac{(4 \times \text{Age at next birthday} + 20)}{100} \times \text{Adult dose}$$

BASTEDO'S RULE

$$\text{Dose} = \frac{\text{Age} + 3}{30} \times \text{Adult dose}$$

COWLING'S RULE

$$\text{Dose} = \frac{\text{Age at next birthday}}{24} \times \text{Adult dose}$$

DILLING'S RULE

$$\text{Dose} = \frac{\text{Age}}{20} \times \text{Adult dose}$$

FRIED'S RULE

$$\text{Dose} = \frac{\text{Age in mos}}{150} \times \text{Adult dose}$$

MARTINET'S RULE

$$\text{Dose} = \frac{\text{Age} + 1}{20} \times \text{Adult dose}$$

YOUNG'S RULE (FOR PATIENT OVER 2Y/O)

$$\text{Dose} = \frac{\text{Age in yrs}}{\text{Age in yrs} + 12} \times \text{Adult dose}$$

PATIENT WEIGHT DOSING RULE

Dosage calculations based on body weight are more accurate than dosage based on age. However, these methods will not give the absolute dose required.

AUGSBURGER'S PEDIATRIC WEIGHT RULE

$$\text{Dose} = \frac{1.5 \times \text{kg of body weight} + 10}{100} \times \text{Adult dose}$$

CLARK'S PEDIATRIC WEIGHT RULE

$$\text{Dose} = \frac{\text{Weight in lbs}}{150} \times \text{Adult dose}$$

DOSAGE GIVEN IN kg OF BODY WEIGHT

Dose = Dose/kg × Weight of patient in kg

PATIENT'S BODY SURFACE AREA DOSING RULES

Dosage based on the total body surface area of the patient is preferred & appears to give the most reliable calculations. The total body surface area of the patient can be obtained by using the West or some other suitable pediatric or adult nomogram.

A nomogram correlates many variables incl age, height, weight, into a reasonable assumption of body surface area. Once the body surface area is determined, the appropriate dose can be calculated.

CLARK'S PEDIATRIC BODY SURFACE RULE

$$\text{Dose} = \frac{\text{Body surface area in m}^2}{1.73} \times \text{Adult dose}$$

DOSAGE GIVEN IN m^2

Dose = Dose/m^2 × Surface area of patient in m^2

DOSAGE GIVEN IN m^2/kg (AN INCREASING TREND BEING PROVIDED BY THE PHARMACEUTICAL MANUFACTURERS)

Dose = Dose/m^2 × Weight of patient in kg.

Pound and kilogram equivalents

lb	kg	lb	kg	lb	kg	lb	kg	lb	kg
1	0.454	27	12.2	52	23.6	78	35.4	103	46.7
2	0.908	28	12.7	53	24.0	79	35.8	104	47.2
3	1.3	29	13.1	54	24.5	80	36.3	105	47.6
4	1.8	30	13.6	55	24.9	81	36.7	106	48.1
5	2.2	31	14.0	56	25.4	82	37.2	107	48.5
6	2.7	32	14.5	57	25.8	83	37.6	108	49.0
7	3.1	33	14.9	59	26.7	84	38.1	109	49.4
8	3.6	34	15.4	60	27.2	85	38.5	110	49.9
9	4.0	35	15.8	61	27.6	86	39.0	111	50.3
10	4.5	36	16.3	62	28.1	87	39.4	112	50.8
11	4.9	37	16.7	63	28.5	88	39.9	113	51.3
12	5.4	38	17.2	64	29.0	89	40.3	114	51.7
13	5.9	39	17.6	65	29.5	90	40.8	115	52.2
14	6.3	40	18.1	66	29.9	91	41.2	116	52.6
16	7.2	41	18.6	67	30.4	92	41.7	117	53.1
17	7.7	42	19.0	68	30.8	93	42.4	118	53.5
18	8.1	43	19.5	69	31.3	94	42.6	119	54.0
19	8.6	44	19.9	70	31.7	95	43.1	120	54.4
20	9.0	45	20.4	71	32.3	96	43.5	121	54.9
21	9.5	46	20.8	72	32.6	97	44.0	122	55.3
22	9.9	47	21.3	73	33.1	98	44.4	123	55.8
23	10.4	48	21.7	74	33.5	99	44.9	124	56.2
24	10.8	49	22.2	75	34.0	100	45.3	125	56.7
25	11.3	50	22.6	76	34.5	101	45.8	126	57.2
26	11.7	51	23.1	77	34.9	102	46.2	127	57.6

Pound and kilogram equivalents—cont'd

lb	kg	lb	kg	lb	kg	lb	kg	lb	kg
128	58.1	153	69.4	178	80.8	203	92.1	228	103.5
129	58.5	154	69.9	179	81.2	204	92.6	229	103.9
130	59.0	155	70.3	180	81.7	205	93.0	230	104.4
131	59.4	156	70.8	181	82.1	206	93.5	231	104.8
132	59.9	157	71.2	182	82.6	207	93.9	232	105.3
133	60.3	158	71.7	183	83.0	208	94.4	233	105.7
134	60.8	159	72.1	184	83.5	209	94.8	234	106.2
135	61.2	160	72.6	185	83.9	210	95.3	235	106.6
136	61.7	161	73.0	186	84.4	211	95.7	236	107.1
137	62.1	162	73.5	187	84.8	212	96.2	237	107.5
138	62.6	163	74.0	188	85.3	213	96.7	238	108.0
139	63.1	164	74.4	189	85.8	214	97.1	239	108.5
140	63.5	165	74.9	190	86.2	215	97.6	240	108.9
141	64.0	166	75.3	191	86.7	216	98.0	241	109.4
142	64.6	167	75.8	192	87.1	217	98.5	242	109.8
143	64.9	168	76.2	193	87.6	218	98.9	243	110.3
144	65.3	169	76.7	194	88.0	219	99.4	244	110.7
145	65.8	170	77.1	195	88.5	220	98.8	245	111.2
146	66.2	171	77.6	196	88.9	221	100.3	246	111.6
147	66.7	172	78.0	197	89.4	222	100.7	247	112.1
148	67.1	173	78.5	198	89.8	223	101.2	248	112.5
149	67.6	174	78.9	199	90.3	224	101.6	249	113.0
150	68.1	175	79.4	200	90.8	225	102.1	250	113.5
151	68.5	176	79.9	201	91.2	226	102.6		
152	69.0	177	80.3	202	91.7	227	103.0		

Key: C, Compatible I, Incompatible Blank spaces indicate no data, insufficient data, or conflicting data.	aminophylline	atropine	calcium gluconate	diazepam	diphenhydramine	epinephrine	hydroxyzine	meperidine	metoclopramide	morphine	nalbuphine	pentazocine	pentobarbital	phenobarbital	procainamide	prochlorperazine	promethazine	scopolamine	secobarbital	verapamil
aminophylline	*		C	I	C	I	I	I		I		I	C	I	C	I	I			C
atropine		*		I	C	I	C	C	C	C	C	C	C			C	C	C		
calcium gluconate	C		*	I	C	I									C				I	C
diazepam	I	I	I	*	I	I	I	I	I	I	I	I	I	I	I	I	I	I	I	I
diphenhydramine	C	C	C	I	*			C		C			I	I	C	C	C	C		
epinephrine	I	I	I	I		*									I					
hydroxyzine	I	C		I			*	C	C	C	C	C	I	I		C	C	C		
meperidine	I	C		I	C		C	*	C	I		C	I	I		C	C	C		
metoclopramide		C		I			C	C	*	C		C						C		
morphine	I	C		I	C		C	I	C	*		C		I		I		C		
nalbuphine		C		I			C				*						I	C		
pentazocine	I	C		I			C	C	C	C		*	I	I			C	C		
pentobarbital	C	C		I	I		I	I				I	*			I	I	C		
phenobarbital	I			I	I		I	I		I		I		*		I				
procainamide	C		C	I	C	I									*					C
prochlorperazine	I	C		I	C		C	C		I			I	I		*		C		
promethazine	I	C		I	C		C	C	C		I	C	I				*	C		
scopolamine		C		I	C		C	C	C	C	C	C	C			C	C	*	I	
secobarbital			I	I														I	*	
verapamil	C		C	I											C					*

No distinction was made between compatible or temporarily compatible mixtures because drugs mixed in a syringe or infusion bottle should be used *immediately*. Furthermore, it is the responsibility of the "mixer" to ascertain, by close observation, that the mixture is compatible before administration. Therefore any compatibility chart is not absolute, and the final authority is the dispenser of the mixture.

APPENDIX C: IV compatibility chart

	D_5	D_{10}	D_5		NS	R	LR	Other
			½ S	S				
acyclovir	C							
amikacin	C				C			
amphotericin B	C							
ampicillin	C				C			
aztreonam	C	C			C	C	C	Normosol-R
cefamandole	C				C			
cefazolin	C				C			
cefotetan	C				C			
cefoxitin	C	C			C	C	C	Aminosol
ceftazidime	C		C	C	C	C	C	M/6 sodium lactate
ceftriaxone	C				C			
cefuroxime	C		C	C		C		M/6 sodium lactate
cephalothin	C				C	C	C	M/6 sodium lactate
cephapirin	C				C			
dopamine	C		C	C	C		C	M/6 sodium lactate
doxycycline	C				C			Invert sugar 10%
gentamicin	C				C			Normosol-R
isoproterenol	C			C	C	C		Invert sugar 5% & 10%
kanamycin	C				C			

APPENDIX C: IV compatibility chart—cont'd

	D_5	D_{10}	D_5		NS	R	LR	Other
			½ S	S				
metaraminol	C			C	C	C	C	Normosol-R
metoclopramide	C			C		C	C	
mezlocillin	C	C	C	C	C	C	C	Fructose 5%
netilmicin	C	C		C	C	C	C	Normosol-R
nitroglycerin	C	C			C			
norepinephrine	C	C		C			C	
piperacillin	C			C	C		C	
ritodrine	C							
ticarcillin	C				C		C	
tobramycin	C				C			
vidarabine	C	C			C			

This chart is not inclusive and is based on manufacturers' recommendations.

Key: *D_5*, Dextrose 5%; *D_{10}*, dextrose 10%; *D_5 ½S*, dextrose 5% in saline 0.45%; *D_5S*, dextrose 5% in saline 0.9%; *NS*, sodium chloride 0.9% (normal saline); *R*, Ringer's solution; *LR*, lactated Ringer's solution; *C*, compatible.

Drug:

CATEGORY: Preg Cat:

BRAND NAME **DOSAGE FORMS**

DOSAGE:

USE/ACTION:

SIDE/ADVERSE EFFECTS:

PHARMACOKINETICS:

INTERACTIONS: Drug:
Food:
Lab:

CONTRAINDICATIONS:

CC:

Note: Side/adverse effects: common in *italic;* serious in ***boldface italic.***

*Available in Canada only.

NURSING MANAGEMENT PRIORITIES
ADMINISTRATION:

NOTES:

EVALUATION:

EDUCATION:

OVERDOSE MANAGEMENT:

B

J

K

O

S

T

U

V

W

X

Y

Z

Drug:

CATEGORY: Preg Cat:

BRAND NAME **DOSAGE FORMS**

DOSAGE:

USE/ACTION:

SIDE/ADVERSE EFFECTS:

PHARMACOKINETICS:

INTERACTIONS: Drug:
Food:
Lab:

CONTRAINDICATIONS:

CC:

Note: Side/adverse effects: common in *italic*; serious in ***boldface italic***

*Available in Canada only

NURSING MANAGEMENT PRIORITIES

ADMINISTRATION:

NOTES:

EVALUATION:

EDUCATION:

OVERDOSE MANAGEMENT: